Vertebrate Hormones

Hormone	Molecular Weight
Melatonin (*N*-acetyl-5-methoxytryptamine)	232
Mesotocin	1007
Methionine enkephalin (Met-enkephalin)	574
Motilin	2670 (p)
MSH release-inhibiting factor (MIF)	
Müllerian regression factor (MRF)[b]	
Nerve growth factor (NGF)	
Neurotensin (NT)	1673
Norepinephrine (NE)	103
Oxytocin	1007
Pancreatic polypeptide (PP)	4221 (b)
Parathormone (PTH)	
Platelet-derived growth factor (PDGF)[b]	
Progesterone	314
Prolactin-inhibiting factor (PIF)	
Prostacyclin I_2 (PGL$_2$)	353
Prostaglandin E_2 (PGE$_2$)	
Prostaglandin $F_{2\alpha}$ (PGF$_{2\alpha}$)	355
Relaxin	
Secretin	3055 (p)
Serotonin (5-hydroxytryptamine, 5-HT)	176
Serum thymic factor (STF)	876
Somatostatin (SS); somatotropin release-inhibiting hormone (SRIH)	1639
Somatotropin (STH) (Growth hormone, GH)	
Substance P (SP)	1347 (b)
Testosterone	288
Thromboxane A_2 (TXA$_2$)	
Thymopoietin	
Thymosin$_{\alpha 1}$	
Thymosin$_{\alpha 4}$	
Thyrotropin; thyroid-stimulating hormone (TSH)	
Thyrotropin-releasing hormone (TRH)	362
Thyroxine (T$_4$)	777
Triiodothyronine (T$_3$)	651
Urogastrone[c]	
Vasoactive intestinal peptide (VIP)	3326 (p)
Vasotocin	1050
Vitamin D_3(1α,25-dihydroxycholecalciferol)(1α,25-(OH)$_2$D$_3$) (calcitriol)	417

[a] All hormones are of human origin unless otherwise noted (p, porcine; b, bovine; f, frog). The molecular weights (MW) are derived from the constituent amino acids of the peptides. It should be noted that commercially available or synthetically prepared peptides may contain a number of counter ions (e.g., acetate, Na$^+$, etc.) depending on the final purification and isolation procedures. This should be carefully considered when using the dry weight of the lyophilized powder to prepare molar concentrations of peptides.

[b] Structure undetermined.

[c] Probably identical to epidermal growth factor (EGF).

Library of Congress Cataloging-in-Publication Data

Hadley, Mac E.
    Endocrinology / Mac E. Hadley. -- 4th ed.
        p.   cm.
    Includes bibliographical references and index.
    ISBN 0-13-317926-5
    1. Endocrinology   I. Title
QP187.H17   1996
599'.0142--dc20   95-10773
                                                  CIP

Acquisitions editor: David Brake
Editorial/production supervision
    and interior design: ETP Services
Copy editor: Jane Loftus
Cover designer: Bruce Kenselaar
Cover credit: The dopaminergic neuron depicted on the front cover of the
    book has been treated in vitro with G-DNF (glial cell line-derived neuro-
    tropic factor). Compared to control (nontreated) cells (back cover), the
    cell has become more dendritic. The deeper red color also indicates that it
    makes more of a key enzyme for dopamine biosynthesis. G-DNF may hold
    promise in the treatment of Parkinson's Disease. Photographs courtesy of
    Lin et al., Synergen, Inc.
Buyer: Trudy Pisciotti
Editorial assistant: Carrie Brandon

© 1996, 1992, 1988, 1982 by Prentice-Hall, Inc.
Simon & Schuster / A Viacom Company
Upper Saddle River, NJ 07458

Printed in the United States of America

10   9   8   7   6   5

ISBN 0-13-317926-5

Prentice-Hall International (UK) Limited, *London*
Prentice-Hall of Australia Pty. Limited, *Sydney*
Prentice-Hall Canada Inc., *Toronto*
Prentice-Hall Hispanoamericana, S.A., *Mexico*
Prentice-Hall of India Private Limited, *New Delhi*
Prentice-Hall of Japan, Inc., *Tokyo*
Simon & Schuster Asia Pte Ltd., *Singapore*
Editora Prentice-Hall do Brasil, Ltda., *Rio de Janeiro*

This text is dedicated to my wife, Trudy, in appreciation for her constant encouragement and assistance during the preparation of this book, and to my daughter,

Martha **S**haron **H**adley

Contents

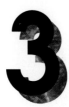

Endocrine Methodologies   34

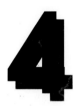

General Mechanisms of Hormone Action   55

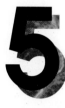

Pituitary Hormones 83

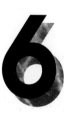

The Endocrine Hypothalamus 102

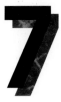

7 Neurohypophysial Hormones 127

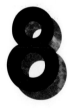

8 The Melanotropic Hormones 153

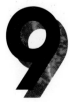

9 Hormonal Control of Calcium Homeostasis 177

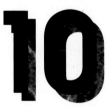

Gastrointestinal Hormones   204

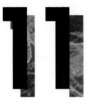

Pancreatic Hormones and Metabolic Regulation   231

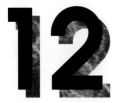

Growth Hormones   257

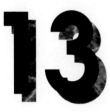

Thyroid Hormones 290

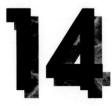

Catecholamines and the Sympathoadrenal System 314

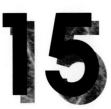

Adrenal Steroid Hormones 338

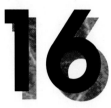

Endocrinology of Sex Differentiation and Development   370

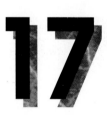

Hormones and Male Reproductive Physiology   392

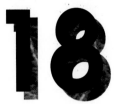

Hormones and Female Reproductive Physiology

412

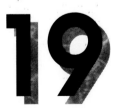

Endocrinology of Pregnancy, Parturition, and Lactation

438

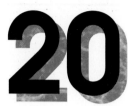

Endocrine Role of the Pineal Gland   458

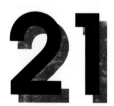

Neurohormones   477

Bibliography   503

Index   507

Preface

The central theme of this text is the role of chemical messengers, or hormones, whether they are of endocrine or neural origin, in the control of physiological processes. Although endocrine physiology has been separated from neurophysiology in the past, it is now amply documented that hormones may originate from either endocrine or neural tissue. Thus has emerged the field of neuroendocrinology. Several eminent endocrinologists have been awarded Nobel Prizes in Physiology/Medicine for their monumental efforts leading to the discovery and elucidation of the chemical structure of several brain neuropeptides (neurohormones); this clearly emphasizes the importance of the concept of neuroendocrine physiology. It is now also realized that the so-called "classical" hormones are produced in many sites throughout the body and may be released either directly into the blood, into neuronal synapses, or into the immediate intercellular space to affect adjacent cellular activity. This more inclusive definition of "hormone" has, therefore, been employed, as suggested by the Nobel laureate, Roger Guillemin. The important point emphasized in this definition is that it is both the method of delivery as well as the source of the hormone that is of greatest physiological significance.

In INTRODUCTION TO ENDOCRINOLOGY a short chronology of endocrine research is presented. The concept of homeostasis is then discussed with special reference given to the roles of chemical messengers in the control of homeostatic systems. The reader is then provided with a general description of THE VERTEBRATE ENDOCRINE SYSTEM, wherein an initial working vocabulary is established. Included here is a discussion of the general classes of chemical messengers and other cellular regulators (steroid and peptide hormones, neurohormones, chalones, growth factors, eicosanoids, pheromones); the cellular synthesis of chemical messengers and their secretion, delivery, and metabolism; and a general overview of the physiological role of hormones. In consideration of the various methodologies used in present-day endocrine research, it was considered necessary to add a chapter on ENDOCRINE METHODOLOGIES early in the text. Classical surgical and histological techniques are discussed, as are more recent methods including radioimmunoassay, radioreceptor assay, radioisotope enzyme assay, autoradiography, and recombinant-DNA methodologies. It was also considered important to provide, early in the book, a discussion of GENERAL MECHANISMS OF HORMONE ACTION, because these concepts are a necessary component of each of the following chapters. Included within this chapter is a discussion of cellular receptors, cyclic nucleotides as second messengers, prostaglandins (and prostacyclins, thromboxanes, and leukotrienes), stimulus-response coupling, calmodulin (a cellular calcium receptor), and phosphorylated proteins as physiological effectors.

The source, synthesis, chemistry, and general role of the PITUITARY HORMONES in the control of endocrine physiology are discussed next, because the pituitary gland is a major source of hormones regulating many other endocrine glands. More specific details of the roles and actions of these hormones are provided in subsequent chapters. Because the secretion of each of the pituitary hormones is controlled by hypophysiotropic hormones of hypothalamic origin, a chapter on the role of THE ENDOCRINE HYPOTHALAMUS is provided. The evidence supporting the neurovascular hypothesis is emphasized.

Chapter 7, NEUROHYPOPHYSIAL HORMONES, provides a complete coverage of the source, synthesis, chemistry, secretion, metabolism, biological actions, and mechanisms of action of the posterior pituitary hormones, oxytocin and vasopressin. The evolution of hormone structure is emphasized under the comparative endocrinology of neurohypophysial hormones. Chapter 8, THE MELANOTROPIC HORMONES, emphasizes the recent discovery that pro-opiomelanocortin is the precursor protein of α-melanotropin, adrenocorticotropin, and human's own analgesic hormones, the endorphins (opiatelike peptides). The author has done considerable research in the field of melanotropins and vertebrate pigmentation, particularly in relationship to the control of melanocyte-stimulating hormone secretion and the mechanisms of action of the melanotropins. Because the secretion and actions of most all hormones involve the calcium ion, the roles of parathormone, calcitonin, and vitamin D in the HORMONAL CONTROL OF CALCIUM HOMEOSTASIS are discussed early in the book (Chap. 9).

The next six chapters are grouped together because they all relate to aspects of metabolic endocrinology. The GASTROINTESTINAL HORMONES play important roles in the control of foodstuff movement through the gastrointestinal tract and its transport through the intestinal mucosa and into the general circulation. The chapter on PANCREATIC HORMONES AND METABOLIC ENDOCRINOLOGY discusses the roles of the endocrine pancreas in the storage and utilization of metabolic substrates. The contrasting roles of insulin and glucagon are explored, as are the possible roles of the newer pancreatic hormones, somatostatin and pancreatic polypeptide. In a chapter on GROWTH HORMONES, the varied roles of the somatomedins and other peptide growth hormones, such as nerve growth factor, epidermal growth factor, erythropoietin, and the thymic growth factors, as well as growth inhibitory factors (chalones) are discussed, in addition to an in-depth coverage of pituitary somatotropin (growth hormone).

In the chapter on THYROID HORMONES evidence is marshaled demonstrating that triiodothyronine is the physiologically relevant thyroid hormone at the cellular level. An up-to-date review of a model of thyroid hormone action is provided. A discussion of the integrated functional aspects of CATECHOLAMINES AND THE SYMPATHOADRENAL SYSTEM provides recent data on the developmental biology of catecholamine biosynthesis within adrenal chromaffin tissue and sympathetic neurons. The physiological roles of catecholamines as mediated through adrenergic receptors (adrenoceptors) is discussed, and the pharmacology of the autonomic nervous system, particularly the sympathoadrenal system, is reviewed. The chapter on the ADRENAL STEROID HORMONES completes the general discussion of the roles and actions of hormones in the control of metabolic homeostasis. Steroid hormone structure and nomenclature are reviewed. The roles of cortisol, a glucocorticoid, and aldosterone, a mineralocorticoid, are discussed in detail. The pathophysiology of adrenocortical dysfunction provides an in-depth view of the etiological bases for endocrine pathophysiology.

The next five chapters deal with the endocrinology of vertebrate reproductive systems, mostly mammalian systems. In the ENDOCRINOLOGY OF SEX DIFFERENTIATION AND DEVELOPMENT, the role of the Sry/SRY gene and its product, the testes-determining factor, in the regulation of gonadal differentiation is discussed. The early organizational roles of gonadal steroids in the development of neural centers (e.g., dimorphic nucleus) within the central nervous system, and the activation roles of steroids in CNS function in the adult animal are reviewed. In HORMONES AND MALE REPRODUCTIVE PHYSIOLOGY, as in HORMONES AND FEMALE REPRODUCTIVE PHYSIOLOGY, the origin, synthesis, chemistry, secretion, metabolism, biological roles, and mechanisms of actions of the male and female reproductive hormones are reviewed. A discussion of the pathophysiology of reproductive function in the human male and female provides an insight into the many genetic and congenital defects that affect normal growth and development of the human reproductive systems. In ENDOCRINOLOGY OF PREGNANCY, PARTURITION, AND LACTATION, the roles of hormones in the fertile period of the female are reviewed. Next is included a chapter on the ENDOCRINE ROLE OF THE PINEAL GLAND, which reviews its putative role in reproductive physiology. This chapter is long overdue; the pineal gland is clearly an endocrine organ.

A final chapter devoted to NEUROHORMONES emphasizes the emerging understanding of the importance of neuropeptides to endocrine system function. For example, the discovery and physiological roles of the endorphins, the opiatelike peptides, or "analgesic hormones," are discussed. The role of other newly discovered brain peptides in the control of behavior, including cholecystokinin (or related peptide), is discussed. The recent discovery that certain gases (e.g., nitric oxide, carbon monoxide) are novel neurohormones is reviewed. The neuroendocrinology of extrinsic sensory perception is discussed, particularly as it provides similarities to hormone receptor transduction mechanisms. A general overview of neuroendocrine pathophysiology is provided to emphasize the molecular basis for the endocrinopathies in general. Lastly, the evolution of endocrine systems is discussed.

Generally, each chapter is subdivided as follows: (1) Introduction (which provides a historical perspective to the particular topic), (2) Source, (3) Synthesis, (4) Chemistry, (5) Secretion, (6) Metabolism, (7) Physiological Roles, (8) Mechanism of Action, (9) Pathophysiology (of endocrine dysfunction), and (10) Comparative Endocrinology. Due to space limitations and other considerations the coverage of neuroendocrine physiology generally has been restricted to vertebrates, mainly mammals, particularly the human. Therefore this book should be of special appeal to preprofessional students in medicine, dentistry, pharmacology, nutrition, nursing, and other related medical or animal sciences. Within each chapter, however, where appropriate, is included a short coverage of comparative endocrinology.

References are provided with each chapter, but, because space limitations place a premium on those selected, the most recently available were used. These references will provide the reader with most of the important earlier studies related to a particular topic. The author therefore acknowledges the unreferenced contributions of many investigators in the field of neuroendocrine physiology. The author appreciates the very informative figures that have been provided for this fourth edition by leading authorities in the field of endocrine physiology. I am particularly grateful to my past students, both in the classroom and the research laboratory, who provided me with an opportunity to develop the thoughts that are now presented in this textbook of endocrinology. The author is indebted to Ms. Danielle (Dani) Camacho for the superb effort she provided in helping formulate this much revised fourth edition.

Helpful criticisms, corrections, or other comments are most welcome and may be addressed to the author.

MAC E. HADLEY
University of Arizona
College of Medicine
Department of Cell Biology & Anatomy
Tucson, Arizona 85724

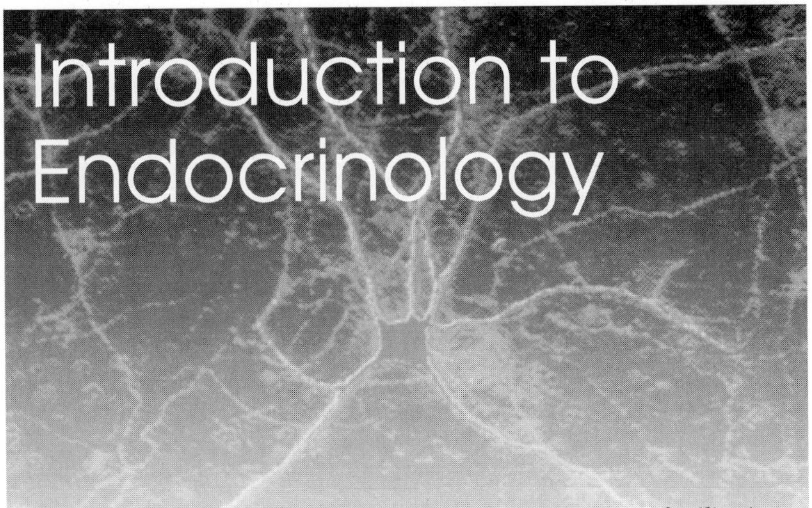

Introduction to Endocrinology

1

*Development of a multicellular organism commences upon fertilization and subsequent division of the egg. Further development is then dependent on continued cell proliferation, growth, and differentiation, including histogenesis and organogenesis. The integration of these developmental events, as well as the coordination of such physiological processes as metabolism, respiration, excretion, movement, and reproduction, are dependent on chemical cues, substances synthesized and secreted by specialized cells within the animal. The role of these **chemical messengers** in the growth and regulation of cellular function in the vertebrate is the topic of this book.*

*Endocrinology is a subdiscipline of the broader field, physiology, and is concerned with the study of chemical messengers, **hormones**, substances secreted by cells of endocrine glands (ductless glands) and tissues that regulate the activity of other cells in the body. Besides the obvious study of the physiological roles of hormones, endocrinologists also study the cellular source, biosynthesis, chemistry and storage of hormones, the factors and mechanisms controlling hormonal secretion, the cellular mechanisms of hormone action, and the pathophysiology of endocrine system dysfunction. The comparative endocrinologist is particularly interested in the study of the endocrine systems of vertebrate as well as invertebrate species [3].*

HISTORICAL PERSPECTIVE

Endocrinology is a relatively infant science that began with the first recorded endocrine experiment published by Berthold (1849) [5]. No other truly significant discoveries were made until about 50 years later (1889–1902). The pace quickened after 1910, and the outlines of vertebrate and invertebrate endocrine systems were generally complete by 1950. From then on, chemistry played a most important role in the development of the science and many advances in the field were made. Molecular biology is now advancing the field at an ever more rapid pace. The elucidation of the gene structure for hormones and their receptors is providing important insights into the evolutionary history of endocrine systems.

An Endocrine Chronology

The history of endocrinology progressed, as one might expect, from simple observations to complex experimentation. Early medical writings described the general symptoms of many endocrine dysfunctions long before the pathophysiology of any of the now well-characterized *endocrinopathies* were understood. In the age of the great European

1

microscopists of the nineteenth century, most tissues and organs of the vertebrate body were described in great detail, but the functional significance of what we now refer to as endocrine glands was not evident. Clinical correlations between tissue or organ abnormalities, such as atrophy or enlargement, and a change in a particular physiological state were occasionally noted. This led to the study of the possible effects of tissue or organ removal from animals and subsequent alteration in physiological function. The use of organ transplants or extracts in replacement therapy for the absent tissue or organ then followed. Successful replacement therapy led to the purification of these physiologically active extracts and ultimately to the identification of the hormonal substances concerned.

Berthold, a French scientist, in the earliest endocrinological study on record, noted that if he castrated cockerels they failed to develop their comb and wattles, and they also failed to exhibit male behavior [5]. Replacement of the testes (one or both) back into the abdominal cavity of the same or another castrated bird resulted in normal development of the comb and wattles, and the birds exhibited male behavior, which involved an interest in hens and aggressive action toward other males. The transplanted testes were functional and therefore not dependent on any direct nervous innervation for their activity. Berthold even observed that a transplanted single testis was larger than either testis of the host when both were present together in the bird. Thus he discovered, but may not have appreciated, what is now referred to as *compensatory hypertrophy*, an increase in the size of an organ to compensate functionally for the activity of the other lost organ. His results also demonstrated that an organ from one (donor) animal could be transplanted to another (host) animal where it became functional (Fig. 1.1).

Berthold concluded that the testes secreted something that conditioned the blood, and he speculated that the blood then acted on the body of the cockerel to cause the development of male characteristics. Actually these experiments only demonstrated the need for the presence of the testes to maintain male characteristics. The testes could maintain such behavioral and physiological functions by a number of possible means: (1) activation or transformation of one or more constituents of the blood into active agents, hormones, (2) removal of an inhibitory substance from the blood or, as is now known, (3) release of a hormone into the circulation. That the testes produce a substance that is released into the blood to affect masculine features and behavior was not proven until many years later when it was shown that extracts of the testes could functionally replace the testes of a castrated animal. The hormone of the testes, testosterone, was finally obtained in pure crystalline form in 1935.

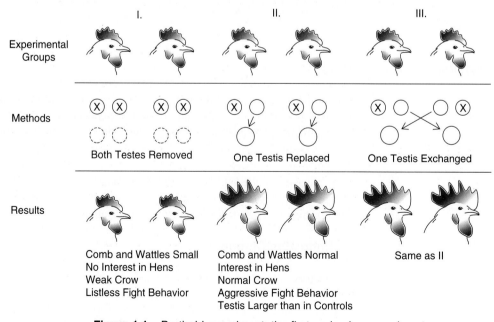

Figure 1.1 Berthold experiment: the first endocrine experiment.

In 1902 the first critical experiment, the *experimentum cruces*, demonstrating the existence of a hormone was reported [2]. Bayliss and Starling, Canadian physiologists, discovered that a substance was liberated by the mucosa of the small intestine that stimulates the flow of pancreatic juice. It was known that the acid present in chyme stimulated pancreatic secretion after it entered into the small intestine from the stomach. Introduction of acid into an isolated (denervated) but vascularized section of the jejunum caused a similar flow of pancreatic juice. This observation supported the view that the control of pancreatic enzyme secretion was mediated by humoral rather than nervous stimulation. Extracts of jejunal epithelium produced similar effects on pancreatic secretion. The active substance was given the name *secretin* and was further shown to be localized only to those regions of the small intestine that could be stimulated by acid to induce pancreatic fluid flow. Starling (1905) introduced the term *hormone* (from the Greek for I arouse to activity or I excite) for this humoral factor [20].

In 1889 Von Mering and Minkowski showed by surgical methods that removal of the pancreas from dogs led to symptoms similar to those characteristic of human *diabetes mellitus*. In these dogs, as in diabetic humans, blood sugar levels were remarkably elevated; this suggested that diabetes mellitus might result from a defect of carbohydrate metabolism due to lack of pancreatic function. Banting and Best [1] concluded from other investigations that the islets of Langerhans, rather than the pancreatic acini, which make up the bulk of the pancreas, are essential in the control of carbohydrate metabolism. They suggested that the pancreatic islets regulate blood glucose levels by producing an internal secretion, rather than by modifying the blood. In 1922 they successfully obtained extracts of the pancreatic islets and showed that these preparations caused a dramatic drop of blood glucose levels when administered to diabetic dogs [6]. This hormone of the pancreas was named insulin by Schaefer in 1912.

Although many hormones are released from cells into the general circulation to mediate their effects on distant target cells, an equally large number of chemical messengers are released from neurons into close proximity to the effector cells that they regulate. These chemical messengers of neural origin play important roles in *central nervous system* (CNS) and *automatic nervous system* (ANS) function. Walter Cannon was the first physiologist to stress the role of the ANS in the "self-regulation of physiological processes" [7]. As is described in Chap. 14, the ANS regulates the activity of such so-called "autonomic" activities as: gastrointestinal (GI) smooth muscle contraction and relaxation; GI secretions (including hormone secretions from the stomach and gut); cardiovascular muscle contraction and relaxation; and adipose tissue metabolism.

That nerves release chemical messengers to control effector cell activity was first demonstrated in 1921 by Otto Loewi [14]. A frog heart with its attached vagus nerve was incubated in physiological saline solution, and after residing therein for a period of time, the solution was removed and used to bathe a second heart. There was no effect of the solution on the *inotropic* (amplitude of beat) or *chronotropic* (rate of beat) characteristics of the incubated heart. If, on the other hand, the vagus nerve innervating an incubated heart was stimulated a number of times and the saline solution then trasnferred to another beaker containing another frog heart, a decreased (negative) inotropic and chronotropic activity was noted. These diminished myotropic responses could be blocked by addition of the drug atropine, which was known to be inhibitory to vagal nerve-induced relaxation of the heart. The atropinized heart preparations did, however, respond to saline solution taken from vagus nerve-stimulated hearts by an increased rate and strength of contraction. These experiments demonstrated that the vagus nerve released substances that affect the relaxation and contraction of cardiac muscle. For this work Loewi received a Nobel Prize. The "vagustuff" (vagal substance) was identified as *acetylcholine* and the accelerator substance as *norepinephrine*. These two neurohormones play very important roles in endocrine physiology (Chap. 14).

In 1953, Sanger established the amino acid sequence for the protein hormone insulin [18]. For this crucial work in the characterization of hormone structure he received a Nobel

Prize. By his methods the structures of most peptide hormones have been elucidated. At the same time Vincent du Vigneaud carried out the first laboratory syntheses of peptide hormones by synthesizing oxytocin and a vasopressin. For this work he, too, received a Nobel Prize. Most interestingly, he also synthesized a related structure (analog) of oxytocin, which turned out to be a hormone found in the pituitaries of most vertebrates. Thus he synthesized the structure of a hormone (vasotocin) before it was actually discovered (Chap. 7).

The Discovery of Cyclic AMP

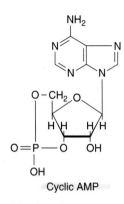

Figure 1.2
Structure of cyclic AMP, a second messenger of hormone action.

In 1962 Earl Sutherland and his colleagues presented a number of papers describing the presence of adenosine 3′, 5′-monophosphate (*cyclic AMP, cAMP*) in biological materials. These papers also dealt with adenylate cyclase, the enzyme responsible for the cellular production of this cyclic nucleotide. Sutherland and his coworkers had previously demonstrated that hormones could stimulate broken cell membrane preparations to activate liver phosphorylase, the enzyme responsible for the normal breakdown of liver glycogen. These workers established that when certain hormones were incubated with a particulate (cell membrane) fraction of liver cells, a factor was produced that could, in turn, activate the phosphorylase enzyme present in the supernatant fraction of the tissue homogenate. This substance was identified by Sutherland as cAMP (Fig. 1.2).

For this monumental discovery Sutherland received a Nobel Prize in Physiology/Medicine in 1971 [21]. Cyclic AMP, the so-called *second messenger* of hormone action, is now implicated in the actions of many hormones and other stimuli on cellular physiological processes [13]. The importance of this cyclic nucleotide to biochemistry, pharmacology, physiology, and medicine is enormous. Much of this book is, in fact, a discussion of the role of cAMP in hormone action and in normal and abnormal cellular function. More recently, a number of other diverse hormonal messengers have been discovered.

Neuropeptides and Nobel Prizes

Another crucial discovery was the demonstration that the pituitary gland, the so-called "master gland" of the body, was controlled by the brain, specifically the area known as the *hypothalamus*. Geoffrey Harris had provided data suggesting that the release of the pituitary hormones was controlled by humoral factors, probably of hypothalamic origin [11]. A number of workers then showed that extracts of the hypothalamus contained substances that affected the release of pituitary hormones [19]. The "race to Stockholm" was then on [15, 24]. Andrew Schally and Roger Guillemin, working independently of each other, began purification of hypothalamic extracts from porcine and ovine sources. After the extraction of about 250,000 pig hypothalami, Schally and his group were able to provide the structure of the factor that stimulates the release of thyroid stimulating hormone (TSH) from the pituitary gland. The structure of this thyrotropin releasing hormone (TRH) (Fig 1.3) was similar to that of the same factor isolated from sheep brains by Guillemin and reported at about the same time. This work was followed by the isolation and structural identification of several other hypothalamic hormones that control the secretion of pituitary hormones [22].

Schally and his collaborators were also able to provide the chemical structure of porcine gonadotropin releasing hormone (GnRH), which controls the release of the gonadotropins from the pituitary. Guillemin and his group then revealed that sheep GnRH was identical in structure. Understanding the structure of GnRH is of immense importance. With this knowledge it may now be possible to control fertility in humans and domestic animals with synthetic GnRH. It is also possible to improve on the structure of the natural GnRH to provide analogs that enhance gonadotropin secretion from the pituitary, which may enhance the probability of conception. On the other hand, antihormone analogs may also be produced, which may then be used as contraceptive agents.

Guillemin and his colleagues were the first to discover and report the structure of a peptide, somatostatin, that was inhibitory to pituitary somatotropin (growth hormone)

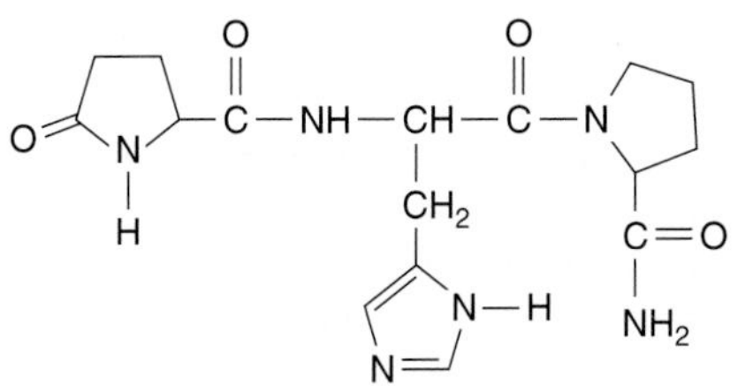

Figure 1.3 Structure of thyrotropin releasing hormone (TRH), a neurohormone.

secretion. Somatostatin, also found in other regions of the brain as well as in the pancreas, inhibits a number of hormone secretions, including the pancreatic hormones glucagon and insulin. The implications of this discovery for medicine may be vast. Already there is hope that somatostatin or related analogs may be used in the treatment of diabetes mellitus, a major endocrine dysfunction of humans.

For their contribution to the isolation and determination of the structures of the hypothalamic regulatory peptides, Guillemin and Schally received a Nobel Prize in Physiology/Medicine in 1978 [9, 19]. Certainly the pioneering work of Geoffrey Harris and many others provided the great impetus for the important accomplishments of Schally and Guillemin, as they have acknowledged. Many other chemists and endocrinologists provided important discoveries that contributed to the determination of the structures and roles of hypothalamic peptide hormones. Understanding the structures and functions of these hypothalamic regulatory hormones is of the greatest importance for the welfare of humanity. As discussed later, other hypothalamic factors are being discovered and their roles in endocrine physiology explained (Chaps. 6 and 21).

The ability to isolate and chemically characterize the hypothalamic factors was enhanced by the development of the radioimmunoassay (RIA). By the use of RIAs it is possible to detect the presence of hormones in the blood or in tissues at minute concentrations. Future possibilities for other uses of RIAs appear to be limitless [25]. For the development of the RIA, Rosalyn Yalow received a Nobel Prize in Physiology/Medicine in 1978, along with Schally and Guillemin.

More recently the Nobel Prize for Physiology/Medicine was awarded to Rita Levi-Montalcini and Stanley Cohen for their discoveries of several factors that control cell growth and development [16]. Levi-Montalcini discovered *nerve growth factor* (NGF, Chap. 12), a peptide hormone required for the growth, development, and maintenance of certain nerve cells of the peripheral nervous system, as well as in the brain. Cohen discovered *epidermal growth factor* (EGF), a peptide hormone that stimulates differentiation and growth of a variety of epithelial and other cells (Chap. 12). These discoveries have opened up a vast field of research on NGF and EGF, as well as numerous other growth factors. The biological actions of these peptide hormones are providing important insights for an understanding of normal and abnormal cell growth.

Important new information in endocrine physiology is being reported at a rapid rate. Certainly knowledge of the molecular mechanisms of peptide and steroid hormone action are being defined in exquisite detail. One might predict that future Nobel Prizes will be awarded in the exciting field of *neuroendocrine physiology*.

THE SCIENCE OF ENDOCRINOLOGY

Endocrine glands secrete their hormones into the immediate extracellular space; from here the hormones enter the circulatory system. These ductless glands differ from *exocrine glands* (e.g., salivary glands) whose products are released into ducts that lead to the digestive tract and then to the exterior of the body. Endocrinology is, therefore, the study of the ductless glands or tissues and their hormonal products. Hormones were originally considered to be synthesized within specific endocrine organs and then secreted into the bloodstream to act on specific target tissues some distance away to evoke a specific physiological response. These definitions of endocrine glands and their hormones are too restrictive and must therefore be modified to be of any instructive value. For example, Bayliss and Starling clearly demonstrated that secretin is released from the small intestine, specifically the jejunum. Secretin is actually produced and secreted by individual cells distributed individually throughout the epithelial lining of the jejunum. The GI tract is the source of other hormones and could well be considered the largest endocrine organ of the body. Cholecystokinin (CCK) travels by way of the blood to act on the pancreas to induce pancreatic secretion, but it also has many other sites of action and produces a number of other effects. CCK or a related peptide may also be released from nerve cells within the brain to act on adjacent or nearby neurons. In this case, the hormone does not travel from its source of origin to its site of action by way of the bloodstream.

Comparative Endocrinology

Much of what is known about the endocrine physiology of humans derives from data obtained from patients manifesting signs of endocrine dysfunction. Research on other animals, particularly the rat and the mouse, has also provided a wealth of information on the endocrine system of mammals, including that of humans. One should appreciate, however, the contributions that comparative endocrinology has provided for a broader evolutionary view of the endocrine system [3, 8, 13].

Although the chemical structures of most human hormones have been elucidated, this information obviously does not provide an understanding of the evolution of these hormones. Once the structures of the related hormones of other vertebrates are determined, however, it becomes possible to trace the changes in the structure of the hormones that have evolved over time. In comparing the amino acid sequences of similar peptide structures from primitive and more recent vertebrates, one can determine the approximate rates of evolutionary change in hormones and when particular chemical changes probably occurred in earth history. The structures and phylogenetic distribution of the neurohypophysial hormones has been particularly well documented (Table 7.1).

Knowledge of how hormones work owes much to studies on the large chromosomes from salivary glands of such dipteran flies as *Drosophila* and *Chironomus*. The action of hormones on genes can be visualized using the large chromosomes from these glands. Certain insect hormones cause so-called "puffs" in the chromosome structure that represent areas where DNA has become exposed and RNA synthesis is increased (see Fig. 3.4). One can follow completely the puffing patterns of these large chromosomes during the larval development of the insects. Therefore, the genomic actions of hormones that relate to the temporal aspects of developmental changes can be precisely delineated. Knowledge of invertebrate hormone structure and mechanisms of action provides a potent tool in the fight against disease-carrying or crop-damaging insects. Understanding the endocrine system of other vertebrate and invertebrate species provides important information that may be essential to animal husbandry and to the culture and raising of species such as shrimp and other edible crustaceans or mollusks [3, 8].

Clinical Endocrinology

Understanding comparative hormone structure allows one to synthesize related structural analogs with possible predictions on biological activity. This is important because some hormones are not available in large enough quantities to supply the medicinal needs of humans. A lack of growth hormone (GH) results in a failure of growth in humans. GH is commercially available and normal growth and body stature can be attained following continued administration of the hormone. Introduction of the human GH gene into bacteria by recombinant-DNA techniques provides a means for the large-scale production of the hormone (Chap. 3). The discovery and elucidation of the hypothalamic GH releasing factor (GHRH) structure has allowed production of this peptide for the stimulation of pituitary GH secretion.

THE CONCEPT OF HOMEOSTASIS

Claude Bernard, a nineteenth-century French physiologist, first formulated the concept of homeostasis [4, 10]. He pointed out that an individual lives within two environments: the exterior environment that surrounds us, and, more important, a *milieu interieur*. This internal environment is the fluid compartment within which the cells of our body are bathed. Bernard noted that this fluid is produced and controlled by the organism. He believed that organisms become more independent from changes in the outer world by maintaining constant their own internal environment. He emphasized that "it is the fixity of the milieu interieur which is the condition of free and independent life" and that "all the vital mechanisms, however varied they may be, have only one objective, that of preserving constant the conditions of life in the internal environment" [4].

This internal fluid environment bathes the cells with nutrients and inorganic and organic ions of critical importance to normal cell functioning. The blood carries important metabolites to all the cells in the body: metabolic substrates, such as sugars, fatty acids, and amino acids; cofactors, such as the vitamins needed for enzyme function; and electrolytes, such as calcium, sodium, and potassium ions, which are necessary for stability of the electrical properties of cells.

Walter Cannon [7] later stated that "the coordinated physiological processes which maintain most of the steady states in the organism are so complex and so peculiar to living beings—involving, as they may, the brain and nerves, the heart, lungs, kidneys and spleen, all working cooperatively that I have suggested a specific designation for these states, homeostasis." Mammals, for example, maintain a very stringent control over the concentration of glucose, Ca^{2+}, and Na^+, and other constituents of the body fluids. Only small fluctuations in these important fluid components are tolerated or the animal will suffer immediate and often fatal consequences. Homeostatic settings, however, are not invariant; they depend on the time of day, time of year, stage of development, age, and reproductive status of an animal. It is the ability to maintain a constant internal environment in the face of adverse environmental conditions that has undoubtedly favored the wide distribution of mammals to all types of environmental habitats. Many poikilothermic vertebrates, on the other hand, are restricted to narrow environmental niches. The price that homeotherms must pay for maintenance of the homeostatic state is a need for a constant food supply. Many poikilotherms hibernate or estivate until more favorable climatic conditions occur, when they become active again. They are, nevertheless, successful in their particular niches as they need not always depend on a continuous supply of metabolic substrates.

Feedback Systems

How does the body maintain precise control over the concentrations of such fluid components as glucose, and calcium and sodium ions? Certain sensory and endocrine cells in the body, either individually or functioning as a unit, seem to possess a definite set point (like a thermostat) for monitoring the concentrations of these substances. If the plasma concentration of a metabolite is diminished, for example, by loss through the urine or by perspiration, these receptive cells respond by releasing a substance, in this context, a hormone, which then acts on other cells to release their stores of the needed metabolite or to prevent its loss from the body. These responses to hormonal stimulation elevate the levels of such factors as Na^+ or glucose in the blood to a point where, for example, the cellular osmostat or glucostat shuts off release of its chemical messenger. Increased metabolite availability therefore functions as a *negative feedback* stimulus (Fig. 1.4).

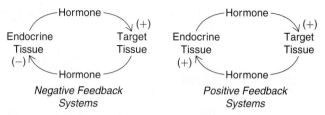

Figure 1.4   General scheme of negative and positive feedback systems.

Many such systems within the vertebrate body have been discovered, and there are even examples of *positive feedback* where rising concentrations of a hormone cause another gland to release a second hormone, which is then stimulatory to an increased output of the first hormone (Fig. 1.4). A positive feedback system must have some mechanism of shutting off release of the first hormone or the system would increase continuously in amplitude. In the primate, estradiol, a gonadal estrogen, increases the release of pituitary hormones, which, in turn, stimulate ovarian estrogen production. Consequently estrogen levels as well as gonadotropin levels increase concomitantly. The monthly demise of the ovarian follicle, the source of estradiol, results in a subsequent fall in plasma estrogen and gonadotropin levels (Chap. 18). Presently there are only a few recognized examples of positive feedback.

In a number of feedback systems an increase in the plasma levels of one hormone may be stimulatory to the release of a metabolite (e.g., glucose) from a target tissue. Elevated plasma levels of the metabolite may then be stimulatory to the release of a second hormone, which has an inhibitory effect on the release of the metabolite from the target tissue. The lowered level of the metabolite would, in turn, be the stimulus to the release of the first hormone (Fig. 1.5). Some specific examples of the roles of hormones in plasma metabolite homeostasis will now be discussed.

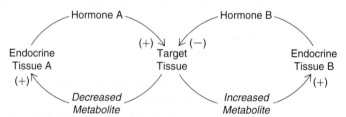

Figure 1.5   General scheme of two-hormone feedback systems.

HORMONES AND HOMEOSTASIS

Maintenance of a constant internal environment is necessary for the normal functioning of the various cellular components of tissues and organs. Nerve cells, for example, must be bathed in an extracellular fluid of a definite electrolyte composition and concentration. If the concentration of monovalent cations, such as Na^+ or K^+, or the divalent cation, Ca^{2+}, is altered, the activity of the neurons will also be affected, which will lead to depressed or hyperactive neuronal activity. The following three examples illustrate the homeostatic control of metabolic and mineral constituents of the blood.

Glucose Homeostasis

Blood glucose in normal humans is maintained at a precise concentration. Many factors affect the circulating levels of glucose such as food intake, rate of digestion, metabolism, excretion, exercise, psychological state, and reproductive state. These influences, individ-

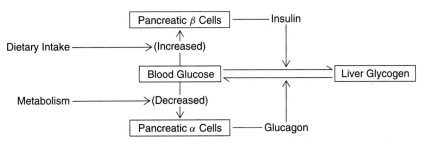

Figure 1.6   Hormonal control of glucose homeostasis.

ually or in combination, constantly affect the physiological processes that regulate plasma glucose levels. The glucose level may drop momentarily due to muscular activity, especially if food intake is limited. The diminished level of blood glucose is in some way recognized by certain cells in the pancreas, specifically the *alpha (α) cells* of the *islets of Langerhans*. These cells then release glucagon, a hormone that acts on cells of the liver to cause the release of glucose. Thus the blood glucose level is brought back to normal. If, on the other hand, blood glucose is elevated, as occurs usually after a meal, other pancreatic islet cells, *beta (β) cells*, release the hormone insulin. Insulin induces the uptake of glucose from the blood into the liver and other cells. Thus the glucose level of the blood is lowered to the normal circulating concentration. There is greater likelihood of developing hyperglycemia than there is of developing hypoglycemia, since most hormones, if they affect metabolism, have a hyperglycemic effect. Lack of insulin, therefore, results in a serious inability to lower blood glucose, which results in diabetes mellitus. The feedback control of blood glucose is shown schematically in Fig. 1.6.

Calcium Homeostasis

Calcium is required by all cells of the body for a variety of functions. The calcium ion (Ca^{2+}) is needed for clotting of the blood, and it is a requirement for cellular secretory processes. This divalent cation is also required for muscle contraction [17] and is undoubtedly required for many other more subtle cellular functions. In most mammals the concentration of Ca^{2+} in the blood is maintained within very narrow limits. Any deviation from this set point will cause homeostatic mechanisms to bring the concentration of Ca^{2+} back to this level. If Ca^{2+} levels fall, this is perceived by cells in the parathyroid glands and they secrete parathormone (Chap. 9). This hormone then (1) acts on bone to release stored Ca^{2+}, (2) stimulates Ca^{2+} absorption from the gut, and (3) enhances resorption of Ca^{2+} from the urine by the kidney. All these actions tend to bring the concentration of the cation back to normal. Lack of parathormone, on the other hand, leads to a lowering of serum Ca^{2+}, which may lead to tetanic convulsions and death.

If serum Ca^{2+} becomes elevated, as it may after a meal, then other cells release a hormone, calcitonin, which lowers the level of circulating Ca^{2+}. In mammals this hormone is released from parafollicular cells within the thyroid gland (Chap. 9). Somehow these cells are capable of detecting elevated levels of Ca^{2+}. Calcitonin causes deposition of Ca^{2+} into bone, and it may have other actions on the gut and kidney to prevent Ca^{2+} uptake and resorption. The hormonal homeostatic mechanisms controlling serum Ca^{2+} levels are shown in Fig. 1.7.

Sodium Homeostasis

Although the sodium ion (Na^+) is the major electrolyte in body fluids, Na^+ is continuously being lost from the body in urine and sweat. Specialized cells in the walls of certain blood vessels within the kidney act as *osmoreceptors* and continuously monitor the Na^+ concentration of the blood. If a drop in osmolarity is noted, these cells release a substance, renin, which, acting as an enzyme, is able to split a plasma protein into a smaller peptide. This

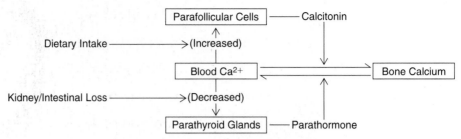

Figure 1.7 Hormonal control of calcium homeostasis.

peptide is then acted upon by yet another enzyme to release a still smaller peptide, angiotensin II, a hormone. Angiotensin II then stimulates certain cells of the adrenal cortex to release aldosterone, another hormone. This hormone then acts on certain collecting tubules of the kidney to cause resorption of Na^+ from the urine. Thus a complex set of hormonal actions are brought into play to maintain the proper levels of blood Na^+ (Fig 15.10).

The Heart as an Endocrine Gland.   Atrial distension due to blood volume expansion is a stimulus to renal salt and water diuresis. In the past it was generally held that the cardiac atria served to sense the fullness of the intravascular fluid compartment. The resulting "reflex" diuresis resulting from atrial stretch receptors was thought to result from activation of neural stretch receptors located within the atrial subendocardium.

The pioneering work of De Bold [23] revealed that saline extracts of atria, but not of ventricles, provoked a marked increase in urinary salt and water excretion when injected into rats. An *atrial natriuretic factor* (ANF) extracted from atria is a polypeptide whose structure has been elucidated, synthesized, and biologically characterized [23]. This cardiac hormone may be a major regulator of the physiological responses to volume overload. The homeostatic regulation of ANF release and volume regulation is depicted in Fig. 15.15. The therapeutic potential of this newly discovered hormone is of obvious clinical importance, as will be discussed at length in Chap. 15.

NEUROENDOCRINE INTEGRATION IN HOMEOSTASIS

A variety of stimuli of both *extrinsic* (environmental) and *intrinsic* (within the body) origin affect physiological processes within an animal. The body must interpret changes in environmental temperature and day length. The recognition of odors produced by members of the opposite sex may be important in the control of reproductive behavior. Changes in fluid electrolyte levels or metabolic substrate levels must be monitored. Pain stimuli, whether of extrinsic or intrinsic origin, must be perceived. The recognition of these factors is accomplished by cellular sensory elements (receptors), which may be referred to as mechanoreceptors, chemoreceptors, osmoreceptors, or baroreceptors, depending on which modality is monitored. These sensory elements may be cellular components of glands, such as the pancreas, or they may be neural elements of the eye, nasal (olfactory) epithelium, or other tissues. These sensory cells respond to sensory cues by releasing a hormone directly into the blood or by transmitting a nerve impulse to other neurons or cellular elements that then release one or more chemical messengers. After the stomach contents (chyme) are released into the small intestine, hydrogen ions (protons from hydrochloric acid) interact with specific cells of the gut epithelium, which results in the release of the hormone, secretin. Secretin then enters the blood stream and interacts with cells of the pancreas to release a fluid secretion that neutralizes the acid within the small intestine. This is the classical example of a hormone, as first described by Bayliss and Starling [2], and a further example of a homeostatic mechanism (Fig 10.6).

The release of most hormones is not as simple as that seen in the example of secretin. Sensory cues are often transmitted from one neuron to one or more other neurons, which may ultimately result in the release of a hormone. Therefore the nervous system, working through the endocrine system, plays an important role in the homeostasis of a number of such physiological processes as water balance, temperature regulation, and even feeding behavior. The following examples of neuroendocrine integration are discussed in more detail in Chap. 21.

Control of Water Balance

If water is lost and not replaced, dehydration results. The hyperosmolality and hypovolemia are detected by *osmoreceptors* and *baroreceptors*, sensory cells that monitor changes in Na^+ concentration or volume (pressure), respectively, of the blood. Baroreceptor neurons, located within the carotid sinus, for example, relay information to specific sites within the brain. Integration of this information within the hypothalamus results in the release of a hormone, vasopressin, from neurons that are components of the posterior pituitary gland. This antidiuretic hormone (ADH) is released into the blood and acts on certain cells of the kidney's collecting tubules to cause water reabsorption. Vasopressin also causes contraction of certain smooth muscles of the vasculature, which results in partial restoration of blood pressure. In addition sensory neurons within the brain may also monitor fluid osmolarity, and, under dehydrating conditions, neurohormones are released to act within the brain to initiate drinking (*dipsogenic*) behavior. The complexity of this neuroendocrine control of water balance is discussed more fully in Chap. 7.

Control of Body Temperature

The temperature of the body, at least that of humans, is maintained at a precise level, although it does exhibit a circadian (daily) variation. Hormones and neuronal mechanisms are crucial in temperature regulation. Alterations in body temperature are monitored by sensory neurons within the brain. These neurons release neurotransmitter substances that stimulate other neurons to initiate physiological processes that lead to warming or cooling of the body back to the normal state. Under cooling conditions where body heat is lost, neurons within the brain release one or more neurohormones that increase metabolic activity and heat production within the body. Specifically, a hormone (Fig. 1.3) released from nerves within the hypothalamus of the brain stimulates the release of a thyroid stimulating hormone (TSH) from the pituitary. This hormone released into the circulation stimulates cells of the thyroid gland to release one or more thyroid hormones, thyroxine and triiodothyronine, which then stimulate metabolism within various cells of the body with resulting heat production [12]. In addition neurohormones released within the brain also activate the *sympathetic nervous system* and the adrenal gland to release hormones that also affect metabolic processes by causing the release of glucose from the liver; this can then be utilized as a metabolic substrate for heat production. The sympathetic nervous system will also release hormones that cause vasoconstriction, which will result in decreased heat loss from the skin. These are only a few of the neuroendocrine mechanisms involved in the complex physiological processes that maintain body temperature.

Control of Feeding Behavior

Blood glucose not only triggers the direct release of pancreatic hormones to restore normal blood sugar levels, but cellular *glucostats* within the brain may also monitor glucose levels and set into motion complex physiological processes to restore the normal blood glucose concentration. These glucostats are located in the basal hypothalamus (*satiety center*) of the brain. Neurons from this center apparently maintain a tonic inhibitory control over neurons in the lateral hypothalamus (*feeding center*). Under conditions of low blood glucose, satiety center neurons no longer inhibit the feeding center neurons.

Neuronal pathways from the feeding center then activate other neuronal centers concerned with the sensation of hunger. This leads to food intake and the restoration of blood glucose back to normal levels (Chap. 21).

HORMONES AND BEHAVIOR

Besides the behaviors associated with water and food intake to maintain volume and nutrient homeostasis, hormones regulate many other behaviors necessary for survival.

Sexual Behavior.   Hormones regulate courtship, mating, and maternal behaviors that are necessary for reproductive success and perpetuation of the species. Libido in the human male is critically dependent upon hormones (androgens) produced by the gonads, which then manifest themselves through actions on the brain. Libido in the human female may be "encephalized" and less dependent upon a hormonal directive. In other mammals, however, female behavior is acutely affected and directed by the hormonal milieu of the animal.

Hormones and Homosexuality.   To what extent, if any, are hormones responsible for sexual behaviors that might be considered by some to differ from the norm? If there is a biological (hormonal) basis for these anomalous sexual behaviors, then how can such actions be viewed as "deviant?" Some evidence suggests that the anatomy of the brain of some homosexual males may be somewhere between the male and female anatomical construct. If true, then we may have to accept that certain sexual activities may therefore be biologically driven and not due to some societal directive (Chap. 17).

HORMONES, GROWTH REGULATION, AND CANCER

Just as hormones regulate glucose, Ca^{2+}, and Na^+ balance, a number of hormones also control the growth of the cellular components of tissues and organs. Growth factors are now known to be involved in homeostasis of body growth and function. A major discovery in cancer research is the finding of a relationship between normal growth regulation by growth factors and by *oncogenes*, proto-oncogenes that acquire cancerous (oncogenic) characteristics. Proto-oncogenes, which are postulated to control normal cellular growth, particularly in early development, may themselves become uncontrolled (mutated) and produce growth factors or growth factor receptors that activate cellular mechanisms leading to uncontrolled (abnormal) cell growth, or cancer. These hormonelike peptides may even be products of cancer-causing viruses and may be responsible for tumor formation (Chap. 12).

REFERENCES

[1]   Banting, F. G., and G. H. Best. 1922. The internal secretion of the pancreas. *J. Lab. Clin. Med.* 7:241–66.

[2]   Bayliss, W. M., and E. H. Starling. 1902. Mechanisms of pancreatic secretion. *J. Physiol.* 28:325–53.

[3]   Bern, H. A. 1990. The "new" endocrinology: its scope and its impact. *Amer. Zool.* 30:877–85.

[4]   Bernard, C. 1965. *Introduction a l'étude de la mèdicine experimentale.* Paris: J. B. Ballière et Fils.

[5] Berthold, A. A. 1849. Transplantation der Hoden. *Arch. Anat. Phsiol. Wiss. Med.* 16:42–6.

[6] Bliss, M. 1989. J. J. R. Macleod and the discovery of insulin. *Quart. J. Exp. Physiol.* 74:87–96.

[7] Cannon, W. B. 1960. *The wisdom of the body.* New York: W. W. Norton & Co., Inc.

[8] Gorbman, A., W. W. Dickhoff, S. R. Vigna, N. B. Clark, and C. L. Ralph. 1983. *Comparative endocrinology.* New York: John Wiley & Sons, Inc.

[9] Guillemin, R. 1978. Peptides in the brain: the new endocrinology of the neuron. *Science* 202:390–402.

[10] Guillemin, R., and L. Guillemin, translators. 1974. Claude Bernard. *Lectures on the phenomena of life common to animals and plants.* Springfield, Ill.: Charles Thomas, Publisher.

[11] Harris, G. W. 1955. *Neural control of the pituitary gland.* London: Edward Arnold, Ltd.

[12] Ismail-Beigi, F. 1988. Thyroid thermogenesis: regulation of (Na^++K^+)-adenosine triphosphatase and active Na,K transport. *Amer. Zool.* 28:363–71.

[13] Kaltenbach, J. C. 1988. Endocrine aspects of homeostasis. *Amer. Zool.* 28:761–73.

[14] Loewi, O. 1921. Uebertragbarkeit der Herznervenwirkung. *Pflüger's Arch. ges Physiol.* 189:239–42.

[15] Marx, J. L. 1986. The 1986 Nobel Prize for physiology or medicine. *Science* 234:543–4.

[16] Marx, J. L. 1988. The 1988 Nobel Prize for physiology or medicine: three researchers are honored for developing drugs that combat some of mankind's most common diseases. *Science* 242:516–7.

[17] Rasmussen, H. 1989. The messenger function of Ca^{2+}: from PTH action to smooth muscle contraction. *Bone Miner.* 5:233–48.

[18] Sanger, F. 1959. Chemistry of insulin. *Science* 129:1340–4.

[19] Schally, A. V. 1978. Aspects of hypothalamic regulation of the pituitary gland. *Science* 202:18–28.

[20] Starling, E. H. 1905. The chemical correlation of the functions of the body. *Lancet* 1:340–1.

[21] Sutherland, E. 1972. Studies on the mechanisms of hormone action. *Science* 177:401–8.

[22] Vance, M. L. 1990. Growth-hormone-releasing hormone. *Clin. Chem.* 36:415–20.

[23] Vesely, D. L. 1991. *The atrial peptides.* Prentice Hall Endocrinology Series. Englewood Cliffs, N.J.: Prentice Hall, Inc.,

[24] Wade, N. 1978. Guillemin and Schally. *Science* 200:279–82; 411–14; 510–3.

[25] Yalow, R. S. 1978. Radioimmunoassay: a probe for the fine structure of biologic systems. *Science* 200:1236–45.

2

The Vertebrate Endocrine System

After fertilization of the vertebrate egg, a number of inductive process-es ensue that cause the zygote to divide and develop into an embryo. The chemical messengers regulating early embryonic differentiation and development are only now being clarified. The fetus will grow, develop, use metabolic substrates, respire, move, and excrete various waste products. The extent to which these physiological processes are regulated by hormones of fetal or maternal origin is also poorly understood. Whether the embryo will develop in a male or female direction is, however, determined by early endocrine influences (Chap. 16). The fetus will be liberated from the environment of the womb at parturition; the infant will continue to grow and develop, and new physiological functions and morphological changes will occur during growth and development of the young animal. The adolescent will develop into an adult and the adult may bear offspring of its own. A large number of hormones are required to control and coordinate these various physiological activities. Some hormones may only func-tion during specific developmental stages, and their physiological roles may even change in time. Growth hormone and thyroid hor-mones, for example, are necessary for normal bone growth in the young animal; these same hormones assume new or additional func-tions in the adult.

Some hormones cause rapid responses after being secreted, such as milk release and uterine contraction in response to oxytocin. Epinephrine, a hormone of the adrenal medulla, causes an almost instantaneous change in the rate and force of the heart beat. Other hor-mones, such as gonadal steroids, initiate a slower response, for instance, protein synthesis within muscle and other tissues. Testosterone or one of its metabolites affects the development of the brain at an early developmental period, but these effects may not become manifest until the animal approaches sexual maturity. In some animals this may occur many years later. Some hormones, for example corticotropin (ACTH), may only control a few physiological functions; others like testosterone may affect physiological processes in many target tissues. A large and diverse number of hormones are required for coordinating the complex physiological events associated with reproductive processes, especially in the female. These may include differentiation of the gonads, germ cell maturation, development of secondary sexual characteristics, milk pro-duction, labor at parturition, and sexual behavior.

In this chapter the general characteristics of the vertebrate endocrine system are considered. Each endocrine gland or tissue and its hormones will be discussed in greater detail later in the text.

ENDOCRINE GLANDS AND THEIR HORMONES

Tissues are composed of one particular cell type, and a number of tissues usually function together to form an organ. An endocrine gland, for example, is composed of a prominent mass (parenchyma) of secretory cells, as well as connective tissue, blood vessels, and nerves. Endocrine glands (ductless glands) secrete their products directly into the bloodstream. This is in contrast to exocrine glands (e.g., salivary glands), which release their products into ducts leading into the lumen of other organs, such as the intestine, or to the outside of the animal. The hormones of the adrenal steroidogenic tissue are synthesized within a compact mass of tissue, but some hormones are secreted by individual cells or groups of cells found distributed within other nonendocrine tissue. The pancreatic islets, for example, which are the source of insulin and glucagon, are found embedded within the much larger exocrine pancreas. Gastrointestinal hormones are produced by individual isolated cells, distributed diffusely throughout the endothelial lining of the stomach and gut [21]. A few endocrine glands are transient in nature. For example, hormones are produced by the placenta during pregnancy; the placenta and its endocrine tissue are lost during parturition but return, de novo, during a subsequent pregnancy. Endocrine glands usually secrete more than one hormone, but the parathyroids may be an example where an endocrine organ secretes but one hormone.

The pituitary gland is the source of a large number of hormones. The anterior lobe, or pars distalis, contains at least six well-characterized hormones and a number of other hormonal candidates (Chap. 5). The pars intermedia (the intermediate lobe of the pituitary) contains one or more hormones, and the posterior lobe, or neurohypophysis, contains at least two hormones. Although the pituitary gland was once considered the master gland of the body, its function is subservient to the brain, in particular, the hypothalamus (Chap. 6). The secretion of the pituitary principles of the pars distalis and pars intermedia is under the control of hypothalamic releasing and inhibiting hormones [18, 20]. Some of these hypothalamic factors have not yet been chemically characterized and are only considered as candidate hormones; they are often referred to as factors rather than hormones (e.g., prolactin releasing factor, PRF). Numerous other hormones are also present within the hypothalamus and other parts of the brain; the brain is one of the richest sources of hormones. The hormones of the hypothalamus and pituitary (Table 2.1), as well as hormones from other sources (Table 2.2), are listed with a brief statement of their functions.

HORMONES DEFINED

Bayliss and Starling [3] discovered that the small intestine is the source of a substance released into the bloodstream that acts on cells of the exocrine pancreas, causing the fluid (bicarbonate) secretion necessary to neutralize the acid present within the chyme. This substance, secretin, was subsequently referred to as a hormone. Hormones are generally considered to be chemical messengers that are released from cells into the bloodstream to exert their action on target cells some distance away. These bloodborne messengers of the endocrine system originally were distinguished from *neurotransmitters*, the chemical messengers released from neurons into a synapse between the nerve and its *effector cells*, such as secretory cells, muscle cells, or other neurons. It was discovered that the posterior pituitary gland mainly consisted of axonal endings of neurons that stored the hormones oxytocin and vasopressin. These hormones are released upon appropriate stimulation into the bloodstream to regulate target tissues of the mammary gland, uterus, and kidney. These peptide hormones of neural origin were referred to as *neurosecretions* to distinguish them from such neurotransmitter substances as acetylcholine, norepinephrine, and serotonin [27].

It has been discovered that many peptide hormones, adrenocorticotropin (ACTH), cholecystokinin (CCK), and others, which function in the classical sense as bloodborne

TABLE 2.1   Vertebrate Hypothalamic and Pituitary Hormones

Source of hormone			Major physiological roles [a]
Hypothalamus			
Gonadotropin releasing hormone	GnRH	↑	FSH and LH secretion
Thyrotropin releasing hormone	TRH	↑	TSH secretion
Corticotropin releasing hormone	CRH	↑	ACTH secretion
Prolactin inhibiting factor	PIF[b]	↓	Prolactin secretion
Melanocyte stimulating hormone (MSH) release inhibiting factor	MIF[b]	↓	MSH secretion
Somatostatin (somatotropin release inhibiting hormone)	SRIF	↓	GH secretion
Somatocrinin (growth hormone releasing hormone)	GHRH	↑	GH secretion
Pituitary Gland			
Posterior Lobe[c]			
Oxytocin		↑	Milk secretion; uterine contraction
Vasopressin (arginine vasopressin) (antidiuretic hormone)	AVP ADH	↑	Renal water absorption; vasoconstriction
Melanin concentrating hormone	MCH	↑	Melanosome aggregation (teleost fishes)
Pars Intermedia			
Melanocyte stimulating hormone	MSH	↑	Integumental melanogenesis; melanosome dispersion
Pars Distalis			
Follicle stimulating hormone (follitropin)	FSH	↑	Female: ovarian follicle growth; estradiol synthesis
		↑	Male: spermatogenesis
Luteinizing hormone (lutropin)	LH	↑	Female: ovulation; ovarian estradiol and progesterone synthesis
		↑	Male: testicular androgen synthesis
Prolactin	PRL	↑	Milk synthesis; corpus luteum progesterone synthesis in some species
Thyrotropin (thyroid stimulating hormone)	TSH	↑	Thyroid hormone (T_4 and T_3) synthesis and secretion
Corticotropin (adrenal cortical stimulating hormone)	ACTH	↑	Adrenal steroidogenesis
Somatotropin (growth hormone, GH)	STH	↑	Hepatic somatomedin biosynthesis

[a]The effect of each hormone on either an increased or stimulated (↑) or a decreased or inhibited (↓) physiological response is indicated.

[b]There is some evidence for putative PRL and MSH releasing factors.

[c]See Chap. 7 for other vertebrate neurohypophysial hormones.

hormones, are also synthesized within specific neurons in the central and peripheral nervous system. There is evidence that some of these peptide hormones may function as neurotransmitters within the nervous system. On the other hand, dopamine, which has always been considered a classic example of a neurotransmitter, is released from nerves within the brain (hypothalamus) into the bloodstream (hypophysial portal system) and carried to the pituitary gland where it functions in the control of prolactin and α-MSH secretion. Here, then, is an example of a neurotransmitter functioning as a classical hormone. One can no longer separate the endocrine and nervous system into unrelated physiological systems. The hypothalamus, for example, is the richest source of chemical messengers and should be considered the "endocrine hypothalamus" (Chap. 6).

Based simply on anatomical considerations, hormones derived from nerve cells may be called *neurohormones*, a specific subclass of hormones; they may be *neuropeptides* or nonpeptidergic in nature (e.g., dopamine). Although neurohormones may be secreted into the bloodstream, they also regulate neuronal function within the nervous system as neurotransmitters or as *neuromodulators*. In contrast to the rapid actions of neurotransmitters, neuromodulatory substances are considered to exert slower, but more sustained, neurotropic

TABLE 2.2 Some Other Vertebrate Hormones

Source of hormone			Major physiological roles [a]
Thyroid			
Thyroxine	*outer glomerulosa → faciculata → reticularis*	T_4 ↑	Growth; differentiation; calorigenesis (↑ metabolic rate and oxygen consumption)
Triiodothyronine		T_3	Same as for thyroxine
Adrenal steroidogenic tissue			
Cortisol *adrenal cortex*		↑	Carbohydrate metabolism; sympathetic function
Corticosterone		↑	Carbohydrate metabolism; sympathetic function
Aldosterone *glomerulosa*		↑	Sodium retention
Adrenal chromaffin tissue			
Epinephrine		E	Multiple ↑ and ↓ effects on nerves, muscles, cellular secretions, and metabolism
Norepinephrine		NE	Generally same physiological roles as epinephrine
Ovary (preluteal follicle)			
Estradiol		E_2 ↑	Female sexual development and behavior
Ovary (corpus luteum)			
Progesterone		↑	Uterine and mammary gland growth; maternal behavior
Relaxin		↑	Relaxation of public symphysis and dilation of uterine cervix
Placenta			
Chorionic gonadotropin (choriogonadotropin)		CG ↑	Corpus luteum progesterone synthesis
Placental lactogen		PL ↑	Possibly fetal growth and development, mammary gland development in the mother
Testes (Leydig cells)			
Testosterone		↑	Male sexual development and behavior
Testes (Sertoli cells)			
Inhibin		↓	Pituitary FSH secretion
Müllerian regression factor		MRF	Müllerian duct regression (atrophy)
Pineal (epiphysis)		↓	Gonadal development (antigonadotropic action)
Melatonin			
Thymus gland			
Thymic hormones		↑	Proliferation and differentiation of lymphocytes
Pancreatic islets			
Insulin		↓	Blood glucose; ↑ protein, glycogen, and fat synthesis
Glucagon		↑	Blood glucose; gluconeogenesis; glycogenolysis
Somatostatin		SRIF ↓	Secretion of other pancreatic islet hormones
Pancreatic polypeptide		PP ↑↓	Secretion of other pancreatic islet hormones
Gastrointestinal tract			
Gastrin		↑	HCl secretion
Secretion		↑	Pancreatic acinar cell fluid (bicarbonate) secretion
Cholecystokinin		CCK ↑	Pancreatic acinar cell enzyme secretion; gall bladder contraction
Gastric inhibitory peptide		GIP ↓ ↑	Gastric acid (HCl) secretion, Insulin secretion
Vasoactive intestinal peptide		VIP ↑	Intestinal secretion of electrolytes; smooth muscle relaxation
Glucagonlike peptide		GLP-1 ↑	Insulin secretion
Motilin		↑	Gastric acid secretion; villous motility
Neurotensin		NT	Enteric neurotransmitter
Substance P		SP	Enteric neurotransmitter
Gastrin releasing peptide		GRP ↑	Gastrin secretion; decreased gastric acid secretion
Parathyroid glands			
Parathormone		PTH ↑ ↓	Blood calcium (Ca^{2+}) Blood phosphate (PO_4^{-3})
Thyroid parafollicular cells (or ultimobranchial glands)			
Calcitonin		↓	Blood Ca^{2+}

TABLE 2.2 Some Other Vertebrate Hormones (*Continued*)

Source of hormone			Major physiological roles [a]
Skin, liver, kidney			
Vitamin D_3		↑	Blood Ca^{2+}; intestinal Ca^{2+} absorption, renal Ca^{2+} reabsorption
Plasma angiotensinogen			
Angiotensin II	AII	↑	Vasoconstriction; aldosterone secretion; thirst (dipsogenic) behavior)
Kidney			
Erythropoietin (erythrocyte stimulating factor, ESF)	EP	↑	Erythropoiesis
Most all tissues			
Prostaglandins (PGs)	PGE_2	↑	Second messenger formation
	$PGF_{2\alpha}$	↑	Second messenger formation
Prostacyclins	PGI_2	↑	Second messenger formation
Thromboxanes	TXA_2	↑	Second messenger formation
Leukotrienes	LTE_4	↑↓	Second messenger formation
Various tissues			
Epidermal growth factor	EGF	↑	Epithelial cell proliferation
Fibroblast growth factor	FGF	↑	Fibroblast proliferation
Nerve growth factor	NGF	↑	Neurite development
Somatomedins	IGF-I	↑	Cellular growth and proliferation
Endorphins (e.g., enkephalins)		↑	Opiatelike activity
Heart			
Atrial natriuretic factor (atriopeptin)	ANF	↑	Renal salt and water diuresis

[a]The major effect of each putative chemical messenger on either an increased or stimulated (↑) or a decreased or inhibited (↓) physiological response is indicated.

actions [16, 34]. Their actions are believed to enhance or inhibit (and therefore modulate) the response of neurons to neurotransmitters. Neuromodulatory hormones may also originate from nonneuronal sources. For example, adrenocortical steroids, such as cortisol, or androgens and estrogens of gonadal origin may modulate central nervous system activity and therefore play an important role in sexual and other behaviors (Chap. 16) [35].

Some cells within the gastrointestinal epithelium and other tissues of the body secrete peptide hormones and neurotransmitter substances (e.g., serotonin) locally to regulate adjacent cells. Here are examples of neurotransmitter substances acting nonsynaptically and hormones acting locally rather than by a bloodborne route. Growth inhibitory substances, *chalones*, may represent other examples of local hormones [7, 19]. Some chemical messengers are released to the exterior of animals where by air convection or water dispersal they interact with cells (e.g., nasal olfactory epithelium) of other members of the same species to evoke a response; these substances are referred to as *pheromones* [22].

In consideration of the multiple sources of peptide hormones, within glandular cells or within neurons, and the observation that classical neurotransmitters may function as a local hormone, neurotransmitter, or neuromodulatory substance, a broader definition of a hormone is required. Guillemin suggested that a hormone be defined as "any substance released by a cell and which acts on another cell near or far, regardless of the singularity or ubiquity of the source and regardless of the means of conveyance, blood stream, axoplasmic flow, or immediate intercellular space" [14]. In this book the term hormone will be used in this generic context, but such terms as neurotransmitter, neuromodulator, or neurohormone may be used to indicate specific examples of hormones (Table 2.3). Endocrinology is, by this definition, the study of hormones derived from the classical endocrine glands (e.g., pituitary, thyroid, adrenal, gonads) or from other cells or tissues such as the brain or GI tract. Some teachers and students may prefer to restrict the use of the term hormone in the classical sense and may use the more cumbersome term, chemical messenger, to include neurohormones, pheromones, and so on.

One problem arising from the recognition of the varied distribution of hormones is one of relating to the physiological roles of a hormone. If one wants to know the func-

TABLE 2.3 Hormone Terminology

Chemical messenger:	Any substance produced by a cell of endogenous or exogenous origin that plays a physiological role in the control of the activity of another cell.
Hormone:	Any substance elaborated by one cell to regulate another cell (used here synonymously with chemical messenger). May be delivered by: endocrine, neuroendocrine, neurocrine, paracrine, autocrine, or even pheromonal route.
Neurohormone:	A hormone produced by a nerve cell.
Neuropeptide:	A peptidergic neurohormone (e.g., substance P).
Nonpeptidergic neurohormone:	Any nonpeptidergic neurohormone, such as acetylcholine, histamine, norepinephrine and serotonin.
Neurotransmitter:	A neurohormone that acts transynaptically.
Neuromodulator:	A hormone that modulates the response of a neuron to a neurotransmitter or other hormone.
Pheromones:	Chemical messengers released to the exterior of one animal to stimulate a response in another member of the same species.
Lumones:	Chemical messengers released into the lumen of the GI tract.
Chalones:	Putative cellular mitotic inhibitors.
Growth factors:	Mitogenic peptides that may, in time, become established hormones.

tional role of a specific hormone, it is necessary to inquire as to which source of the hormone is being discussed. For example, the hormone somatostatin is released from specific neurons in the brain to regulate the release of somatotropin and possibly other hormones from the pituitary gland (Chap. 6). This peptide hormone is also present in other neurons within the CNS where it may function as a neurohormone (neurotransmitter or a neuromodulator). Somatostatin is also found within the gut epithelium and the pancreas, and it undoubtedly functions in these sites by a local mechanism to regulate gastrin, glucagon, and insulin secretion (Chap. 11). Portal plasma levels of somatostatin are elevated after a meal; the peptide may function in this example as a bloodborne chemical messenger (hormone in the classical sense) as it does in the regulation of pituitary STH secretion. Somatostatin eventually may be shown to have as many functions as the particular neurons or cells within which it is localized. Like the neurotransmitter dopamine, which is distributed widely within the brain and which subserves many functions, the localization of peptide hormones to specific neurons suggests that they, too, probably regulate a diverse number of functions.

GENERAL CLASSES OF CHEMICAL MESSENGERS

Although there are many vertebrate hormones, they may be conveniently categorized into groups that bear structural and/or functional similarities. Generally these groupings also imply some major differences in cellular source and synthesis of the particular chemical messengers that comprise the group. Peptide hormones, thyroid hormones, and all neurotransmitters are of neuroectodermal or endodermal origin, whereas steroid hormones are of mesodermal origin.

Peptide Hormones

As implied by the subgroup classification, these hormones are composed of amino acids. There may be as few as 3 amino acids (as in thyrotropin releasing hormone, TRH, Fig 1.3) or as many as 180 or more in the pituitary gonadotropins. Although the individual hormones could be referred to as peptide, polypeptide, or protein in nature, depending on their specific chain length, for the sake of brevity here they are referred to as peptide hormones. Peptide hormones may be composed of a linear chain, as in α-MSH or angiotensin II, or may contain a ring structure due to bridge formation through disulfide bonds, as in the *neurohypophysial hormones* oxytocin and vasopressin (see Fig. 7.2) or somatostatin (see Fig. 6.6). Some of the larger protein hormones are composed of two chains, as in insulin (see Fig. 11.5), thyrotropin (TSH), and the gonadotropins (follicle stimulating hormone, FSH, and luteinizing hormone, LH). The dimeric (quaternary) structure of insulin is held together by interchain disulfide bonds. Intrachain disulfide bonds are also present in insulin and in prolactin (PRL), growth hormone (GH), and in some other hormones. These covalent bonds may be important for establishing the tertiary structure necessary for producing the active site (conformation) within these peptides or, in some instances, for protecting the hormones from enzymatic degradation [4, 10].

In some hormones tyrosine is sulfated (e.g., gastrin, see Fig. 10.1), and the glutamic acid moiety may be cyclized into a pyrrole structure (as in TRH, see Fig. 1.3). Because peptide hormones are composed of a linear sequence of amino acids, there is usually an amino (NH_2)- or N-terminal and a carboxy (COOH)- or C-terminal group present in the structure. In some peptides the C-terminal end may be amidated (to a carboxamide) and the N-terminal group may be acetylated (as in α-MSH, see Fig. 8.1). Some of the larger peptides (FSH, LH, TSH, and hCG) are *glycoproteins*, that is, they are conjugated to one or more carbohydrate residues.

The amino acid sequence (primary sequence) of a hormone may differ between species (for example, ACTH and calcitonin, see Figs. 5.8 and 9.4, respectively). Two or more isoforms of a peptide hormone may be present within a single species of animal. Isoforms of hormones can arise from differential splicing of mRNA, or as products of separate genes or as post-transcriptional or post-translational modifications (sulfation, glycosylation, etc.) of the peptide. Knowledge of such species differences in primary sequence provides information on the evolution of the hormone. Single amino acid substitutions may even lead to the evolution of new hormone structures within an individual species [9, 23]. Although oxytocin and vasopressin are closely related structurally and presumably evolutionarily, they play entirely different physiological roles within an individual animal. Based on similarity of structure, one can group hormones into families of peptides that undoubtedly are derived from a common evolutionary precursor. The insulin family of peptides includes nerve growth factor (NGF), relaxin, and one or more of the somatomedins. The melanotropin family of peptides includes ACTH, α-MSH, and possibly other melanotropins (see Fig. 8.1). Invariant sequences of amino acids within the primary structure of a peptide may suggest that such sequences are components of the active site of the hormone.

Thyroid Hormones

The thyroid gland synthesizes two hormones, thyroxine (T_4) and triiodothyronine (T_3), from the precursor amino acid tyrosine (see Fig. 13.1). These two iodinated hormones have a diverse number of functions within and between members of the different vertebrate classes. These hormones are unique in that an inorganic ion is incorporated into their structures. These hormones are indispensable for normal growth and development.

Steroid Hormones

produced in adrenal glands

Steroid hormones are produced by steroidogenic tissue of adrenal or gonadal origin. The adrenal steroidogenic tissue produces *glucocorticoids* (e.g., cortisol, corticosterone, and cortisone) and *mineralocorticoids* (e.g., aldosterone). These corticosteroids play important roles in carbohydrate metabolism and electrolyte balance, respectively. The pathway of steroid biosynthesis is complex, and many steroid precursors are formed in the synthetic pathway of any particular steroid hormone (e.g., see Fig. 15.3). Under abnormal conditions of biosynthesis the production of these metabolites may increase and exert undesirable physiological effects [2, 17, 31]. Figure 2.1 shows the structures of three adrenal steroid hormones.

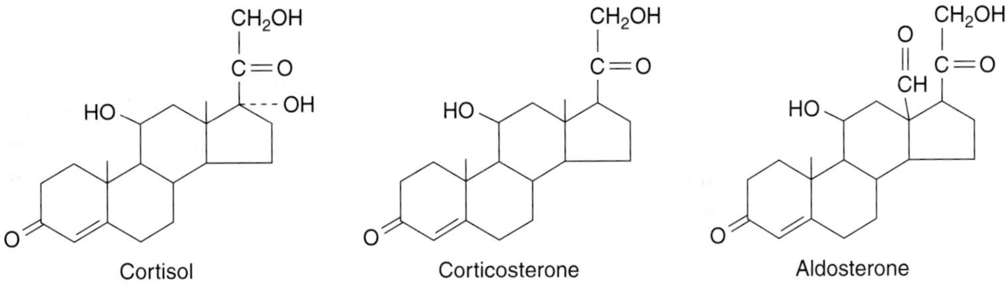

Figure 2.1 Examples of adrenal steroid hormones.

The steroidogenic tissue of the gonads produces a number of sex (gonadal) steroids: *androgens* (masculinizing), *estrogens* (feminizing), and *progestins* (related to pregnancy, gestation). The testes produce testosterone; in the ovary estradiol and progesterone are the main steroids synthesized and secreted. During pregnancy the placenta is an additional source of estrogens and progestins (progestogens). Under certain developmental conditions the adrenal steroidogenic tissue may be an important additional source of androgens and estrogens. Figure 2.2 shows the structure of three important gonadal steroid hormones.

Figure 2.2 Examples of gonadal steroid hormones.

Neurotransmitters

Neurohormones are synthesized by neurons and are usually released into a specialized structure, the synaptic cleft, adjacent to the cell to be regulated (effector/target cell). Neurotransmitters regulate another nerve cell, a muscle cell, or a secretory cell (e.g., salivary gland cell). The common neurotransmitters are acetylcholine, norepinephrine, dopamine, and serotonin (5-hydroxytryptamine, 5-HT), but there are a number of other putative neurotransmitters (Chaps. 6 and 21). Dopamine released from hypothalamic neurons of the brain may also function as a bloodborne hormone to regulate pituitary hormone secretion. Figure 2.3 shows the structures of three important neurotransmitters. A number of other biogenic amines (see Fig. 6.12), including amino acids (see Fig. 6.13) themselves, also function as neurotransmitters within the central and peripheral nervous systems.

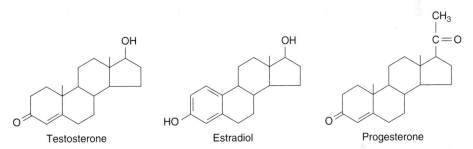

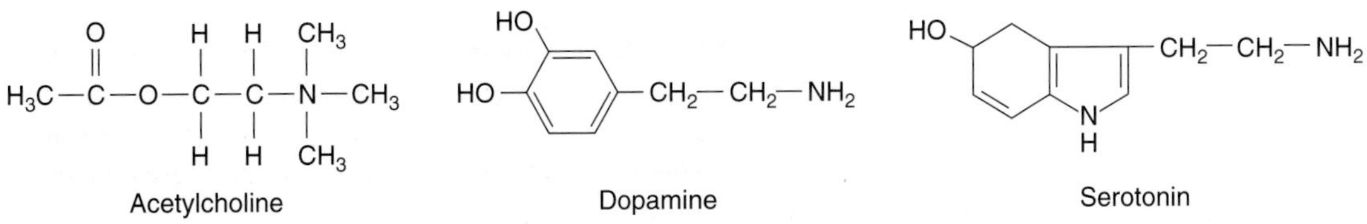

Figure 2.3 Examples of neurotransmitters.

Neuropeptides

Many of the peptide hormones have been found in the brain where they are synthesized by specific neurons and localized to specific nerve tracts [27]. Such a discrete localization argues strongly for a function of these neuropeptides within the nervous system. It is speculated that these hormones act as neuroregulators, either as neurotransmitters (to conduct information synaptically between neurons) or as neuromodulators (to affect the response of a neuron to neurotransmitters released from other neurons). Some neuropeptides are distributed widely throughout the central nervous system. The *endorphins*, for example, may function as neuroregulators to act on so-called opiate receptors and, in humans at least, function as analgesic hormones. Methionine enkephalin and leucine enkephalin and β-endorphin are examples of endorphins (see Fig. 21.3).

Chalones

Endogenous mitotic inhibitors are referred to as chalones [7]. These growth factors are usually capable of inhibiting the mitotic activity of a given cell type. Only a few cytostatic regulators of cell growth are presently known. Transforming growth factor-beta [19], TGF-β, may be the most readily accepted candidate growth inhibitory peptide (Chap. 12).

Peptide Growth-stimulating Factors

A number of peptides of diverse origin possessing growth-promoting activity have been identified. In some cases the structural characteristics of the molecules have been partially or fully determined. The thymus may produce one or more *thymosins*, which are believed to induce maturation of white blood cells that then function in the immune response. Nerve growth factor (NGF) is responsible for neuron maturation in developing systems. These and other growth-stimulating peptides, such as erythropoietin (erythrocyte-stimulating factor) epidermal growth factor (EGF), fibroblast growth factor (FGF), and the somatomedins (insulinlike growth factors) will be discussed in Chap. 12.

Eicosanoids

Prostaglandins are one class of chemical messengers known as eicosanoids. Although discovered relatively recently, they are ubiquitous and affect the activity of many physiological processes. Prostaglandins are synthesized from fatty acid substrates (e.g., arachidonic acid) within the membranes of cells. Their generic name was derived because they were first discovered within seminal fluid. They are composed of a 20-membered fatty acid carbon skeleton folded into a hairpinlike structure by incorporating a 5-membered ring at the bend of the molecule. The thromboxanes, prostacyclins [32], and leukotrienes are related chemical messengers that may prove to play significant roles in many physiological processes (Chap. 4). Figure 2.4 shows the structure of two important prostaglandins.

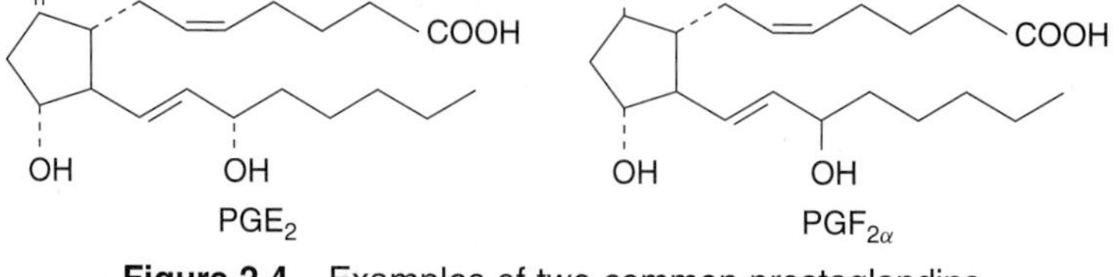

Figure 2.4   Examples of two common prostaglandins.

Pheromones

Most hormones act on cells within the animal in which they are produced. Chemical signals are also used for transmitting information between individuals of the same species [11, 13, 33]. The term pheromone denotes a chemical substance that is liberated by one animal and that causes a relatively specific behavior modification in a recipient animal following its chemoreception [33]. This chemical communication is implied to function within a species, but may also affect some unrelated species. Pheromones are classified into two types, a *signaller* (or *releaser*) pheromone, which brings about a prompt behavioral reaction, and a *primer* pheromone, which causes a slower effect, such as an alteration of the endocrine and reproductive systems. These effects are produced through neuroendocrine mechanisms for which the primary stimulus is olfactory. Pheromones play important roles in insects and other invertebrates. Pheromones are generally aliphatic, thus facilitating their volatilization and subsequent transport by air. The structure of the vertebrate pheromone civetone (from the civet) and the invertebrate pheromone bombykol (from the silk-worm moth) are shown (Fig. 2.5). Pheromones may also be delivered (dispersed) within an aquatic environment. The structures of these pheromones are therefore hydrophilic in nature.

Other Cellular Regulators

Besides the well-recognized classes of hormones, other substances play important roles as chemical messengers controlling cellular function. The simplest such messenger is the hydrogen (H^+) ion (proton). Hydrochloric acid present within chyme is responsible for stimulating secretin release from cells of the duodenal epithelium (see Fig. 10.6). Because other acids will similarly stimulate secretin release, it can be presumed that interaction of the hydrogen ion with specific cellular components of secretin-producing cells elicits release of this hormone. Osmoreceptors also monitor sodium ion (Na^+) levels within the plasma. These chemoreceptor cells undoubtedly have special recognition sites for this monovalent cation (Chap. 15). The divalent calcium (Ca^{2+}) ion is an important regulator of parathormone and calcitonin secretion from the parathyroid glands and parafollicular cells, respectively. These cells have specific recognition sites (Ca^{2+} sensing receptors) for this important cation (Chap. 9, Fig. 9.13).

Glucose is a specific stimulus for insulin secretion from the beta (β) cells of the pancreatic islets. Glucose is also inhibitory to glucagon secretion from the alpha (α) cells of the pancreatic islets. Glucose is bound and transported into cells by plasmalemmal structural elements referred to as glucose transporters (Chap. 11). Glucostats are apparently present within the hypothalamus where these cells may function as the receptive units of the so-called *satiety center*. These cells must have special sensory elements for recognizing this metabolic substrate or one or more of its metabolites [24].

Certain amino acids (e.g., arginine) may function as specific stimulants of insulin secretion from the pancreatic islets. Certain neurons within the hypothalamus also monitor

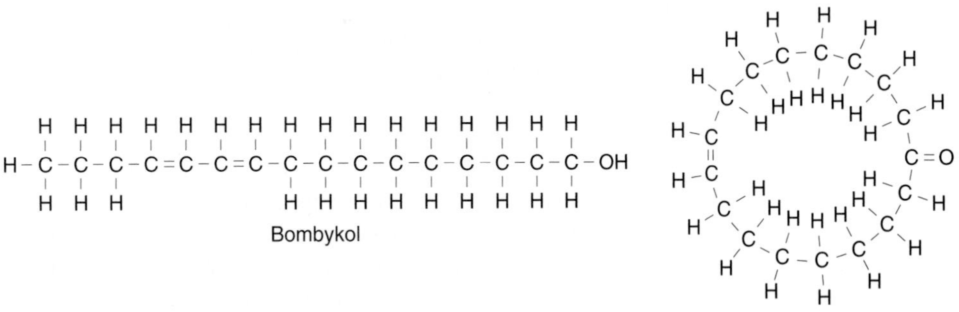

Figure 2.5 Examples of vertebrate and invertebrate pheromones.

the levels of certain circulating amino acids; these sensory elements may then regulate the release of pituitary somatotropin. The simplest amino acid, glycine, probably functions as a neurotransmitter within the brain. Glutamate, a derivative of glutamic acid, also functions as a chemical messenger within the CNS. Other as yet unrecognized metabolic substrates or end products may also play important roles in cellular regulation (Chap. 21).

HORMONE SYNTHESIS

Because of the diversity of hormone structures, a number of interesting synthetic processes are involved in hormone biosynthesis. The simplest of hormones are amino acids themselves or derivatives thereof (see Fig. 6.13). For example, glycine and glutamic acid (glutamate) are certainly implicated as neurotransmitters within the brain. The amino acids phenylalanine and tyrosine (a derivative of phenylalanine) are precursors for the synthesis of dopamine, norepinephrine, and epinephrine, which function as neurotransmitters or as bloodborne chemical messengers. Tyrosine is also the substrate for biosynthesis of the thyroid hormones, triiodothyronine and thyroxine (see Fig. 13.1). The amino acid tryptophan, is the precursor for the formation of serotonin, a CNS neurotransmitter, and melatonin, a pineal hormone (see Fig. 20.2).

Peptide Hormones

Most vertebrate hormones are peptide in nature and are therefore composed of amino acids. Like other proteins, they are synthesized on ribosomes where their specific amino acid sequence is determined (*translated*) by a specific messenger RNA sequence (codon). The nucleotide sequences of the mRNA are dictated (*transcribed*) from specific nucleotide sequences (genes) in the DNA of chromosomes. The nascent proteins are then released and transported into the cisternae of the rough endoplasmic reticulum and then to the Golgi elements where they may be altered (e.g., sulfated or combined with carbohydrate moieties). Vesicles containing the hormone and possibly other products (e.g., proteolytic enzymes) are then pinched off the terminal cisternae of the Golgi apparatus. These secretory vesicles are distributed within the cytoplasm in patterns generally characteristic of the cell type involved. Abnormal control of gene expression and protein synthesis is characteristic of most neoplastic cells.

Steroid Hormones

Steroid hormones are synthesized within elements of the smooth endoplasmic reticulum. Steroid-secreting cells are easily identified by the large amounts of smooth endoplasmic reticulum present within them. However, a complex multiple-enzyme system is required for the synthesis of steroids. These enzymes are present within the mitochondria as well as the cytoplasm. Steroid hormone synthesis can, therefore, be blocked by protein synthesis inhibitors. Because of the great number of enzymes involved in the biosynthesis of any one steroid hormone, mutations leading to faulty enzymes may result in one or a number of pathophysiological states (Chap. 15).

Thyroid Hormones

These iodinated hormones are synthesized on a proteinaceous substrate (thyroglobulin), which is extracellular (intraluminal). They are then taken up by endocytosis and transported through the follicular cells of the thyroid gland where they are enzymatically released from the carrier protein prior to secretion (Chap. 13). Thyroid hormone (thyroxine and triiodothyronine) production and secretion within the thyroid gland is a unique process that provides important clues for understanding cellular function.

Neurotransmitters

Neurotransmitters are synthesized within the axonal endings of neurons (Chap. 14). The enzymes needed for the many neurotransmitter production steps are, however, synthesized on ribosomes in the perikarya (cell bodies) of neurons and are subsequently transported by axoplasmic flow to the neuron terminals. The secreted neurotransmitter (e.g., norepinephrine) may then be taken back up into axon terminals for further use (Fig. 14.5). Acetylcholine is inactivated by enzymatic cleavage after secretion, but the constituent moieties (acetate and choline) are then taken up for resynthesis of the hormone.

Neuropeptides

The peptide neurohormones (e.g., oxytocin and vasopressin) are synthesized in neuronal perikarya and are transported within vesicles for long distances for storage in the axon terminals (see Fig. 7.1). Numerous other neuropeptides are synthesized within discrete neurons in the brain by genomic mechanisms of transcription and translation.

Prohormones

Oxytocin —
9 AA

Some peptide hormones are composed of only a small number of amino acids. Oxytocin and other neurohypophysial hormones, for example, contain only nine amino acids (nonapeptides). These hormones are not coded directly by the DNA. Rather, sequences of about one hundred amino acids and longer (e.g., neurophysins) are initially synthesized (Chap. 7). These proteins are then packaged within secretory vesicles along with proteolytic enzymes. These enzymes (endopeptidases) then cleave the protein into one or more smaller peptides, in some cases the definitive hormone. A number of cleavage events may, however, take place during posttranslational processing before the definitive hormone is produced. Thus some hormones are derived indirectly by way of a prohormone. The prohormone itself may be derived from a preprohormone (Fig. 2.6). Some large plasma proteins also serve as prohormones for hormone production. Renin, an enzyme released from the juxtaglomerular cells of the kidneys, acts on angiotensinogen, a substrate protein produced by the liver, to convert it to a smaller fragment. This fragment, angiotensin I, is then converted by another enzyme to the active hormone, angiotensin II. Large precursor plasma proteins, kininogens, are converted by certain serine proteases, referred to as kallikreins, to kinins, such as bradykinin, an important hormone in regulating blood flow in certain vascular beds (Chap. 15). Bradykinin and

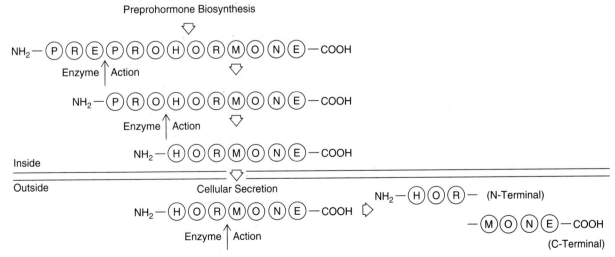

Figure 2.6   General scheme for hormone production from a precursor peptide.

angiotensin II are examples of hormones that are released from liver cells as larger pro-hormones to be converted into active hormonal peptides within the blood.

Certain steroids serve as prohormones in the production of other definitive steroid hormones. For example, certain cells possess the enzyme 5α-reductase that converts testosterone to dihydrotestosterone, the effector molecule for activating these cells (see Fig. 16.8). Within the brain, testosterone is also aromatized within certain neurons to estradiol, which is the biologically active steroid structure required for activation of these cells.

CONTROL OF HORMONE SECRETION

Hormones are synthesized within cells and, except for the thyroid and steroid hormones, are packaged within secretory vesicles until released. Stimuli of both an intrinsic (inter-nal) or extrinsic (light, sound, smell, temperature, etc.) nature affect hormone secretion. Stimulation of hormone-secreting cells results in vesicular fusion with the plasma membrane and *exocytosis* of the granule contents. Hormones often stimulate hormone secretion from other endocrine glands. For example, pituitary hormones, such as TSH, FSH, LH, and ACTH, stimulate target tissue cells of the thyroid, gonads, and adrenal gland, respectively, to secrete their own respective hormones: thyroxine, gonadal steroids, and adrenal glucocorticoids (see Fig. 6.15). Hormone-secreting cells of the neurohypophysis, the adrenal medulla (*chromaffin tissue*), and the pineal gland are reg-ulated by direct neural innervation. Stimulation of hormone secretion by nerves is referred to as *neuroendocrine transduction* [1, 25]. Metabolic substrates (glucose, amino acids, FFAs) and inorganic ions also provide a selective stimulus to hormone secretion by some cells.

Calcium ion levels are monitored directly by parathormone- and calcitonin-secret-ing cells. Thus the hormone-secreting cells that regulate Ca^{2+} levels do so by sensing the extracellular Ca^{2+} concentration [7]. Glucose concentration is monitored by the glucagon- and insulin-secreting cells of the pancreatic islets. These cells regulate blood glucose lev-els by sensing the circulating glucose concentration. Somatotropin stimulates tissue uptake of amino acids, and the amino acids that are present in the blood at increased lev-els after a meal provide cues to growth hormone secretion.

The pituitary hormones, FSH, LH, TSH, and ACTH, stimulate hormone secretion from the gonads, thyroid, and adrenal, respectively, and are controlled through negative feedback mechanisms. Target organ hormones, gonadal steroids, and thyroxine or adren-al glucocorticoids feed back to the hypothalamus and pituitary to inhibit further secretion of pituitary hormones (see Fig. 6.15). Examples of positive feedback have also been described (Chap. 18). Some hormones exert a negative feedback on the cells within which they are synthesized by a so-called *autoinhibition*.

The factors that stimulate cellular secretion, whether they are hormones or metabo-lites, interact with cellular receptors of the secretory cells. For example, epinephrine, a bloodborne hormone, or norepinephrine, a neurotransmitter, interact with cell membrane adrenergic receptors (Chap. 14). Hormone interaction with some membrane receptors results in membrane *depolarization*. This stimulates the movement of Ca^{2+} into the cells, which results in secretory vesicle exocytosis (so-called *stimulus-secretion coupling*). Some chemical messengers are inhibitory to cellular secretion, and their effects are medi-ated by cell membrane *hyperpolarization*. Changes in cellular secretion are generally cor-related with changes in levels of intracellular cyclic nucleotides or other second messen-gers. Secretion is often correlated with elevation of cyclic adenosine monophosphate (cAMP) levels.

Most hormone-secreting cells only exhibit minimal (basal) secretion in the absence of stimulatory cues. Prolactin- and MSH-secreting cells of some species are unique as hormone-secreting cells, in that they spontaneously secrete their hormones when placed in vitro or when the pituitary is transplanted to an ectopic site in the animal. These cells are normally under tonic inhibition by the brain, and they spontaneously depolarize and secrete their hormones in the absence of such inhibitory input (Chap. 8).

HORMONE DELIVERY

Chemical messengers are delivered from the cell of origin to their target cells by one of several routes [12, 14]: (1) *endocrine*, where the messenger substance is bloodborne (the classical definition of a hormone); (2) *neurocrine*, where a neuron contacts its target cells by axonal extensions and then releases the hormone into a synaptic cleft between the two cells; (3) *neuroendocrine*, where the hormone released by a nerve is bloodborne; and (4) *paracrine*, where the released hormone diffuses to its adjacent target cells through the immediate extracellular space; or even (5) *lumonal*, where the hormone is released into the lumen of the gut. Chemical messengers may also be released into the environment by a pheromonal route [14]. Following the release of a hormone it may also feed back on the cell of origin by a so-called *autocrine* mechanism [15] (Fig. 2.7). Somatostatin is an example of a hormone that may be delivered to its target tissue by all these routes. It is delivered to the pituitary by way of the hypophysial portal system (neuroendocrine route) to regulate somatotropin secretion. Somatostatin is localized within other specific neurons of the CNS and controls target tissue neurons by a neurocrine mechanism. Somatostatin regulates pancreatic islet function by a local paracrine mechanism [26], and in the gut the peptide may also function as a local hormone and control gastrin secretion by a paracrine mechanism. Portal blood somatostatin levels are increased after a meal, suggesting an additional endocrine method of delivery to undetermined target sites.

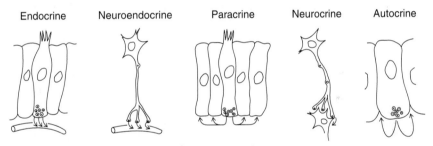

| Endocrine | Neuroendocrine | Paracrine | Neurocrine | Autocrine |

Figure 2.7   Methods of hormone delivery. Modified from [12].

Hormones achieve selectivity of target cell activation by several means. Neurotransmitters may be delivered (by a neurocrine mechanism) only to those target cells being innervated. Some selectivity of hormone action is achieved by delivery through specialized circulatory routes, such as the hypophysial portal system linking the hypothalamus to the pituitary. The specificity of target tissue receptors also assures that these cells will respond only to certain hormones. Under certain pathological states, overproduction of a hormone and its excessive release results in undesirable target tissue responses due to excess amounts of the hormone. Most neurons in the brain are protected from systemic endocrine influences by a *blood-brain barrier*.

HORMONE CIRCULATION AND METABOLISM

Hormones are secreted from endocrine cells to initiate immediate target tissue responses or to set in motion more long-term effects. In either case, hormones must be continuously inactivated or the cellular response cannot be terminated. Both intracellular and extracellular mechanisms function in the cessation of hormone-mediated responses.

Peptide Hormones

Peptide hormones have short half-lives. The half-life of a hormone or other active agent is defined as the amount of time required for half the molecules to become inactivated or cleared from the circulation. Shorter peptides such as MSH and oxytocin have particularly short half-lives (possibly 2 to 30 min.). The large protein hormone TSH is reported to have a half-life of about 60 min., and this may be one example of a long half-life. Peptidases, the enzymes responsible for metabolizing peptides, play an essential role in biologic regulation because of the close involvement of peptide messengers in the maintenance of homeostasis. Proteolytic enzymes are intimately concerned with all stages in the life of a biologically active peptide, from synthesis in the ribosomes to ultimate hydrolysis to individual amino acids. The initial proteolytic events occur within the secretory cell in a highly organized and compartmentalized manner and involve conversion of large gene products to smaller secretory forms of the peptide. Once secreted from a nerve ending or an endocrine cell, a peptide will encounter peptidases associated with cellular membranes and soluble in tissue fluids. The postsecretory metabolism of peptides may inactivate the peptide or convert it to forms with different biologic activities. Such transformation is of considerable physiologic importance in view of the essential role of peptide hormones and neurotransmitters in the regulation of cellular metabolism [8].

Enzymes inactivate peptide hormones by splitting the molecules at specific peptide bonds. *Exopeptidases*, both *carboxypeptidases* and *aminopeptidases*, cleave off the C-terminal or N-terminal amino acids, respectively. Peptide hormones may also be inactivated by simple deamination at either the N- or C-terminal (if amidated) ends of the molecule. *Endopeptidases* split the molecule at other specific peptide bonds within the molecule. The sites of internal cleavage are quite specific, for example, often between repeating sequences of certain basic amino acids, such as Lys-Lys, Arg-Lys, Lys-Arg, Arg-Arg, Arg-Lys, Lys-Arg, as found in β-LPH (see Fig. 8.4). The clinical use of some peptides has been limited because of their short half-lives. Understanding biodegradation mechanisms may facilitate the preparation of appropriate peptide hormone analogs with longer lasting actions.

Insulin is composed of two chains held together by a pair of disulfide bonds. The hormone is inactivated by a so-called insulinase, an enzyme complex that inactivates the hormone by reduction of the interchain disulfide bonds, thus splitting the hormone into two individual inactive chains. A hypothetical model for the action of various proteolytic enzymes on hormone degradation is shown (Fig. 2.8).

Steroid and Thyroid Hormones

Most steroid hormones are bound to plasma proteins that are specific for each hormone. The half-life of steroid hormones is apparently enhanced by their ability to be bound to these plasma proteins. Aldosterone, a steroid that is not readily bound, has a shorter half-life than other steroid hormones with specific carrier (transport) proteins. In the liver both adrenal and gonadal steroids usually are conjugated to glucuronic acid or they are sulfated (Fig. 2.9). These structural modifications may render them inactive and more soluble so they can be more readily excreted in the urine. Some of the glucuronide salts are secret-

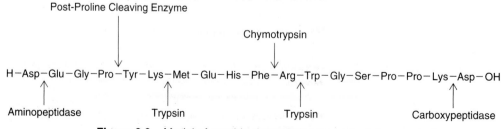

Figure 2.8 Model of peptide degradation by proteolytic enzymes.

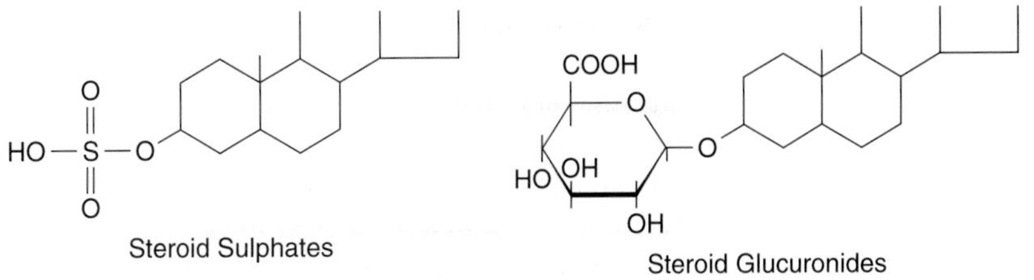

Steroid Sulphates

Steroid Glucuronides

Figure 2.9 Steroid hormone sulfation and glucuronide formation.

ed with the bile salts and may be reabsorbed into the blood. Thyroxine and triiodothyronine are deiodinated in many tissues. These hormones are also conjugated in the liver to form sulfates and glucuronides that enter the bile to pass into the intestine where they are reabsorbed or eliminated from the bowel.

Adrenal Catecholamines and Neurotransmitters

The metabolism of circulating catecholamines occurs mainly in the liver by orthomethylation and oxidative deamination by catechol-0-methyl transferase (COMT) and monoamine oxidase (MAO), respectively (see Fig. 14.4). Neurotransmitter action within synapses is terminated rapidly by a number of enzymatic or other processes. Norepinephrine and dopamine are inactivated in the synapse by COMT. These neurotransmitters are also taken back into the presynaptic axon to be used again or to be inactivated by MAO. Acetylcholine liberated into the synapse from cholinergic neurons is split into choline and acetate by the enzyme acetylcholinesterase. The reaction products, choline and acetate, are also taken back into the presynaptic axon to be resynthesized into acetylcholine.

PHYSIOLOGICAL ROLES OF HORMONES

Hormones control the activity of probably all cells in the body. The vast number of effects produced by hormones can, however, be reduced to a few general processes.

1. Hormones affect cellular synthesis and secretion of other hormones within other endocrine glands and in neurons. Hormones affect the secretion of digestive tract products, such as enzymes, hydrochloric acid, and bile salts. They also affect epithelial mucus and milk synthesis and secretion, as well as integumental sebum and sweat production and release. Hormones also affect the production and secretion of pheromones and probably other odoriferous substances [28].

2. Hormones affect metabolic processes, both *anabolic* and *catabolic*, in most cells. The synthesis and degradation of carbohydrates, lipids, and proteins are controlled by hormones to meet the specific energy or growth needs of the individual.

3. Hormones affect contraction, relaxation, and metabolism of muscle. They cause contraction and relaxation of vascular and gastrointestinal smooth muscle, as well as genital tract musculature such as the uterus and oviducts. Hormones also affect cardiac and skeletal muscle contractile properties. Some steroid hormones profoundly affect anabolic and catabolic processes within muscle.

4. Hormones control reproductive processes, such as gonadal differentiation, maturation, and gametogenesis.

5. Hormones are stimulatory or inhibitory to cellular proliferation, thus affecting growth. Recent evidence suggests that hormones may play regulatory roles in the earliest aspects of cell division and differentiation of the fertilized egg.

6. The excretion and reabsorption of inorganic cations and anions is regulated by hormones. Sodium, potassium, calcium, and phosphate ions are particularly affected.

7. Hormones have a permissive action on the effects of other hormones: the effectiveness of certain hormones is often considerably enhanced by the action of another hormone. The permissive hormone may be without any noticeable effect of its own, but it may be an absolute requirement for the actions of the other hormone.

8. Hormones play important roles in animal behavior. Sexual and aggressive behaviors are affected by hormones, particularly during certain phases of the reproductive cycle. Maternal behavior is controlled by gonadal hormones and by pituitary hormones. Group behavior may even be affected by the release of chemical messengers (pheromones) into the environment [28].

Hormones may control certain physiological functions at one stage in life and certain others at a later developmental stage. Some hormones are secreted on an off-and-on basis to control fluctuations in serum constituents, such as glucose and calcium. Some hormones are secreted spasmodically to meet particular needs; oxytocin, for example, is generally secreted at parturition and during suckling of the breast. Adrenal catecholamines, on the other hand, are usually secreted under conditions of stress. The continuous secretion of hormones (e.g., cortisol) under prolonged stress may debilitate an organism [2, 17, 30]. Some hormones are not secreted in large amounts until a later stage in development. The gonadotropic hormones, for example, increase in secretion after puberty to stimulate the gonads and subsequent growth and development of the secondary sex characteristics.

Some hormones may come into existence only a few times in the life of an individual. Human chorionic gonadotropin and other peptide hormones are made by the placenta and therefore are only produced during pregnancy. Some hormones lose their function with time; after menopause, for example, FSH secretion is enhanced, but the ovary no longer responds to the hormone [5, 29]. Thyroid hormone secretion and/or effectiveness is diminished with age, and this results in a decreased capacity for thermogenesis (as noted in the elderly).

GENERAL MECHANISMS OF HORMONE ACTION

The physiological processes regulated by hormones result from interaction of the hormone with specific constituents of the cell, referred to as *receptors*. All peptide hormones, as well as nonpeptidergic neurotransmitters, act on membrane receptors. Stimulation of membrane receptors leads to activation of cyclizing enzymes, which initiate the production of a cyclic nucleotide, either cAMP or cGMP. These and other so-called second messengers generally activate one or more specific protein phosphorylation events within the cell. Addition of a phosphate group to a protein, an enzyme for example, by a phosphoprotein kinase may result in its activation. Phosphorylation of another protein might enhance its contractile activity. Protein substrate phosphorylation may, in contrast, also inactivate an enzyme. Phosphoprotein phosphatases, on the other hand, remove phosphate groups from proteins, and this can result in either inactivation or activation of the particular protein (see Fig. 7.13).

Steroid hormones, unlike most other chemical messengers, interact with intracellular receptors. These receptors within the nucleus interact with the chromatin (DNA) of specific chromosomes, which initiates mRNA synthesis (transcription) and protein synthesis (translation, see Figs. 4.12, 9.10, and 9.11). Thyroid hormones also interact with intracellular receptors to activate protein synthetic processes (see Fig. 13.10).

The cellular response to membrane receptor activation may be instantaneous as in nerve-nerve or nerve-muscle communication. The ultimate physiological response of cells to steroid or thyroid hormones is obviously much slower as the genomic and synthetic events require more time to be consummated.

ENDOCRINE PATHOPHYSIOLOGY

Endocrine glands release their hormones in response to bodily needs. The released hormones exert their effects on target tissues and are rapidly degraded and excreted. Failure of a gland or tissue to secrete enough hormones can lead to fatal consequences. For example, in the absence of insulin, elevated blood glucose (hyperglycemia) adversely affects other physiological processes. Individuals with diabetes mellitus may go into coma and die, or they may ultimately succumb to destructive alterations of other physiological processes. Lack of parathormone leads to hypocalcemia and results in tetanic convulsions and death. Failure to secrete vasopressin will result in severe water loss (*diabetes insipidus*) and dehydration.

underproduction (Addison's)

Failure to secrete enough hormone may result from destruction of the endocrine gland, as can happen to the adrenal cortex due to tuberculosis. Failure to secrete cortisol (*Addison's disease*) may result from destruction of the adrenal cortex or failure of the pituitary to secrete ACTH, which is responsible for stimulation of adrenal cortisol formation. Failure to secrete ACTH can result from pituitary gland dysfunction or failure of the hypothalamus to secrete corticotropin releasing hormone (CRH). Diabetes insipidus may result from a lack of vasopressin, but, if the kidney fails to respond to the hormone, this also results in *nephrogenic diabetes insipidus*.

overproduction (Cushing's)

Overproduction of hormone secretion, on the other hand, can also lead to pathophysiological states and possible death. Excess cortisol secretion (*Cushing's syndrome*) can cause altered carbohydrate, fat, and protein metabolism [2]. This usually leads to hyperglycemia and pancreatic beta cell exhaustion resulting in diabetes mellitus. Oversecretion of aldosterone may lead to severe hypertension because of the hypervolemia (increased blood volume) caused by the hypernatremia (increased blood Na^+) characteristic of *hyperaldosteronism*.

Many endocrinopathies of excess hormone secretion result from neoplasms where the tumor produces an excess of a hormone. Adrenal cortical tumors may secrete tremendous amounts of cortisol (Cushing's syndrome). Insulinomas secrete excessive amounts of insulin, which results in lowered blood glucose levels. The resulting hypoglycemia may cause rapid coma and death since nerve cells must have a constant supply of glucose to function.

mutation

Endocrine disorders can result from a number of events related to hormone-target cell interaction. For example, the structure of a peptide hormone may be altered due to a mutation (nucleotide base change) in the gene coding for the hormone, as in one form of familial hyperinsulinemia. In the *testicular feminizing syndrome*, target tissues lack receptors for testosterone, and the body may then differentiate along the direction of the female phenotype. In pseudohypoparathyroidism, although blood Ca^{2+} levels are low, there is an excess of parathormone. The target tissue of the hormone, the kidney, apparently lacks functional receptors responsible for the production of cAMP; therefore, the cells fail to respond to the hormone. Other examples of endocrine dysfunction are discussed in Table 2.4 and in more detail within the following chapters (Chap. 21).

COMPARATIVE ENDOCRINOLOGY

Most information on the vertebrate endocrine system is derived from experiments on mammals, particularly rats and mice. Endocrine dysfunction in humans has, of course, contributed immensely to understanding the role of hormones in normal physiological processes. Primates, the closest relatives of humans, provide important experimental model systems for understanding the roles of hormones.

Much less is known about the endocrinology of nonmammalian forms. Studies on these vertebrates have, however, provided particularly interesting insights into the specialized aspects of endocrine regulation. Thyroid hormones, for example, are required for the metamorphic change necessary for the emergence of some amphibians (e.g., frogs, toads, salamanders) from the aquatic to the terrestrial environment. The hormonal form of vitamin D, because of its crucial role in Ca^{2+} homeostasis, is of special importance to egg laying in the bird. Prolactin is necessary for successful transition of certain species of fishes from the saline (marine) to the freshwater environment. Prolactin is required for brood-patch development in some birds. Melanocyte-stimulating hormone plays an important role in regulating color changes of the integument of many vertebrates. Understanding the diverse roles of each of the vertebrate hormones provides interesting insights into the evolution of hormone structure and function.

TABLE 2.4   Some Examples of Endocrinopathies

Disease	Etiology	Symptoms
Diabetes mellitus	Lack of insulin (β – pancreatic)	Hyperglycemia, glucosuria
Diabetes insipidus		
Pituitary	Lack of AVP (ADH)	Water loss, hypovolemia, dehydration
Nephrogenic	Renal unresponsiveness to AVP (ADH)	Water loss, hypovolemia, dehydration
Addison's disease		
Primary	Adrenal cortical destruction (lack of all adrenal steroids)	Altered carbohydrate metabolism, salt-losing syndrome
Secondary	Lack of ACTH secretion	Altered carbohydrate metabolism
Cushing's syndrome		
Primary	Adrenal tumor (excess cortisol secretion)	Protein catabolism, hyperglycemia
Secondary	Pituitary adenoma (excess ACTH secretion, excess cortisol secretion)	Protein catabolism, hyperglycemia
Cretinism (infantile hypothyroidism)	Lack of T_4–T_3 secretion	Lowered BMR, decreased mentation, growth failure
Myxedema (adult hypothyroidism)	Lack of T_4–T_3 secretion	Lowered BMR, decreased mentation
Hyperthyroidism (thyrotoxicosis)	Excess T_4–T_3 secretion	Enhanced BMR, hyperexcitability
Hypoparathyroidism	Parathyroid gland destruction	Lowered blood Ca^{2+} levels
Hyperparathyroidism	Parathyroid gland tumor or hypertrophy (increased PTH secretion)	Elevated blood Ca^{2+} levels
Pseudohypoparathyroidism	Lack of renal response to PTH	Lowered blood Ca^{2+} levels
Testicular feminizing syndrome	No androgen receptors	Genital tract feminization in the male
Hyperaldosteronism (Conn's disease)	Adrenocortical tumor (excess aldosterone secretion)	Sodium retention (hypernatremia), hypervolemia, hypertension

REFERENCES

[1]   Armstrong, S. M. 1989. Melatonin and circadian control in mammals. *Experientia* 45:932–8.

[2]   Aron, D. C., J. W. Findling, and J. B. Tyrrell. 1987. Cushing's disease. *Endocrinol. Metab. Clin. N. Amer.* 16:705–30.

[3]   Bayliss, W. M., and E. H. Starling. 1902. The mechanism of pancreatic secretion. *J. Physiol.* 28:325–53.

[4]   Beebe, J. S., K. Mountjoy, R. F. Krzesicki, F. Perini, and R. W. Ruddon. 1990. Role of disulfide bond formation in the folding of human chorionic gonadotropin beta subunit into an alpha beta dimer assembly–competent form. *J. Biol. Chem*. 265:312–7.

[5]   Brenner, P. F. 1988. The menopausal syndrome. *Obstet. Gynecol.* 72:6S–11S.

[6]   Brown, E. M., G. Gamba, D. Riccardi, M. Lombardi, R. Butters, O. Kifor, A. Sun, M. A. Hediger, J. Lytton, and S. C. Herbert. 1993. Cloning and characterization of an extracellular Ca^{2+}-sensing receptor from bovine parathyroid. *Nature Lond.* 366:575–80.

[7]   Bullough, W. S. 1975. Mitotic control in adult mammalian tissue. *Biol. Rev.* 50:99–127.

[8]   Bunnett, N. W. 1987. Release and breakdown. Postsecretory metabolism of peptides. *Amer. Rev. Respir. Dis.* 136:S27–34.

[9]   Castrucci, A. M. L., M. E. Hadley, M. Lebl, C. Zechel, and V. J. Hruby. 1989. Melanocyte stimulating hormone (MSH) and melanin concentrating hormone (MCH) may be structurally and evolutionarily related. *Reg. Pept.* 24:27–35.

[10] Combarnous, Y. 1988. Structure and structure-function relationships in gonadotropins. *Reprod. Nutr. Develop.* 23:211–28.

[11] Cutler, W. B., G. Preti, A. Drieger, G. R. Huggins, C. R. Garcia, and H. J. Lawley. 1986. Human axillary secretions influence women's menstrual cycles: the role of donor extract from men. *Horm. Behav.* 20:463–73.

[12] Dockray, G. J. 1979. Evolutionary relationship of the gut hormones. *Fed. Proc.* 38:2295–301.

[13] Dulka, J. G., N. E. Stacey, D. W. Sorenson, and G. J. Van Derokraav. 1987. A steroid sex pheromone synchronizes male–female spawning readiness in goldfish. *Nature* (Lond.) 325:251–3.

[14] Guillemin, R. 1977. The expanding significance of hypothalamic peptides, or, is endocrinology a branch of neuroendocrinology. *Rec. Prog. Horm. Res.* 33:1–28.

[15] Karlson, P. 1982. Was sind Hormone? Der Hormonbegriff in Geschichte und Gegenwart. *Naturwissenschaften* 69:3–14.

[16] Kow, L.-M., and D. W. Pfaff. 1988. Neuromodulatory actions of peptides. *Annu. Rev. Pharm. & Toxicol.* 28:163–88.

[17] Lebedev, N. B., and I. V. Osokina. 1989. Precocious puberty syndrome in a boy with hormone-producing tumor of the liver. *Pediatria* 11:96–8.

[18] Lechan, R. M. 1987. Neuroendocrinology of pituitary hormone regulation. *Endocrinol. Metab. Clin. N. Amer.* 16:475–501.

[19] Lyons, R. M., and J. L. Moses. 1990. Transforming growth factors and the regulation of cell proliferation. *Eur. J. Biochem.* 187:467–73.

[20] Maclean, D. B., and I. M. Jackson. 1988. Molecular biology and regulation of the hypothalamic hormones. *Baillière's Clin. Endocrinol. Metab.* 2:835–68.

[21] Makhlouf, G. M. 1990. Neural and hormonal regulation of function in the gut. *Hosp. Pract.* 25:79–98.

[22] Nishimura, K., K. Utsumi, M. Yuhara, Y. Funitani, and A. Iritani. 1989. Identification of puberty-accelerating pheromones in male mouse urine. *J. Exp. Zool.* 251:300–5.

[23] Ohta, T. 1989. Role of gene duplication in evolution. *Genome* 31:304–10.

[24] Rajan, A. S., L. Aguilar-Bryan, D. A. Nelson, G. C. Yaney, W. H. Hsu, D. L. Kunze, and A. E. Boyd III. 1990. Ion channels and insulin secretion. *Diabetes Care* 13:340–63.

[25] Rosbash M., and J. C. Hall. 1989. The molecular biology of circadian rhythms. *Neuron* 3:387–98.

[26] Samols, E., and J. I. Stagner. 1988. Intra-islet regulation. *Amer. J. Med.* 85:31–5.

[27] Scharrer, B. 1987. Neurosecretion: beginnings and new directions in neuropeptide research. *Annu. Rev. Neurosci.* 10:1–17.

[28] Schneider, D. 1992. 100 years of pheromone research. *Naturwissenschaften* 79:241–50.

[29] Segal, J. 1988. Aging: a non-regulated process. *Med. Hypo.* 25:197–207.

[30] Selye, H. 1976. *The stress of life.* New York: McGraw-Hill Book Company.

[31] Simpson, E. R., and M. R. Waterman. 1988. Regulation of the synthesis of steroidogenic enzymes in adrenal cortical cells by ACTH. *Annu. Rev. Physiol.* 50:427–40.

[32] Smith, W. L. 1989. The eicosanoids and their biochemical mechanisms of action. *Biochem. J.* 259:315–24.

[33] Stoddart, D. M. 1976. *Mammalian odours and pheromones.* London: Edward Arnold, Ltd.

[34] Strange, G. P. 1988. The structure and mechanism of neurotransmitter receptors. Implications for the structure and function of the central nervous system. *Biochem. J.* 249:309–18.

[35] Warren, M. P., and J. Brooks-Gunn. 1989. Mood and behavior at adolescence: evidence for hormonal factors. *J. Clin. Endocrinol. Metab.* 69:77–83.

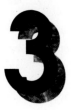

Endocrine Methodologies

Some of the methods presently used in endocrinological studies were developed for more practical purposes. In many cultures castration was practiced as a form of punishment. In the Middle and Far East castration was performed to provide servants (eunuchs) for harems; in Italy castrated young boys were trained to be adult sopranos. Castration is presently used to improve the flavor of meat from some domestic animals (e.g., castrated chickens produce capons). These "practical" operations were the forerunners of the gonadectomies of present-day endocrinological studies.

The idea that glands contained humors or substances that could act as replacement therapy for a lost function of a gland was first entertained seriously by a French physician, Charles Brown-Séquard. He injected himself with extracts from dog, guinea pig, and rabbit testicles and proclaimed that the extracts had remarkable rejuvenating effects. Brown-Séquard even recommended that extracts be obtained from the mature calf to give to men the vigor of horses and other larger animals. It is now believed that these extracts had only a placebo effect. Nevertheless, glandular extraction, purification, and injection into animals have become important methods in elucidating the hormonal role of particular tissues and organs.

Although hormones control a large variety of physiological events, their basic function is to act at the level of the cell to stimulate cellular physiological processes inherent in the cell. Melanocytes, for example, synthesize the pigment melanin. Melanocyte stimulating hormone (MSH) enhances melanin formation by increasing the activity of the rate-limiting enzyme tyrosinase. Cortisol is a hormone produced by adrenal steroidogenic tissue. Corticotropin (ACTH) activation of adrenocortical enzyme activity leads to elevated cortisol biosynthesis. Thus effects of hormones are reflected in physiological processes in the many cell types present within an organism. This chapter summarizes some of the methods employed by endocrinologists to study endocrine glands and the target cells and tissues that they regulate.

GENERAL CONSIDERATIONS

The methods now employed to study endocrine systems are highly diverse. They include surgical manipulations, tissue extract preparation for hormone isolation and identification, histological methods for the localization of hormones, and numerous assay methods. The techniques described below will be mentioned in more detail in later chapters.

Following discovery of a hormone, endocrine studies usually focus on the following investigations (not necessarily in the order delineated):

1. *Source.* The distribution of the hormone will be determined. The hormone may be found in more than a single organ, tissue, or cellular source. For example, several gastrointestinal hormones are also found within the central nervous system.

2. *Structure determination and synthesis.* Depending on the type of hormone, the structure will be determined by any of a variety of methods. In the case of a peptide hormone, the primary (amino acid) sequence will be determined. From this information the peptide will then be synthesized and its biological activity, compared to the purified extract, will be determined. This will establish the substance and structure as the authentic hormone.

3. *Biosynthesis.* The biosynthetic pathway of hormone production should be delineated. Knowledge of the primary structure of a peptide hormone can be used to predict the complementary cDNA structure responsible for mRNA and subsequent protein synthesis. This information will usually predict the prohormone structure and possible enzymological events related to production of the mature hormone.

4. *Control of secretion.* The extrinsic or intrinsic factor(s) regulating the control of hormone secretion must then be determined. Endogenous stimuli may involve negative or positive feedback effects of the hormone, or the circulating products (other hormones, metabolic substrates), or consequences (blood volume, water and/or electrolyte composition of the blood) of its actions. The nervous system may directly or indirectly regulate hormone secretion from endocrine organs or tissues.

5. *Cellular mechanisms of secretion.* Once the first messengers regulating hormone secretion have been determined, it is then necessary to determine the nature of the second messengers and structural elements (ion channels, cytoplasmic organelles) that participate in the process of hormone release (secretion).

6. *Circulation and metabolism.* It is important to determine the half-life of the hormone in the systemic circulation. Steroid or peptide hormones may be noncovalently bound to circulating proteins. Fluctuations in the levels of the "binding" proteins may affect the total amount of hormone available in the circulatory system and therefore available for hormone action. The half-life of the hormone in the circulation may be affected by degradation or other alterations of the hormone by serum enzymes. The retention time of the hormone in the circulation may also be affected by processes of filtration by the kidney.

7. *Biological actions and roles.* Removal of the hormone from the body by one or more methods usually will result in physiological effects in the animal that will predict one or more functions for the hormone. Administration of the hormone (replacement therapy) or related analog to the animal should confirm one or more roles for the hormone. Studies on other species of animals may suggest additional or alternate roles for the hormone.

8. *Mechanisms of action.* Following administration of the hormone, in vivo and in vitro cellular changes in biochemical processes and products should indicate one or more second messengers involved in hormone action. The receptor and signal transduction mechanisms involved in hormone action should define the temporal aspects between receptor activation and cellular response. Structure-activity studies will determine the essential features of the hormone required for hormone action, in the case of a peptide, the "message sequence."

HISTOLOGICAL-CYTOLOGICAL STUDIES

The early endocrine studies were, as expected, anatomical and purely descriptive in nature. The light microscope was used to determine the histological nature of the endocrine glands. Many early observations were made on these tissues even before their endocrine role was suspected. Much of this work was accomplished by the great German, Italian, and other European cytologists of the nineteenth century. Although light microscopic methods are still important, the electron microscope is now the tool in the investigation of cellular function at the ultrastructural level. The scanning electron microscope has now bridged the gap between light and electron microscopy.

Gross observations of endocrine tissue provide only general details of anatomical localization, organ size, vascularization, and innervation. Severe alterations from the normal in organ size may provide clues to an underlying pathophysiology. The thyroid gland, for example, may become enlarged or goitrous under certain conditions of hyperstimulation. At the histological level, one is able to discern the cytological characteristics of endocrine tissues. The cells may be *hypertrophic* (enlarged) or *atrophic* depending on whether they are hyperactive or hypoactive, respectively. Hypertrophic cells contain an abundance of endoplasmic reticulum and Golgi bodies, as these organelles function in many cellular synthetic processes. Atrophic cells, on the other hand, lack this synthetic machinery and contain a much diminished cytoplasmic mass. Endocrine cell hypertrophy is usually accompanied by *hyperplasia*, an increase in cell number.

Histological stains are available to provide further information on chemical components of cells. Hematoxylin and eosin are two popular dyes for staining cells for routine histological observation. Hematoxylin, a basic dye, interacts with acidic components of the cell, such as the phosphoric acid of DNA and RNA. These components are said to be *basophilic* or to exhibit basophilia. On the other hand, eosin, an acidic dye, interacts with the basic components of the cell, which are then said to be *acidophilic* or to exhibit acidophilia. Used in combination, hematoxylin and eosin usually stain the nucleus and cytoplasm blue and pink, respectively.

By the use of a battery of histological stains one can characterize each cell present in the pituitary. With hematoxylin and eosin it is only possible to separate the basophils from the acidophils and chromophobic (non-staining) cells (*chromophores*). Other histological stains are needed to further differentiate the several types of basophils. Certain stains can also be used to demonstrate the presence of specific organic constituents, such as glycoproteins, in such cells as the gonadotrophs of the pituitary, or glycogen in hepatocytes.

Immunocytochemistry

In techniques using immunocytochemistry, antibodies to peptide or protein hormones are conjugated to a fluorescent dye and used to identify hormone-producing cells [35]. After the tissue is placed on a microscope slide, a solution of the antibody conjugate is added to the tissue, and the excess solution is then rinsed from the slide several times. Microscopic observations usually reveal that the fluorescent antibody is deposited only in those cells that produce the hormone, the antigen (see Fig. 10.8). Specificity is determined by prior treatment with the nonfluorescent antibody, which interacts with the cellular antigen and thus prevents ("swamps out") the fluorescent antibody from binding to the antigen.

In immunoenzyme histochemistry an antibody to a hormone is conjugated to an enzyme, such as peroxidase. The antibody-enzyme conjugate is then allowed to interact with the tissue slice. When substrate for the enzyme is added, the conjugated enzyme catalyzes very localized reactions that yield a color or opaque product in the vicinity of the antigen (the hormone). By this immunoperoxidase method and use of the electron microscope, it is even possible to localize the site of the enzyme activity to the secretory vesicles of a cell, which provides strong evidence that these organelles contain the hormone under investigation.

SURGICAL METHODS

Surgical removal of a putative endocrine gland or tissue from an animal is followed by subsequent assessment of physiological alterations [43]. A change in functional activity of suspected target organs (i.e., atrophy) suggests an endocrine function for the extirpated tissue. One might also monitor changes in blood or urinary levels of certain metabolites or electrolytes. Removal of the adrenals, for example, would result in lowered circulating levels of adrenal steroids and catecholamines and a reduction in the plasma Na^+ concentration. Transplanting an organ back into the same or different animal also provides information on the functional role of the organ. In mammals transplantation of an organ from a donor to a host is usually done in genetically related (inbred) strains of animals so that the transplant is not rejected by immunological processes. Endocrine organs can be transplanted to an *ectopic* (abnormal) site in the animal, usually beneath the kidney capsule or within the eye, where rapid vascularization often occurs. Removal of the pituitary is referred to as a *hypophysectomy*. The pituitary target organs of "hypox" animals become atrophic due to the absence of hormonal stimulation. In a few examples endocrine tissue is normally under a tonic inhibitory control; the tissue becomes hypertrophic when transplanted to an ectopic site within the animal or when incubated in vitro.

Removal of both members of paired (bilateral) target organs (for example, adrenal glands or gonads) usually leads to complete loss of dependent tissue/organ functions. If only one of the pair (unilateral) is removed, the remaining organ usually undergoes *compensatory hypertrophy*. In other words, there is an increase in cell size and number in the remaining organ to compensate functionally for the loss of hormone secretion from the ablated organ (see Fig. 1.1).

Certain experimental animals can be sutured together and their vascular systems joined. Under these conditions if the endocrine (or other) organs of one *parabiosed* animal are removed, the organs of the other animal hypertrophy (Fig. 3.1). Obviously, some form of chemical communication must be transferred between the parabiotic animals to produce this compensatory hypertrophy. Castration of one of the animals, either orchidectomy in the male or ovariectomy (spaying) in the female, would be expected, for example, to partially remove a negative feedback to the hypothalamus, since the total circulating levels of gonadal steroids of both animals would be decreased compared to that of a pair of intact animals. This would result in enhanced gonadotropin secretion from the pituitary of both animals and compensatory growth of the remaining gonads of the non-gonadectomized animal.

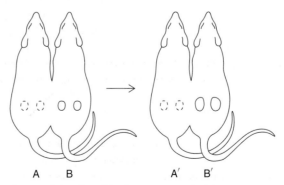

A   B   A′   B′

Figure 3.1 Parabiosis accompanied by compensatory organ hypertrophy after removal of the same organs from one of the parabiotic animals.

Other examples of endocrine ablations include pinealectomy (epiphysectomy), adrenalectomy, thyroidectomy, and thymectomy. The diverse nature of such endocrine tissues as the gastrointestinal hormone-secreting cells prevents such a surgical procedure. The pancreatic islets are similarly impossible to remove without removing concomitantly the exocrine tissue that comprises most of the mass of the pancreas. Islet ablation, however, can be accomplished by the use of alloxan or streptozotocin, drugs that specifically destroy the insulin-secreting cells of the islets. Cobalt chloride is similarly effective in the elimination of the glucagon-secreting cells of the pancreatic islets.

HORMONE REPLACEMENT THERAPY

The undesirable effects of hormone loss following surgical ablatement or loss due to certain disease states can often be adequately reversed by administration of the needed hormone or related analog [31]. At menopause, for example, many women experience bone mineral loss (osteoporosis) due to declining levels of ovarian estrogens. Estrogen (contraceptive steroid) replacement therapy is important in preventing the increased risk of bone fractures in these women [7, 24]. Children lacking somatotropin (growth hormone) can maintain normal stature (growth) when given this hormone, thus avoiding dwarfism, which is the result of the absence of the hormone.

IMMUNOLOGICAL NEUTRALIZATION OF HORMONE ACTIVITY

Antibodies can be prepared against most of the peptide hormones. Injected into the intact animal, these antibodies neutralize the biological activity of the endogenous hormones. This methodology may have clinical applications, since such an immunological approach may be useful for contraception in both the male and the female. For example, the mammalian zona pellucida, which surrounds growing oocytes and ovulated eggs, is a potential immunogen for a contraceptive vaccine. Immunizing mice with sera against the zona produces reversible contraception in the mouse without obvious side effects [23]. Many experimental uses of this methodology can be foreseen. For example, injections of antibodies to nerve growth factor (NGF, Chap. 12), a hormone required for growth and development of the sympathetic nervous system, result in failure of this system to develop. The injected animals are effectively immunosympathectomized (Chap. 14).

TISSUE EXTRACTS AND PURIFICATION

Crude extracts of endocrine or other tissues were used by some early investigators to determine whether these materials could replace the excised endocrine tissue. With improved chemical techniques, the hormonal entities contained within the extracts were purified. This led eventually to the preparation of pure substances that were, and still are in many cases, marketed by pharmaceutical houses for medicinal or experimental use. Replacement therapy with these preparations can lead to full restoration of target organ function or even to hypertrophy, an overshoot, if too much of the preparation is provided. Many diabetics must receive daily injections of exogenous insulin to augment insufficient quantities produced endogenously by the pancreatic islets. Until recently the only source of peptide/protein hormones, such as insulin, that are too large to synthesize was generally from endocrine glands obtained from the abattoir (slaughterhouse). Generally, the hormones extracted are of *bovine* (cattle), *ovine* (sheep), *porcine* (pig), or even *equine* (horse) origin. Often these foreign proteins are immunologically neutralized within the body following administration, therefore necessitating a change in the type (source) of the hormone used.

CHEMICAL IDENTIFICATION AND SYNTHESIS

Next, a purified hormone must be chemically identified. The simplest analysis of the hormonal entity may yield only information relative to the percentage of carbon, hydrogen, oxygen, nitrogen, sulfur, or other atoms present and thus provide only an empirical formula. Further analysis of a protein, for example, may then indicate the number and nature of amino acids present (an amino acid analysis). This may be followed by a determination of the *primary sequence* (exact amino acid sequence) of the peptide or protein under study. This is not easy if a large protein hormone is being studied. Nevertheless, one may obtain information on the N-terminal or C-terminal sequences of these large protein hormones. Recently primary sequences of a number of large proteins have been determined by analyzing the nucleotide sequences of the DNA that code for the molecules. Secondary (helical) and tertiary (intrachain bonding) structures may often be implied from such information as the distribution of basic or acidic amino acids or the presence of sulfhydryl (—SH) groups within the protein. Some peptide hormones, such as insulin, possess a quaternary structure, that is, the hormone is made up of two peptide chains folded together into a three-dimensional structure (conformation). A number of the larger peptide hormones, for example, FSH, LH, and TSH, are composed of two chains, the so-called α- and β-subunits of their structures.

Chemical analysis may indicate that proteins are modified through sulfation or conjugation to carbohydrate moieties. The pituitary hormones, FSH, LH, and TSH, are examples of *glycoproteins* (Chap. 5). Determination of steroid or other hormone structures requires different chemical and physical methods of analysis. After determination of the putative hormone structure, it is necessary to synthesize the proposed structure and demonstrate that the natural and synthetic structures are identical with respect to chemical, physical, and biological characteristics. One can then synthesize related structural analogs of the hormone to determine the structural basis for the biological activity of the hormone.

BIOASSAYS

The physiological activity of a hormone was originally determined by bioassay. Although some assays have been replaced by more modern methods, in some instances the only method available is bioassay [43]. In a bioassay, the activity of a hormone is studied on living cells, tissues, or organs. Physiological responses such as muscle contraction and relaxation or glandular secretion are monitored. The assay may be performed in vitro or in vivo (in situ) depending on the assay used. Usually a tissue or organ selected is naturally responsive to the hormone. These biological preparations are usually responsive to hormones in the nanomolar (10^{-9} M) to picomolar (10^{-12} M) range [34]. Other hormones may also affect these tissues, but usually in pharmacological (micromolar, 10^{-6} M) doses.

The frog skin bioassay for melanocyte-stimulating hormone (MSH) is simple, specific, and exquisitely sensitive. Melanin granules within melanophores of frog skin disperse in response to the hormone, causing the skin to turn from light green to dark brown (Chap. 8). This change can be measured in a number of ways, but one objective method is to monitor changes in light reflectance off the surface of the skin [34]. The toad bladder, and such epithelial structures as frog skin and the mammalian renal nephron, have been used in vitro to study the actions of vasopressin on transport of water and other components, such as Na^+ and urea, across these organs. Studies of ion transport in the toad bladder have contributed detailed information of the mechanisms involved in vasopressin action (Chap. 7).

The steroid-primed uterus of the rat has been used in vitro to study the mechanisms of oxytocin-induced contraction of this organ. Mammary tissue from the lactating mouse is used in vitro to determine milk-ejecting potency of oxytocin and related analogs. Other bioassays include in vitro adrenal steroidogenesis and secretion in response to ACTH: prostate and seminal vesicle growth in vivo in response to testosterone in the castrated male rodent; measurement of iodine uptake by the thyroid after exogenous TSH injections; measurement of epiphyseal (cartilage) plate growth in the young rat in response to growth hormone. Because of animal rights concerns, many investigators are turning to cell culture systems.

STRUCTURE-ACTIVITY STUDIES

Bioassays determine whether a putative hormone or hormone analog possesses biological activity. Structure-activity studies determine the amount of activity, usually compared with some standard hormone. The minimal effective dose (MED) and maximal activities within the particular assay are usually determined first. Then, intermediate concentrations of the hormone between the two extremes (maximum and minimum) can be utilized to provide a dose-response curve. Usually, the half-maximal activity of the hormone is compared with a similar half-maximal control response (e.g., to the parent hormone or to an analog) and expressed as a potency ratio. The hormone or hormone analog may possess one or more times greater or lesser activity (potency) than the native hormone (see Fig. 8.18).

Site-directed Mutagenesis

Although the primary sequence of many hormone receptors is known, how the receptors function can not readily be discerned from the amino acid sequence. One would like to know the sequence(s) responsible for ligand (hormone) binding and the sequence(s) responsible for signal transduction leading to a cellular response. Such questions can be answered by "reverse" genetics [6, 26]. A mutant receptor can be synthesized from the original normal receptor cDNA and the mutated DNA introduced into "immortalized" (usually cancer) cells. Then, a functional response to a hormone by these cells containing mutated DNA can be measured. For example, one can measure changes in levels of a second messenger, such as cAMP, following addition of the hormone to the cells. Single base changes, multiple base changes, additions, or deletions (subtracting amino acids) can be made (Chap. 19) [6].

RADIOISOTOPE STUDIES

A number of endocrine methods use the radioactive isotopes of various elements (e.g., ^{125}I, ^{45}Ca, ^{35}S, ^{32}P, ^{23}Na, ^{14}C, ^{3}H) to determine physiological and biochemical responses within a cell. The half-life of a hormone, for example, can be ascertained by radiolabeling the hormone and then determining its distribution, excretion rate [4], and metabolism within the body of an animal. Iodide [^{125}I] is taken up by thyroid cells and incorporated into thyroid hormones (T_4 and T_3). Radiometric methods can be used to measure uptake of radioactive iodide atoms by the thyroid. Information obtained often reflects the biosynthetic activity of the thyroid gland, and this method is also used to localize hyperplastic thyroid tissues.

The radioisotope of carbon [^{14}C] can be incorporated synthetically into the structure of a molecule such as glucose. Subsequent metabolism of glucose with the concomitant evolution of radioactive carbon dioxide [^{14}C]O$_2$ is a measure of the metabolic activity of the cell. Insulin, for example, increases release of radioactive CO_2 by stimulating the uptake of radiolabeled glucose into diaphragm muscle where it is metabolized. This is also a good example of a bioassay. Tritium, a radioisotope of hydrogen [^{3}H], is widely used in autoradiography and in enzyme assays. The tritium isotope is generally used as a component of some organic structures, such as an amino acid or nucleotide (e.g., thymidine). The sodium radioisotope [^{23}Na] is most often used to measure Na$^+$ uptake into nerve or muscle cells during studies on transmembrane potential changes in response to chemical messengers or other stimuli. Radioactive calcium [^{45}Ca] is often used to measure uptake of this divalent cation during muscle contraction and relaxation, nerve stimulation, or cellular secretion. Moreover, this isotope can localize Ca^{2+} sequestration within mitochondria or in the sarcoplasmic reticulum. Incorporation of sulfur [^{35}S] into the amino acid cysteine has been particularly productive in the study of neurohypophysial hormone synthesis because neurohypophysial peptides contain a high percentage of this amino acid. Such labeling of newly synthesized neurophysins and neurohypophysial hormones has greatly advanced studies on the movement of these proteins by axoplasmic transport down the neuronal secretory axons (Chap. 7).

Radioactive phosphorus [^{32}P] in the form of phosphate can be used to monitor protein phosphorylation as induced, for example, by hormonal stimulation of cells (see Fig 4.16). A variety of assays use radioisotopes to determine the concentration of a hormone in an endocrine tissue, in the blood, or in the urine. Radioisotope assays can also be used to determine enzyme activation or inhibition by a hormone. In each of these assays specialized equipment capable of measuring the decay of the isotope is used (liquid scintillation counters or gamma counters, for example).

Radioimmunoassays

The development of the radioimmunoassay (RIA) has allowed the detection of hormones in minute concentrations and with a high degree of specificity [42]. RIA has provided greatly increased diagnostic accuracy of pathologic states characterized by hormonal excess or deficiency (see Fig. 9.13). These assays are routinely employed to determine the concentration of hormones and other molecules in blood or other body fluids (see Figs. 6.14 and 7.12). Antibodies against the antigenic principle (e.g., hormone) are usually raised in rabbits or other animals. The hormone is then iodinated or tritiated; in peptide hormones or in other proteins the tyrosine moiety incorporates iodide. The radiolabeled ligand (e.g., hormone) can then be shown to combine with a given quantity of antibody in a dose-related manner to provide a standard curve. Unknown samples containing native (unlabeled) hormone compete with labeled hormone for the antibody, and the concentration of the hormone is then determined. Because the native and labeled hormones compete equally well (sometimes an assumption) for the antibody, the decreased binding of the labeled hormone to the antibody is a reflection of the amount of the native hormone bound to the antibody (and therefore present in the sample). Cyclic nucleotides and many other nonprotein substances are also measured by radioimmunoassay. They are, however, usually conjugated to an antigenic principle to produce antibodies for their assay.

Radioreceptor Assays

In the radioreceptor assay, plasma membranes or intact cells are carefully prepared and a dose-related binding of radiolabeled hormone to the membranes is then demonstrated. Instead of an antigen-antibody reaction, the assay employs interaction between hormone and natural membrane receptors. The detailed mechanisms are, nevertheless, similar to those described for the radioimmunoassay. The specificity of the binding is determined by the ability of the cold, native hormone to compete (swamp out) with the radiolabeled hormone for receptor. Other cold or radiolabeled hormones or other ligands can be used to determine the specificity of the hormone for its receptor. Both ACTH, as well as prostaglandins, for example, interact with adrenal cortical cell membranes to initiate steroidogenesis. Radiolabeled ACTH can be displaced from its receptor by cold ACTH, but not cold prostaglandin. Cold prostaglandin, but not cold ACTH, will displace radiolabeled prostaglandin from the membrane preparation. These results

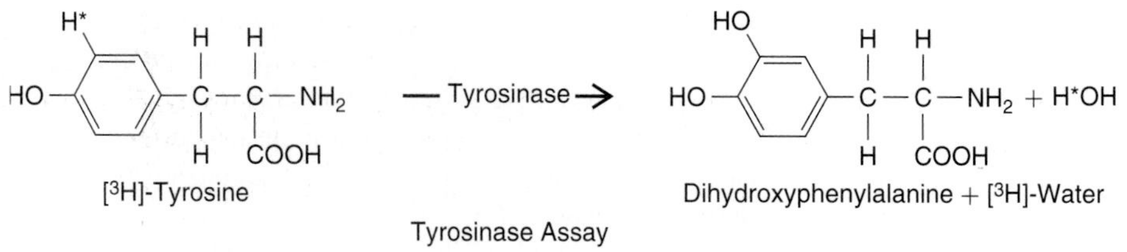

Figure 3.2   Radioisotope enzyme assay; tyrosinase assay.

demonstrate that the receptors for these active agonists are separate because each agonist can be specifically blocked while the integrity of the other receptor is uncompromised.

Enzyme Assays

Enzyme activity can also be measured by radioisotope methods. Adenylate cyclase or guanylate cyclase are measured by quantitation of the conversion of an appropriately radiolabeled precursor, ATP or GTP, respectively, to radiolabeled cyclic nucleotide. This is a true measure of cyclizing activity of the membrane fractions, as measurements of cyclic nucleotide levels in the cell fail to indicate how the nucleotide levels are altered. Cyclic AMP levels, for example, may be altered by a number of processes, such as increased or decreased phosphodiesterase activity, which are unrelated to cyclase activity and cAMP formation. Measurement of tyrosinase activity of melanocytes is monitored by production of radiolabeled water from the appropriately labeled precursor, tyrosine (Fig. 3.2).

Autoradiography

This technique determines the cellular site of a radiolabeled substrate incorporation [6, 15, 16]. A radioisotope is injected into an animal or added to the medium within which cells are grown. A sample of tissue/organ from the animal or the cell culture is then placed on a microscope slide, as is done for routine microscopy. In the darkroom the slide is now immersed in a photographic emulsion and kept in the dark for a period of time. Decay of the isotope (usually tritium) leads to reduction of the silver bromide in the overlying emulsion to silver crystals. Because the *beta* particles released by the tritium travel only a short distance, the silver grains directly over the emulsion are preferentially exposed, since they are closest to the source of isotope decay. The tissue with emulsion is then placed in developer and stained, if desired. By this method, for example, one can determine the incorporation of tritium-labeled thymidine into DNA [16]. This nucleotide is generally used to determine the mitotic activity of tissue cells. After orchidectomy, for example, there is enhanced hypothalamic activation of pituitary gonadotrophs (due to lack of negative feedback inhibition by testosterone). This leads to increased incorporation of radiolabeled thymidine into the DNA of these cells, which can be visualized by autoradiographic methods.

The action of steroid hormones involves interaction with nuclear DNA. Autoradiography using tritium-labeled steroids provides a method for demonstrating the cellular site of these hormones' action (Fig. 3.3). Radiolabeled peptide hormones can be used to determine the topographical localization of hormone receptors in an organ or tissue (see Fig. 7.7). Some hormones mediate their effects through stimulation of RNA synthesis. This is demonstrated by the use of tritium-labeled uracil, which is incorporated specifically into RNA rather than DNA. Using giant chromosomes of the dipteran fly (midge), *Chironomus*, for example, it is possible to localize tritium uptake to specific Balbiani rings (large "puffs") of the chromosomes [1], sites known to be responsible for very active RNA synthesis (Fig. 3.4).

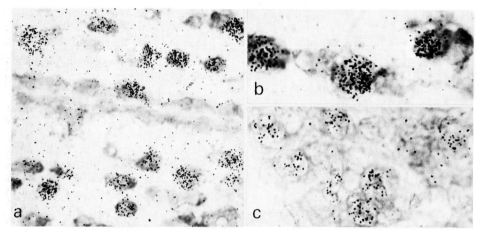

Figure 3.3 (a) Heavily labeled cells in the medial preoptic nucleus of the mouse after injection with [³H]estradiol; ×850. (b) Labeled neurons, at a higher magnification, showing the concentration of silver grains over the cell nuclei; ×1,360. (c) Guinea pig anterior pituitary cells; radioactivity is retained in nuclei of certain cells after injection of [³H]estradiol; ×1,360. (From Warembourg [40], with permission.)

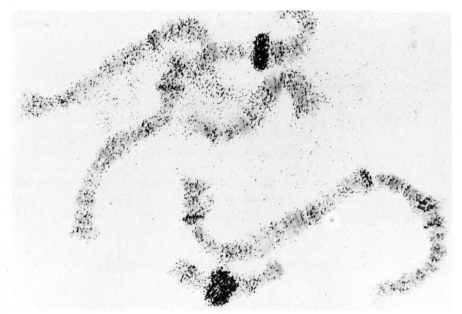

Figure 3.4 Pattern of [³H]uridine incorporation into RNA produced by larval salivary chromosomes of a dipteran fly. Note intense labeling of Balbiani rings 1 and 6. (From Beermann [1], with permission.)

Hybridization Studies

Hybridization, or annealing, involves pairing of complementary strands of nucleic acids. Hybrids can form between DNA-DNA, DNA-RNA, or RNA-RNA strands. DNA is analyzed on a solid support such as a membrane (Southern hybridization) and RNA can be analyzed on such a support (Northern hybridization). The powerful technique used to localize mRNA involved in hormone synthesis is beautifully demonstrated in Fig. 8.5 [39].

The nucleotides can also be localized within cells and tissues by in situ hybridization (Fig. 3.5). The principal advantage of in situ hybridization methods over total RNA hybridization methods is the cellular resolution afforded by in situ hybridization. With in situ hybridization, it is possible to address questions regarding differential gene regulation within different nuclei in a given brain region or within different cell populations in a specific nucleus. This level of resolution can reveal subtleties of gene regulation that cannot be detected with Northern or Southern hybridization methods. Moreover, it is also possible to determine if specific colocalized genes are coordinately regulated in brain nuclei in which some or all of the neurons display such colocalization. The principal disadvantages of in situ hybridization methods are that they are time and labor intensive and that absolute quantification cannot be ensured [5].

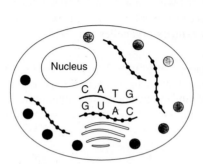

Figure 3.5 In situ hybridization. The probe (RNA or DNA) is labeled with a radioactive or nonradioactive detection system. The DNA probe in this example (5′-CATG-3′) is hybridizing with the messenger RNA associated with the rough endoplasmic reticulum. After hybridization to cells or tissue sections, the RNA or DNA of interest can be detected by autoradiography or nonisotopic methods. Advantages of in situ hybridization include more precise intracellular localization of the RNA or DNA of interest and direct visualization of positive cells in relationship to surrounding cells and tissues (From Lloyd [17], with permission. *Endocrine Pathophysiology* 4:64–72, 1993.)

ELECTROPHYSIOLOGICAL METHODS

Most cells are excitable, that is, they will respond to stimuli by becoming depolarized or hyperpolarized, which results, for example, in relaxation or contraction, respectively. These potential transmembrane changes can be monitored by intracellular or extracellular microelectrodes. The response of the cells to hormonal or other stimuli can therefore be detected. Most stimuli depolarize cells, but some chemical messengers—for example, gamma aminobutyric acid (GABA), a central nervous system neurotransmitter—hyperpolarize cells. Chemical messengers can be applied to the surface of a cell by *microiontophoresis* and resulting transmembrane potential changes recorded downstream by microelectrode recordings. Electrophysiological methods have been important in studying electrical properties of the neurosecretory neurons of the neurohypophysis (see Fig. 7.3) and the response of pituitary cells to hormones (see Fig. 6.18).

PHARMACOLOGICAL METHODS

Many exogenous substances interact with molecular components of cells, and they therefore can be used to study the physiological activity of cells or the mechanism by which chemical messengers stimulate or inhibit such activity [10]. For example, at the level of the plasmalemma, cardiac glycosides, such as ouabain, are used to inhibit the Na^+/K^+ pump. Certain hormone secretions are enhanced or inhibited by ouabain, and this suggests that active transport (Na^+/K^+ ATPase) systems may be involved in the secretion mechanism of these hormones.

Many agents are inhibitors of intracellular enzyme activity. Of particular interest are the methylxanthines, such as theophylline (from tea) and caffeine (from coffee), which are phosphodiesterase inhibitors. These drugs mimic the actions of many hormones because they elevate intracellular cAMP levels (see Fig. 4.6).

There are a number of metabolic inhibitors that affect utilization of substrates for ATP formation. Iodoacetic acid blocks glycolysis, dinitrophenol (DNP) uncouples oxidative phosphorylation, and oligomycin prevents mitochondrial phosphorylation of ADP to ATP. The false substrate, 2-deoxyglucose, can be used to slow down glucose utilization within cells. These inhibitors provide information on the degree to which the glycolytic (Embden-Myerhof) pathway or the citric acid cycle (Krebs cycle) contributes to cellular function.

Colchicine, a plant alkaloid, inhibits microtubule assembly by binding with tubulin, the protein subunit of these intracellular filaments. Inhibition of hormone action by colchicine or related microtubule inhibitors (vincristine and vinblastine) might suggest, therefore, that the hormone works through a cellular mechanism in which microtubules are involved. Insulin secretion is inhibited by colchicine, suggesting that microtubules may function in the secretion of this hormone. Cytochalasin B is a fungal metabolite that specifically interferes with microfilament function and is without effect on microtubule integrity. Cytochalasin B is inhibitory to the secretion of a number of hormones, suggesting that these filamentous organelles may be involved in the secretory process of these hormones.

At the level of the nucleus, actinomycin D inhibits RNA production. Puromycin and cycloheximide, on the other hand, inhibit protein synthesis. Thus inhibition of hormone action by actinomycin D implies that the hormone works through a transcriptional process of RNA synthesis. Inhibition of hormone action by puromycin or cycloheximide, in contrast, is interpreted to implicate a translational process of protein synthesis in the action mechanism of the chemical messenger.

Rather specific cation *ionophores* have been discovered and synthesized. These organic cation transport molecules specifically incorporate certain cations into their structure. They cross biological membranes and carry ions into cells. Ionophore A23187, for example, is specific for Ca^{2+} and, because many hormones activate cells by a calcium ion mechanism, this ionophore is in some systems hormone-mimetic. Valinomycin is an ionophore with relatively high specificity for K^+ transport. Some agents, on the other hand, are specific inhibitors of ion transport into cells. Verapamil, a Ca^{2+} channel antagonist, blocks Ca^{2+} entry into cells [18]. Used concomitantly with a hormone, verapamil's inhibitory action may suggest that a particular hormone action is Ca^{2+} dependent. Local anesthetics, such as procaine and tetracaine, may also block the action of some hormones by their antagonism of Ca^{2+} flux into cells.

Phospholipid vesicles (liposomes) have proved to be suitable carriers for many biologically active molecules. These transport vehicles fuse with and become incorporated into the plasma membrane, thereby transferring their contents into the cytoplasm. Liposomes loaded with Ca^{2+}, for example, are incorporated into the mast cell plasma membrane, which results in localized cell surface secretion of histamine [37]. Liposomes therefore provide a novel method of studying mechanisms of stimulus-secretion coupling, particularly as it relates to the release of a chemical messenger such as histamine.

Some agents are hormone receptor agonists, although in some cases they may not appear to bear any structural similarity to the true receptor agonist, the hormone. Certain ergot alkaloids, for example, stimulate dopamine receptors and inhibit MSH and prolactin secretion, thus providing some evidence that dopamine may be the natural hypothalamic inhibitor of these hormones. Certain structures related to acetylcholine (e.g., carbachol) exhibit intrinsic cholinergic activity, and they are of particular usefulness because they have a longer duration of activity as they are more resistant to enzymatic degradation.

Hormone action can be blocked by compounds that specifically act with hormone receptors but lack intrinsic agonistic activity [3, 13, 20]. For example, chlorpromazine and related antidepressant drugs block dopamine receptors. Acetylcholine action can be blocked by atropine (on smooth muscle) and curare (on skeletal muscle) and other cholinergic receptor antagonists. Cimetidine is a specific inhibitor of histamine (H_2) receptors and markedly inhibits histamine-stimulated gastric acid secretion. Cyproterone acetate and spironolactone are specific antagonists (antihormones) of testosterone and aldosterone receptors, respectively. Cyproterone acetate is a valuable tool in the treatment of cancer or hyperplasia of the prostate, hirsutism in the female, and precocious puberty in both sexes, as these maladies are often due to excess androgen secretion and action [2].

Synthetic analogs of peptide hormones may be used to block receptor occupancy by the native hormone. Hormone antagonists might prove useful in blocking the actions of excessive amounts of the native hormone in certain disease states (e.g., Cushing's disease) [13, 20, 31]. So called "beta blockers," for example, have proved clinically useful in reducing the activity of the heart [3]. In women, the steroid hormone, progesterone, plays a central role in the establishment and maintenance of pregnancy (Chap. 19). A synthetic progesterone analog has been developed that possesses antiprogesterone activity (see Fig. 19.10). It has been used successfully as a medical alternative for early pregnancy interruption and other clinical applications.

As mentioned earlier, cobalt chloride and alloxan can be used specifically to destroy the alpha (glucagon-secreting) or beta (insulin-secreting) cells, respectively, of the pancreas. Monosodium glutamate (MSG) administered neonatally causes degeneration of neurons of the arcuate nucleus of the hypothalamus [11]. The neurotoxicity of MSG appears to be useful for investigative purposes because it is difficult to produce such lesions by electrolytic and radiofrequency methods without damage to other neurons or fiber tracts. The use of MSG, therefore, offers the opportunity to study the endocrine and morphological manifestations of destruction of specific neurons within the brain. Some pharmaceutical agents used in endocrine studies are described in Table 3.1.

TABLE 3.1   Some Pharmaceutical and Other Agents Used in Cell Physiology Studies

Agent	Application
Actinomycin D	Inhibits RNA synthesis (transcription)
Alloxan	Destroys beta (insulin-secreting) cells of pancreatic islets
Chlorpromazine	Dopamine receptor antagonist
Cobalt chloride	Destroys alpha (glucagon-secreting) cells of pancreatic islets
Colchicine	Disrupts microtubules
Cycloheximide	Inhibits protein synthesis
Cyproterone acetate	Testosterone receptor antagonist
Cytochalasin B	Disrupts microfilaments
2-Deoxy-D-glucose	Metabolic inhibitor: inhibits glucose uptake and utilization
Dexamethasone	Synthetic glucocorticoid agonist
Dinitrophenol	Metabolic inhibitor: uncouples oxidative phosphorylation
Ergot alkaloids (e.g., ergocryptine)	Dopamine receptor agonist (inhibits prolactin secretion)
Iodoacetic acid (or iodoacetamide)	Metabolic inhibitor: inhibits glycolysis
Ionophore A23187	Calcium (Ca^{2+}) transport carrier (ionophore)
Liposomes	Drug carriers
Local anesthetics (procaine, tetracaine)	Inhibit cellular uptake of Ca^{2+}
Methylxanthines (theophylline, caffeine)	Phosphodiesterase inhibitors (elevate cAMP)
Spironolactone	Aldosterone receptor antagonist
Saralasin	Angiotensin II receptor antagonist
Thiouracil	Inhibits thyroid iodide uptake and T_4–T_3 synthesis
Valinomycin	Potassium transport carrier (ionophore)
Verapamil	Inhibits cellular uptake of Ca^{2+}
Puromycin	Inhibits protein synthesis (translation)
[3H]Thymidine	Studies on DNA synthesis
[3H]Uracil	Studies on RNA synthesis
Oligomycin	Metabolic inhibitor: inhibits phosphorylation of ADP to ATP

MONOCLONAL ANTIBODIES AND OTHER PROTEINS

Although the RIA is used extensively in diagnostic laboratories for a variety of purposes, including measurement of hormone levels in blood and other tissues, these assays have always been plagued by the heterogeneity of the antibodies generated to the "pure" antigen utilized. Recent studies have led to a technology for the production of large quantities of homogeneous antibodies against a wide variety of antigens, including hormones [23]. These monoclonal antibodies recognize only one antigenic determinant, thus improving the quality and discriminating power of diagnostic methods for the detection and localization of hormones and their receptors [14, 19, 21, 22, 28].

The production of monoclonal antibodies against partially purified preparations of steroid hormone receptors has been a major step in the study of these important regulatory proteins [23]. Monoclonal antibodies provide important probes for many other receptor-related studies [25]. Immunoblotting allows for study of their structure and, to some extent, of their concentration. Immunocytochemistry at the cellular, and in the near future at the ultrastructural, level will allow for the determination of the distribution of receptors in various cells and their localization inside these cells. Immunoaffinity chromatography allows rapid and complete purification of receptors in high yields for new structural and functional studies.

Cloning of receptor genes provides important insights into the nature and structure of hormone receptors. For example, the cloned DNA for a particular receptor can be introduced into an immortalized cell line where the receptor is then transcribed, translated into a polypeptide/protein, which is then inserted into the cell membrane. Hormones or related analogs can then be added to the cells cultured in vitro to determine the structural requirements for hormone action as determined by measurement of second messenger production.

RECOMBINANT-DNA TECHNIQUES

Hormones play important roles in regulating the activity of most cells of the body; indeed, some hormones are necessary for life. Parathormone and aldosterone, two hormones that regulate the electrolyte composition of the body fluids, are examples. Growth hormone is necessary for growth, and its absence in the young animal results in dwarfism. Failure of the pancreas to produce insulin results in diabetes mellitus. Insulin replacement therapy requires obtaining these hormones from other animal sources, but some individuals develop antibodies to these nonhuman sources of the hormone. In the case of GH, only pituitaries obtained from human cadavers or primates can be used, since GH from other animals is ineffective.

Recombinant-DNA techniques offer the hope that a number of human hormones can be synthesized by bacteria in large amounts and at reasonable prices. Recombinant-DNA techniques are essentially in vitro extensions of natural phenomena [8]. These methods involve purification or synthesis of genetic material and its insertion into a bacterial host. Several bacterial strains have been constructed that can produce human hormones, and genetically engineered bacteria now provide important sources of peptide hormones [30]. Two methods have been used to provide the genetic material to be cloned. For shorter peptides (e.g., insulin, somatostatin), DNA synthesis is used to make a gene of the desired hormone. In the case of the two chains of insulin, the 21-amino-acid A chain and the 30-amino-acid B chain are made in separate bacterial strains as tails on a larger precursor protein, the enzyme β-galactosidase. The individual insulin chains are then clipped from the precursor proteins and, after purification of the separate insulin chains, they are joined by air oxidation (Fig. 3.6). The method used for larger proteins utilizes mRNA and reverse transcriptase to make a DNA copy that is then inserted into the bacterial genome and cloned [12]. For example, cDNA for proinsulin is inserted into *Escherichia coli* cells, which are then grown by fermentation to produce proinsulin. The

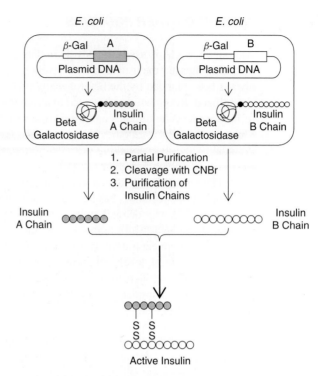

Figure 3.6 Recombinant-DNA technique for the microbial production of insulin. (From Riggs et al. [30], with permission.)

connecting peptide is then cleaved enzymatically from proinsulin to produce human insulin [36].

GENETIC ENGINEERING

The possibility of introducing foreign genes into mammalian embryos provides a powerful tool for use in endocrine research. It is now feasible to introduce foreign DNA into the mammalian genome by microinjection of DNA molecules of interest into pronuclei of fertilized cells, followed by the implantation of the eggs into the reproductive tracts of recipient mothers. The integration of the foreign DNA into one of the host chromosomes at an early stage of embryonic development results in the development of a transgenic animal. Microinjection of the structural gene for rat growth hormone into the pronuclei of fertilized mouse eggs resulted in the development of some offspring that grew significantly larger than their littermates (Fig. 3.7). This methodology has important implications for studying the biological effects of growth hormone as a way to accelerate animal growth, as a model for gigantism, and possibly as a means of correcting genetic disease [9, 27].

Transgenic technologies have been studied in several fish species with emphasis on growth enhancement as a strategy to shorten long production cycles. For the production of transgenic Pacific salmon, an "all-salmon" genetic construct consisting of a metallothionein-β promotor fused with the full-length type-1 growth-hormone gene was developed. The pOnMTGH1 DNA was injected into coho salmon eggs with extraordinary results (Fig 3.8). On average, the transgenic salmon were more than elevenfold heavier than the nontransgenic controls. Most interesting was the observation that the transgenic fish precociously developed a silver body coloration typical of salmon undergoing the physiological preadaptation (smoltification) necessary for the spring migration from fresh water to the marine environment.

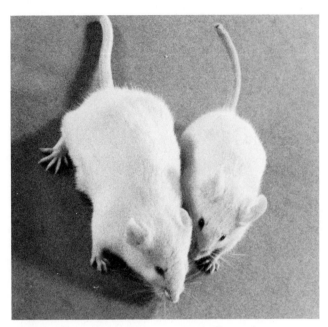

Figure 3.7 Photograph of gigantism produced in the mouse by injection of metallothionein-growth hormone fusion genes into the pronucleus of the fertilized egg followed by implantation within the uterus of a recipient mother [27]. Giant mice (left) became almost twice as heavy as littermates (not bearing the GH gene). (Reprinted by permission from *Nature*, 300 [5893]:611–15. ©1982 by Macmillan Journals, Limited.)

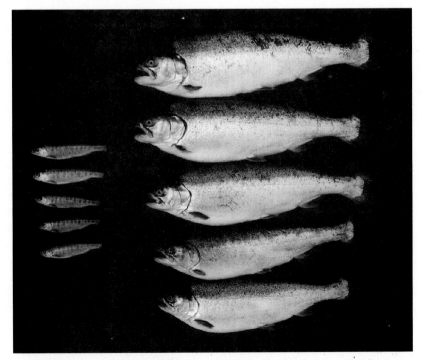

Figure 3.8 Nontransgenic (left) and transgenic (right) coho salmon siblings at 14 months old showing size difference and silver appearance of transgenic individuals, indicative of transformation to seawater adaptability. Length of top large fish (fork length), 41.8 cm. Used by permission from Devlin et al. "Extraordinary salmon growth." *Nature* 371:209–10, 1994.

ANIMAL MODELS FOR RESEARCH

Both vertebrate and invertebrate animals are used as model systems for endocrine research. A few examples of vertebrate models are discussed.

Cyclostomes

These most primitive vertebrates, which include the hagfish and lampreys, have not been extensively studied. These eel-shaped animals spend their lives in both marine and freshwater environments and therefore most likely possess a complex endocrine system as in other more evolved ("higher") vertebrates.

Cartilaginous Fishes

These ancestors of the bony fishes include sharks and rays and, although prevalent in numbers and readily available, they have not been the subject of much endocrine research.

Bony Fishes

These fish represent the largest and most diverse group of vertebrates. They have evolved adaptive features that enable them to survive in a multitude of ecological niches. Many of their specialized physiological functions are under endocrine regulation [29]. Migration to and from the sea by some species requires unique roles for some hormones. Prolactin, for example, is essential for survival in some fish transferred from salt to fresh water (as happens in salmon migrations). The control of color change in fish is much more complex than in other vertebrates and may, in some species, use a recently discovered melanin-concentrating hormone, whose function may be limited to more recent (teleost) fishes (Chap. 8). The corpuscles of Stannius are also unique to certain bony fishes and produce a hormone, teleocalcin, not found in other vertebrate species. The urotensins derived from the urophysis of certain species provide another example of hormones whose roles may be restricted to certain bony fishes (Chap. 7).

Amphibians

Amphibians include urodeles (salamanders, e.g., "mudpuppies," newts) and anurans (frogs and toads), as well as less well-known representatives. Their ready availability, their relatively small size, and the fact that they go through a dramatic metamorphic change from larval to adult life has made them important models for endocrine research. Our understanding of the roles of the thyroid gland and its hormones in endocrine physiology has been greatly influenced by studies on amphibians (Chap. 13). The amphibian egg has always been an important model for an understanding of early vertebrate development. More recently these eggs have provided evidence for roles of hormones (growth factors and steroid hormones) during the earliest developmental stages [33].

Reptiles

Snakes, lizards, turtles and tortoises, as well as the crocodilians and related species, compose this vertebrate group. There has been relatively little research done on these animals, but important information on some unique reproductive strategies under endocrine control have been discovered (see Fig. 7.12).

Birds

These descendants of the reptiles include a large variety of birds that occupy a great diversity of ecological niches. It is not surprising, therefore, that these animals have evolved some unique endocrine strategies. Both wild and domesticated birds (chicken, quail) are available in substantial numbers for experimental studies. The endocrine control of egg laying is a particularly interesting challenge to the endocrinologist. Birds have also provided unique models for understanding the neuroanatomical substrates controlling behavior (e.g., bird song, courtship). The role of the kidney in vitamin D hormone production has been best studied in birds due to the important relationship between the hormone and the control of Ca^{2+} metabolism necessary for eggshell formation (Chap. 9).

Nonprimate Mammals

The mouse, rat, and guinea pig have been particularly important animals for the advancement of our knowledge of endocrinology. The hamster has proved to be a particularly useful model for understanding the role of the pineal gland and its hormone, melatonin, in the control of reproductive cycles (Chap. 20). The nude mouse has been a useful model for supporting the growth of human tumors, since it lacks an active immune system necessary to reject the transplants. The Brattleboro rat lacks the hormone vasopressin and therefore is a unique model of "diabetes insipidus" (Chap. 7).

Primates

Monkeys, because of their close evolutionary relatedness to humans, have played important roles in understanding the human endocrine system. For example, our knowledge of the structure and function of the corpus luteum of the ovary has been aided by use of primate models.

ANIMAL WELFARE

Most endocrinologists would probably strongly agree that studies in animals have been essential for the progress of endocrinology. Surgical removal of various organs has provided key insights into the existence and origin of hormones. Most endocrinologists would also probably agree that animals are still absolutely essential for basic studies in endocrinological research. Only recently, for example, an atrial natriuretic factor (ANF) was isolated from the heart of rats. This atrial peptide probably plays a pivotal role in the pathophysiology of several disease states. Nevertheless, most endocrinologists would probably agree that not all animals have always been treated humanely and, in many cases, the numbers of animals used may have been in excess of the actual numbers needed. The past indiscretions are being remedied at most or all research centers.

Molecular biology has now provided a variety of nonanimal model systems wherein the actions of hormones can be studied in vitro using cell cultures [37, 41]. Although these methods will not entirely supplement studies on living animals, they will provide some alternate methods of study.

PERSPECTIVES

As in other subdisciplines of biology, endocrinological research faces some interesting issues.

Fetal Tissue Transplants

The fetal tissue transplant controversy is similar to that of other bioethical debates, but with a novel twist because of the contested status of the fetus and abortion. Fetal tissue transplants hold great hope for many patients. Extensive work with animal models has shown that human fetal brain cells transplanted into the substantia nigra of monkeys with exogenously produced Parkinson's disease have had beneficial effects. Researchers think that the time has come for expanded clinical trials. Clinical trials, conducted either abroad or with private funding, are already showing that fetal tissue implants can significantly improve the symptoms of Parkinson's disease in some individuals. Transplantation of fetal brain cells from 6- to 8-week old fetuses into multiple sites on each side of the patient's brain resulted in an increase in brain dopamine production and, more importantly, symptoms were greatly reduced for a considerable period of time [38]. Experimental evidence is also strong that fetal islet cell transplants will restore normal insulin function in diabetics. And fetal thymus and liver transplants may have utility for blood and immune system disorders. Many other examples could be cited to document the urgent need of fetal tissues for use in clinical medicine. Unfortunately "respect for the needs of such patients appears to conflict with respect for prenatal human life and larger societal concerns" [32].

REFERENCES

[1] Beermann, W. 1973. Direct changes in the pattern of Balbiani ring puffing in *Chironomus*: effects of sugar treatment. *Chromosoma* 4:297–326.

[2] Biffignandi, P., and G. M. Molinatti. 1987. Antiandrogens and hirsutism. *Horm. Res.* 28:242–9.

[3] BLACK, J. 1989. Drugs from emasculated hormones: the principle of syntropic antagonism. *In Vitro Cell. Develop. Biol.* 25:311–20.

[4] Burgoyne, R. D., and A. Morgan. 1993. Regulated exocytosis. *Biochem. J.* 293:305–16.

[5] Camp, P., A. Sahu, G. Sanacora, P. Ponsalle, and J. D. White. 1992. Gene expression of peptidergic signals: effects of steroids. *Neuroprotocols* 1:67–76.

[6] Chirguin, J. M. 1990. Molecular biology for nonmolecular biologists. *Diabetes Care* 13:188–97.

[7] Ettinger, B. 1988. Prevention of osteoporosis: treatment of estradiol deficiency. *Obstet. Gynecol.* 72:12S–7.

[8] Flodh, H. 1986. Human growth hormone produced with recombinant DNA technology: development and production. *Acta Paediatr. Scand.* 325:1–9.

[9] Fukamizu, A. 1993. Transgenic animals in endocrinological investigation. *J. Endocrinol. Invest.* 16:461–73.

[10] Gilman, A. G., L. S. Goodman, and A. Gilman. 1990. *Goodman and Gilman's the pharmacological basis of therapeutics.* New York: Macmillan, Inc.

[11] Holzwarth, M. A., J. R. Sladek, Jr., and K. M. Knigge. 1976. Monosodium glutamate induced lesions of the arcuate nucleus. *Anat. Rec.* 186:197–205.

[12] Johnson, I. S. 1983. Human insulin from recombinant DNA technology. *Science* 219:632–7.

[13] Kinter, L. B., W. F. Huffman, and F. L. Stassen. 1988. Antagonists of the antidiuretic activity of vasopressin. *Amer. J. Physiol.* 23:F165–77.

[14] Kobilka, B. K., H. Matsui, T. S. Kobilka, T. L. Yang-Feng, U. Francke, M. G. Caron, R. J. Lefkowitz, and J. W. Regan. 1987. Cloning, sequencing, and expression of the gene coding for the human platelet α_2-adrenergic receptor. *Science* 238:650–6.

[15] Kuhar, M. J., E. B. DeSouza, and J. Unnerstall. 1986. Neurotransmitter receptor mapping by autoradiography and other methods. *Annu. Rev. Neurosci.* 9:27–59.

[16] Leblond, C. P. 1991. Time dimension in cell biology. A radioautographic survey of the dynamic features of cells, cell components, and extracellular matrix. *Protoplasma* 160:5–38.

[17] Lloyd, R. V. 1993. Introduction to molecular endocrine pathology. *Endocr. Pathol.* 4:64–72.

[18] Loutzenhiser, R., and M. Epstein, 1987. Calcium antagonists and the kidney. *Hosp. Pract.* 22(1): 63–76.

[19] Lund, T., J. Olsen, and J. F. Rehfeld. 1989. Cloning and sequencing of the bovine gastrin gene. *Mol. Endocrinol.* 3:1585–8.

[20] Manning, M., and W. H. Sawyer. 1989. Discovery, development, and some uses of vasopressin and oxytocin antagonists. *J. Lab. Clin. Med.* 114:617–32.

[21] McDonald, J. D., F. K. Lin, and E. Goldwasser. 1986. Cloning sequencing and evolutionary analysis of the mouse erythropoietin gene. *Mol. Cell. Biol.* 6:842–8.

[22] Milgrom, E. 1985. Monoclonal antibodies to steroid hormone receptors. *Pharmac. Ther.* 28:389–415.

[23] Millar, S. E., S. M. Chamow, A. W. Baur, C. Oliver, F. Robey, and J. Dean. 1989. Vaccination with a synthetic zona pellucida peptide produces long-term contraception in female mice. *Science* 246:935–8.

[24] Mishell, D. R. 1989. Estrogen replacement therapy: an overview. *Amer. J. Obstet. Gynecol.* 151:1825–7.

[25] Mumby, M. E., S. L. Weldon, C. W. Scott, and S. S. Taylor. 1985. Monoclonal antibodies as probes of structure, function and isoenzyme forms of the type II regulatory subunit of cyclic AMP-dependent protein kinase. *Pharmac. Ther.* 28:367–87.

[26] Oksenberg, D., S. A. Marsters, B. F. O'Dowd, H. Jin, S. Havlik, S. J. Peroutka, and A. Ashkenazi. 1992. A single amino-acid difference confers major pharmacological variation between human and rodent 5-HT$_{1B}$ receptors. *Nature* 360: 161–3.

[27] Palmiter, R. D., R. L. Brinster, R. E. Hammer, M. E. Trumbauer, M. G. Rosenfeld, N. C. Birnberg, and R. M. Evans. 1982. Dramatic growth of mice that develop from eggs microinjected with metallothionen-growth hormone fusion genes. *Nature* 300:611–5.

[28] Parmentier, M., F. Libert, C. Maenhaut, A. Lefort, C. Gerard, J. Perret, J. Van Sande, J. E. Dumont, and G. Vassart. 1989. Molecular cloning of the thyrotropin receptor. *Science* 246:1620–2.

[29] Powers, D. A. 1989. Fish as model systems. *Science* 246:352–58.

[30] Riggs, A. D., K. Itakura, R. Crea, T. Hirose, A. Kraszewski, D. Golddel, D. Kleid, D. G. Yansura, F. Bolivar, and H. L. Heyneker. 1980. Synthesis, cloning, and expression of hormone genes in *Escherichia coli. Rec. Prog. Horm. Res.* 36:261–76.

[31] Robertson, G. L., and A. Harris. 1989. Clinical use of vasopressin analogues. *Hosp. Pract.* 24:114–39.

[32] Robertson, J. A. 1988. Rights, symbolism, and public policy in fetal tissue transplants. *Hastings Ctr. Rpt.* 5–12.

[33] Rosa, F., A. B. Roberts, D. Danielpour, L. L. Dart, M. B. Sporn, and I. B. Dawid. 1988. Mesoderm induction in amphibians: the role of TGF-β_2-like factors. *Science* 239:783–5.

[34] Shizume, K., A. B. Lerner, and T. B. Fitzpatrick. 1954. In vitro bioassay for melanocyte stimulating hormone. *Endocrinology* 54:553–60.

[35] Spicer, S. S. 1993. Advantages of histochemistry for the study of cell biology. *Histochem. J.* 26:531–47.

[36] The, M.-J. 1989. Human insulin: DNA technology's first drug. *Amer. J. Hosp. Pharm.* 46:S9–11.

[37] Theoharides, T. C., and W. W. Douglas. 1978. Secretion in mast cells induced by calcium entrapped within phospholipid vesicles. *Science* 201:1143–5.

[38] Thompson, L. 1992. Fetal transplants show promise. *Science* 257:868–70.

[39] Tong, Y., J. Covet, J. Simard, and G. Pelletier. 1990. Glucocorticoid regulation of proopiomelanocortin mRNA levels in rat arcuate nucleus. *Mol. Cell. Neurosci.* 1:78–83.

[40] Warembourg, M. 1976. Detection of diffusible substances. *J. de Microscopie et de Biologie Cellulaire* 27:277–80.

[41]   Weiss, J. and J. L. Jameson. 1993. Perifused pituitary cells as a model for studies of gonadotropin biosynthesis and secretion. *TEM* 4:265–70.

[42]   Yalow, R. S. 1978. Radioimmunoassay: a probe for the fine structure of biologic systems. *Science* 200:1236–45.

[43]   Zarrow, M. X., J. M. Yochim, J. L. McCarthy, and R. C. Sanborn. 1964. *Experimental endocrinology: a sourcebook of basic techniques.* New York: Academic Press, Inc.

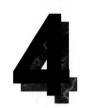

General Mechanisms of Hormone Action

*Some hormones, often referred to as first messengers, interact with the cell membrane to increase the production of intracellular second messengers, which are more directly responsible for activation of the cell [16]. The second messenger is often a cyclic nucleotide, either **cyclic adenosine monophosphate (cyclic AMP, cAMP)** or **cyclic guanosine monophosphate (cyclic GMP, cGMP)**. This first messenger–second messenger model of hormone action now must be expanded to include other messengers in the temporal sequence of hormone action. For example, some hormones require calcium for activation of cyclic nucleotide formation. In some cells the first messenger, acting through induction of an inward Ca^{2+} flux, may activate prostaglandin (PG) biosynthesis. The newly synthesized PG activates the production of cAMP or cGMP. These cyclic nucleotides actually mediate their actions through stimulation of cellular enzymes, kinases, which phosphorylate cell-specific proteins; these phosphorylated proteins then function as the ultimate physiological effectors in the cell. Other first messengers (steroid and thyroid hormones) interact with intracellular constituents (receptors) of a cell to mediate slower, but more sustained actions.*

CELLULAR RECEPTORS AND HORMONE ACTION

Hormones regulate specific target tissues, not all cells in the body. One might ask what mechanism or characteristic of a cell determines whether it will be responsive to a particular hormone. Molecular components of cells, so-called *receptors*, provide the specificity for hormone-cell interaction. The receptor concept originated early in this century with the work of Langley [21]. Receptors may be components of the plasma membrane or they may be cytosolic or nuclear elements. Receptors provide the means by which hormones initially interact with cells. If each type of cell did not possess specific hormone receptors, all cells might be expected to respond to all chemical messengers. If this were the case, each time a single hormone was released, all cells in the body would respond, and this would result in uncoordinated muscle contraction and relaxation and the uncontrolled secretion of numerous cellular products, such as hormones and enzymes. Therefore, cells do not possess receptors for all hormones, but rather only a limited number of receptor types. Certain cellular elements may exhibit specific affinities for nonhormonal agents, such as narcotics or other drugs; these affinities provide the basis for medicinal drug therapy. Some drugs interact with hormone receptors, which may result in activation of the cell, or, if the ligand (receptor-binding substance) lacks intrinsic biological activity, it may act as an antagonist to block the binding of a hormone.

Oxytocin and vasopressin (AVP) are related in structure, and both hormones stimulate uterine smooth muscle contraction and activate renal tubular cAMP production. Uterine receptors are, however, more sensitive to oxytocin than to AVP, whereas renal receptors are more sensitive to AVP than to oxytocin. Thus at normal circulating concentrations, each neurohypophysial hormone will only activate its appropriate target cell receptor. Vascular smooth muscle neurohypophysial hormone receptors are generally less sensitive to oxytocin or AVP than are uterine or renal tubular cells. During severe hemorrhage, however, large quantities of AVP are released from the neurohypophysis; the hormone may then be able to induce vasoconstriction and serve an important role in hemostasis.

Some hormones stimulate a number of tissues, which implies that each of these diverse tissues possesses receptors for the hormone. Insulin stimulates glucose uptake by hepatocytes, fat cells, and certain muscle cells, and interacts with many other cell types. Thus insulin is able to rapidly lower extracellular glucose levels, which is one of its major functions. If more than one tissue responds to a particular hormone at one time, it might be expected that all these different physiological responses would complement the physiological process being regulated. For example, parathormone elevates serum Ca^{2+} levels by releasing Ca^{2+} from bone, stimulating Ca^{2+} uptake from the gut and preventing Ca^{2+} loss from the kidney. Each of these individual responses is important in elevating serum Ca^{2+} levels.

At normal physiological levels each hormone interacts with its own specific cellular receptor. Estradiol, for example, interacts with estrogen receptors, not with other steroid receptors, such as those for cortisol or progesterone. Therefore hormone receptors possess a recognition function that must then be converted into an action function. Receptors recognize differences in hormone structure and thus provide receptor specificity. Norepinephrine and epinephrine are structurally similar (see Fig. 14.3), but norepinephrine preferentially interacts with certain types of adrenergic receptors, whereas epinephrine interacts more specifically with other adrenoceptor types (Chap. 14) [22]. The pharmaceutical industry capitalizes on receptor specificity to provide hormone analogs that can be used medicinally to activate or inhibit certain tissue-specific receptors.

PLASMA MEMBRANE HORMONE RECEPTORS

With the exception of steroid and thyroid hormones, other hormones stimulate cells by an initial interaction with specific plasma membrane receptors. This initial receptor interaction results in *transduction* of signals to the cytoplasmic side of the membrane where enzymes are activated, resulting in production of one more intracellular second messengers. These membrane receptors are conceptually visualized as macromolecules, usually glycoprotein in nature, which display a high affinity for a specific hormonal ligand. Most receptors studied thus far, such as those for insulin, LH, and TSH, contain carbohydrate moieties. Peptide hormone receptors are localized, at least partially, to the outer surface of the cells, as shown by a number of experimental techniques. For example, ACTH covalently linked to a large polymer is still able to stimulate cAMP-mediated adrenal steroidogenesis. Other hormones have also been linked to sepharose beads, which are also too large to enter cells, and in all cases the hormones still activate cAMP production in a variety of cells. In addition, specific antisera to peptide hormones rapidly terminate their actions, again indicating that the site of action of the hormones is extracellular.

Regulation of Receptor Number

Receptors are not static components of the plasmalemma; indeed, receptor number is in a constant state of flux and may change with the cell cycle or with the state of cellular differentiation. A cell may therefore become more or less responsive to a hormone depending on its specific developmental or differentiated state. Cells may even lose their capacity to respond to a certain hormone, but gain the ability to respond to another, presumably because of the differentiated loss and gain of membrane receptors. Hormones may even regulate the number of their own (*homospecific*) or other (*heterospecific*) receptors. Homospecific receptor regulation may be negative or positive, resulting in so-called "down" or "up" regulation, respectively. Prolactin, for example, induces the appearance of PRL receptors (up regulation) in the liver and certain other tissues. Continuous exposure of lymphocytes to insulin results in decreased binding (down regulation) of the hormone to the cells. Some obese individuals have high concentrations of insulin in their blood, even though their blood sugar level is normal. Theoretically glucose levels should be diminished in the presence of insulin. The cells of these obese individuals apparently possess fewer insulin receptors. When obese individuals diet, which lowers blood glucose and insulin levels, their cells are able to bind increased amounts of insulin due to restoration of receptor number.

Most hormones, like insulin, produce the same effect (e.g., down or up regulation) on receptors in the various tissues that they regulate. Angiotensin II, however, appears to increase or decrease receptors depending on the particular cell type involved. For example, AII increases the number of its receptors on adrenal glomerulosa cells, but decreases its receptor population on certain smooth muscles. TRH acts on pituitary thyrotrophs to release TSH, which then stimulates thyroid hormone (T_4 and T_3) production by the thyroid gland. Thyroid hormones then decrease the sensitivity of thyrotrophs by stimulating a loss of TRH receptors, a good example of negative feedback. Glucocorticoids, on the other hand, increase the number of pituitary TRH receptors. The latter two examples of heterospecific receptor regulation demonstrate both down and up regulation. Changes in receptor number may provide an important mechanism for preventing hyperstimulation of cells to hormones under pathological states of hormone oversecretion. Receptor modulation may also provide a mechanism by which hormones act in sequence to amplify or diminish responses to other hormones. The gonadotropins, FSH and LH, are secreted and act on the ovaries in a sequential manner; it appears that LH action is dependent on induction of LH receptors by FSH.

Receptor Cooperativity and Hormone Action

Hormone receptor studies suggest that mechanisms of hormone-receptor interaction are compatible with negative or positive models of *cooperativity*. There are two major events that govern the response elicited by a hormone: hormone binding, and the coupling between the binding event and the first biochemical signal elicited. The binding event can be described as being *noncooperative, positively cooperative*, or *negatively cooperative*. These terms describe how binding of a hormone to its receptors affects its subsequent binding to other receptors possessed by the cells. Although it was originally believed that binding to one site did not affect binding to others, it is now realized that subsequent binding events can also be affected in a positive or negative manner. Positive cooperativity is the phenomenon observed where the initial binding of the hormone to its receptor enhances the affinity of other receptors to the hormone. This may be an important mechanism for sensitizing a cellular system when hormone levels are low and occupy only a few of the available receptors. Negative cooperativity, where binding of the hormone reduces the affinity of receptors for subsequent binding events, may provide a mechanism for desensitizing cells to abnormal concentrations of a hormone. The kinetics of negative and positive cooperativity in hormone binding depart from the typical law of mass action behavior. The affinity of insulin receptors, for example, is not fixed, but decreases as occupancy increases.

Spare Receptors

In most cells a maximum biological response is achieved when only a small percentage of receptors is occupied. For example, maximal stimulation of steroidogenesis by Leydig cells of the testis occurs when only about 1% of LH receptors are occupied. The additional receptors are referred to as *spare receptors* and are considered to be fully functional. The role of this receptor reserve may be to increase the sensitivity of target cells to activation by low levels of hormone. It is recognized, however, that the term spare is used in a relative sense, as the degree of receptor excess differs according to the particular biological response measured. Generally, the magnitude of adenylate cyclase activation is closely correlated with the degree of receptor occupancy, but the more distal physiological response, such as muscle contraction or hormone secretion, is evoked when only a small percentage of the receptor population is occupied.

Separate Receptors for Hormone Action

The hormones epinephrine and glucagon stimulate glycogenolysis and the release of glucose by liver cells. Because glucagon and epinephrine are not similar in structure, they would not be expected to mediate their effects through the same receptor, although they both activate hepatic adenylate cyclase activity. This can be demonstrated by the use of antagonists that are specific for a receptor. Propranolol, a β-adrenergic receptor blocking agent, antagonizes epinephrine-induced liver glycogenolysis, but not the glycogenolytic action of glucagon (Chap.14). The action of glucagon, but not epinephrine, on the other hand, is blocked by specific antagonists of glucagon. Present evidence indicates that hormones with similar actions do not stimulate separate cyclases. Maximal production of cAMP produced by one hormone is not augmented by the addition of another hormone. If individual cyclases were linked to each receptor, it would be expected that the maximal effects of each hormone would be additive (Fig. 4.1).

One might wonder why one cell, such as the hepatocyte (liver cell), possesses two separate receptors that activate the same ultimate physiological response. The reason is that different hormones, such as glucagon and epinephrine, are released under different physiological states of an animal. Glucagon released from the pancreatic islets regulates the moment-by-moment breakdown of liver glycogen whenever blood glucose levels become slightly depressed (hypoglycemic). Under conditions of stress, however, epinephrine is released from the adrenal chromaffin tissue. This hormone not only stimulates hepatic glycogen breakdown into glucose, but it also increases vascular blood flow, respiratory rate, and many physiological processes associated with the stress response. Continuous stress would, over time, be detrimental to the welfare of the individual; thus each hormone plays a specific temporal role in maintaining blood glucose levels (Chap.14).

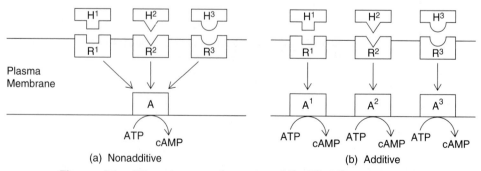

Figure 4.1 Although many hormones (H^1, H^2, H^3) mediate their effects through separate membrane receptors (R^1, R^2, R^3), transduction of their signals is funneled through only one adenylate cyclase (a), *not* through different cyclases (A^1, A^2, A^3) linked separately to each receptor (b).

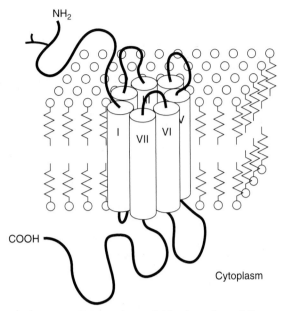

Figure 4.2   Schematic model for insertion of G-protein-coupled receptors in the plasma membrane. From Strosberg [38], with permission.

Receptor Structure

There are four main classes of membrane-bound receptors: (1) receptors that are also enzymes (tyrosine protein kinases or guanylate cyclase; (2) receptor channels; (3) receptors coupled to G (GTP-binding) proteins; and (4) receptors with unknown transduction mechanisms. The majority of receptors for peptide hormones and neurotransmitters are linked to G proteins. The G protein-coupled receptors contain a recognition site for the agonist (ligand) and a recognition site for a particular G protein (see discussion later in this chapter). These receptors are made up of a single chain consisting of 400 to 600 amino acid residues. The amino terminus contains sites for N-linked glycosylation whereas the carboxy terminus has sites for phosphorylation by one or more protein kinases (e.g., protein kinase A, PKA). Seven stretches of 22–28 hydrophobic conserved residues, separated by hydrophilic segments, are characteristic structural features of these receptors [38]. These transmembrane segments presumably form closely packed helical bundles crossing the membrane (Fig. 4.2).

The N-terminal region, by virtue of its glycosylation, is extracellular and the carboxy-terminal domain is intracellular. The various portions between the seven hydrophobic stretches are either extra- or intracellular. The third intracellular segment and the carboxy-terminal segments display an extensive variability in length and sequence, which has led to the hypothesis that these parts of the receptors are responsible for the selective interaction with various regulatory G proteins required for information transfer [38].

SECOND MESSENGERS OF HORMONE ACTION

Many hormones acting as first messengers manifest their actions by stimulating the production of intracellular second messengers that then effect a physiological response.

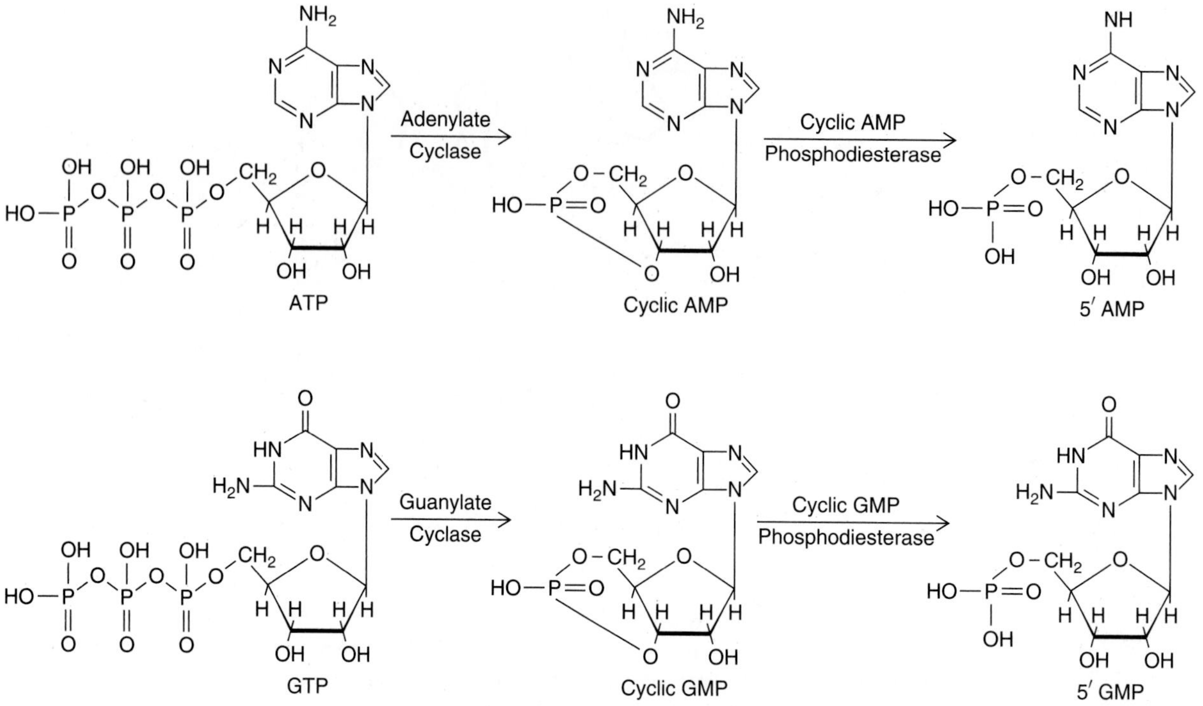

Figure 4.3 Cyclic nucleotide synthesis and inactivation.

Cyclic Nucleotides and Hormone Action

Receptors provide the recognition site for hormone-cell interaction. This binding event must be translated into a cellular response. Binding of hormone to its membrane receptor often results in the activation of one or more nucleotide-cyclyzing enzymes located on the inner surface of the membrane. Best studied is the enzyme adenylate cyclase, which, upon stimulation by a chemical messenger, converts ATP (adenosine triphosphate) to 3′,5′-cyclic adenosine monophosphate, cyclic AMP (cAMP). A complex and not-well-understood signal transduction process was envisioned by Rodbell and coworkers as a key to the conversion of the hormone-binding signal into increased adenylyl cyclase activity. Borrowing from information transfer theory, they coined the terms "discriminator" for the role played by receptor, "amplifier" for the role of the cAMP forming enzyme, and "transducer" for the role of the intervening process [1]. Some hormones, on the other hand, activate guanylate cyclase that converts guanosine triphosphate (GTP) to cyclic cGMP [46, 47]. Enzyme cleavage of the cyclic ring of the nucleotides by *phosphodiesterase* results in the production of inactive 5′AMP or 5′GMP (Fig. 4.3).

Each of the cyclic nucleotides produced intracellularly combines with a specific *cyclic nucleotide–dependent protein kinase*. Cyclic AMP-dependent protein kinase (PKA), for example, is composed of two components, a *regulatory subunit* and a *catalytic subunit*. Interaction of cAMP with the regulatory subunit results in the release of the catalytic unit (Fig. 4.4). The catalytic unit is now free to function as a *kinase*, that is, a phosphorylating enzyme. Cyclic nucleotides therefore function by causing phosphorylation of some cellular component (substrate protein) of the cell (Fig. 4.5), structural or enzymatic [5, 33]. Enzyme phosphorylation leads to a cascade phenomenon, whereby activation by phosphorylation of the first enzyme allows this enzyme to act as a kinase to phosphorylate a second enzyme, which may then phosphorylate another enzyme. At each step amplification occurs; thus, relatively few first-messenger molecules acting on a limited number of receptors may produce a response several orders of magnitude greater. This cascade phenomenon has been studied in detail in the liver cell (see Fig.11.11), but may be common to a number of cellular systems.

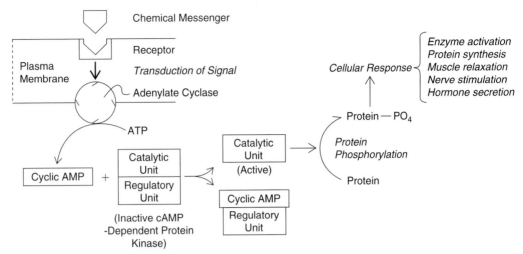

Figure 4.4   Cyclic AMP production and action.

Cyclic nucleotides produced by hormone action are rapidly metabolized. Cyclic AMP- and cGMP-specific phosphodiesterases cleave the cyclic bonds within cAMP and cGMP to produce inactive 5′AMP and 5′GMP, respectively. *Phosphoprotein phosphatases* within the cell then dephosphorylate the proteins that were phosphorylated by the cyclic nucleotide-dependent protein kinases. Thus, cellular activity is rapidly returned to basal level.

Methylxanthines inhibit cAMP- and cGMP-dependent phosphodiesterase activity. Caffeine, theophylline, and theobromine are methylxanthines derived from coffee, tea, and cocoa, respectively (Fig. 4.6). Theophylline is the most potent of the three (but is less concentrated in tea than caffeine is in coffee). In the presence of relatively low concentrations of methylxanthines, hormones that stimulate adenylate cyclase are potentiated, as the cAMP generated by the hormones is not degraded by phosphodiesterase. At high concentrations (e.g., 10^{-3} M) theophylline or caffeine alone may evoke a maximal response in a particular tissue. This suggests that adenylate cyclase is always active, but that the cAMP generated is continually being destroyed.

Sutherland was the first to demonstrate that extracellular chemical messengers, first messengers, activate production of intracellular cAMP, the so-called second messenger of hormone action [40]. Because many hormones interact with receptors to activate adenylate cyclase, which then causes a physiological response, Sutherland and his colleagues suggested criteria that should be satisfied before concluding that a particular effect of a hormone is mediated through cAMP.

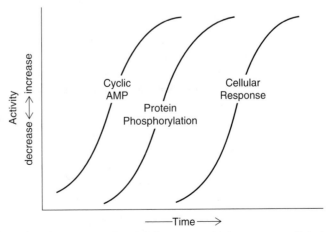

Figure 4.5   Temporal cellular events in hormone-mediated cyclic AMP production and action.

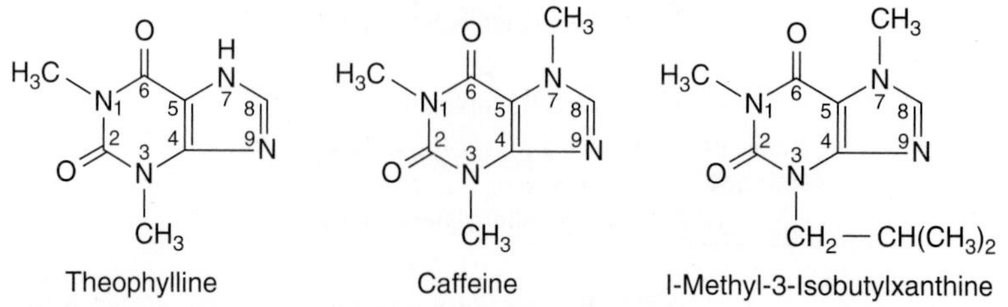

Figure 4.6 Methylxanthine structures: theophylline, caffeine, and I-methyl-3-isobutylxanthine (a synthetic xanthine analog).

1. The hormone should stimulate adenylate cyclase in broken cell preparations.
2. Physiological levels of the hormone should elevate cAMP before or concurrently with the physiological response (Fig. 4.5).
3. There should be a correlation between the activity of hormone analogs that elevate cAMP and their ability to activate the particular cellular response.
4. Methylxanthines or other drugs that inhibit phosphodiesterase activity should potentiate and, at high concentrations, mimic the hormone response.
5. Exogenous cAMP or its analogs should mimic the effect of the hormone.

The criteria have been satisfied for many cells studied. There is no convincing reason, however, that the first criterion should be met as, in the intact cell, information is generated from the receptor on the outer side of the plasmalemma to adenylate cyclase on the inner surface. The ionic environments of these two compartments are not similar and cannot be duplicated in vitro for both compartments at any one time. Calcium, for example, is inhibitory to adenylate cyclase, but may be necessary for transduction of signal from receptor to cyclase. It is difficult in vitro to provide Ca^{2+} for receptor binding or receptor signal transduction and, at the same time, not inhibit adenylate cyclase. The second criterion has been claimed not to have been satisfied in some systems. It is possible, however, that small changes in cAMP are undetectable or that in some tissues the increase in cAMP is compartmentalized to a few cells. Thus, changes in cyclic nucleotide levels are not perceived among the larger cyclic nucleotide pool. The third and fourth criteria generally have been demonstrated in all cellular systems where cAMP plays a role as second messenger.

Cyclic AMP added to an in vitro preparation may induce the physiological response characteristic of the tissue, but only at very high concentrations. Apparently, this is because the nucleotide does not easily enter cells through the plasmalemma. To satisfy the fifth criterion, certain lipophilic analogs of cAMP (e.g., $(Bu)_2cAMP$) have been synthesized; they may produce a maximal response at relatively low concentrations in some tissues, but only at high levels in others (Fig. 4.7).

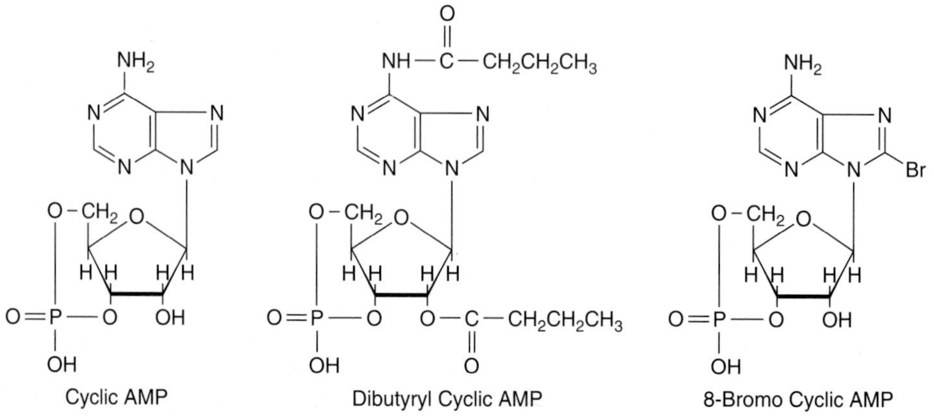

Figure 4.7 Cyclic AMP and related analogs.

Genomic Actions of Cyclic AMP

Many actions of second messengers initiate immediate cellular responses, such as opening or closing ion gates, stimulating cellular secretion, and stimulating muscle contraction or relaxation. Some of the actions are slower in commencement, but are more enduring. In some cells the actions of cAMP are mediated at the level of the genome since the actions of some hormones that elevate intracellular cAMP levels are blocked by the actions of actinomycin D and cycloheximide, inhibitors of transcription and translation, respectively. Cyclic AMP mediates its action by way of PKA, which can phosphorylate a number of proteins depending on the particular cell type. One such protein common to the genomic actions of cAMP is the CRE (cAMP responsive element)-binding protein, CREB. This *transcription factor* is phosphorylated by cAMP-activated PKA. Phosphorylation of CREB by PKA allows the transcription factor to interact with the CRE (a DNA sequence) to activate transcription of a cell-specific mRNA for protein synthesis [32]. Some genes do not have the CRE consensus sequence, yet their expression is regulated by the level of cAMP. For example, PKA also phosphorylates some structural proteins associated with chromatin to modify their interactions with DNA [36].

RECEPTOR SIGNAL TRANSDUCTION

Hormone binding to receptors located on the outer side of the plasmalemma often results in an immediate activation of adenylate cyclase on the inner membrane of the cells. How does receptor occupation by hormonal ligands result in enzyme activation on the opposite side of the cell membrane? Receptor and enzyme were once thought to be structurally coupled, and binding of the hormone to the receptor then induced a conformational change in the enzyme, thus activating it. Actually, this model may be true in one instance; a membrane guanylate cyclase is apparently the receptor for certain hormones (e.g., atrial natriuretic factor, Chap. 15) [46, 47]. Receptors may be "freely floating" in the membrane and in the unoccupied state may possess negligible affinity for the enzymatic unit. Upon hormone binding, however, a conformational change occurs in the receptor, resulting in transduction of signal across the membrane to activate second messenger production. Hormone receptors are discrete units, not components of the inner membrane nucleotide cyclyzing enzymes. Fusion of cells, which lack receptors but possess adenylate cyclase activity, to a different species of cell, which possesses receptors but no adenylate cyclase activity, results in a hybrid cell that synthesizes cAMP in response to hormone stimulation.

G Proteins and Dual Control of Adenylate Cyclase

In some cells transduction of signal from receptor to adenylate and guanylate cyclases involves the participation of monovalent and divalent cations, as well as PG biosynthesis. In addition, one or more regulatory proteins may be components of the transduction signal. One such regulatory protein is a guanylyl nucleotide regulatory protein that exhibits GTPase activity (converts guanosine triphosphate to guanosine diphosphate) in the activated state. Receptor signal transduction involves the mobilization and interaction of this protein with the hormone receptor, an event that would then be requisite to adenylate cyclase activation [2, 10, 15].

G proteins act as transducers by coupling membrane-bound receptors to intracellular effectors. G proteins are heterotrimers and dissociate to liberate a nucleotide-bound α subunit and a complex of β and γ subunits when the α subunits are activated by the binding of GTP. Functional characterization provided the first basis for classification of G proteins: G_s is the G protein that activates adenylyl cyclase, and G_t (transducin) is the

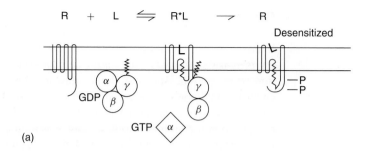

(a)

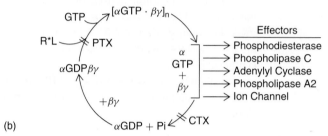

(b)

Figure 4.8 Receptor G protein-mediated signal transduction.
(a) Receptor (R) associates with a specific ligand (L), stabilizing an activated form of the receptor (R^*), which can catalyze the exchange of GTP for GDP bound to the α subunit of a specific G protein. The $\beta\gamma$ heterodimer may remain associated with the membrane through a 20-carbon isoprenyl modification (ξ) of the γ subunit. The receptor is desensitized by specific phosphorylation ($-P$).
(b) The G protein cycle. Pertussis toxin (PTX) blocks the catalysis of GTP exchange by the receptor. Activated α subunits (αGTP) and $\beta\gamma$ heterodimers can interact with different effectors. Cholera toxin (CTX) blocks the GTPase activity of some α subunits fixing them in an activated form. (Used by permission from Simon et al., "Diversity of G proteins in signal transduction," *Science* 260:1072–1073, 1993. © 1993 by the American Association for the Advancement of Science.)

retinal G protein that activates a guanosine 3',5'-monophosphate-specific phosphodiesterase. In each of these cases, the dissociated GTP-α subunit complex activates the effector enzyme (cyclase or phosphodiesterase). Thus the concept arose that each G protein oligomer contains a functionally specific α subunit in association with mixtures of a small number of different β and γ subunits. Nearly 20 distinct α subunits have now been described, as well as four β subunits and a similar number of γ polypeptides [42]. A model of the G protein cycle is shown (Fig. 4.8).

The functional role of specific α subunits is not obvious from their structural classification [18]. One of the most effective tools for implicating G proteins in specific functions in intact cells has been the use of pertussis toxin (PTX). The toxin uncouples the receptor from its G protein and thus blocks signal transduction by receptors that cause decreases in cAMP, that regulate ion channels, and that activate phospholipases [43]. Members of the Gi class of α subunits contain sites susceptible to modification by PTX and are therefore expected to mediate activation of the PTX-sensitive processes. Activated Gα_i subunits lower intracellular cAMP levels and Gα_o has been implicated in increasing phosphoinositide release [34].

Not all hormone receptor/G-protein interactions involve effects on intracellular second-messenger production (e.g., increased cAMP or decreased cAMP) as a component of signal transduction. Receptor/G-protein interaction may result in the direct activation of membrane ion channels (e.g., K^+, Ca^{2+}). Indeed, the $G\alpha_i$ and $G\alpha_o$ subtypes have been shown to function in regulating ion channels. The transmembrane movement of ions may then lead to depolarization or hyperpolarization of the cell membrane, resulting in a cellular response (Chap. 21).

Receptor Crosstalk

Agonist activated transduction pathways and second-messenger formation are not entirely separate. Changes in concentration of one second messenger often lead to change in concentration of another—"crosstalk" [15]. Activation of a single receptor type may be able to activate G proteins of more than one family. The effect of a particular G protein might be attenuated by the activation of another G protein, which would provide free $\beta\gamma$ subunits. Because $\beta\gamma$ subunits can combine with different α subunits, they would displace the equilibrium toward the trimeric inactive form of the G proteins [7].

Birnbaumer [1, 2] has succinctly summarized the landmarks in our understanding of the nature and roles of G proteins in signal transduction [1, 2]. Further details on receptor-G protein interaction and signal transduction are discussed later (Chap. 21).

MULTIPLE MEMBRANE MESSENGERS

Other messengers are involved in cellular regulation besides cyclic nucleotides. *Phosphoinositides* are phospholipids present within the plasma membrane of all eukaryotic cells. Some function as storage forms for potential messenger molecules and, in response to agonists, the phosphoinositides break down to liberate intracellular second messengers [9, 24]. At least three different messenger molecules are known to be produced from phospholipids: (1) *arachidonic acid* (a precursor to certain eicosanoids), (2) inositol triphosphate (IP$_3$), and (3) *diacylglycerol* (*DG* or *DAG*). Arachidonate is oxygenated to form several messengers, which include: prostaglandins, prostacyclins, thromboxanes, and leukotrienes, as will be discussed later.

G Proteins and IP$_3$ and DG Formation

Many hormones stimulate cellular processes through activation of G proteins whose α subunit (Ga_o) activates a specific phospholipase (PLC) that hydrolyzes the phosphodiester bond of phosphatidylinositol 4,5-biphosphate, providing the two messenger molecules $Ins(1,4,5)P_3$ and 1,2-diacylglycerol. The water-soluble $Ins(1,4,5)P_3$ diffuses to intracellular Ca^{2+} stores where it induces the release of Ca^{2+} by binding to Ca^{2+}-channel-linked IP$_3$ receptors. Diacylglycerol, being highly lipophilic, remains in the plasma membrane matrix where it activates protein kinase C (PKC). Two downstream signal cascades are thus initiated, involving both elevation of the cytosolic Ca^{2+} activity resulting in modulation of Ca^{2+}-sensitive response elements and Ca^{2+}/PKC-promoted protein phosphorylation. Removal of the agonist from the agonist-receptor complex results in the cessation of PLC-mediated $PtdIns(4,5)P_2$ hydrolysis. Both IP$_3$ and DG are rapidly metabolized in cells, so in the absence of de novo synthesis the cellular levels of these two messengers rapidly decline; PKC is inactivated and cytosolic Ca^{2+} levels are brought back to resting levels by the membrane-associated Ca^{2+} transport systems [8].

The Role of Protein Kinase C in Signal Transduction

Protein kinase C (PKC) is a multifunctional enzyme present within the plasma membrane [30]. This Ca^{2+}-activated, phospholipid-dependent enzyme has been shown in many tissues to be linked to signal transduction. Multiple subspecies of PKC have been described. These subspecies show subtle differences in enzymological properties, differential tissue expression, and specific intracellular localization. Many growth factors (Chap. 12) are stimulatory to cell proliferation, and PKC plays a role as a component of the factors acting on cellular differentiation and proliferation. In one model, hormone receptor activation results in the production of IP$_3$ (see above), as well as in an increase in intracellular Ca^{2+}. The intracellular Ca^{2+} may be derived from one or several sources, either from sequestration within the endoplasmic reticulum or from the extracellular compartment. In this model, PKC is activated by diacylglycerol in the presence of Ca^{2+}. A model of hormone action involving IP$_3$ and DG is shown in Fig. 4.9 and summarized here:

1. Activation of the membrane receptor is coupled to phospholipase C (PLC) through guanylyl nucleotide-binding (G) proteins.

2. This leads to hydrolysis of phosphoinositol (PIP2) and formation of two key metabolites, diacylglycerol (DG) and inositol triphosphate (IP3).

3. IP3, which is released into the cytoplasm, mobilizes intracellular Ca^{2+} from stores within the endoplasmic reticulum (ER) and, possibly, from transmembrane transport of Ca^{2+} into the cell.

4. During the initial phase of cell activation two signals, the rise in DG content of the plasma membrane and the rise in the Ca^{2+} concentration in the cell cytosol, act synergistically to cause binding of PKC to the plasma membrane.

5. The resulting association of the kinase with the membrane leads to its conversion to a Ca^{2+}-sensitive form.

EICOSANOIDS AND HORMONE ACTION

In the early 1930s, it was noted that human semen and extracts of seminal vesicles from animals caused uterine tissue to contract or relax. The purified substance was given the name *prostaglandin* (*PG*), although it is now realized that the prostate glands are not a major source of PGs. The PGs belong to a family of chemically related substances, eicosanoids, that are produced by cells in response to a variety of extrinsic stimuli [35]. They may be produced by cells in response to some hormones and can, therefore, be con-

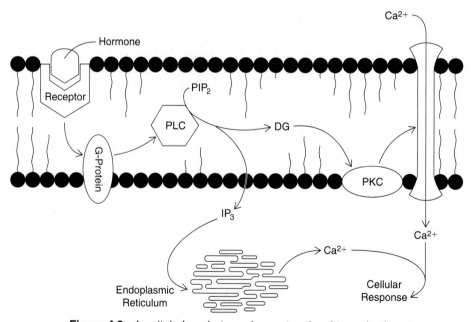

Figure 4.9 Inositol phosphate and receptor signal transduction.

sidered as intracellular second messengers in the actions of these hormones. The Nobel Prize in Physiology/Medicine for 1982 was awarded to Bergstrom, Samuelsson, and Vane for their "discoveries concerning prostaglandins and biologically related substances" [17, 26].

Eicosanoids are produced exclusively within the plasma membrane of cells and are derived mainly from arachidonic acid released from phospholipids by the action of phospholipase A_2 (PLA_2) [39]. Arachidonic acid is formed from the essential fatty acid linolenic acid, by elongation and desaturation. Hormones and other stimuli (e.g., local hypoxia) may activate phospholipase activity and liberate arachidonic acid to serve as substrate for eicosanoid biosynthesis. The arachidonic acid may be used in one or more different pathways, depending on the tissue concerned and particular nature of the extrinsic stimulus. In one pathway arachidonic acid is converted to unstable endoperoxide intermediates by a group of enzymes termed the cyclooxygenase system (Fig. 4.10). Then, depending on the action of other tissue-specific enzymes, these intermediates may be converted to one of a number of related products: prostaglandin E_2 (PGE_2), prostaglandin $F_{2\alpha}$ ($PGF_{2\alpha}$), prostacyclin I_2 (PGI_2), or thromboxane A_2 (TXA_2) (Fig. 4.10).

In some cells arachidonic acid metabolism follows a second pathway to produce a group of biologically active *leukotrienes*. Leukotrienes are formed by the enzyme 5-lipoxygenase, which converts arachidonic acid to 5-hydroperoxy-6,8,11,14-eicosatetraenoic acid (5-HPETE). 5-HPETE is then converted to the epoxy acid, LTA_4, which is subsequently changed to LTB_4 by the addition of water, or to LTC_4 by the addition of glutathione [28]. LTD_4 is then formed by the loss of glutamic acid and LTD_4 is converted to LTE_4 by the loss of the glycine residue (Fig. 4.10).

Each of these definitive products of arachidonic acid metabolism may then act on nucleotide cyclases within the plasma membrane to stimulate cyclic nucleotide formation. PGE_2 and PGI_2 invariably stimulate adenylate cyclase. The second-messenger system activated by occupation of the $PGF_{2\alpha}$ receptor is still unknown. In cultured rabbit endometrial cells, $PGF_{2\alpha}$ exerts no effect on the levels of cAMP or cGMP; however, phosphatidic acid and phosphoinositide turnover can be stimulated by $PGF_{2\alpha}$. $PGF_{2\alpha}$ receptors may be associated with a specific guanine nucleotide regulatory protein linked to activation of PLC [12]. Leukotrienes and PGI_2 and TXA_2 are released from their cells of origin to act as humoral hormonal messengers (Fig. 4.11).

Aspirin and indomethacin inhibit cyclooxygenase activity, but not that of the lipoxygenase system. Therefore, these drugs may be used selectively to inhibit PG, prostacyclin, and thromboxane formation without a concomitant effect on leukotriene formation.

Steroidal anti-inflammatory agents, such as cortisone, block the release of precursor fatty acids and thus the formation of all eicosanoids. Nonsteroidal anti-inflammatory agents, such as aspirin, inhibit cyclooxygenase and prevent the production of prostanoids. It is also possible to modulate the precursor fatty acid component in cell membrane phospholipids by dietary means, which in turn can alter the types of eicosanoids formed endogenously. Some food constituents, such as vitamin C, vitamin E, garlic, onion, ginger, and alcohol, can affect the production of eicosanoids. Dietary manipulation may serve as a long-term strategy to favorably modify endogenous eicosanoid production [31].

Prostaglandins

Prostaglandins were the first of the arachidonic acid products to be discovered [17, 28]. All the PGs are variants of a basic 20-carbon carboxylic fatty acid (prostanoic acid) that is bent back on itself in the shape of a hairpin and is conformationally restricted by a five-membered cyclopentane ring. The number of double bonds present within the side chains determines whether the PG belongs to the 1, 2, or 3 series. Two particularly important PGs

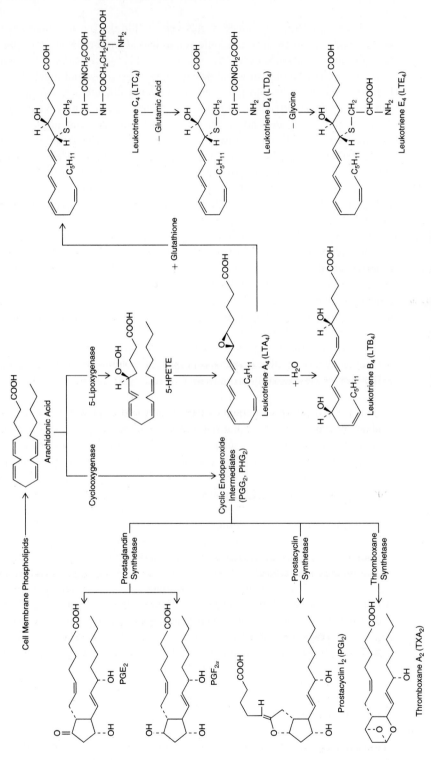

Figure 4.10 General scheme for prostaglandin, prostacyclin, thromboxane, and leukotriene biosynthesis.

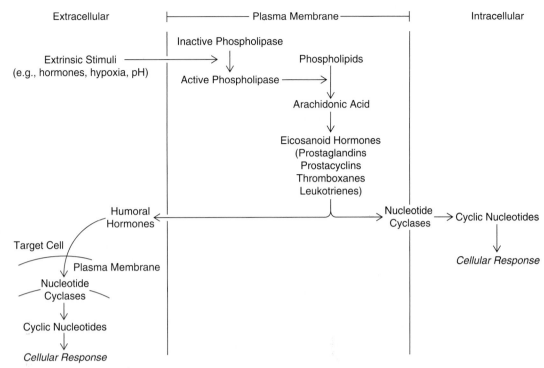

Figure 4.11   General scheme of eicosanoid biosynthesis and mechanisms of action.

of the E and F series are $PGF_{2\alpha}$ and PGE_2 which differ by the presence of a hydroxyl or a keto-group, respectively, at carbon 9 within the cyclopentane ring (see Figs. 2.4 and 4.10).

A major physiological role of PGE_2 and $PGF_{2\alpha}$ is the control of vascular smooth muscle activity. Hormones that regulate smooth muscle relaxation or contraction stimulate the production of PGE_2 or PGI_2 and $PGF_{2\alpha}$ respectively. In response to tissue hypoxia, PGE_2 production may lead to a localized hyperemia in skeletal muscle. Thus PGs, by their localized actions on the microcirculation, adjust local blood flow in response to changing metabolic requirements of the tissue.

Prostacyclins

Prostacyclins (PGI_2) are produced by the blood vessel wall (endothelial cells), and PGI_2 is the most potent natural inhibitor of blood platelet aggregation known. PGI_2 binds to a specific platelet receptor and activates adenylate cyclase. Increased intracellular levels of cAMP are then inhibitory to platelet aggregation. The vascular endothelium can therefore be considered as an endocrine tissue that produces a humoral hormone, PGI_2, whose role may be to prevent blood platelet aggregation and to maintain vascular flow through its action as a local vasodilator. Whether PGI_2 is released into the general circulation to function as a hormone on more distant blood platelets and vascular endothelia is presently unresolved.

Thromboxanes

Thromboxane A_2 is a specific product of the blood platelet [12]. In response to stimuli known to induce clotting (collagen substrate, thrombin, epinephrine), platelet TXA_2 levels are elevated, as are cGMP concentrations. It is believed that TXA_2 may act in some way as a Ca^{2+} ionophore to translocate this divalent Ca^{2+} from the extracellular environment or from sequestered intracellular organelles. The free cytosolic Ca^{2+} may then be responsible for inducing the cellular shape changes associated with the platelet aggregation phenomenon. As noted, PGI_2 is inhibitory to platelet aggregation through its action on increasing platelet cAMP levels. Inhibition of platelet aggregation may result from protein substrate phosphorylation and the subsequent uptake of Ca^{2+} into vesicular components of the cell. It is hoped that selective inhibitors of thromboxane synthesis will be developed so that the tendency toward platelet aggregation is reduced, while permitting normal rates of formation of the other PGs.

Leukotrienes

Leukotrienes are so named because they are made by leukocytes and contain three conjugated double bonds [28]. The subscript indicates the total number of double bonds in the molecule (Fig. 4.10). Leukotrienes are extremely potent in causing vascular contraction and inducing vascular permeability. Migratory leukocytes function in local inflammatory responses by releasing leukotrienes at the site of injury in response to noxious stimuli. The anti-inflammatory actions of glucocorticoids (Chap. 15) may be because these steroids inhibit phospholipase activity and, therefore, restrict the availability of arachidonic acid for leukotriene formation. Certain leukocytes may be considered as wandering endocrine cells that release chemical messengers, leukotrienes, at sites of injury or invasion by foreign proteins to induce inflammatory or allergic responses. Increased leukotriene production appears to be implicated in the pathophysiology of tissue trauma. There are increased concentrations of leukotrienes in blood plasma and bile subsequent to tissue injury [28].

Leukotrienes are a family of bioactive lipids that have a constellation of pharmacologic effects on respiratory, cardiovascular, and gastrointestinal systems. They produce smooth muscle spasm, cause myocardial depression, increase vascular permeability, enhance mucous production, decrease mucociliary transport, and have the chemotactic property to attract leukocytes to a site of cellular injury. The overwhelming evidence suggests that leukotriene synthesis and subsequent release in experimental animals and in humans are associated with certain pathophysiological events. Disorders such as asthma, adult respiratory distress syndrome, chronic bronchitis, cystic fibrosis, septic shock, psoriasis, inflammatory bowel disease, and myocardial ischemia have all been reported to be associated with increased levels of leukotrienes.

LTD_4/LTE_4 receptors appear to be linked to the turnover of inositol phosphates via activation of phospholipase C. Regulation of the activity of PLC appears to be coupled to the receptor via a G protein. Since the response to LTD_4 is inhibited by pertussis toxin, the G protein may be of the G_i (inhibitory) class. In a variety of tissues and cell culture systems, LTD_4/LTE_4 and agonist analogs produced a rapid increase in inositol phosphates after stimulation, an effect that was blocked stereoselectively by receptor antagonists. The agonist-induced increases in inositol phosphates correlated directly with the generation of lipoxygenase products and smooth muscle contraction. Current data support the hypothesis that, at least for LTD_4/LTE_4 receptors, phosphoinositide hydrolysis with subsequent Ca^{2+} mobilization constitute important transduction mechanisms [8].

CYTOSOLIC HORMONE RECEPTORS

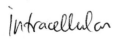

In contrast to many polypeptide hormones, steroid and thyroid hormones initiate their actions by combining with intracellular receptors. The mechanisms by which these hormones cross the plasmalemma are unknown. It is likely that these hormones enter all cells, but only manifest their action in those cells that possess receptors. Steroid hormones, for example, bind to specific cytoplasmic receptors of a proteinaceous nature, and the steroid-receptor complex then migrates to the nucleus, where it interacts with specific chromosomal proteins and DNA.

Steroid/Thyroid Hormone Receptors

A recent consensus suggests that steroid hormones may interact with unoccupied receptors within the nucleus, rather than being transported by receptors from the cytosol to the nucleus. Nevertheless, a two-step mechanism is involved, wherein the activated nucleoplasmic receptor must be translocated to the chromatin. The binding of the receptor-steroid complex to chromatin (DNA and associated proteins) results in derepression of a specific DNA sequence and increased messenger RNA synthesis. The mRNA then codes for proteins specific to that cell type; in uterine muscle (myometrium), for example, estradiol induces the synthesis of actin and myosin, proteins necessary for the contractile machinery of uterine myometrial cells.

Each steroid hormone has its own specific intracellular receptor. Estrogens, but not androgens, bind at physiological concentrations to uterine receptors. Thus, for membrane receptors, receptor specificity determines whether a particular cell type will respond to the steroid. The synthesis of mRNA and the subsequent production of proteins require a matter of hours or days to be fully manifested (Chap. 18). The actions of most hormones are on membrane receptors and, in contrast, result in an immediate production of one or more second messengers followed by rapid protein phosphorylation and a subsequent cellular response.

The effects of steroid and steroidlike hormones are mediated by specific receptors that belong to a superfamily of transacting "zinc finger" proteins. After binding of the specific ligand, these receptor proteins (so-called "ligand-induced transcription factors") influence gene expression via association with specific DNA elements, known as hormone-responsive elements (HREs). Specific HREs are known for estrogen-, thyroid hormone-, progesterone-, and glucocorticoid-responsive genes. The estrogen-response element (ERE) is similar to, but distinct from, the glucocorticoid-responsive element (GRE) and the thyroid hormone-responsive element (T_3RE). The progesterone- and glucocorticoid-responsive elements are so similar as to be functionally identical. $1,25(OH)_2D_3$ affects cellular replication and function in many cells and tissues through a typical steroidal hormone receptor and exerts its effects through a vitamin D-responsive element (VDRE) [14]. It is not clear whether opposing effects on gene expression by different steroidal hormones are elicited through the same or different HREs.

In summary, the sequential steps in steroid hormone action involve the following [13]:

1. The hormone enters into target cell by simple diffusion.
2. The steroid hormone binds to its cytoplasmic/nuclear protein receptor. These intracellular receptors exist as dimers complexed with a nonsteroid-binding heat shock protein. The receptor binds the ligand with high affinity and with a high degree of specificity.
3. Activation of the receptor into a DNA-binding form (transcription factor) results, following binding with the steroid hormone.
4. Receptor/steroid hormone translocates into the nucleus of the cell if it is not already in the nucleoplasm.
5. The receptor/steroid complex binds to DNA hormone-responsive elements (HREs) and mRNA synthesis (transcription) results.
6. mRNA is translated into cell-specific protein synthesis.

More specific details of this model (Fig. 4.12) are discussed in Chap. 9. It is recognized that this model is an oversimplification of a much more complex mechanism of steroid/thyroid hormone action.

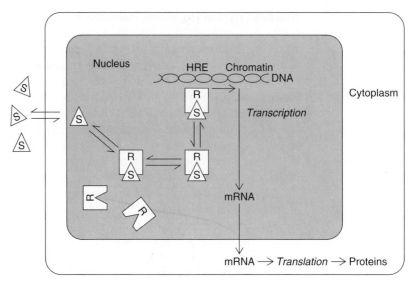

Figure 4.12   Mechanisms of steroid hormone action.

Direct Membrane Actions of Steroid Hormone

The classical model of steroid action involves their binding to intracellular receptors that are members of a superfamily of ligand-induced transcription factors. The hormone receptor complexes then modulate the expression of target genes by binding to specific DNA sequences, the so-called hormone response elements (HREs). There is increasing evidence for rapid, actinomycin-D and cycloheximide-insensitive (therefore presumably non-genomic) effects of some steroid hormones. For example, in rats, short-term exposure to the gonadal steroid progesterone is associated with rapid changes in behavior, and this effect occurs in the absence of new protein synthesis. Gonadal and steroid hormones can alter neuronal firing activity in certain neurons within milliseconds to minutes after administration [27].

PERMISSIVE ACTION OF HORMONES

Some hormones exert a permissive action, that is, they must be present for other hormones to exert their effects. Because the majority of peptide hormones stimulate cells through activation of cAMP, one would not expect that the action of one peptide hormone could enhance the action of another peptide hormone, other than in an additive manner. Rather, it might be expected that for one hormone to potentiate the activity of another, the mechanisms of action of the two hormones would be different. The permissive effects of hormones are restricted mainly to the actions of steroid or thyroid hormones, where the ligands enhance the action of each other or they enhance the action of other hormones working through membrane receptors. The following mechanisms, among others, could account for the permissive actions of steroid or thyroid hormones:

1. These hormones, through their actions on specific mRNA synthesis, could cause an increase in the number of membrane receptors, which might increase the production of cyclic nucleotides, thus leading to an increased cellular response to hormones acting on the plasmalemma.

2. Thyroid or steroid hormones could increase or decrease the amount of cyclic nucleotide-dependent protein kinases or the amount of substrate available for phosphorylation by cAMP- or cGMP-dependent protein kinases.

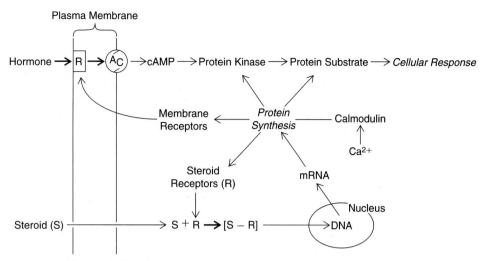

Figure 4.13 General scheme for the permissive actions of steroid hormones.

3. Thyroid and steroid hormones could enhance the synthesis of a protein that could act as an inhibitor of another protein (e.g., phosphoprotein phosphatase) whose action is antagonistic to cyclic nucleotide action (Fig. 4.13).

Synergism is a term often used to describe the physiological response of a tissue to a combination of two hormones that greatly exceeds the individual actions of either hormone. For example, FSH has no detectable effect on enzyme activity of testicular interstitial tissue and LH only minimally stimulates such activity. However, in the presence of FSH, the actions of LH are greatly enhanced. This might be caused by an FSH-induced increase in LH receptors known to occur in other steroid-synthesizing tissue in response to these two gonadotropins. Methylxanthines, when used at low concentrations, may only slightly increase the basal activity of cells. Used at a low concentration, a hormone might also have a minimal effect. When used in combination, however, a hormone and a methylxanthine may produce a dramatic response. The action of the hormone is to increase cyclic nucleotide levels, whereas the action of the methylxanthine is to inhibit degradation of cAMP by phosphodiesterase.

In summary, the action of one hormone may require the action of one or more other hormones that individually are relatively inactive, a phenomenon referred to as the permissive action of hormones. Synergism, on the other hand, occurs when a tissue's response to two or more hormones in combination is greater in magnitude than the sum of the individual actions of the hormones. The permissive and synergistic actions of a hormone may not easily be separated into distinct physiological entities.

STIMULUS RESPONSE COUPLING

Most membrane-mediated hormone actions involve changes in the transmembrane potential. Because of the unequal distribution of ions between the extracellular and intracellular environments of a cell, a cell is generally 60 to 90 mv (millivolts) negative on the inside. The unequal charge distribution across the plasmalemma causes the cell to be electrically excitable. Muscle and nerve cells are particularly excitable, as are some secretory cells. The excitability of certain cells is of pivotal importance in hormonal control of cellular function [23]. In response to hormonal stimuli, cells may become *depolarized* or *hyperpolarized*. Acetylcholine, for example, depolarizes skeletal muscle cells, which leads to contraction. Interaction of acetylcholine with membrane receptors causes Na$^+$ ion flow into the cell, thus depolarizing the muscle. Sodium ion flux into the cell is linked to an increase in cytosolic Ca^{2+}; Ca^{2+} interacts with the contractile proteins of the muscle and contraction ensues. This event is referred to as *stimulus-contraction coupling*. A similar *stimulus-secretion coupling* is responsible for hormone-induced cellular secretion. These phenomena are collectively termed *stimulus-response coupling*.

Substitution of Na$^+$ by other monovalent cations, such as Li$^+$ (lithium), provides information on the specificity of the cation requirement for hormone action. Magnesium (Mg^{2+}) or barium (Ba^{2+}) ions are often substituted for Ca^{2+} to determine the divalent cation specificity for hormone action. Their failure to substitute is considered to mean that Ca^{2+} is the specific divalent cation required for hormone action. Although Ca^{2+} is of prime importance to stimulus-response coupling, this ion undoubtedly plays other more subtle roles in cellular responses to hormones [29]. Calcium modulates adenylate cyclase and cyclic nucleotide phosphodiesterase activities. Ca^{2+} is also required in some cellular systems for coupling between hormone receptors and nucleotide cyclase activity. Melanocyte-stimulating hormone (MSH) action, for example, requires Ca^{2+} for activation of adenylate cyclase; this is a receptor-specific requirement, as prostaglandin and epinephrine stimulation of melanocyte adenylate cyclase is without such a requirement. In a number of cellular systems Ca^{2+} may also be specifically required for hormone activation of guanylate cyclase [25].

Calmodulin—An Intracellular Calcium Receptor

Calcium, a divalent cation, is required for the actions of many hormones [11]. Calcium may be essential for hormone activation of phospholipase A$_2$ and thus prostaglandin biosynthesis. Calcium may be directly required for transduction of signal between hormone receptor and adenylate or guanylate cyclase. Hormones may translocate Ca^{2+} into the cytosol to function in such processes as enzyme activation or cellular contraction. However, the precise mechanism of action of Ca^{2+} was for a long time an enigma. Ca^{2+} is now known to interact with its own cellular receptor, a protein referred to as *calmodulin* (*CaM*), or calcium-dependent regulatory protein [11]. This ubiquitous protein is found in all eukaryotic cells and therefore in plants.

Calmodulin exists as a monomer of 148 amino acid residues. The primary sequence of CaM has been stringently conserved throughout phylogeny; for example, there are only seven conservative amino acid substitutions between vertebrate CaM and that of a marine coelenterate. A distinctive feature of the protein is that the amino group of lysine 115 is posttranslationally trimethylated. CaM possesses four Ca^{2+}-binding sites, and the amino acid sequences within each domain contain a high degree of homology (Fig. 4.14). It is suggested that CaM may have evolved from a smaller precursor (which bound a single Ca^{2+}) by gene duplication. The homology is greatest between domains 1 and 3, and 2 and 4; it is possible that CaM may have arisen by two successive doublings or a primordial gene coding for a Ca^{2+}-binding domain. CaM is structurally related to troponin C, found in skeletal and cardiac muscle.

The binding of Ca^{2+} to CaM results in a conformational change of the protein that may be required for the interaction of CaM with its substrate. It has been concluded that at physiological ionic strength, the Ca^{2+}-binding sites on CaM are not filled in a sequentially ordered fashion. Further, investigators have examined a number of CaM-mediated proteins and their dependence on Ca^{2+} for activation and concluded that CaM needs only three atoms of Ca^{2+} per molecule of protein for activation. The binding of the fourth atom of Ca^{2+} is apparently neither necessary nor inhibitory. Activation of CaM by Ca^{2+} is apparently an all-or-none process. When CaM has three or four Ca^{2+} ions bound, it is active; when it has fewer than three it is inactive.

Three major roles of CaM are regulation of intracellular Ca^{2+} levels, enzyme activation, and control of cellular filamentous organelle activity. The actions of CaM

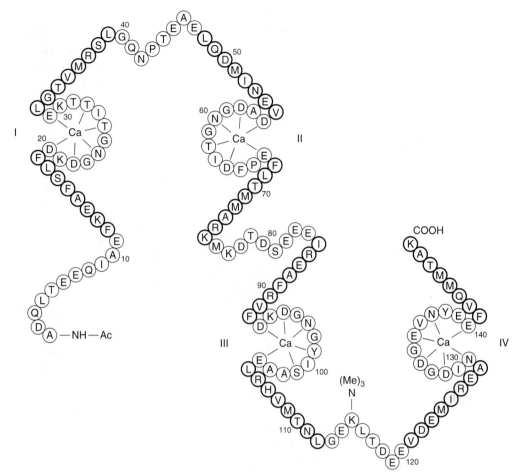

Figure 4.14 Primary structure of calmodulin (CaM), an intracellular calcium receptor. The following are one-letter codes for amino acid residues: A, Ala; D, Asp; E, Glu; F, Phe; G, Gly; H, His; I, Ile; K, Lys; L, Leu; M, Met; N, Asn; P, Pro; Q, Gln; R, Arg; S, Ser; T, Thr; V, Val; Y, Tyr. (Reproduced with permission, from *The Annual Review of Biochemistry*, Klee, et al., "Calmodulin." Vol. 49, pp. 480–515. © 1980 by Annual Reviews, Inc.)

are direct and indirect; for example, CaM may activate an enzyme directly or indirectly through prior activation of another enzyme. A number of peptide and steroid hormones have been shown to be without effect on cellular levels of CaM; levels of the Ca^{2+} regulatory protein apparently remain constant, regardless of the hormonal environment.

As an intracellular Ca^{2+} receptor, CaM may play a pivotal role in cellular Ca^{2+} homeostasis [11]. The levels of Ca^{2+} within cells fluctuate due to fluxes of Ca^{2+} across the plasma membrane from or into storage depots within mitochondria and smooth endoplasmic reticulum, each of these pathways being of more or less importance, depending on the cell type. In each case CaM stimulates a Ca^{2+}-Mg^{2+}-dependent ATPase (Ca^{2+} pump) in the membranes of these organelles. In the presence of excessive cytosolic Ca^{2+}, CaM would become activated and would subsequently stimulate one or more of these membrane Ca^{2+} pumps, which would bring Ca^{2+} levels back to normal.

Calmodulin may play an important role in the control of cyclic nucleotide levels. CaM is stimulatory to adenylate cyclase and phosphodiesterase. Although these two actions of CaM may first appear to be opposed, the sensitivities of the two enzymes to CaM may differ considerably. In fact, cAMP increases the affinity of phosphodiesterase for CaM, which may provide a cellular homeostatic mechanism involving an initial activation of cAMP production, followed by a mechanism for the degradation of the cyclic nucleotide. In addition to a role for a cytosolic CaM in the control of adenylate cyclase activity, CaM may function by a Ca^{2+}-dependent mechanism in the transduction of signal between receptor and adenylate cyclase. Thus CaM can be envisioned to function at a number of sites in the control of cAMP levels.

Calmodulin regulates a variety of cellular contractile or motile processes. Actin and myosin are the major proteins responsible for cell motility, and they are present in both muscle and nonmuscle cells. Calcium is required for muscle contraction, and in smooth muscle it is now known that Ca^{2+} activates CaM that then binds to a regulatory subunit of an enzyme, myosin light chain kinase, whose catalytic domain phosphorylates the light chain protein of myosin (see Fig.7.13). Activation of myosin ATPase provides the stimulus for formation of the actomyosin complex leading to the contractile process. In skeletal muscle an elevation of cytosolic Ca^{2+} is the stimulus to the contractile process resulting from actin and myosin interaction. Binding of Ca^{2+} to troponin C (which is structurally related to CaM) results in a conformational change in the troponin-tropomyosin-actin complex that causes actomyosin formation.

Microtubules are filamentous components of cells and are involved in cellular activities involving motile processes, such as chromosome movement, axoplasmic flow, and neurite extension. Most interesting is the apparent role of CaM in chromosomal movement during mitosis. There is a major shift of CaM from a diffuse distribution within the cell during interphase to high local concentrations within the mitotic apparatus during mitosis. In this process CaM may perform such roles as regulating the concentration of Ca^{2+} in the microenvironment and thus affect microtubular assembly/disassembly. In addition CaM may activate other proteins or enzymes that may be involved in the mitotic machinery.

In skeletal muscle CaM regulates the activity of the enzyme phosphorylase kinase, which causes glycogen degradation to provide the glucose substrate necessary for mitochondrial ATP production. CaM is an integral regulatory subunit of phosphorylase, as the enzyme is completely dependent on Ca^{2+} for activity. Phosphorylase kinase is composed of four different subunits, α, β, γ, and δ, and the δ subunit is CaM. In liver, skeletal, and cardiac muscle, phosphorylase kinase plays a dual role in the control of glycogen metabolism. It activates the enzyme phosphorylase, which splits glycogen into its glucose subunits, and it may function as glycogen synthetase kinase, an enzyme that inactivates glycogen synthetase through phosphorylation of the enzyme.

A general model for the action of CaM is shown in Figure 4.15. Interaction of Ca^{2+} with CaM results in a conformational change in an associated affector protein, which then induces a physiological response. The affector protein would differ in each cell type. For example, one of the subunits of skeletal muscle phosphorylase kinase would be considered to function as the affector protein. The affector molecule associated with troponin, for example, might be tropomyosin.

PHOSPHORYLATED PROTEINS AS PHYSIOLOGICAL EFFECTORS

The membrane actions of most hormones involve generation of an intracellular cyclic nucleotide as second messenger. The immediate acceptor site for the action of cAMP is the regulatory subunit of cAMP-dependent protein kinase (PKA). Two forms of the enzyme with slightly different regulatory properties have been isolated and are referred to as type I and type II. Both consist of two regulatory (R) and two catalytic (C) subunits. The regulatory units may differ in structure, but the catalytic units are believed to be iden-

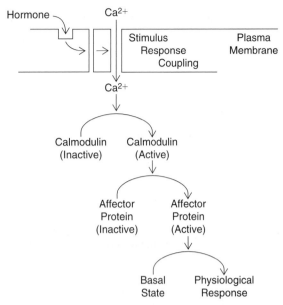

Figure 4.15 Model for the mechanism of action of calmodulin.

tical. Cyclic AMP acts as the positive effector and causes the dissociation of the oligomeric protein and an activation of the enzyme according to the following scheme:

$$R_2C_2 \text{ (inactive)} + 4 \text{ cAMP} \rightleftarrows (R\text{-cAMP}_2)_2 + 2 \text{ C (active)}$$

The complete amino acid sequences of the catalytic and regulatory subunits of bovine cardiac muscle cAMP-dependent protein kinase have been elucidated [19, 41]. The crystal structure of the catalytic subunit of cAMP-dependent protein kinase (PKA) has been solved.

Within each cell type one or more specific proteins act as substrate for phosphorylation by PKA. For example, the amino acid serine is a substrate for protein kinase action (Fig. 4.16). Specific nuclear histone proteins may be the targets of the enzyme within hepatocytes. Within smooth muscle and nerve, specific membrane proteins become phosphorylated through the actions of cAMP or cGMP. In neurons these substrate proteins may control the permeability of the postsynaptic membrane to ion flux [20]. In smooth muscle, phosphorylation of specific membrane substrate proteins, in response to cAMP or cGMP generated by receptor-specific agonists, may be related to the phenomena of membrane hyperpolarization and depolarization that accompany smooth-muscle relaxation and contraction, respectively.

Cyclic nucleotide-independent substrate phosphorylation may be important in the actions of certain hormones (insulin and other growth factors). The intracellular effector

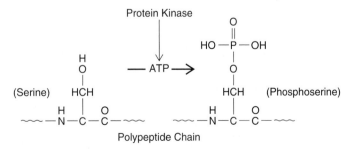

Figure 4.16 Protein kinase phosphorylation of a protein substrate.

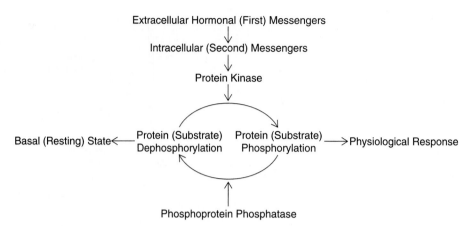

Figure 4.17   Role of protein kinases and phosphoprotein phosphatases in hormone action.

molecules that activate the kinases involved in these substrate phosphorylations remain undetermined. Ca^{2+} may be shown to be a major stimulus to cyclic nucleotide-independent substrate phosphorylation. Once complexed with Ca^2, CaM binds to and activates a wide variety of proteins, including a number of protein kinases and calcineurin, a phosphoprotein phosphatase. Initial characterizations of Ca^{2+}/CaM-dependent protein kinases in tissue extracts used a variety of exogenous protein substrates. A number of enzymes, including phosphorylase kinase, myosin light chain kinase (MLCK) (see Fig.7.13), and Ca^{2+}/CaM-dependent protein kinases I, II and III (CaMK-I, II and III, respectively) were resolved. Among these enzymes CaMK-II is unique in that it can phosphorylate a wide range of proteins in vitro and is widely distributed. These properties suggest that CaMK-II regulates many physiological responses to agonists that elevate intracellular Ca^{2+}. For this reason it is also called the multifunctional Ca^{2+}/CaM-dependent protein kinase, or CaM-dependent multiprotein kinase. Thus, CaMK-II plays a role in Ca^{2+}-mediated regulation analogous to the roles of cAMP-dependent protein kinase (PKA) and protein kinase C (PKC) in the cAMP- and diacylglycerol-mediated systems, respectively [6].

Protein Phosphatases: Role in Cellular Regulation

It is becoming clear that in addition to protein kinases, *protein phosphatases* are also important targets for cellular regulation [5, 45]. The steady-state level of cellular protein phosphorylation is dependent on the balance of the activities of several protein phosphatases that act on protein substrates (Fig 4.17). Protein phosphatases reverse the action of protein kinases by hydrolyzing phosphoryl groups from proteins. It has been thought that only kinases required regulation and that they activated one another in sequence to overwhelm phosphatase activity in order to produce a temporary increase in phosphate content of key target proteins. However, some kinases critical to cell growth have sites for phosphorylation that cause inactivation, as well as activation. Therefore, the action of a protein phosphatase can be required to bring about increased phosphorylation of proteins. It is possible that not only kinases, but also some protein phosphatases, are probably involved in activating cellular responses to extracellular signals [4].

TERMINATION OF HORMONE ACTION

Hormones that act at the plasmalemma are degraded within the blood by serum enzymes. The declining circulating level of a hormone would result in a decrease in further stimulation of membrane adenylate or guanylate cyclase activities. In the absence of cyclic nucleotide production, the residual intracellular cyclic nucleotides would be destroyed

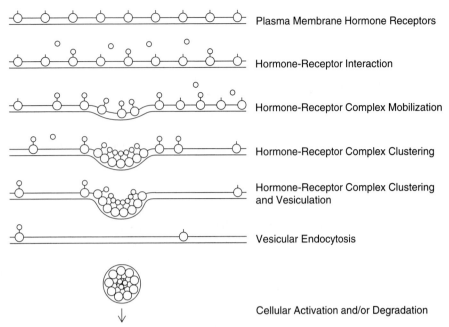

Figure 4.18 Scheme for hormone-receptor clustering and vesicular endocytosis.

rapidly by cytosolic phosphodiesterase action, and cellular activity would return to basal levels. Effects of steroid and thyroid hormones and some peptide hormones may be of longer duration. The actions of these hormones involve DNA, RNA, and protein synthesis. In the absence of further hormone stimulation the newly synthesized RNA species and proteins are degraded by cytoplasmic enzyme actions.

After the initial stage in hormone-plasma membrane interaction, the hormone-receptor complexes cluster at specific sites on the cell membrane. Clustering of hormone-receptor complexes apparently triggers vesiculation of the plasma membrane hormone-receptor complex, followed by cellular internalization by endocytosis (Fig 4.18). What is unclear is whether the contents of the vesicle are degraded by lysosomal or other enzymes, or whether plasmalemmal vesiculization and endocytosis provide a mechanism for hormone transport to intracellular target sites. Both events may be operative, depending on the particular hormone and cellular species.

PATHOPHYSIOLOGICAL CORRELATES OF HORMONE ACTION

Syndromes of hormone deficiency are often associated with increased sensitivity to the missing hormone, and this is correlated with increased concentrations of receptors for the hormone. Conversely, exposure of cells to elevated levels of a hormone may result in a decrease in target tissue receptors for the hormone. Clinical evidence suggests that receptor modulation by circulating hormone concentrations is an important physiological adaptation. There are examples of heterospecific receptor modulation that can lead to adverse physiological responses. Thyroxine, for example, increases the number of β-adrenergic receptors in cardiac muscle and vascular tissues, as well as having a direct effect on the heart. This accounts for the enhanced sympathetic nervous activity that is usually a symptom of hyperthyroidism (Chap. 14).

Myasthenia gravis is an example of an *autoimmune disease* where antibodies to cholinergic receptors have been developed within the body. The antibodies block acetylcholine receptors at the neuromuscular junction. This, of course, leads to muscle dysfunction. In patients with Graves' disease there are circulating immunoglobulins that bind to thyrotropin receptors in the thyroid gland. This immunoglobulin, the so-called thyroid-stimulating antibody (TSAb), enhances T_4–T_3 production, which results in hyperthyroidism (Chap. 13). A large number of human endocrinopathies are related to defects in hormone-receptor interaction. The hormone may be defective in structure, receptor number may be decreased, increased, or blocked as described, or there may be a defect in receptor-signal transduction. *Cholera* is a disease characterized by an enormous secretion of water and electrolytes by intestinal mucosal cells and often leads to death from dehydration. The affliction is caused by the cholera vibrio (*Vibrio cholerae*). The pathogen secretes a toxin (an antigen) that irreversibly binds to the guanylyl nucleotide regulatory protein [44]. This leads to the continuous production of cAMP and abnormal secretion of water and electrolytes.

That mutations of G-proteins are involved in some pathological states is becoming increasingly clear [37]. It has been discovered that a subset of somatotropin (STH)-secreting human pituitary tumor carries somatic mutations that inhibit the GTPase activity of the α_s subunit. This results in an increase in cAMP production by these cells and cell proliferation (Chap. 21). Thus, mutated G proteins may behave as oncogenes in some specific cell types [3]. The importance of understanding the role of G proteins in normal and abnormal cellular function is evident by the fact that two researchers won the Nobel Prize in Medicine/Physiology in 1994 for their discoveries of G proteins and their role in ligand activated cellular signal transduction.

REFERENCES

[1]   Birnbaumer, L. 1990. Transduction of receptor signal into modulation of effector activity by G proteins: the first 20 years or so. *FASEB J.* 4:3068–78.

[2]   ———. 1991. On the origins and present state of the art of G protein research. *J. Receptor Res.* 11:577–85.

[3]   Bockaert, J. 1991. Coupling of receptors to G proteins, pharmacological implications. *Therapie* 46:413–20.

[4]   Brautigan, D. L. 1992. Great expectations: protein tyrosine phosphatases in cell regulation. *Biochim. Biophys. Acta* 1114:63–77.

[5]   Cohen, P. 1988. Protein phosphorylation and hormone action. *Proc. Royal Soc. London, Series B* 234:115–44.

[6]   Colbran, R. J. 1992. Regulation and role of brain calcium/calmodulin-dependent protein kinase II. *Neurochem. Int.* 21:469–497.

[7]   Deckmyn, H., C. Van Geet, and J. Vermylen. 1993. Dual regulation of phospholipase C activity by G proteins. *NIPS* 8:61–3.

[8]   Drøbak, B. K. 1992. The plant phosphoinositide system. *Biochem. J.* 288:697–712.

[9]   Exton, J. H. 1990. Signaling through phosphatidylcholine breakdown. *J. Biol. Chem.* 265:1–4.

[10] Gilman, A. G. 1984. G. proteins and dual control of adenylate cyclase. *Cell* 36:577–79.

[11] Gnegy, M. E. 1993. Calmodulin in neurotransmitter and hormone action. *Annu. Rev. Pharm. Toxicol.* 33:45–70.

[12] Hanley, R. M., and A. L. Steiner. 1989. The second-messenger system for peptide hormones. *Hosp. Pract.* Aug. 59–70.

[13] Harrison, R. W., and S. S. Lippman. 1989. How steroid hormones work. *Hosp. Pract.* Sept. 63–76.

[14] Haussler, M. R., D. J. Mangelsdorf, K. Yamaoka, E. A. Allegretto, B. S. Komm, C. M. Terpening, D. P. McDonnell, J. W. Pike and B. W. O'Malley. 1988. Molecular characterization and actions of the vitamin D hormone receptor. *Steroid Horm. Action* 247–62.

[15] Hille, B. 1992. G protein-coupled mechanisms and nervous signalling. *Neuron* 9:187–95.

[16] Kaltenbach, J. C. 1988. Endocrine aspects of homeostasis. *Amer. Zool.* 28:761–73.

[17] Kirtland, S. J. 1988. Prostaglandin E_1: a review. *Prost. Leuk. Essen. Fatty Acids* 32:165–74.

[18]   Kleuss, C., H. Scherubl, J. Hescheler, G. Schultz, and B. Wittig. 1993. Selectivity in signal transduction determined by gamma subunits of heterotrimeric G proteins. *Science* 255:832–4.

[19]   Knighton, D. R., J. Zheng, L. F. Ten Eyck, V. A. Ashford, N.-H. Xuong, S. S. Taylor, and J. M. Sowadski. 1991. Crystal structure of the catalytic subunit of cyclic adenosine monophosphate-dependent protein kinase. *Science* 253:407–14.

[20]   Kolb, A., S. Busby, H. Buc, S. Garges, and S. Adhya. 1993. Transcriptional regulation by cyclic AMP and its receptor protein. *Annu. Rev. Biochem.* 62:749–95.

[21]   Langley, J. N. 1906. On nerve endings and on special excitable substances. *Proc. Roy. Soc. B* 78:170–94.

[22]   Levitzki, A. 1988. From epinephrine to cyclic AMP. *Science* 241:800–806.

[23]   Lincoln, T. M., T. L. Cornwell, and A. E. Taylor. 1990. cGMP-dependent protein kinase mediates the reduction of Ca^{2+} by cAMP in vascular smooth muscle cells. *Amer. J. Physiol.* 258:C399–407.

[24]   Monaco, M. E., and M. C. Gershengorn. 1992. Subcellular organization of receptor-mediated phosphoinositide turnover. *Endocr. Rev.* 13:707–18.

[25]   Nakatsu, K., and J. Diamond. 1988. Role of cGMP in relaxation of vascular and other smooth muscle. *Can J. Physiol. Pharmacol.* 67:251–62.

[26]   Oates, J. A. 1982. The 1982 Nobel prize in physiology or medicine. *Science* 218:765–68.

[27]   Oichinik, M., T. F. Murray, and F. L. Moore. 1991. A corticosteroid receptor in neuronal membranes. *Science* 252:1848–51.

[28]   Parker, C. W., and W. F. Stenson. 1989. Prostaglandins and leukotrienes. *Curr. Opin. Immunol.* 2:28–32.

[29]   Rasmussen, H. 1989. The messenger function of Ca^{2+}: from PTH action to smooth muscle contraction. *Bone Miner.* 5:233–48.

[30]   Sando, J. J., M. C. Maurer, E. J. Bolen, and C. H. Grisham. 1992. Role of cofactors in protein kinase C activation. *Cell. Signalling* 4:595–609.

[31]   Sardesai, V. M. 1992. Biochemical and nutritional aspects of eicosanoids. *J. Nutr. Biochem.* 3:562–79.

[32]   Schmid, W., D. Nitsch, M. Boshart, and G. Schutz. 1993. Role of cyclic AMP in the control of cell-specific gene expression. *TEM* 4:204–9.

[33]   Schuchard, M., J. P. Landers, N. P. Sandhu, and T. C. Spelsberg. 1993. Steroid hormone regulation of nuclear proto-oncogenes. *Endocr. Rev.* 14:659–69.

[34]   Simon, M. E., M. P. Strathmann, and N. Gautam. 1991. Diversity of G proteins in signal transduction. *Science* 252:802–8.

[35]   Smith, W. L. 1989. The eicosanoids and their biochemical mechanisms of action. *Biochem. J.* 259:315–24.

[36]   Spaulding, S. W. 1993. The ways in which hormones change adenosine 3′,5′-monophosphate-dependent protein kinase subunits, and how such changes affect behavior. *Endocr. Rev.* 14:632–50.

[37]   Spiegel, A. M., A. Shenker, and L. S. Weinstein. 1992. Receptor-effector coupling by G-proteins—implications for normal and abnormal signal transduction. *Endocr. Rev.* 13:536–65.

[38]   Strosberg, A. D. 1991. Structure/function relationship of proteins belonging to the family of receptors coupled to GTP-binding proteins. *Eur. J. Biochem.* 196:1–10.

[39]   Sumida, C., R. Graber, and E. Nunez. 1993. Role of fatty acids in signal transduction: modulators and messengers. *Prost. Leuk. Essen. Fatty Acids* 48:117–22.

[40]   Sutherland, E. W. 1972. Studies on the mechanism of hormone action. *Science* 177:401–408.

[41]   Takio, K., S. B. Smith, E. G. Krebs, K. A. Walsh, and K. Titani. 1982. Primary structure of the regulatory subunit of type II cAMP-dependent protein kinase from bovine cardiac muscle. *Proc. Natl. Acad. Sci. USA* 79:2544–48.

[42]   Tang, W.-J., and A. G. Gilman. 1991. Type-specific regulation of adenylyl cyclase by G protein $\beta\gamma$ subunits. *Science* 254:1500–3.

[43]   Taussig, R., J. A. Iniguez-Liuhi, and A. G. Gilman. 1993. Inhibition of adenyl cyclase by $G_{i\alpha}$. *Science* 261:218–21.

[44]   Vaughan, M. 1982. Cholera and cell regulation. *Hosp. Pract.* June: 145–52.

[45]   Walton, K. M., and J. E. Dixon. 1993. Protein tyrosine phosphatases. *Annu. Rev. Biochem.* 62:101–20.

[46]   Wong, S. K.-F., and D. L. Garbers. 1992. Receptor guanylyl cyclases. *J. Clin. Invest.* 90:299–305.

[47]   Yuen, P. S. T., and D. L. Garbers. 1992. Guanylyl cyclase-linked receptors. *Annu. Rev. Neurosci.* 15:193–225.

Pituitary Hormones

The pituitary has often been referred to as the master endocrine gland of vertebrates. This perceived importance may have arisen because the pituitary is located near the brain and controls such important endocrine glands as the adrenals, thyroid, and the gonads. The pituitary gland is now known to be subservient to hormonal stimuli derived from the brain and other endocrine glands [3].

The pituitary gland of the human male is somewhat smaller than the tip of the little finger and weighs between 0.5 to 1.0 g; its size in the human female becomes larger during pregnancy. The pituitary is recessed within the sella turcica of the sphenoid bone, beneath the hypothalamus near the optic chiasm. In this position the pituitary is one of the most inaccessible of the mammalian endocrine glands. Early anatomists considered the pituitary to be a part of the brain and, in fact, the gland does possess a neural component.

In 1886 Marie made an important observation that acromegaly often occurred along with a tumorous condition of the pituitary [13]. Other physicians noted that the pituitary gland of the male and the female often became enlarged following gonadectomy. Cushing was the first to note the association between basophil tumors of the pituitary and the resultant disease that bears his name. Much later it was established that pituitarigenic Cushing's disease was associated with elevated secretion of corticotropin. Cushing showed in 1909 that partial removal of the anterior pituitary of an acromegalic patient resulted in rapid recovery.

Smith [13] noted that hypophysectomy of the rat resulted in complete stasis of growth and a rapid regression of the size of the adrenals (mainly the steroidogenic cortex), the thyroid, and the gonads. Ablation of the posterior lobe of the pituitary alone failed to produce these effects. Smith also observed that daily intramuscular injections of fresh rat or bovine anterior pituitary homogenates into hypophysectomized rats brought about a nearly normal growth rate. In addition this replacement therapy caused a partial restoration of the size of the adrenals, thyroid, and gonads. Evans and Long [13] noted that extracts of bovine pituitaries enhanced the growth rate of intact rats over that of their littermates. Treatment of rats with such extracts for 9 months or more resulted in the production of experimental gigantism. This exaggerated increase in growth was due to generalized overgrowth of the skeleton and to an enlargement of most tissues and organs. These results provided experimental evidence for the existence of a growth hormone (somatotropin) of hypophysial origin.

Smith and Allen, working independently, demonstrated that growth and metamorphosis of larval amphibians (frog tadpoles) were prevented by extirpation of the anlage (tissue primordium) of the epithelial (non-neural component) pituitary [13]. The larval animals were also light in color compared to normal intact tadpoles. These early experiments provided evidence for the existence of a pituitary thyroid-stimulating hormone and a melanocyte-stimulating hormone. Subsequently, other researchers provided evidence for the existence of other pituitary hormones regulating adrenal and gonadal function and numerous other physiological processes. This chapter will discuss the nature and endocrine role of the pituitary hormones.

ANATOMY OF THE PITUITARY GLAND

The pituitary gland (also known as the hypophysis) is composed of tissues that are derived from two diverse origins [12]. An understanding of the origin and development of the pituitary is critical to an understanding of the structure-function relationships of this endocrine gland. Early anatomists believed that the structural components of the pituitary (from the Latin, *pituita* or phlegm) gland were concerned with the removal of phlegm or mucus from the cavities of the brain. The comparative anatomy of the pituitary of many vertebrates has been reviewed in an important monograph by Holmes and Ball [15]. The ultrastructural characteristics of the anterior pituitary cells have been described in detail elsewhere [10].

Developmental Anatomy

The human pituitary is composed of an *adenohypophysis* (glandular or epithelial hypophysis) and a *neurohypophysis* (Fig. 5.1). The former derives from an inward invagination of the oral ectoderm of the stomodeum (primitive mouth cavity) known as Rathke's pouch (Fig. 5.2). The neuronal component arises from the neural ectoderm of the floor of the forebrain. Rathke's pouch elongates and becomes constricted at its attachment to the oral epithelium. A remnant of the connection between Rathke's pouch and the stomodeal ectoderm may persist as a "pharyngeal" pituitary. An infundibular process develops as a diverticulum of the floor of the diencephalon. The infundibulum increases in size because of neuroepithelial cell proliferation. Nerve fibers grow into the infundibulum from hypothalamic nuclei. The neuroepithelial cells then differentiate into *pituicytes* (neuroglial-like elements), which are dispersed between the neuronal endings within the infundibulum.

Cells of the anterior wall of Rathke's pouch proliferate to give rise to the pars distalis or anterior pituitary [10]. Continued proliferation of these cells leads to reduction of the lumen of Rathke's pouch to a *residual cleft* and a separation of the cells of the posterior wall from the anterior pituitary. Those cells adjacent to the infundibulum may proliferate to give rise to a pars intermedia of considerable size in some species. Failure of the

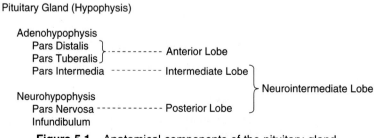

Figure 5.1   Anatomical components of the pituitary gland.

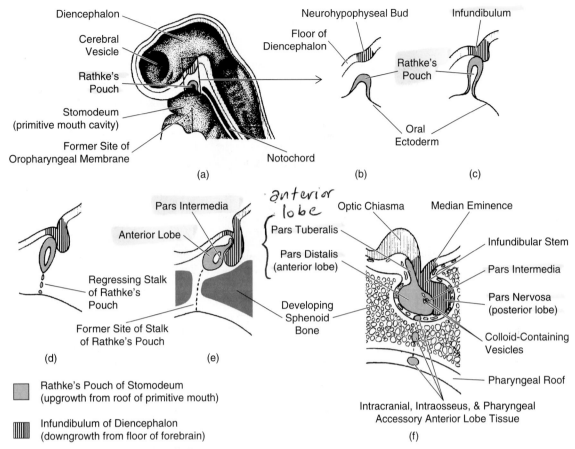

Figure 5.2 Developmental anatomy of the pituitary. (From K. L. Moore [19], *The Developing Human*. "Clinically Oriented Embryology," 2nd ed., 1977. Courtesy of W. B. Saunders Company.)

adenohypophysis to contact the developing neurohypophysis results in the inability of the pituitary cells to form a pars intermedia. In birds the adenohypophysis is separated from the neurohypophysis by a layer of connective tissue and a pars intermedia does not develop. In humans the fetal pars intermedia regresses and is absent in the adult (see Chap. 8). Dorsal extensions of the anterior pituitary surround the infundibular stalk to give rise to the *pars tuberalis*. The pars tuberalis may provide an important anatomical link between the pars distalis and the hypothalamus. The definitive pituitary in many species consists of the pars distalis, the pars intermedia, the pars tuberalis, and the pars nervosa (Fig. 5.3). The intimate anatomical relationship between the pituitary gland and the overlying brain provides an important clue to understanding the essential functional relationship of the components of the brain-pituitary axis [14, 20].

Lobation, Vascularization, Innervation

The size of each lobe of the pituitary gland varies between different species; the size of the gland may be related to the particular environmental niche occupied by the species [12]. Animals that rapidly change color may possess a relatively large pars intermedia, the pars nervosa of aquatic species may be small, but relatively large in land-dwelling species, particularly those inhabiting arid climates. These size differences in pituitary gland components reflect the hormonal output of the glands required for successful adaptation to a particular habitat.

The pituitary gland receives its blood supply from the superior and inferior hypophysial arteries. The anterior and posterior branches of the superior hypophysial

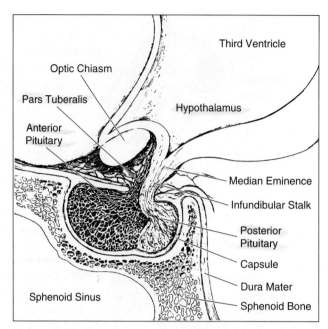

Figure 5.3 The pituitary gland of humans. In the adult human, unlike most mammals, the pars intermedia is absent. (From R. Guillemin and R. Burgus [14], "The Hormones of the Hypothalamus," with permission. ©1972 by *Scientific American*, Inc. All rights reserved.)

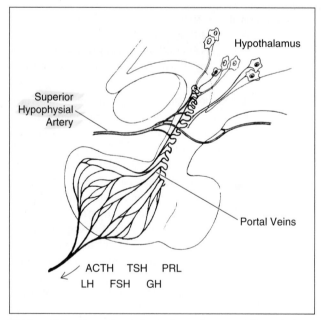

Figure 5.4 Vascular connections between the pituitary gland and the hypothalamus. (From R. Guillemin and R. Burgus [14], "The Hormones of the Hypothalamus," with permission. ©1972 by *Scientific American*, Inc. All rights reserved.)

artery penetrate the hypophysial stalk, as well as the hypothalamus (Fig. 5.4). The pars distalis is vascularized by hypophysial portal vessels that arise from the capillary beds within the median eminence of the hypothalamus. This hypophysial portal system provides an important link for carrying hormonal information from the CNS to the pituitary (Chap. 6). Whether the anterior lobe receives blood exclusively from the portal circulation, or whether some additional direct arterial blood supply is available, is unresolved. The pars nervosa receives a separate blood supply from the inferior hypophysial artery. The pars intermedia, if present, is relatively avascular. Physiologists have generally assumed that all hormones produced by the adenohypophysis are released directly into the efferent portal veins to be carried through the systemic circulation to distant target tissues. There is evidence that some adenohypophysial venous blood may be shunted to the neurohypophysis [3]. This circular path of blood flow may permit adenohypophysial venous blood to be carried up the infundibular process to the brain. This observation carries the important implication that pituitary hormones might be able to modify CNS function.

Except for neurovascular elements, there is no evidence that neurons innervate or otherwise directly influence the cell activity of the human pars distalis or that of most other mammals. Neuronal elements may affect cellular hormone secretion within the pars distalis of some teleost fishes. The cells of the pars intermedia of amphibians and some mammals are surrounded by a plexus of catecholaminergic neurons that regulate MSH secretion from the melanotrophs (MSH-secreting cells). Such a direct neuronal innervation is absent from the pars intermedia of some reptiles. The pars nervosa is composed of axonal endings of neurons whose cell bodies are located in hypothalamic nuclei, and in mammals, the paraventricular and supraoptic nuclei (Fig. 5.5).

The gross morphology of the pituitary differs considerably between the vertebrate classes and often between species of the same class. At the cytological level the individual cell types may be intermingled to varying degrees (as in tetrapods) or separated into zones (as in most teleost fishes). There is no distinct neural lobe in fishes. The neural lobe is, however, characteristic of tetrapods, and this may be related to the terrestrial manner of life of these vertebrates, where one or both neurohypophysial hormones may be of adaptive importance (see Fig. 8.2). The size of the pars intermedia varies considerably between species, and all birds lack a pars intermedia. This is not a unique feature, as the pars intermedia is not present in some mammals (elephants, whales, adult humans).

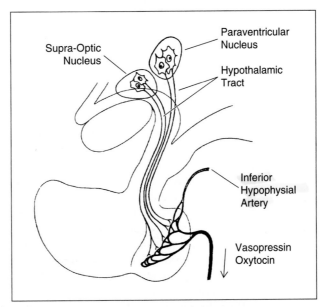

Figure 5.5 Neural components of the pituitary gland of humans. (From R. Guillemin and R. Burgus [14], "The Hormones of the Hypothalamus," with permission. ©1972 by *Scientific American*, Inc. All rights reserved.)

TABLE 5.1 Histochemical Classification of Pituitary Pars Distalis Cells

Cell type	Hormone	Staining characteristic
Corticotroph[a]	Corticotropin (ACTH)	Basophil
Thyrotroph	Thyrotropin (TSH)	Basophil
Gonadotroph		
FSH-gonadotroph	Follitropin (FSH)	Basophil
LH-gonadotroph	Lutropin (LH)	Basophil
Lactotroph (mammotroph)	Prolactin (PRL)	Acidophil
Somatotroph	Somatotropin (STH)	Acidophil

[a]Cytological classification uses either the suffix -troph or -trope (e.g., corticotrope).

Cytology

The cells of the pituitary are referred to as *acidophils, basophils,* or *chromophobes,* depending on their affinity for certain dyes used in histological stains (Table 5.1). Histochemical and immunocytochemical methods have provided definitive information on the specific cellular sources of each pituitary peptide hormone [31]. The cells of the pars distalis have been differentiated into somatotrophs, lactotrophs (mammotrophs), corticotrophs, thyrotrophs, and gonadotrophs. These terms relate to the particular hormonal product synthesized by each of these cells. Somatotrophs and lactotrophs are acidophils, whereas the thyrotrophs and the gonadotrophs are basophils. The corticotrophs are basophils but are often referred to as chromophobes. The cells of the mammalian pars intermedia are also considered to be chromophobes. The extent to which a cell exhibits acidophilia, basophilia, or chromophobia may depend on the granular content (hormone-containing vesicles) of the cell, which often varies with the temporal secretory activity of the cell. These secretory vesicles may become depleted after continued secretory activity of the cells; in contrast, these granules may accumulate, at least transiently, if the cells stop releasing hormone. Granule synthesis may eventually decline if the cell is no longer stimulated to secrete its hormonal product. Except for the sparse pituicytes (glial-like cells), the pars nervosa contains only neuronal axonal endings.

Nongranulated, presumably nonsecretory cells are also present in the pars distalis, pars intermedia, and neurohypophysis. These elements have been referred to as glial cells, glial-like cells, stellate cells, and follicular cells. The processes of these cells often separate one pituitary cell from contact with another. In some species they may form the lining of minute ductules or follicles within the adenohypophysis. A variety of putative functions have been suggested for these cells, and it is possible that they modulate pituitary hormone secretion in response to regulatory cues [26].

The utilization of peroxidase-labeled antibodies for the ultrastructural localization of hormones provides an identification method for the specific hormone-producing cells of the pituitary and the intracellular sites of hormone synthesis. Antibodies to each of the pituitary peptides (antigens) are linked to the enzyme horseradish peroxidase. Thin sections of tissue are then exposed to the antibody-peroxidase conjugate and rinsed. The antibody interacts with its specific antigen (hormone), which is localized within the appropriate pituitary cells. The peroxidase is then localized histochemically by providing a substrate (peroxide) and a dye. The peroxidase reacts with the peroxide to yield molecular oxygen, which then produces a particular color depending on the dye present. Different dyes provide differently colored end products. By this method one can note that the reaction product is specifically localized to the secretory granules of the cells. One cell can be differentiated from another by the sequential addition of different antibody-peroxidase conjugates and by the use of different dyes. Differentiation of one gonadotroph from another uses antisera raised specifically against the β subunit of follitropin or of lutropin.

Although each of the pituitary hormones is localized to a particular cell type, as determined by ultrastructural and immunocytochemical analysis, most gonadotrophs (human, rat, quail, frog) contain lutropin and follitropin. Nevertheless, subpopulations of gonadotrophs contain only one of the gonadotropins. This may account for the nonparallel release of gonadotropins in response to certain stimuli (see Fig. 18.11). Individual gonadotrophs vary in their staining intensity for labeled antibodies to each of the gonadotropins, suggesting that gonadotrophs may represent a fluid, heterogeneous population of cells capable of synthesizing and storing both or one of the hormones. Immunocytochemical observations have revealed that all cell types of the pars distalis are present within the pars tuberalis of the human and monkey. The hormonal function of the pars distalis therefore may be augmented by secretory contributions from the pars tuberalis.

HORMONES OF THE PITUITARY

A number of peptide hormones are produced by the pituitary. These hormones regulate such target organs as the gonads, the adrenals, and the thyroid gland. The mammary glands, uterus, kidneys, and other tissues are also controlled by hypophysial hormones. Two gonadotropins are present: *follicle-stimulating hormone* (FSH), or *follitropin,* and *luteinizing hormone* (LH), or *lutropin.* A *thyroid-stimulating hormone* (TSH), or *thyrotropin,* and an *adrenal cortical-stimulating hormone* (ACTH),.or *adrenocorticotropin* (*corticotropin*), regulate thyroid and adrenal activity, respectively. A *somatotropin* (STH), or *growth hormone* (GH), which has generalized growth-promoting effects, and a *prolactin* (PRL), which has more specific growth-promoting action on the mammary glands, are also present in some species. A melanocyte-stimulating hormone (α-MSH, α-melanotropin) is produced by cells of the pars intermedia, or possibly by cells within the pars distalis (of birds). The neurohypophysial hormones, *oxytocin* and the *vasopressins,* are elaborated within neurons of the neurohypophysis, whose cell bodies originate within the hypothalamus. A melanin-concentrating hormone is also present within the neurohypophysis of teleost fishes [4] (see Chap. 8). The pituitary hormones are released into the bloodstream where they circulate to interact with their target organs.

Families of Pituitary Hormones

The hormones of the pituitary can be classified into four groups based on their structural similarity and presumed evolutionary origin. Somatotropin and prolactin possess numerous similar sequences of amino acids within their individual structures, and they are also structurally related to placental lactogen (also known as somatomammotropin) [28]. Thyrotropin, follitropin, and lutropin are glycoproteins and are related in structure to each other and to chorionic gonadotropin (choriogonadotropin), a hormone of placental origin. α-Melanotropin and corticotropin contain a sequence of amino acids in common, which accounts for their overlapping actions and suggests a related evolutionary origin. Two neurohypophysial hormones are present in the neurohypophysis, and they are structurally related to each other.

Growth Hormone and Prolactin

These hormones of the pituitary exert profound effects on body growth. In the young animal GH plays an essential role in general body growth, whereas PRL stimulates the growth of specialized tissues such as the mammary gland during pregnancy and lactation.

Growth Hormone. The existence of a hormone that is responsible for general somatic growth was suggested by the early experiments of Evans and Long (1922) and Smith (1926) [13]. Hypophysectomized young rats failed to grow to adult size, but extracts of the pituitary stimulated growth in these rats and in rats of normal growth. Human GH is also effective in promoting linear growth in children with congenital GH deficiency. In young animals the epiphyses of the long bones are separated from the shaft of the bones by an epiphyseal cartilaginous plate. Chondrogenesis is accelerated by GH, which results in a widening of the epiphyseal plates as more extracellular matrix (chondroitin sulfate) is synthesized and released by chondrocytes. This widening has been used as a bioassay for GH (tibia test).

Somatotropin accounts for 4% to 10% of the wet weight of the anterior pituitary in the human adult (5 to 10 mg per gland). GH circulates in the plasma complexed to one or more binding proteins, and basal (resting or nonstressed) levels of immunoassayable GH in the plasma range from 1 to 5 ng per milliliter. The circulating levels of the hormone decline during the first 2 or 3 weeks after birth to then reach the basal levels characteristic of the adult human. Age-related changes in total 24-hour secretion of GH have been described. Although GH levels remain rather constant during the period of accelerated growth in early childhood, there is an appreciable increase during the period of maximal growth in adolescence. Interestingly, a substantial part of the 24-hour secretion of GH occurs during the first 90 minutes of nocturnal sleep. In every mammalian species studied so far, spontaneous episodes of GH secretion occur several times over a 24-hour period. Particularly in the rat, GH release follows a rhythm with high-amplitude GH secretory bursts occurring at regular 3.3 hour intervals. In the intervening trough periods, basal plasma GH levels are undetectable. Both a hypothalamic growth hormone-releasing hormone (GHRH), somatocrinin, as well as an GH release-inhibiting factor (SRIF, somatostatin) control GH secretion (see Tannenbaum [30]).

Somatotropin is a polypeptide synthesized by certain acidophils (somatotrophs) of the pars distalis. GH is derived from a prohormone in the pituitary cells but is rapidly converted to GH by proteolysis. The human hormone consists of 191 amino acids with two intramolecular disulfide bonds. The hormone is strikingly similar in structure to PRL and placental lactogen. The latter molecule also contains 191 amino acids and possesses S—S bonds in exactly the same locations as in GH; in 161 positions the amino acids are identical. The structural homologies between GH, PRL, and placental lactogen suggest a single progenitor molecule that arose early in vertebrate evolution (see Fig 12.12).

GH is a protein anabolic hormone in that it enhances amino acid incorporation into muscle protein and stimulates extracellular collagen deposition (Chap. 12). Thus it produces a positive nitrogen and phosphorus balance and a concomitant fall in blood urea nitrogen and amino acid levels. Urinary excretion of Na^+ and K^+ is also decreased, probably due to the increased uptake of these ions by growing tissue. These effects of GH on protein metabolism and electrolyte balance are mediated indirectly through the actions of somatomedins released from the liver in response to GH stimulation of hepatocytes. These somatomedins (insulinlike growth factors, IGFs) stimulate cellular growth in a variety of tissues and organs (see Fig. 12.3).

The absence of GH secretion leads to dwarfism (short stature) in the young child, whereas overproduction of GH during early postnatal development leads to gigantism [25]. In the adult excess GH secretion leads to acromegaly. Dwarfism may result from a pituitary failure of GH production (hypopituitary dwarfism) or from a failure of the liver to respond to GH and synthesize somatomedins (Laron syndrome). The pathogenesis of acromegaly has been explained by a "pituitary" or a hypothalamic hypothesis. In the former view overproduction of GH may result from GH-secreting tumors of the adenohypophysis (intrasellar tumors). The hypothalamic hypothesis implicates the defect as residing within the central nervous system, possibly from an overproduction of somatocrinin or an underproduction of somatostatin [30]. The secretion of either of these factors is controlled by other neural inputs (e.g., dopaminergic neurons) that may contribute indirectly to the etiology of acromegaly. Nevertheless, the vast majority of patients with acromegaly have identifiable pituitary tumors, but whether these tumors arise from long-term overstimulation by the hypothalamus or are independent of hypothalamic influence, possibly due to cellular mutagenesis of somatotrophs or a related stem cell, is still unclear [9, 21, 22].

The acromegalic characteristics of GH overproduction probably result from the direct effects of GH on target tissues, as well as growth effects mediated through the somatomedins. The growth changes in bones and soft tissues are most noticeable in the hands, feet, and face. Proliferation of connective tissue and interstitial fluid results in thickening of the skin and in an increase in subcutaneous tissues. The viscera and related organs, the lungs, liver, heart, and kidneys, are usually enlarged. Acromegalics may display increased metabolic rates, and the lipolytic actions of GH on adipose tissue combined with anti-insulin actions on other tissues result in hyperglycemia as a symptom of a developing diabetes mellitus.

The etiology of GH deficiency may also relate to a pituitary or hypothalamic dysfunction [9]. Intrasellar tumors or other destructive processes, as well as familial (genetic) or congenital (birth) defects, may result in a lack of GH production that could lead to dwarfism if initiated at a young age. Lack of GH secretion may be accompanied by a total lack of pituitary hormone production (panhypopituitarism) or may be an example of an isolated GH deficiency of unknown etiology. Dwarfism may also result from pituitary deficiency secondary to hypothalamic dysfunction, possibly related to an absence of somatocrinin. Suprasellar (CNS) lesions may also result in GH deficiency, and there are even examples of psychosocial dwarfism. GH of mammalian origin is active in many species, but human subjects are responsive only to human or primate GH. However, GH has become available commercially for the treatment of short stature by gene-splicing techniques within bacteria (see Chap. 3).

Prolactin. Mammary growth and development and lactogenesis in the human female are regulated, in part, by a lactotropic hormone from the pituitary. Prolactin plays diverse roles in other vertebrates [16]. In fact, no other known peptide hormone has such a repertoire of biological actions. Because the varied effects of this hormone usually bear some relationship to physiological responses essential for reproductive success, PRL has been referred to as the "hormone of maternity." Only recently has a role for PRL in the male and nonpregnant female been recognized (Chaps. 17 and 18).

In 1928 Stricker and Grueter discovered that an extract of the anterior pituitary gland could stimulate milk secretion in rabbits. The control of mammary gland development and the stimulation of milk synthesis are complex processes that involve the participation of many hormones. The mammotropic action of PRL requires the participation of several hormones, which, in some species, include estrogens, insulin, glucocorticoids, progesterone, and GH. The direct action of PRL on the mammary gland was shown in ovariectomized rabbits first given estrogen and progesterone to produce lobuloalveolar growth (see Chap. 19). When PRL was injected into the individual ducts of the mammary gland, only the alveoli connected to the injected duct produced milk. Riddle, Bates, and Dykshorn discovered that a specific fraction of bovine pituitary extracts, which they named prolactin, stimulated crop sac growth in pigeons [24].

During pregnancy or in the postpartum lactational period prolactin cells comprise as much as 50% of the acidophil population of the pituitary. Production of PRL by lactotrophs in the pituitary is affected by estrogens, and during pregnancy and lactation serum PRL levels rise substantially. Estrogens stimulate PRL secretion by the anterior pituitary gland and stimulate PRL synthesis by a direct effect on PRL gene transcription. Estrogens increase mitotic activity and cell number of pituitary lactotrophs. Hyperprolactinemia and PRL-secreting pituitary tumors are relatively common in women of reproductive age, and this has raised the question of the role of endogenous estrogens in their pathogenesis.

Serum PRL levels increase at puberty, but only modestly compared to the rise in FSH and LH concentrations that also occur. Estrogen infusions are stimulatory to PRL secretion, which may explain the increase in PRL secretion at puberty, a time when ovarian steroid biosynthesis is enhanced. During pregnancy there is a progressive increase in serum PRL concentrations reaching maximal values at term. In mothers who do not nurse their young, the postpartum concentrations of PRL rapidly fall back to normal by three weeks, unless breast feeding is commenced. Concentrations of PRL in the amniotic fluid exceed those in the maternal or fetal circulation early in pregnancy and at term. By biological, chemical, and immunological criteria, human amniotic fluid PRL is similar or identical to that in the pituitary hormone. The chorion-decidua may be the source of amniotic lactogen, but the possible physiological function, if any, of the placental PRL is unknown.

PRL is luteotropic in some mammalian species, and it may act in concert with LH or FSH on the corpus luteum to stimulate progesterone biosynthesis and secretion. Progesterone production by the ovarian corpus luteum is required for growth and development of the uterus and for suppression of further ovum maturation and ovulation (Chap 19). PRL has a profound effect on the growth, differentiation, and function of a number of integumental structures: hair and sebaceous glands in mammals; brood patch and feather development in certain birds; epidermal sloughing in lizards; and integumental mucous gland secretion in certain teleosts. Because the mammary gland is an integumental derivative and is considered to be phylogenetically related to sweat glands, one may conclude that the highly specialized mammotropic action of PRL in humans and most mammals may have evolved from the more generalized action of PRL on a variety of integumentary functions.

In certain birds (pigeons and doves) PRL controls the production of a so-called crop sac "milk." In response to PRL the epithelium of the two lateral lobes of the crop wall thicken in both the male and the female at the time the eggs are hatched. The epithelium proliferates, and the cells accumulate lipid and begin to degenerate. The layers of cells are sloughed off to form a mass of material that is regurgitated to feed the young birds. Besides its effect on the integument, PRL controls many other physiological processes. Considering its versatility, the name given to the hormone, prolactin, is obviously restrictive and only refers to one of its many roles.

Although the major role of PRL in humans is the control of lactation, evidence suggests that PRL may control testicular function, at least in some rodents. Hypophysectomy of adult rats causes a loss of testicular LH receptors and this, as expected, is associated with a loss in testicular responsiveness to LH. Inhibition of LH or FSH secretion from the pituitary is not, however, associated with a loss of LH receptors. Inhibition of pituitary PRL release, on the other hand, is associated with a loss of testicular LH receptors. Thus PRL may be essential for the maintenance of LH receptors. This view is substantiated by the observation that PRL treatment increases LH receptor number in the gonads of dwarf male mice and in atrophic testes of light-deprived hamsters (see Chap. 20). Prolactin also stimulates growth of the testosterone-stimulated prostate gland of the castrated rat.

Plasma levels of PRL in humans are slightly higher in females than males, although there is considerable overlap of the ranges of PRL concentration in the two sexes. PRL is secreted episodically and has a half-life in the blood of about 15 to 20 minutes. There is a nighttime surge of PRL secretion, which, like GH, is associated with sleep (Fig. 5.6). The times of onset and duration of the PRL peak are not identical to those of GH. The most potent stimulus to PRL secretion is nursing. Release of the hormone is mediated by cutaneous sensations arising from the breast and nipple, not by psychic factors associated with the presence of the infant. Breast stimulation of the human male has no effect on PRL release. Secretion of PRL from the pituitary is controlled by a PRL inhibiting factor, PIF. This inhibitory control is somehow diminished during late pregnancy and lactation. The existence of PRL-releasing factor has been suggested in mammals, and PRL secretion in birds is mainly under a stimulatory control (Chap. 6).

Studies using [^{125}I]-labeled PRL reveal that mammary aveolar cells possess plasmalemmal PRL receptors. Antibodies prepared against mammary gland cell receptors block the binding of PRL to these receptors and also selectively block PRL-stimulated casein synthesis and amino acid transport into mammary tissue in culture. These results

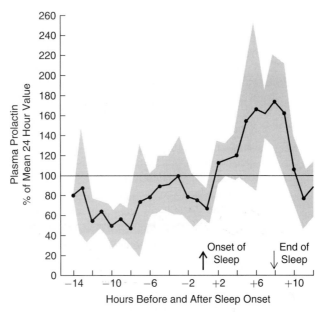

Figure 5.6 Human plasma levels of PRL during a 24-hour period. (Reprinted by permission of *The New England Journal of Medicine*, Frantz, A. G. [11]. "Prolactin," vol. 298, pp. 201–207, 1978.)

support a functional role for PRL receptors in mediating some actions of the hormone on lactogenesis.

Although PRL and GH share structural similarity [18, 32], their physiological actions in humans are discrete. Acromegalic patients with elevated GH levels only occasionally develop galactorrhea; individuals with galactorrhea or women who are breast-feeding have normal serum GH concentrations. Some patients with a hereditary form of isolated growth hormone deficiency lactate normally, although GH is absent.

The Glycoprotein Hormones

Three hormones of the anterior pituitary are glycoproteins [6, 17]. Thyrotropin (TSH), follicle-stimulating hormone (FSH), and luteinizing hormone (LH) contain covalently bound carbohydrate moieties at one or more positions within their structures. Each of these pituitary glycoproteins is composed of two chains, so-called α and β subunits. The α subunits of the three pituitary glycoproteins within a species are identical to each other, whereas the β subunit of each hormone is structurally distinct [27]. The α subunit consists of a polypeptide of 92 residues in humans and 96 residues in the other mammalian species studied. Although α subunits exhibit identical amino acid sequences in a given species, their N-linked oligosaccharide chains are generally different [29]. The amino acid sequence is very similar between different mammalian species. Seventy-one of the 96 positions are occupied by the same amino acid residue in most mammals. Ten of the half-cystine residues of these molecules are conserved, which suggests that the five disulfide bridges are likely to be identical, thus leading to a common conformation in all α subunits [2]. This hypothesis is strengthened by the observation that hybrid heterodimers can be obtained with α and β subunits from different species [7].

Although related in structure, the β subunits exhibit different amino acid sequences within and between species. The β subunits are composed of 110–111 residues (LHs), 112–118 residues (TSHs), 117–121 residues (LHs), or 145 residues (hCG). Each subunit possesses 12 Cys residues at highly conserved positions among species. The six disulfide bridges within the β subunits probably result in similar overall three-dimensional structures [7].

Amino acid sequences that are identical in the glycoprotein β subunits represent intersubunit contact sites, whereas the nonidentical residues contribute to interaction with target tissue receptors and therefore provide hormonal specificity. The α and β subunits of the glycoprotein hormones are independently synthesized; some pituitary tumors, for example, exhibit isolated or unbalanced α-subunit secretion. Also, isolated or unbalanced ectopic secretion of α or β subunits of choriogonadotropin by malignant uterine neoplasms has been noted. Two separate mRNA species have been identified from mouse thyrotropic tumors, each coding for a different subunit of the hormone. A single gene per haploid DNA complements codes for the α subunits of the glycoprotein family of hormones in any one species. The peptide component of the glycoproteins is first synthesized under direct genetic control. Glycosylation, the attachment of carbohydrate moieties, is a postribosomal event controlled by glycosyltransferase enzymes localized in the Golgi cisternae of the cells [29].

The constituent sugars of glycoprotein hormones are D-mannose, D-galactose, L-fucose, N-acetyl neuraminic acid, D-glucosamine, and N-acetylated D-galactosamine [17]. All α subunits contain two oligosaccharides that are N-linked to asparagines. All pituitary glycoprotein hormones may contain O-sulfated (attached through serine to the peptide chain) hexosamines [29]. The carbohydrate moieties of the α subunit in the gonadotropic hormones are important for biological function. Their specific removal, without affecting the polypeptide primary structure, causes an uncoupling of the receptor-adenylate cyclase system in target cells of the testis. The integrity of the carbohydrate in the α subunit is directly or indirectly involved in receptor signal transduction. Removal of 70–75% of the total carbohydrate in gonadotropins leads to derivatives that are still able to bind to their specific receptors, but are unable to stimulate adenylate cyclase. It has been shown for oLH, bLH, hCG, oFSH that deglycosylated gonadotropins specifically antagonize the action of the corresponding native hormones. The protein and carbohydrate components of gonadotropins clearly have different roles in the expression of biological activity. The role of the glycosylated α subunit in signal transduction could be of evolutionary significance, as there is a high degree of structural conservation of the α subunit among different species, and an identical α subunit is used in the assembly of the three glycoprotein hormones in all species [2].

One may question the individual role of each glycoprotein hormone's subunit in cellular interaction. It has been suggested that the α subunit endows the β subunit with a conformation necessary for binding to the receptor and that the α subunit itself is necessary for stimulation of adenylate cyclase. It has also been proposed that domains in the α subunit, in combination with domains in the β subunit, are responsible for interaction with receptors. In the latter case conformational changes contributing to the specificity of binding could also be induced in an α subunit by the β subunit [17]. Molecular hybridization studies involving recombinations of α subunits with β subunits demonstrate that hormonal specificity is conferred upon the hybrid by the β subunit (Fig. 5.7).

Thyrotropin. The early work of Allen and of Smith [13] demonstrated that thyroidectomy resulted in failure of tadpoles to metamorphose into frogs. This effect could also be duplicated by hypophysectomy of tadpoles. Metamorphosis of thyroidectomized tadpoles could be accomplished, however, by addition of thyroid gland extracts to the water in which the larvae swam. Pituitary extracts stimulated metamorphosis of hypophysectomized, but not thyroidectomized, tadpoles. These observations suggested that the pituitary gland might be the source of a substance that was stimulatory to thyroid production of a metamorphic hormone. Thyroxine and triiodothyronine are the hormones produced by the thyroid (Chap. 13). A thyroid-stimulating hormone (TSH, thyrotropin) has been isolated from the pituitary and its structure determined in a number of mammalian species. Thyroid-stimulating activity has also been found in pituitaries of all vertebrates examined. Thyrotropin is synthesized within basophilic thyrotrophs of the pars distalis. The number of secretory granules present within the thyrotrophs is increased if animals are treated with thyroxine, suggesting that thyroid hormones exert a negative feedback to TSH secretion.

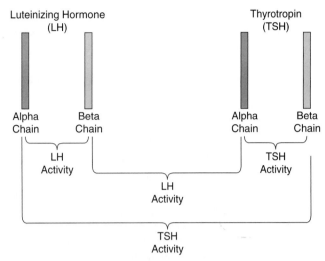

Figure 5.7   Glycoprotein subunit hybridization studies.

As the name implies, the most important role of TSH is the control of thyroid gland function. By its action on the thyroid to liberate thyroid hormones, TSH is responsible for the control and coordination of many biological processes. In the amphibian, for example, TSH is responsible for inducing metamorphosis; in the mammal TSH plays an important role in thermogenesis. Thyrotropins of mammalian origin stimulate thyroid activity in all vertebrates except cyclostomes, and pituitary extracts of nonmammalian vertebrates stimulate mammalian thyroid glands. The amino acid composition of turtle TSH is strikingly similar to that of bovine TSH. Purified lutropin of mammals possesses intrinsic TSH activity when tested on teleost thyroid glands. This observation supports the suggestion that the primitive glycoprotein may have been an LH-like molecule that became modified during evolution into a TSH-like molecule.

Lutropin.   The gonads—the ovaries and the testes—secrete steroid hormones that regulate the growth and development of a variety of target tissues. In many animals hypophysectomy leads to atrophy of the gonads, and extracts of the pituitary cause recrudescence of the gonads of hypophysectomized animals. These experiments implicate the pituitary gland in the control of gonadal function. Originally two pituitary fractions possessing gonadotropic activity were obtained. One of these stimulated follicular growth in the ovaries and increased spermatogenic activity in the testes. This hormone is now referred to as follicle-stimulating hormone (FSH) or follitropin. The other factor, referred to as luteinizing hormone (LH) or lutropin, stimulated corpora lutea formation and ovulation in the female and stimulated testosterone secretion and development of secondary sexual characteristics in the male.

LH stimulates testosterone synthesis by the interstitial cells of Leydig of the testes. The action of LH is dependent on FSH induction of Leydig cell LH receptors. Indirectly LH stimulates spermatogenesis by way of its effect on testosterone biosynthesis, which is required for maturation of the germ cells. In the human female LH induces ovulation and is necessary for the initial development of the corpus luteum (Chap. 18 and 19).

Follitropin.   After many initial difficulties, a gonadotropic hormone separate from LH was obtained. FSH is responsible for the early development of the ovarian follicle in the female and for the initial steps of spermatid maturation in the male. The role of FSH in the male is twofold: to increase the LH receptor population of testicular Leydig cells so that they are sensitive to the actions of LH and to act in concert with LH to stimulate spermatogenesis. Specifically FSH stimulates synthesis of a testicular (Sertoli cell) androgen-binding protein. FSH interacts with granulosa cells of the developing follicle, and its actions are mediated through cAMP. The biological roles and mechanisms of action of FSH are discussed later (see Chaps. 17 and 18).

Pro-opiomelanocortin: Corticotropin and Melanotropin

Corticotropin and α-melanotropin are hormones of the pituitary that share some structural similarity. ACTH is localized to corticotroph cells of the pars distalis [5]. The pars intermedia is the major source of a melanotropin that controls integumental melanocyte (melanophore) melanin production in many vertebrates. A β-lipotropin (β-LPH) of pars distalis origin was first described by Li in 1964, but the physiological significance of this polypeptide was not discerned until many years later. β-LPH is now realized to be a component of an even larger precursor molecule referred to as pro-opiomelanocortin, or POMC (see Fig. 8.4). Within the structure of this precursor protein is the amino acid sequence of ACTH and other hormonal peptides. In addition within the molecule of β-LPH is found the amino acid sequence of a so-called β-melanotropin (β-melanocyte-stimulating hormone, β-MSH). There is no evidence, however, that this melanotropic peptide is cleaved from the POMC and plays any normal hormonal role (see Chap. 8). The C-terminal 61–93 sequence of bovine β-LPH is referred to as β-endorphin, and the smaller 61–65 sequence is referred to as methionine enkephalin (see Fig. 21.4). Both β-endorphin and Met-enkephalin function within the nervous system as neurohormones, perhaps as the analgesic hormones of humans (see Chap. 21). In the pars distalis, enzymes within corticotrophs split the ACTH sequence from the precursor protein. In the pars intermedia, on the other hand, enzymes release the tridecapeptide sequence of α-MSH (see Fig. 8.3) from POMC. The remaining components of POMC protein are released along with ACTH or α-MSH during vesicular exocytosis.

Both α-MSH and ACTH possess similar sequences within their structures (see Fig 8.1), which is why each hormone stimulates the target tissues of the other hormone, melanocytes, and adrenal glands, respectively. β-Lipotropin has been isolated from the fin whale pituitary and chemically characterized. The proposed primary structure of whale β-LPH differs from the ovine LPH only at four amino acid residues. The β-endorphin segment (residues 61–91) is identical to that of ovine β-LPH. The total number of residues in β-LPH differs among species: human (89), ovine (91), bovine (93), porcine (91), ostrich (90), fin whale (91).

Corticotropin. The steroidogenic tissues of the adrenal glands secrete a number of steroid hormones that profoundly affect carbohydrate and mineral metabolism. In most mammals steroidal tissue surrounds the adrenal medulla to form the so-called adrenal cortex. Hypophysectomy results in atrophy of the adrenal cortex. The steroidogenic tissue of the hypophysectomized animal is restored in animals receiving replacement therapy with pituitary extracts. Purification of pituitary preparations led to the isolation and structural characterization of an adrenal cortical-stimulating hormone (ACTH), adrenocorticotropin or corticotropin, as it is also designated.

Corticotropin is synthesized within basophils of the pars distalis [5]. Unlike the glycoprotein-containing basophils that synthesize TSH, FSH, and LH, the corticotroph cells are often chromophobic and are sometimes considered to be chromophobes. Certain chromophobic basophils may represent very active corticotrophs that are essentially degranulated. Certain adenoma cells associated with Cushing's disease are, on the other hand, intensely PAS-positive. The glycoprotein present within these cells is not directly related to ACTH but is apparently a component of the precursor molecule of ACTH.

Corticotropin is the smallest peptide hormone of the anterior pituitary and is composed of a single linear chain consisting of 39 amino acids. Thus far this chain length is a consistent feature of all species of ACTH. Structural differences between species are found only between residues 24–33, and these differences in mammals amount to only

```
         5              10             15             20
Ser—Met—Glu—His—Phe—Arg—Trp—Gly—Lys—Pro—Val—Gly—Lys—Lys—Arg—Arg—Pro—Val—Lys—Val—Tyr—Pro┐
```

```
                              35                    30                  25
        Human   Phe—Glu—Leu—Pro—Phe—Ala—Glu—Ala—Ser—Glu—Asp—Glu—Ala—Gly—Asn┘
        Bovine                 —Glu—       —Ser—
        Ovine                  —Gln—       —Ser—
        Porcine                —Glu—       —Leu—
```

Figure 5.8 Comparative primary structures of the adrenocorticotropins.

one or two residue differences (at position 31 and 33) between any two species (Fig. 5.8). A shark (*Squalus acanthias*) corticotropin is also 39 amino acids long but differs at 11 positions from the human hormone. Ostrich (*Struthio camelus*) ACTH is similar in length to other corticotropins and differs from human ACTH at only five residues. The synthesis of a biologically active nonadecapeptide, corresponding to the first 19 amino-terminal residues of ACTH, and the subsequent total synthesis of the porcine ACTH were landmarks in the field of peptide hormone synthesis. $ACTH_{1-24}$ is commercially available and is the form generally used for studies on ACTH action, as the biological activity resides within this invariant 1–24 sequence of the hormone.

As its name implies, the major role of ACTH is to stimulate steroid biosynthesis within adrenal steroidogenic tissue. Cortisol and corticosterone are the major glucocorticoids produced by the adrenal gland in response to ACTH stimulation. These steroid hormones are important in carbohydrate metabolism. Excessive secretion of ACTH in humans leads to Cushing's disease (syndrome), which is characterized by excessive plasma levels of cortisol and, therefore, pathological alterations in glucose metabolism. The absence or diminished secretion of ACTH results in Addison's disease, a disorder characterized by deficits in cortisol production with severe consequences on cellular metabolism. Because the first 13 amino acids are similar to those comprising α-MSH, it is not surprising that ACTH possesses considerable melanotropic activity. Nevertheless there is no evidence that ACTH plays any normal role in the control of integumental melanocyte function. On the other hand, in primary Addison's disease and in Cushing's syndrome of secondary origin, where ACTH is secreted in excessive amounts, hyperpigmentation is also a visually obvious symptom, a so-called "cardinal symptom" of the disease. In these diseases the hyperpigmentation is probably due to the excessive levels of circulating ACTH. The heptapeptide sequence, -Met-Glu-His-Phe-Arg-Trp-Gly-, an active sequence of α-MSH, is mainly responsible for the melanotropic activity of ACTH. In some species ACTH also possesses lipolytic activity, an action shared by other melanotropins. It is doubtful, however, whether this so-called adipokinetic action represents a physiological role of the hormone. Corticotropin is also localized to certain neurons within the brain, where it may function as a neuropeptide in processes related to memory and learning.

Melanocyte Stimulating Hormone. The pars intermedia is the source of a melanocyte-stimulating hormone (α-MSH, α-melanotropin). The pituitary gland of the adult human lacks a pars intermedia, and this is correlated with the absence of α-MSH in the pituitary and plasma in humans. α-Melanotropin is present in the pituitary of other vertebrates and plays an important role in the skin coloration of many animals. α-MSH is composed of 13 amino acids (see Fig. 8.1). The physiological roles of α-melanotropin are discussed in detail in Chap. 8.

Neurohypophysial Hormones

Two nonapeptides, oxytocin and arginine vasopressin (AVP), are present in the neurohypophysis of humans. Each of these hormones is separately synthesized in different neurohypophysial neurons. Each neurohypophysial hormone is derived from a prohormone, oxyphysin or pressophysin, synthesized in cell bodies located within the paired paraventricular and supraoptic nuclei, respectively, of the hypothalamus (Fig. 5.5). Oxytocin- and AVP-containing vesicles travel from the sites of synthesis within the hypothalamic nuclei by axoplasmic flow to axon terminals within the pars nervosa, where they are stored until released.

The neurohypophysial hormones are released into the circulation to travel to their distant target tissues. Oxytocin plays an instrumental role in stimulating milk release from the mammary gland through an action on contractile elements (myoepithelial cells) of the breasts. Oxytocin also stimulates uterine contraction at term and therefore provides a major endocrine stimulus to the process of parturition. Vasopressin plays an essential role in water retention (and therefore blood pressure) by its action on the collecting tubules of the kidney. Two or more neurohypophysial hormones are present in the neurohypophysis of each vertebrate species except cyclostomes (lampreys and hagfishes), which possess but a single such principle, arginine vasotocin (AVT). The structures of the individual neurohypophysial hormones (oxytocin, lysine and arginine vasopressin, vasotocin, mesotocin, isotocin, and others) have been determined from a number of species (see Table 7.1) and the possible pathways of their structural evolution described. The roles and actions of the neurohypophysial hormones are discussed in Chap. 7.

PITUITARY PATHOPHYSIOLOGY

Pituitary dysfunction may involve undersecretion or oversecretion of one or more hypophysial hormones. Table 5.2 summarizes the major physiological defects related to the pathophysiology of the pituitary gland (also see Chap. 21). Hyposecretion of pituitary hormones may result from destruction of normal glandular cells within the pituitary by an expanding tumor, disruption of hypothalamo-pituitary vascular connections, or damage or disease of the hypothalamus. Hypersecretion, on the other hand, may result from neoplasia (pituitary tumors) or from hypertrophy and hyperplasia, resulting from enhanced hypothalamic stimulation of the pituitary. Hypersecretion of α-MSH or PRL could result, plausibly, from loss of a tonic hypothalamic inhibitory input to the pituitary (see Chap. 6).

Panhypopituitarism, which involves total loss of hypophysial hormone secretion, could be due to a congenital dysfunction—failure of the pituitary to develop—or to destruction of the pituitary at a later stage in life. It is also possible that the pars distalis might fail to secrete only one of its many hormones. Hypopituitary (pituitarigenic) dwarfism may result, for example, from the specific failure of the pituitary to secrete GH. Currently, somatotropin is being used in medicine to stimulate growth in GH-deficient patients. Recombinant human GH is quite effective in permitting children to attain normal growth. Its development and application, therefore, have been significant advances in medicine. In the future GH may be used clinically for a wide variety of other applications, such as aiding wound healing, repartitioning fat into muscle, reversing certain aspects of aging, and immunopotentiation in conjunction with vaccines. There is evidence, however, that GH promotes the proliferation of certain types of transformed cells. Furthermore, immunoreactive GH can be found in prostatic tumors, and GH can be elevated in human cancer patients. Other health concerns about the use of growth hormone have been raised, ranging from diabetes to hypertension. Although the use of GH appears to be safe and is actually improving the quality of life for some patients, its use must be monitored to learn whether it causes any significant long-term side effects.

Microadenomas may be responsible for the excess secretion of a particular pituitary hormone. Microadenomas composed of PRL-secreting cells are the most common pituitary neoplasms of rats and humans [33]. Although some patients may have very high levels of serum PRL, not all develop galactorrhea. Other hormones, such as estrogens

TABLE 5.2 Some Examples of Pituitary Pathophysiology

Hormone	Etiology	Symptom
All hormones	No pituitary hormones (empty sella syndrome)	Panhypopituitarism
Somatotropin (STH) *(GH)*	Deficiency (childhood)	Dwarfism
	Excess	
	child	Gigantism
	adult	Acromegaly
Prolactin (PRL)	Deficiency	No disease states reported
	Excess	Hyperprolactinemia: galactorrhea-amenorrhea syndrome
Thyrotropin (TSH)	Deficiency	
	child	Hypothyroidism (cretinism) ✔
	adult	Hypothyroidism (myxedema) ✔
	Excess	Hyperthyroidism (thyrotoxicosis, Graves' disease)
Follitropin (FSH)	Deficiency	Hypogonadism: failure of germ cell maturation
	Excess	No information available
Lutropin (LH)	Deficiency	Hypogonadism: failure of sexual maturation
	Excess	No information available
Corticotropin (ACTH)	Deficiency	Addison's disease
	Excess	Cushing's disease/syndrome (hypercortisolism)
Oxytocin	Deficiency	No information available (necessary for milk secretion)
	Excess	No disease states reported
Vasopressin (AVP, ADH)	Deficiency	Diabetes insipidus (excessive water loss, dehydration)
	Excess	Syndrome of inappropriate ADH secretion (hypertension)

and corticosteroids, along with PRL, are responsible for stimulation of lactogenesis. Amenorrhea, anovulation, and galactorrhea are all common sequelae of excess PRL secretion, and hypogonadism occurs in many hyperprolactinemic adult females. Hypersecretion of PRL is inhibitory to pituitary gonadotropin secretion, which accounts for the loss of gonadal function associated with the galactorrhea-amenorrhea syndrome. If PRL-secreting adenomas are selectively removed by surgical techniques, normal menses return. The pivotal role of PRL in mammary gland growth and differentiation is well established. In addition there is substantial evidence that PRL is a causative factor in mammary gland neoplasia of rodents and possibly of humans. There is evidence that PRL, in conjunction with sex steroids, contributes to accelerated malignant mammary growth as indicated by the more fulminant course of breast cancer during pregnancy.

There are no reported examples of overproduction or underproduction of oxytocin. Vasopressin may, however, be excessively secreted or not secreted at all. In the Brattleboro strain of rats, for example, the animals do not secrete any vasopressin, and this defect is correlated with an absence of AVP within neurons of the neurohypophysis. In the syndrome of inappropriate ADH (AVP) secretion, excess amounts of AVP are secreted without relationship to plasma osmolality (Chap. 7). A common cause of excessive AVP secretion is malignancy, where AVP is secreted ectopically from a carcinoma of the lung.

Although excess secretion of pituitary hormones may result from a defect at the pituitary or hypothalamic level, pituitary hormones may be secreted by tumors of nonpituitary origin. Thus *ectopic* production of excessive amounts of ACTH by certain lung tumors may be responsible for the etiology of Cushing's syndrome, where the adrenal cortex releases excessive amounts of cortisol in response to the ACTH of ectopic tumor origin. Elevated plasma levels of β-LPH and ACTH are frequently observed in blood and tumor tissue of patients with various types of carcinoma. Because β-LPH and ACTH are components of a larger POMC precursor, it is not surprising that these peptides are elaborated by neoplastic tissues.

Tumors of patients with acromegaly may secrete GH and PRL, which suggests that these tumors may represent mixed adenomas. There is no evidence that a common pituitary stem cell persists beyond the prenatal period. When more than one hormone is found within a certain tumor, they are usually those most related structurally, that is, PRL and GH, or TSH, FSH, and LH. During the induction and progression of pituitary neoplasms, secretion of more than one hypophysial hormone is common. Ectopic secretion of PRL occurs from cancers of nonhypophysial origin (e.g., bronchogenic or nephrogenic sources). The molecular basis of pituitary hormone under- or over-secretion are being increasingly better understood [8, 21, 22, 23].

REFERENCES

[1]   Beebe, J. S., J. R. Huth, and R. W. Ruddon. 1990. Combination of the chorionic gonadotropin free beta subunit with alpha. *Endocrinology* 126:384–91.

[2]   Beebe, J. S., K. Mountjoy, R. F. Krzesicki, F. Perini, and R. W. Ruddon. 1990. Role of disulfide bond formation in the folding of human chorionic gonadotropin beta subunit into an alpha beta dimer assembly-competent form. *J. Biol. Chem.* 265:32–7.

[3]   Bergland, R. M., and R. B. Page. 1979. Pituitary-brain vascular relations: a new paradigm. *Science* 204:18–24.

[4]   Castrucci, A. M. L., M. E. Hadley, M. Lebl, C. Zechel, and V. J. Hruby. 1989. Melanocyte stimulating hormone (MSH) and melanin concentrating hormone (MCH) may be structurally and evolutionarily related. *Reg. Pept.* 24:27–35.

[5]   Childs, G. Y. 1992. Structure-function correlates in the corticotropes of the anterior pituitary. *Front. Neuroendocrinol.* 3:271–317.

[6]   Combarnous, Y. 1988. Structure and structure-function relationships in gonadotropins. *Reprod. Nutr. Develop.* 23:211–28.

[7]   ———. 1992. Molecular basis of the specificity of binding of glycoprotein hormones to their receptors. *Endocr. Rev.* 13:670–91.

[8]   Davis, J. R. E., and N. Hoggard. 1993. Towards the pathogenesis of human pituitary tumours. *J. Endocrinol.* 136:3–6.

[9]   De Gennaro Colonna, V., S. G. Cella, V. Locatelli, S. Loche, E. Ghigo, D. Cocchi, and E. E. Muller. 1989. Neuroendocrine control of growth hormone secretion. *Acta Paediatr. Scand.* 349:87–92.

[10]   Dubois, P. M., and F. J. Hemming. 1991. Fetal development and regulation of pituitary cell types. *J. Electron Microscopy Technique* 19:2–20.

[11]   Frantz, A. G. 1978. Prolactin. *New Engl. J. Med.* 298:201–7.

[12]   Green, J. D. 1951. The comparative anatomy of the hypophysis with special reference to its blood supply and innervation. *Amer. J. Anat.* 88:225–311.

[13]   Greep, R. O. 1974. History of research on anterior hypophysial hormones. In *Handbook of physiology,* sec. 7, vol. 4, part 2, eds. R. O. Greep and E. B. Astwood, pp. 1–27. Washington, D.C.: Am. Physiological Soc.

[14]   Guillemin, R., and R. Burgus. 1972. The hormones of the hypothalamus. *Sci. Amer.* 227:24–33.

[15]   Holmes, R. L., and J. N. Ball. 1974. *The pituitary gland.* Cambridge, England: Cambridge Univ. Press.

[16]   Jaffe, R. B., ed. 1981. *Prolactin.* New York: Elsevier North-Holland, Inc.

[17]   Matzuk, M. M., C. M. Kornmeier, G. K. Whitfield, I. A. Kourides, and I. Boime. 1988. The glycoprotein α-subunit is critical for secretion and stability of the human thyrotropin β-subunit. *Mol. Endocrinol.* 2:95–100.

[18] Miyajima, K., A. Yasuda, P. Swanson, H. Kawauchi, H. Cook, T. Kaneko, R. E. Peter, S. Suzuki, S. Hasegawa, and T. Hirano. 1988. Isolation and characterization of carp prolactin. *Gen. Comp. Endocrinol.* 70:407–17.

[19] Moore, K. L. 1973. *The developing human.* Philadelphia: W. B. Saunders Company.

[20] Omeljaniuk, R. J., H. R. Habbi, and R. E. Peter. 1989. Alterations in pituitary GnRH and dopamine receptors associated with the seasonal variation and regulation of gonadotropin release in the goldfish (*Carassius auratus*). *Gen. Comp. Endocrinol.* 74:39–99.

[21] Parks, J. S, E.-I. Kinoshita, and R. W. Pfaffle. 1993. Pit-1 and hypopituitarism. *TEM* 4:81–5.

[22] Pfaffle, R. W., G. E. Dimattia, J. S. Parks, M. R. Brown, J. M. Wit, M. Jansen, H. Vander Nat, J. L. Van Den Brande, M. G. Rosenfield, and H. A. Ingraham. 1992. Mutation in the POU-specific domain of Pit-1 and hypopituitarism without pituitary hypoplasia. *Science* 257:1118–21.

[23] Radovick, S., M. Nations, Y. Du, L. A. Berg, B. D. Weintraub, and F. E. Wondisford. 1992. A mutation in the POU-homeodomain of Pit-1 responsible for combined pituitary hormone deficiency. *Science* 257:115–8.

[24] Riddle, O., R. W. Bates, and S. W. Dykshorn. 1933. The preparation, identification and assay of prolactin—a hormone of anterior pituitary. *Amer. J. Physiol.* 105:191–216.

[25] Sano, T., S. L. Asa, and K. Kovacs. 1988. Growth hormone-releasing hormone-producing tumors: clinical, biochemical, and morphological manifestations. *Endocr. Rev.* 9:357–73.

[26] Semoff, S., and M. E. Hadley. 1978. Localization of ATPase activity to the glial-like cells of the pars intermedia. *Gen. Comp. Endocrinol.* 35:329–41.

[27] Shome, B., A. F. Parlow, W-K Liu, H. S. Nahm, T. Wen, and D. N. Ward. 1988. A reevaluation of the amino acid sequence of human follitropin β-subunit. *J. Protein Chem.* 7:325–39.

[28] Slater, E. P., J. D. Baxter, and N. L. Eberhardt. 1986. Evolution of the growth hormone gene family. *Amer. Zool.* 26:939–49.

[29] Smith, P. L., and J. U. Baenziger. 1988. A pituitary N-acetylgalactosamine transferase that specifically recognizes glycoprotein hormones. *Science* 242:930–2.

[30] Tannenbaum, G. S. 1988 Somatostatin as a physiological regulator of pulsatile growth hormone secretion. *Horm. Res.* 29:70–74.

[31] Tixier-Vidal, A., and M. G. Farquhar, eds. 1975. *The anterior pituitary.* New York: Academic Press, Inc.

[32] Tsubokawa, M., K. Muramoto, and H. Kawauchi. 1985. Primary structure of fin whale prolactin. *Int. J. Pept. Protein Res.* 25:442–48.

[33] Vance, M. L., and M. O. Thorner. 1987. Prolactinomas. *Endocrinol. Metab. Clin. N. Amer.* 16:731–53.

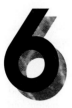

The Endocrine Hypothalamus

In the embryonic development of the pituitary gland, ectoderm from the oral cavity and neuroectoderm from the brain evaginate and move toward each other to form the pituitary gland. There must be some physiological significance that these two different tissues have become integrated into one functional glandular component. As we have noted (see Chap. 5) the pituitary gland is a rich source of hormones that controls a variety of physiological functions. Adrenocorticotropin secretion exhibits a diurnal (daily) rhythm; it is also released in response to a variety of stresses. FSH and LH secretion fluctuates in a predictable pattern throughout the female ovarian cycle and, midway through the cycle, there is a pulsatile burst of LH release that is responsible for initiating ovulation. Oxytocin is released from the pituitary in response to suckling or sometimes during coitus. Pituitary somatotropin (growth hormone) is secreted due to the ingestion of certain metabolic substrates.

Pituitary hormone secretions are clearly adaptive in nature, as hormones play essential roles under conditions of special need. For example, the reproductive cycles of many animals are linked to seasonal changes in day length. The pelage color of the weasel is white in winter and brown the rest of the year. The weasel's coat color is regulated by pituitary melanocyte-stimulating hormone. What are the cues that dictate whether or not a particular pituitary hormone will be secreted? Metabolic substrates, such as glucose, fatty acids, and amino acids, might serve as intrinsic cues to inform the pituitary of circulating levels of these substrates. But in vitro studies reveal that the pituitary is not directly sensitive to these substrates. Cold temperature is a stimulus to TSH secretion, and day length affects pituitary gonadotropin secretion. Obviously these extrinsic stimuli must be initially intercepted by the nervous system. A vast body of experimental data supports the view that the control of secretion of each of the pituitary hormones is regulated by the brain. This would explain the embryological processes related to the early development of the pituitary. In this chapter the evidence for a central nervous system control of pituitary function is reviewed, and the specific roles of the **hypophysiotropic** *hormones that control pituitary hormone secretion are explained.*

THE NEUROVASCULAR HYPOTHESIS

Removal of the pituitary gland leads to atrophy of the adrenal cortex, thyroid, and gonads. Transplantation of the pituitary to an ectopic site in an animal, such as in the eye or under the kidney capsule, leads to a similar end-organ atrophy. Transplantation of the pituitary back under the hypothalamus, however, is followed by revascularization and functional reactivation of the pituitary. Transection of the pituitary stalk or placement of a barrier between the hypothalamus and the pituitary leads to atrophy of the pituitary and its target organs. Subsequent revascularization of the pituitary leads to functional reactivation of the gland and its target organs. From these observations Harris concluded that it is "difficult to escape from the conclusion that the hypophysial portal supply has some specific effect in activating anterior pituitary tissue" [20]. Transplantation of pituitary tissue from young rats under the pituitary stalk of adult female rats resulted in the recurrence of normal, regular estrus cycles at a time when the donor young were still immature. The onset of pituitary-gonadotropic activity, it was concluded, probably depends on a hypothalamic influence rather than a maturation of pituitary or ovarian tissues. Even a pituitary from a young male animal could reactivate the pituitary-gonadal axis when transplanted into a female. According to Harris, the anterior pituitary tissue is plastic in nature and "its pattern of secretory activity is not due to any intrinsic property of the tissue itself, but to some outside 'drive' or stimulus, derived probably from the central nervous system."

These observations led Harris to elaborate the *neurovascular hypothesis*. He suggested that humoral factors released by the hypothalamus were carried by the portal blood vessels to the pituitary to regulate hormone secretion. Extracts of the brain, specifically of the hypothalamus, will stimulate or inhibit secretion from the pituitary whether studied in vivo or in vitro. Lesions of specific areas of the hypothalamus, as induced by electrocautery, lead to specific defects in pituitary hormone secretion. Electrode stimulation of these same anatomical sites within the hypothalamus, on the other hand, leads to the release of a particular pituitary hormone.

Crude extracts of the hypothalamus provided early evidence that the hypothalamus contained factors inhibitory or stimulatory to pituitary hormone secretions. These extracts were further purified to yield subfractions that by bioassay inhibited somatotropin release or stimulated thyrotropin or gonadotropin secretion. Still further purification and physical methods of analysis provided information on the definitive structures of the so-called *hypophysiotropic factors* present in these extracts. The data from these studies have revolutionized the field of endocrinology [17, 26, 28].

STRUCTURE-FUNCTION OF THE ENDOCRINE HYPOTHALAMUS

The hypothalamus is the basal part of the diencephalon lying below the thalamus, as its name implies [44]. The hypothalamus forms the walls and lower part of the third ventricle of the brain (Fig. 6.1). It includes the optic chiasm, the tuber cinereum, the infundibulum, and the mammillary bodies. The tuber cinereum is the part of the third ventricle floor that extends downward toward the infundibulum. The lower part of the tuber cinereum, which is richly supplied with blood vessels that drain into the pituitary stalk and then in turn empty into a secondary plexus in the anterior pituitary, is referred to as the *median eminence*. The vascular link between the median eminence and the pituitary gland is known as the *hypophysial portal system* (Fig. 6.2). Within the hypothalamus are clusters of neurons, *hypothalamic nuclei*, which are symmetrically located around the third ventricle. The supraoptic nuclei (SON) and paraventricular nuclei (PVN), for example, are composed of cell bodies whose axons extend into the median eminence and then into the neurohypophysis (see Fig. 5.5). This particular nerve tract, consisting of neuronal axons from the SON and PVN, is the *supraopticoparaventriculohypophysial tract*. Other major nuclear groups within the hypothalamus include the ventromedial nuclei, arcuate nucleus, lateral tuberal nuclei, and dorsomedial nuclei (Fig. 6.1).

The endocrine hypothalamus consists of *neurosecretory neurons* whose secretory activity provides the neurohormones (hypophysiotropic factors) that regulate adenohypophysial function [6]. These neurons are the elements of the *parvocellular* (from the Latin *parvus* or small) *neurosecretory system* and are distinguished from the *magnocellular*

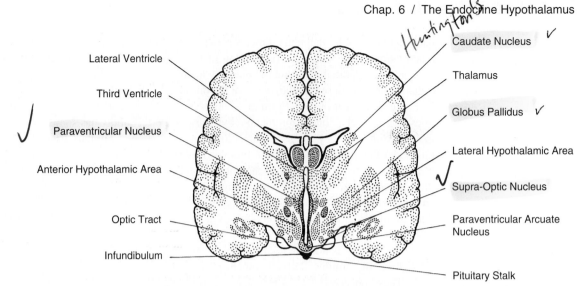

Huntingtons

Lateral Ventricle

Third Ventricle

Paraventricular Nucleus

Anterior Hypothalamic Area

Optic Tract

Infundibulum

Caudate Nucleus

Thalamus

Globus Pallidus

Lateral Hypothalamic Area

Supra-Optic Nucleus

Paraventricular Arcuate Nucleus

Pituitary Stalk

Figure 6.1 Frontal section through the cerebral hemispheres of the human brain, the principal hypothalamic nuclei present within the plane of transect are indicated.

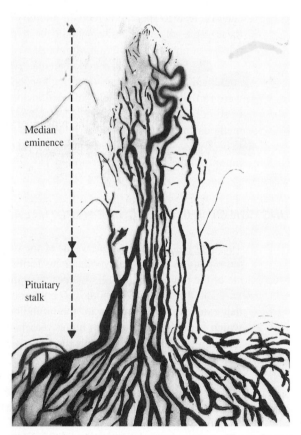

Median eminence

Pituitary stalk

Figure 6.2 Hypophysial portal system. (From Porter et al. [36], with permission.)

system of neurosecretory neurons that compose the supraoptic and paraventricular neurons that synthesize oxytocin and vasopressin. The neurons of the parvocellular neurosecretory system converge toward the pituitary stalk to form the *tuberoinfundibular tract*. These neurons abut on the endothelium of the primary plexus of the portal system of the median eminence. Immunocytochemical methods have demonstrated hypophysiotropic factors (hypophysiotropins) within these neurons [27]. Electron microscopic studies provide evidence that these cells release their chemical messengers into the hypophysial portal system.

When pieces of pituitary tissue were grafted into various regions of the basal forebrain of rats, the *medial basal hypothalamus* (MBH) was capable of maintaining the normal structure and function of the pituitary grafts. Therefore, the MBH was named the *hypophysiotropic area* [19]. Apparently the integrity and secretory activity of pituitary cells implanted within this area is due to the local release of hypophysiotropins from the parvocellular neurons. The hypophysiotropic area extends from the median eminence upward and forward, through the anterior hypothalamus, to the suprachiasmatic region.

The endocrine hypothalamus is connected to the rest of the central nervous system by synaptic contacts from other neuronal elements. Information flow from other brain centers is relayed to hypothalamic parvocellular neurons, which then secrete their hypophysiotropins into the pituitary portal vasculature of the median eminence. The median eminence therefore can be considered the final point of convergence of the CNS upon the peripheral endocrine system. The hypophysial portal system provides a restricted vascular link between the neurosecretory cells of the hypothalamus and the anterior pituitary gland.

The most rigid proof that the hypothalamus does indeed release hormones into the hypophysial portal system to regulate pituitary function would be the demonstration that such hormones are found in the portal vessels in higher concentrations than in the systemic circulation. Elegant methods involving cannulation of the hypophysial portal system and selective collection of portal blood have verified this thesis (Fig. 6.3) [34, 36, 37]. Each of the hypophysiotropins has been demonstrated within portal blood; the concentration of these hormones is increased after stimulation of certain hypothalamic sites. In addition, infusion of hypophysiotropins by portal cannulation induces secretion of pituitary hormones.

To determine the functional relationship of the medial basal hypothalamus to the rest of the brain, a knife was designed by Halász and colleagues to cut all the neural connections between the MBH and the remainder of the forebrain. This knife left the MBH in continuity with the pituitary gland and supposedly left most of the blood supply to the MBH and the pituitary intact. Nevertheless, the hypophysiotropic area remained almost fully functional after this hypothalamic deafferentation. This suggests that the cells of origin of the hypophysiotropins reside mostly, if not entirely, within the MBH [19].

The importance of hypothalamic humoral factors in the control of pituitary function was uniquely demonstrated by ectopic transplantation of the adenohypophysis under the kidney capsule [11]. Although the adenohypophysis becomes well vascularized in this site, most of the gland atrophies due to generalized hypoactivity of most cellular elements of the

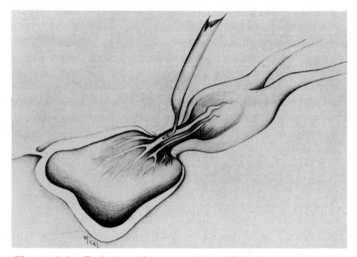

Figure 6.3 Technique for cannulation of the hypophysial portal system. (From Porter et al. [36], with permission.)

gland. The lactotrophs, however, become hypertropic and hyperplastic (increase in size and cell number). The systemic effects of adenohypophysial inactivity include end-organ atrophy of the gonads, adrenals, and thyroid gland. On the other hand, there is "functional reactivation and cytological restoration of pituitary grafts by continuous local intravascular infusion of median eminence extracts." It was concluded that hypothalamic humoral factors of median eminence origin control the structure and function of the pituitary gland.

THE HYPOPHYSIOTROPIC HORMONES

GnRH

TRH
GIH
CRH

vasopressin
son

Stimulatory and inhibitory factors of hypothalamic origin are implicated in the control of pituitary hormone secretion as previously discussed [42]. There is overwhelming evidence for a gonadotropin-releasing hormone, thyrotropin-releasing hormone, somatotropin release-inhibiting hormone, corticotropin-releasing hormone and PRL and MSH release-inhibiting hormones. There is less information available relative to the existence of putative PRL- and MSH-releasing factors. In many cases the distribution of hypophysiotropins within the CNS has been determined by RIA of brain tissue. Brain tissue can be cut in a rostral-caudal direction, as well as laterally from side to side, to provide a series of tissue slices. A small, round (Palkovits) punch is used to obtain small samples of tissue from the brain slices. By RIA one can determine the concentration of hypophysiotropins within these punch biopsies and then map the distribution of the neuropeptides within the brain. Using immunohistochemical methods involving antibodies against neuropeptides, one can also localize hypophysiotropins to specific neurons within the brain.

Thyrotropin-releasing Hormone (TRH)

The structure of the hypothalamic hormone-controlling TSH secretion was determined in 1969 independently by Guillemin and Schally and their colleagues. For this monumental work and the elucidation of the structures of the growth hormone release-inhibiting hormone (somatostatin) and the gonadotropin-releasing hormone (GnRH), they received a Nobel Prize in Physiology/Medicine. The task of elucidating the structure of TRH was not easy, but its eventual determination provided important insights into present-day methods of endocrine research. The episodes relating to the so-called race to Stockholm have been dramatically described [50].

NH$_2$–His–Pro–Glu–OH
NH$_2$–Pro–Glu–His–OH
NH$_2$–Pro–His–Glu–OH
NH$_2$–His–Glu–Pro–OH
NH$_2$–Glu–Pro–His–OH
NH$_2$–Glu–His–Pro–OH

(pyro)–Glu–His–Pro–NH$_2$

Figure 6.4 Six synthetic peptides related to thyrotropin-releasing hormone (TRH).

From about 25,000 ovine and porcine hypothalamic fragments, about 1 mg of TRH was obtained. These purified preparations, extremely potent in stimulating TSH release from the pituitary, both in vivo and in vitro, consisted of a simple peptide composed of three amino acids: glutamic acid, histidine, and proline in equimolar ratios. What was the exact sequence of the amino acids in the peptide? There was not enough material left to answer this essential question. It was decided, therefore, to synthesize the six possible putative isomers of the peptide (Fig. 6.4). Most surprisingly, none of the tripeptides possessed the chromatographic or biologic characteristics of TRH. It was discovered that there was no free N-terminal amino group in the natural tripeptide; in other words, the amino terminal group was protected in some way. The peptides were then treated with acetic anhydride in an effort to protect the NH$_2$-terminus, as in the natural TRH that lacked a free NH$_2$ group (Fig. 6.5). Only one of the peptides, Glu-His-Pro-OH, possessed biological activity, that was, however, lower than that of the natural TRH. This product proved to be pyro-Glu-His-Pro-OH. The α-amino group of glutamic acid had condensed with the carboxyl group of the glutamic acid to give the pyroglutamic acid form of the peptide. This structure, however, was not identical to natural TRH, which was more basic in nature. A more basic, less acidic compound could be obtained by protecting the free carboxyl group of the proline. Amidation of the C-terminal proline then yielded pyro-Glu-His-Pro-NH$_2$, whose activity was indistinguishable from that of natural TRH (Fig. 6.5). The structures of porcine, ovine, bovine, and human TRH proved to be identical. The

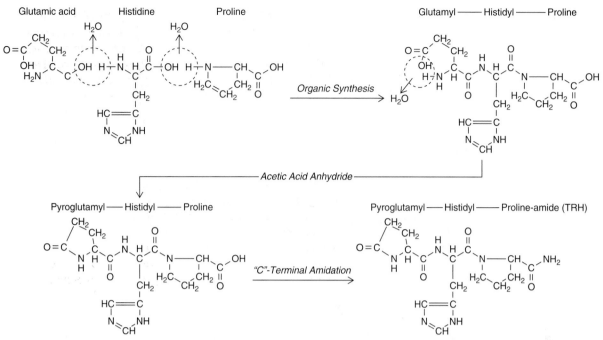

Figure 6.5 Synthesis of thyrotropin-releasing hormone.

arduous task just outlined for determining the structure of TRH illustrates the important contributions of chemistry to the emerging field of neuroendocrinology.

The mode of TRH biosynthesis in the mammalian brain is by post-translational cleavage of a larger precursor protein. Processing proTRH yields several copies of the biologically active peptide. Only the repeated TRH coding units dispersed throughout the precursor are maintained between amphibian and mammalian prohormones. Conservation of this pattern throughout evolution suggests that the ability of a precursor to generate multiple bioactive peptides may be an important mechanism in the amplification of hormone production [26].

TRH immunoactive cell bodies have been localized within the brain. The highest concentration of TRH cells is found in the medial part of the external layer of the median eminence and extends laterally, with high numbers also found in the pituitary stalk. Electrical stimulation of the medial basal hypothalamus of the rat elevates plasma TRH levels, suggesting that there are neural structures within the hypothalamus that release preformed TRH.

TRH also stimulates the release of PRL in humans, cattle, sheep, and rats. TRH stimulates GH secretion in cattle and rats under certain specific conditions and in humans with acromegaly or chronic renal insufficiency. It is not known whether the TRH effect on PRL and GH secretion is physiological. TRH is rapidly degraded by plasma of adult rats, but not by plasma from young (4- to 16-day-old) rats. The development of an active peptidase in rat plasma suggests that this may represent the physiological mechanism for the inactivation of TRH.

Although TRH is present in the CNS of teleosts, this tripeptide has not been clearly demonstrated to have hypophysiotropic activity in fishes. TRH can be detected in neural tissues of most classes of vertebrates, but its ability to promote TSH release is less universal than its occurrence. TRH has been shown to cause PRL release by the adenohypophysis of all tetrapod groups, as well as teleosts and birds. The ability of TRH to stimulate TSH release, on the other hand, appears to be restricted to homeotherms. The ability of thyrotrophs to respond to TRH may be a recent evolutionary acquisition relative to that of the lactotrophs. The TSH-releasing activity of the tripeptide may have emerged coincident with homeothermy.

Ala–Gly–Cys–Lys–Asn–Phe–Phe–Trp–Lys–Thr–Phe–Thr–Ser–Cys

Figure 6.6   Primary structure of mammalian somatostatin.

The amphibian hypothalamus contains large amounts of TRH. In addition TRH circulates in the blood of the frog (*Rana pipiens*) and is present in the skin in concentrations twice those in the hypothalamus. Thus the role of TRH, like other hypothalamic peptides, may not be limited to the central nervous system. TRH is present in the larval lamprey (a cyclostome) and in the head end of amphioxus and has even been localized to the circumesophageal ganglia of a snail. Because the lamprey lacks TSH and the snail and amphioxus a pituitary, it has been proposed that the TSH-regulating function of TRH may be a late evolutionary development, an example where an organism acquires a new function for a pre-existing hormone or chemical substance. In addition, TRH appears to regulate a variety of physiological processes in the CNS; the presence of the peptide in the brain does not, therefore, necessarily restrict its role to TSH secretion and thyroid function (see Chap. 21).

Somatostatin (Somatotropin Release-inhibiting Hormone) (SRIF)

Pituitary GH is secreted episodically in all species, including humans [13]. The pulsatile pattern of GH release from the pituitary gland is the net result of a delicate interplay between two hypothalamic hormones, a stimulatory, GH-releasing factor and a GH release-inhibiting hormone [45]. A hypothalamic peptide that inhibits the release of GH from the anterior pituitary was isolated and its primary sequence determined [28, 45]. This tetra-decapeptide, referred to as somatostatin (SRIF or somatotropin release-inhibiting hormone/factor), has been synthesized and has been determined to be chemically and biologically identical to the hypophysiotropic peptide (Fig. 6.6). The oxidized (ring) and the reduced (linear) forms of the peptide have full biological activity in vitro and in vivo.

Somatostatin has been localized to secretory granules of neurons located within the hypothalamus by electron microscopic immunohistochemistry. Although originally isolated from the hypothalamus, this peptide has been shown to have widespread effects on brain, endocrine and exocrine pancreas, and gut function [15]. Furthermore, SRIF has a widespread distribution in the CNS and is also found localized to the D cells of the gut and the endocrine pancreas. Somatostatin has an inhibitory effect on GH released in response to every known stimulus. The action of SRIF is directly on the pituitary somatotrophs.

A 28-residue prosomatostatin, a putative SRIF precursor from the porcine hypothalamus, has been isolated, chemically characterized, and its primary structure determined (Fig. 6.7). The last 14 amino acids of the precursor are identical in structure to SRIF. After synthesis it was found to be chemically and biologically identical to the prosomatostatin isolated from the brain and gut [41]. This peptide possesses high GH and PRL release-inhibiting activity and may, in time, be shown to be a hormone in its own right.

Somatostatin also inhibits TRH-induced TSH secretion but, at the same time, does not affect the concomitant secretion of PRL triggered by TRH. This suggests that the inhibitory action of SRIF is specifically on the thyrotrophs, not the lactotrophs. A physiologic inhibitory role for SRIF in TSH secretion regulation in some species is supported by

1   14
Ser–Ala–Asn–Ser–Asn–Pro–Ala–Met–Ala–Pro–Arg–Glu–Arg–Lys–

28
–Ala–Gly–Cys–Lys–Asn–Phe–Phe–Trp–Lys–Thr–Phe–Thr–Ser–Cys

Figure 6.7   Primary structure of porcine prosomatostatin.

5   10   15   20

Tyr–Ala–Asp–Ala–Ile–Phe–Thr–Asn–Ser–Tyr–Arg–Lys–Val–Leu–Gly–Gln–Leu–Ser–Ala–Arg–Lys–Leu⎤

25   30   35   40

⎣Leu–Gln–Asp–Ile–Met–Ser–Arg–Gln–Gln–Gly–Glu–Ser–Asn–Gln–Glu–Arg–Gly–Ala–Arg–Ala–Arg–Leu–NH$_2$

Figure 6.8 Primary structure of a somatotropin-releasing hormone (somatocrinin).

the demonstration that anti-SRIF serum administered to rats enhances the release of TSH due to cold or to exogenous TRH. Somatostatin lowers blood glucose levels, and this is associated with an inhibition of glucagon and insulin secretion. Other studies have shown that SRIF also inhibits secretion of the following: renin, parathormone, calcitonin, gastric HCl, acetylcholine, and adrenergic neurotransmitters. Plasma GH levels fall and remain low for several hours after stress. Administration of SRIF antiserum to rats prior to stress partially restores GH secretory pulses. These results indicate that somatostatin plays a role in stress-induced inhibition of GH secretion in the rat.

Somatostatin has been found in the brain and pancreas of the frog, catfish, torpedo (an elasmobranch), and hagfish (a cyclostome). It is also present in the skin and bladder of the frog. Incubation of pituitary glands of the teleost, tilapia (*Sarotherodon mossambicus*), in the presence of synthetic SRIF resulted in a dose-dependent decrease in GH secretion. These results suggest that GH secretion in teleosts may be controlled by SRIF or a SRIF-like peptide, indicating that this action of the molecule has been fully conserved throughout vertebrate evolution.

Somatocrinin (Growth Hormone-releasing Hormone) *44 AA*

A 44-amino-acid peptide was isolated from a human pancreatic tumor that specifically stimulated GH secretion, both in vitro and in vivo, from the rat pituitary gland (Fig. 6.8) [48]. The synthetic replicate had full biological activity and was similar in physicochemical properties to somatocrinin present in hypothalamic tissues [16, 38]. Somatocrinin (growth hormone-releasing hormone, GHRH) possesses sequence homologies to several gut peptides of the secretin-glucagon family of peptides [14]. Somatocrinin-like immunoreactivity has been found in hypothalamo-hypophysial regions of many mammals, amphibians, and a variety of teleost fishes. There is a high degree of sequence similarity in the first 29 residues of somatocrinin from various species. The 1–29 residues possess similar activity as the entire 1–44 sequence. The highly conserved bioactive core of the peptide therefore accounts for the lack of species specificity of the molecule [5].

Gonadotropin-releasing Hormone (GnRH)

A vast amount of experimental evidence has established that the hypothalamus regulates pituitary gonadotropin secretion [8]. GnRH has been detected in the nerve fibers and terminals in proximity to the portal vessels in the median eminence of the hypothalamus. The structure of GnRH was determined from extracts of 250,000 porcine hypothalami. The peptide was subsequently synthesized and found to act in an identical physiological manner to the putative hypothalamic peptide in all animals studied. Mammalian GnRH is a decapeptide whose primary structure appears to be similar between mammalian species (Fig. 6.9).

Deafferentation of the rat hypothalamus causes a marked reduction in the GnRH content of the MBH, which suggests that GnRH arises from, or is controlled by, cells elsewhere in the brain [18, 19]. GnRH has been found in higher concentrations in hypophysial portal blood than in the systemic circulation. Portal GnRH levels are elevated after castration and following electrochemical stimulation of the hypothalamus.

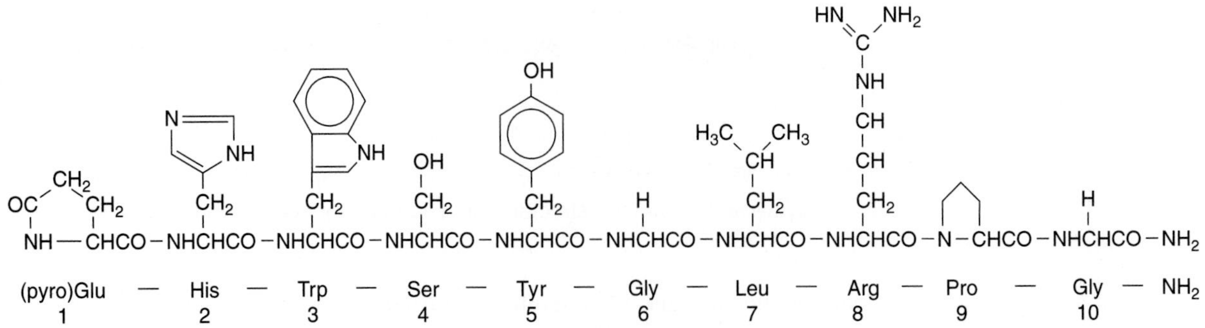

Figure 6.9 Primary structure of mammalian gonadotropin-releasing hormone (GnRH).

The role of GnRH in the control of pituitary gonadotropin secretion was further confirmed by the use of immunization techniques. Injections of antibodies to GnRH are followed by testicular atrophy. Similarly, when GnRH antiserum is injected into female rats on the morning of proestrus, the preovulatory surge of LH release that normally follows in the afternoon does not occur, and ovulation is prevented (see Chap. 18). Furthermore, administration of anti-GnRH serum to normal or castrated rats lowers LH and FSH levels, thus revealing the key role of the hypophysiotropin in maintaining the secretion of both gonadotropins.

In the intact rhesus monkey, GnRH appears to be released in a pulsatile manner [49]. Although intermittent administration of GnRH may be optimal for re-establishing gonadotropin secretion in monkeys with hypothalamic lesions, constant infusions of GnRH fail to do so. Constant GnRH administration may lead to a desensitization or down regulation of the processes responsible for gonadotropin release (see Chap. 18).

Both LH and FSH are synthesized within the same gonadotroph following stimulation with GnRH and modulation by gonadal hormones (steroids and polypeptides). The capacity to synthesize preferentially and secrete one gonadotropin differs in the different sizes of gonadotrophs and can be altered by prior exposure to stimuli or priming. The frequency of the GnRH stimulus may be the major regulator of the relative proportions of FSH and LH synthesized and secreted, with less frequent GnRH pulses leading to preferential FSH secretion and more frequent GnRH pulses to LH secretion. Within the gonadotroph, the rate at which the α and β subunits are synthesized is regulated by the amount of translatable mRNA, and the actual amount of β-subunit mRNA may be the rate-limiting step in gonadotropin synthesis [2].

Synthetic GnRH has significant gonadotropic activity in mammals, birds, and amphibians. In the amphibian, hypothalamic concentrations of GnRH vary with the seasonal reproductive cycle. A physiological role for GnRH has been demonstrated in teleosts. Because GnRH functions in the reproductive processes in mammals, the demonstration of the presence of the peptide in the brain of nonmammalian species need not restrict its function to only a reproductive role.

Multiple molecular forms of the peptide have evolved, but all bear striking structural similarity. The structures of seven different GnRHs have been determined (Fig. 6.10). Molecular biological studies have shown that human GnRH is identical with that of other mammals. Clearly, the forms of GnRH belong to a family of peptides that are structurally related. All the GnRH structures in vertebrates to date are decapeptides with at least 50% sequence identity [43]. Two GnRHs have been isolated from the chicken hypothalamus. The cGnRH II occurs together with a second form of GnRH in most vertebrate species. This implies that cGnRH II arose early in vertebrate evolution and has been conserved, presumably to play some important physiological role(s). The variable form of GnRH is predominant in the hypothalamus where it serves a role in regulating pituitary gonadotropin secretion. The more conserved cGnRH II is more prevalent in extrahypothalamic tissue where it may regulate diverse physiological functions [24].

	1	2	3	4	5	6	7	8	9	10
Mammal	pGlu	His	Trp	Ser	Tyr	Gly	Leu	Arg	Pro	Gly–NH₂
Chicken I	pGlu	His	Trp	Ser	Tyr	Gly	Leu	Gln	Pro	Gly–NH₂
Catfish	pGlu	His	Trp	Ser	His	Gly	Leu	Asn	Pro	Gly–NH₂
Chicken II	pGlu	His	Trp	Ser	His	Gly	Trp	Tyr	Pro	Gly–NH₂
Dogfish	pGlu	His	Trp	Ser	His	Gly	Trp	Leu	Pro	Gly–NH₂
Salmon	pGlu	His	Trp	Ser	Tyr	Gly	Trp	Leu	Pro	Gly–NH₂
Lamprey	pGlu	His	Tyr	Ser	Leu	Glu	Trp	Lys	Pro	Gly–NH₂

Figure 6.10 The primary structures of seven known forms of GnRH [24]. The amino acid residues that differ from the mammal appear enclosed here.

Corticotropin-releasing Hormone (CRH)

The first of the hypophysiotropic hormones to be investigated with great vigor was the putative corticotropin-releasing hormone (CRH) [40]. A peptide with high potency for stimulating the secretion of ACTH from cultured rat pituitaries was isolated from ovine hypothalami and synthesized [40]. The structure of this 41-residue peptide is shown (Fig 6.11) and is partially similar in structure to urotensin I, a peptide found within the spinal cord (urophysis) of certain teleost fishes. Antisera to ovine CRH significantly lowers ACTH levels in adrenalectomized rats, suggesting that an endogenous CRH plays a physiological role in regulating pituitary ACTH secretion [7].

Characterization of CRH from a number of species indicates that its structure is highly conserved; the molecules in humans and rats are identical and differ by seven amino acids from the bovine sequence and by only two amino acids from the porcine structure. CRH shares homologies with a number of peptides found in primitive vertebrates, suggesting a common primal precursor [47].

Prolactin Release-inhibiting Factor (PIF)

There is abundant evidence that PRL secretion from the pars distalis is under an inhibitory control by the hypothalamus. When female rat anterior pituitaries are autotransplanted to extracranial sites, they selectively maintain functional corpora lutea while the remainder of the ovary atrophies, as do the adrenals and thyroid gland [31, 32]. In the rat, PRL is required for functional activation of the corpora lutea and progesterone biosynthesis. These results demonstrate that PRL secretion continues uninterrupted, whereas FSH, LH, and other anterior pituitary hormones are discontinued following ectopic transplantation. If after being autotransplanted under the kidney capsule for a month, pituitaries are retransplanted back into close anatomical relationship with the median eminence, female rats return to normal cycling, which includes ovulation. If these recycling rats are mated, they will successfully carry litters to term.

Patients with pituitary stalk section or hypothalamic lesions also have elevated plasma levels of PRL. In the rat, electrolytic lesions in the median eminence result in a large

```
1                                                                        20
Ser–Gln–Glu–Pro–Pro–Ile–Ser–Leu–Asp–Leu–Thr–Phe–His–Leu–Leu–Arg–Glu–Val–Leu–Glu–Met ┐
                                                                                       │
                                                                                       │
          30                                          41                               │
└Thr–Lys–Ala–Asp–Gln–Leu–Ala–Gln–Gln–Ala–His–Ser–Asn–Arg–Lys–Leu–Leu–Asp–Ile–Ala–NH₂
```

Figure 6.11   Primary structure of a corticotropin-releasing hormone (CRH).

increase in PRL secretion. If anterior pituitary glands are incubated in vitro, PRL secretion commences immediately and continues uninterrupted almost indefinitely. Cytologically the lactotrophs hypertrophy under such conditions. None of the other hormones of the pars distalis is secreted and, with the exception of the lactotrophs, the other secretory elements of the glands atrophy and disappear from the incubated glands. Taken together, all these observations, both in vivo and in vitro, support the hypothesis that the hypothalamus is the source of a prolactin-inhibiting factor (PIF).

The evidence is overwhelming that this PIF is dopamine (DA). The presence of DA in hypophysial portal blood, as well as in the anterior pituitary gland, has been demonstrated. DA inhibits PRL secretion from pituitary glands incubated in vitro. In addition, apomorphine or ergot alkaloids (e. g., ergocryptine), known DA receptor agonists, are inhibitory to PRL secretion in vitro or in vivo. This inhibition by DA and related agonists can be antagonized by chlorpromazine, haloperidol, and other DA receptor antagonists. Injections of DA receptor antagonists result in increased PRL secretion. On the other hand, injections of levodopa, a substrate for DA biosynthesis, are inhibitory to PRL secretion. Bromocriptine, a long-acting dopamine receptor agonist, is highly effective in reducing serum PRL levels in over 90% of patients with hyperprolactinemia, regardless of etiology. This drug has also been found to reduce the size of many prolactinomas.

Prolactin-releasing Factor (PRF)

There is some experimental evidence for the existence of a PRL-releasing factor. TRH, for example, is a potent stimulus to PRL secretion in virtually every vertebrate species studied [26]. It is unclear, however, whether TRH is the physiological PRF; there is evidence for a PRF of hypothalamic origin that is not TRH.

MSH Release-inhibiting Factor (MIF)

The role of the pars intermedia as the source of a melanotropin (α-MSH) that regulates color change in many animals is well established (see Chap. 8). Like PRL, MSH is under an inhibitory control by the hypothalamus. Stalk transection or damage to the hypothalamus results in enhanced MSH secretion. Transplantation of the pars intermedia to an ectopic site in the animal also leads to enhanced MSH secretion. In addition incubation of neurointermediate lobes in vivo results in a sustained secretion of MSH. These results suggest that the hypothalamus exerts a tonic inhibitory control of MSH secretion.

What is the mechanism by which the hypothalamus tonically represses MSH secretion? In many vertebrates (e.g., frog and mouse) the pars intermedia is penetrated by aminergic neurons whose cell bodies are located within the hypothalamus. The axons of these neurons form a plexus around and between the pars intermedia cells. The release of a neurotransmitter, most likely DA, from these neurons is apparently responsible for inhibition of MSH secretion. In vitro, DA is inhibitory of MSH secretion from isolated pituitary glands (see Chap. 8). Present evidence suggests that DA is the physiological MSH release-inhibiting factor (MIF, melanostatin). There is minimal evidence for the existence of any putative hypothalamic MSH-releasing factor (MRF) of peptidergic nature. In some species serotonin may be a factor regulating pars intermedia MSH secretion (see Chap. 8).

CONTROL OF HYPOTHALAMIC/HYPOPHYSIAL HORMONE SECRETION

In response to cold many mammals release TSH, and in response to stress ACTH is secreted from the pituitary gland. Suckling of the mammary glands stimulates PRL and oxytocin secretion, and GH is released in response to intake of certain dietary metabolic sub-

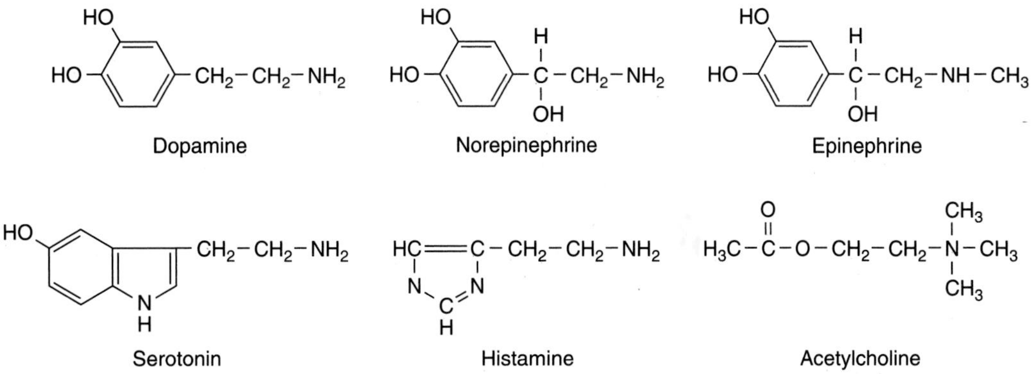

Figure 6.12   The monoamine neurotransmitters.

strates. These pituitary responses are regulated by hypophysiotropic factors. What factors and mechanisms regulate the secretion of the hypophysiotropins? Because the brain is composed mainly of neurons and supporting elements, other neurons within the brain would be expected to regulate the hypophysiotropin-secreting neurons. These other neurons, in turn, are linked to yet other neuronal inputs or to sensory neurons that are receptive to endogenous (intrinsic) and exogenous (extrinsic) cues.

The Role of CNS Neurohormones

Extrinsic and intrinsic stimuli received through sensory neurons are conducted through neuronal routes to the brain where this information may be inhibitory or stimulatory to hypophysiotropic hormone secretion. Conduction of sensory information involves neuronal elements, and each one must release a neurotransmitter to affect synaptic transmission. These neurohormones include the monoamine neurotransmitters (Fig. 6.12) and the amino acid neurotransmitters (Fig. 6.13). There are well-defined aminergic (monoamine) pathways within the brain that are composed of serotonergic, dopaminergic, noradrenergic, and even epinephrine-containing neurons. Axons from these neurons project from extrahypothalamic sites into the hypothalamus where they innervate hypophysiotropic hormone-producing cells. Depending on the nature of the receptors possessed by these neurons, the neurotransmitters may inhibit or stimulate hypophysiotropin secretion from these peptidergic neurons. This will then be reflected in enhanced or inhibited pituitary hormone secretion. For example, inhibitory inputs to hypophysiotropic neurons containing inhibitory factors (MIF, PIF, SRIF) would be expected to enhance pituitary secretion of MSH, PRL, and GH, respectively.

Histamine is synthesized within the brain where it interacts with receptors (H_1- or H_2-type histamine receptors). Whether histamine is derived from histaminergic neurons to act as a neurotransmitter or released from mast cells is unclear. Nevertheless, histamine injected into the brain does affect the secretion of certain pituitary hormones, presumably through its action at the level of the hypothalamus. Serotonergic neurons have a major influence on the regulation of neuroendocrine function. Activation of serotonergic neurotransmission in the hypothalamus leads to increased secretion of adrenocorticotropic hormone (ACTH), PRL, oxytocin, vasopressin, and renin. Serotonergic neurons that innervate the hypothalamus also send collaterals to limbic brain areas where they probably

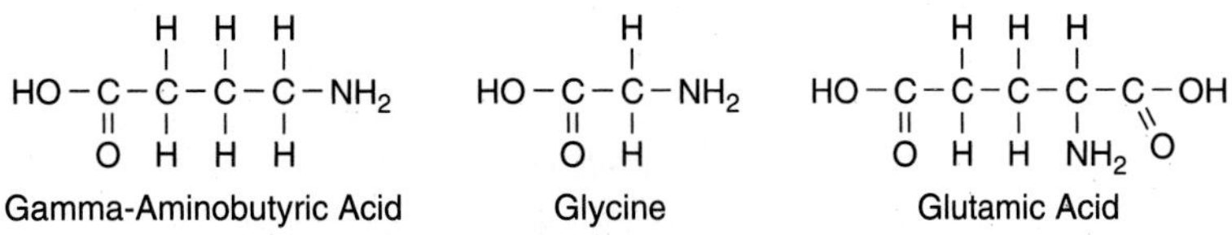

Figure 6.13   The amino acid neurotransmitters.

influence mood. Several new classes of drugs that are specifically targeted to serotonergic neurons and their receptors are successful in the treatment of depression, anxiety, and psychosis.

One method of partially determining the role of various neurotransmitters in the regulation of hypophysiotropin secretion is by *microiontophoresis*. This involves placing microliter quantities of a substance onto a group of neurons. *Single-unit iontophoresis* involves application of the agent onto single neurons.

Neurohormonal Control of Hypophysiotropin Secretion

A brief discussion of the neuroendocrine control of each hypothalamic hypophysiotropin is provided.

Control of CRH Secretion. It is unclear which transmitters and pathways play regulatory roles in ACTH secretion, but there is evidence that a number of different neurotransmitters are involved [47]. Stress is a potent stimulus to ACTH secretion. This response is diminished by atropine implantations at sites within the hypothalamus, thus implicating one or more cholinergic pathways (involving acetylcholine as neurotransmitter) in the control of ACTH secretion. Stimulation of CNS cholinergic structures provokes pituitary ACTH release [33]. Central catecholamines induce release of both CRH and AVP into the portal capillary plexus. These findings support the hypothesis that stress induces release of catecholamines from axons projecting to the paraventricular nucleus, thus activating adrenergic receptors that may selectively stimulate an AVP-containing subpopulation of CRH neurosecretory cells [53].

Control of PIF Secretion. Suckling is the normal stimulus to PRL secretion. This neuroendocrine reflex involves the inhibition of dopaminergic neurons whose release of PIF maintains a tonic inhibition of PRL secretion. A number of neurotransmitters participate in the control of PRL secretion. PRL secretion increases during sleep and is entrained to sleep, as a shift in the sleep cycle will shift the rhythm of PRL secretion (see Fig. 5.6). The nocturnal rise in PRL secretion apparently involves activation of hypothalamic serotonergic (5-HT) neurons because administration of the 5-HT blocking agent, methysergide, blunts the increase in PRL secretion. In addition, inhibitors of serotonin synthesis (e.g., p-chlorophenylalanine) abolish suckling-induced PRL release. There is an increased metabolism of brain 5-HT in suckled female rats, and PRL secretion is enhanced following administration of 5-HT receptor agonists.

Gamma aminobutyric acid (GABA) may also function in the control of PRL secretion. Injections of GABA stimulate or inhibit PRL secretion depending on the concentrations employed. The stimulating effect of large doses of GABA is blocked by the GABA receptor antagonist, bicuculline. Vasoactive intestinal peptide (VIP) has been localized to nerve endings in the hypothalamus and is present in the hypothalamohypophysial portal blood. VIP receptors have been identified in a PRL-secreting tumor; the peptide stimulates cAMP production in the pituitary gland while stimulating PRL secretion. VIP may, therefore, play a physiological role in the control of PRL secretion. There is evidence for the role of the histaminergic system in the regulation of PRL secretion because intraventricular injections of histamine stimulate PRL secretion in rats, whereas blockage of histamine H_1 receptors prevents stimulation of PRL secretion in response to stress or suckling.

Control of Growth Hormone. A variety of stimuli elevate GH secretion, presumably through inhibition of somatostatin secretion or by an enhancement of somatocrinin secretion. The participation of dopaminergic, noradrenergic, and serotonergic systems in the control of GH has been reviewed [10, 13], but the precise relationship of these neurotransmitter systems to somatostatin or to somatocrinin is presently unclear. Some of the GHRH-immunoreactive nerve cell bodies within the arcuate nucleus of the rat hypothalamus possess SRIF binding sites. The finding of SRIF-receptors on GHRH-containing arcuate neurons provides a morphological substrate for the concept of direct "cross-talk" between SRIF and GHRH neuronal systems within the central nervous system. Such intrahypothalamic interactions between these two neuropeptides may be a vital component in the generation and maintenance of the ultradian (cycle more frequent than 24 hours) rhythm of GH secretion [29]. The dynamic role of SRIF (somatostatin) and somatocrinin (GHRH) in the control of GH secretion is depicted (Fig. 6.14).

Control of GnRH Secretion.   Several transmitters and neuropeptides participate in the regulation of gonadotropin secretion [51]. At the hypothalamic level, control of gonadotropin releasing hormone (GnRH) involves noradrenaline, GABA, glutamate, angiotensin II, neuropeptide Y, neurotensin, and 5-hydroxytryptamine, as well as interleukins 1 and 2. Hypothalamic dopaminergic neurons are clearly stimulatory to GnRH secretion from parvocellular neurons. Dopamine secretion itself is inhibited by enkephalinergic neurons. Therefore an enkephalin such as Met-enkephalin, is indirectly in control of GnRH secretion and ultimately FSH and LH secretion (Chap. 21). Ovarian steroids can interfere with gonadotropin regulation by either direct effects on GnRH release or by increasing the sensitivity of anterior pituitary cells to GnRH, thus potentiating the release of pituitary hormones [25].

Control of TRH Secretion.   Apparently noradrenergic neurons stimulate TSH secretion by a stimulatory action on TRH-secreting neurons.

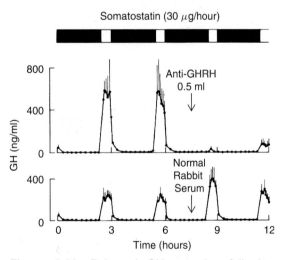

Figure 6.14 Rebound GH secretion following somatostatin withdrawal involves GHRH release. Regular rebound GH secretion can be elicited by intermittent infusions of somatostatin in conscious rats. The figure shows two groups of four animals given intravenous somatostatin infusions interrupted for 30 minutes every 3 hours. The lower panel shows that injection (arrowed) of 0.5 ml normal rabbit serum has no effect on GH rebound release, whereas injection of 0.5 ml antirat GHRH serum in another group of rats (upper panel) greatly attenuates the subsequent GH rebounds. (From Robinson [39], with permission, *Acta Paediatrica Scandinavia* 372:70–8, 1991.)

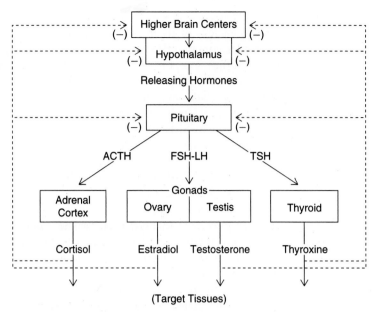

Figure 6.15   Feedback control of pituitary hormone secretion.

Feedback Mechanisms

In response to a hypophysiotropin, adenohypophysial hormones, such as TSH, ACTH, and the gonadotropins, are released into the general circulation where they circulate to their target tissues. Target tissue stimulation results in increased secretion of target tissue hormones, such as thyroid hormones (T_4 and T_3), adrenal glucocorticoids (e.g., cortisol), and gonadal steroids (e.g., estradiol, testosterone, progesterone). These hormones then circulate to their respective target tissues to mediate their actions. The pituitary gland and the hypothalamus are themselves target organs of these steroid or thyroid hormones [12] (Fig 6.15). Three mechanisms of feedback control of hypophysiotropin and hypophysial hormone secretion are recognized. Peripheral target tissue hormones may feed back through a so-called *long-loop* system to act at the level of the pituitary, at the

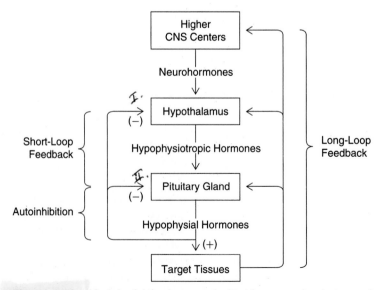

Figure 6.16   Model of long-loop and short-loop mechanisms and autoregulation of pituitary hormone secretion.

level of the hypothalamus, or even at higher brain centers (Fig. 6.16). Hypophysial hormones may also circulate by retrograde portal system blood flow to affect hypothalamic hypophysiotropic hormone secretion by a so-called *short-loop* mechanism. There is even evidence that secreted hypophysial hormones may feed back on their cells of origin to inhibit their own secretion, referred to as *autoinhibition* or *autofeedback inhibition* (Fig. 6.16).

Although some of the pituitary hormones, such as PRL, the neurohypophysial hormones, and α-melanotropin, stimulate peripheral target tissues, these target tissues do not themselves secrete hormones. The secretion of these hypophysial hormones therefore is not controlled by long-loop hormonal feedback mechanisms. The secretion of these hormones may, however, be controlled by reflex mechanisms and other sensory stimuli reaching the hypothalamus from sensory receptors. For example, suckling of the breast by the infant leads to secretion of oxytocin from the neurohypophysis. A decreased blood volume or increase in plasma electrolyte concentration is stimulatory to vasopressin secretion. It is becoming more evident that certain metabolic substrates (e.g., glucose, amino acids, FFAs) may also act at the level of the hypothalamus to affect hypophysiotropin secretion.

Steroid hormones implanted in the hypothalamus also modulate pituitary hormone secretion [28]. It can be demonstrated, using autoradiographic methods, that steroid hormones localize to specific sites within the CNS. These feedback sites for steroid hormones may also represent production sites of the hypophysiotropins. Indeed, immunocytochemical methods have localized hypophysiotropins, such as GnRH and somatostatin, to these same hypothalamic steroid-binding sites.

Corticotropin Secretion.   ACTH stimulates adrenal glucocorticoid production and secretion. Glucocorticoids, such as cortisol and corticosterone, and dexamethasone (a synthetic glucocorticoid) exert a negative feedback on ACTH secretion. Their locus of action is apparently at the level of both the pituitary and the hypothalamus, as determined by the following experiments. Dexamethasone injected into the adenohypophysis inhibits ACTH secretion. Given prior to microinjection of exogenous CRH or hypothalamic extract directly into the pituitary, dexamethasone abolishes ACTH release in response to the hypophysiotropin. Finally CRH stimulation of ACTH secretion from pituitary glands incubated in vitro is inhibited by addition of corticosterone to the medium. CRH levels in the brain are increased after bilateral adrenalectomy; this change can be prevented by administration of exogenous glucocorticoids. Thus glucocorticoids act on the hypothalamus to modulate the turnover of hypothalamic CRH, as well as acting directly on the pituitary.

Gonadotropin Secretion.   Gonadectomy of an animal, such as the rat, results in an increased secretion of gonadotropins. Injections of gonadal steroids—estrogens or androgens—result in decreased circulating levels of gonadotropins in gonadectomized animals. These results suggest that gonadal steroids exert a negative feedback inhibition of gonadotropin secretion. Where are the sites of action of gonadal steroids in this feedback mechanism? This question has been partially answered by the use of radiolabeled gonadal steroids. Injections of [³H]estradiol, for example, result in an accumulation of the ligand within the hypothalamus; autoradiographic studies demonstrate that the hormone localizes over the nuclei of neurons in specific hypothalamic sites (see Fig. 3.3). The radiolabeled hormone localizes to the same hypothalamic neurons that have been implicated in the control of pituitary gonadotropin secretion. These results indicate that gonadal steroids regulate pituitary gonadotropin secretion through long-loop feedback to the hypothalamus. Gonadal steroids may also exert positive and negative feedback effects directly at the level of pituitary gonadotrophs (see Chap. 18).

Implantation of luteinizing hormone (LH) or follicle-stimulating hormone (FSH) into specific sites within the hypothalamus is reported to depress hypophysial LH and FSH secretion. These effects are suggested to be an example of a short-loop feedback mechanism. There is even evidence that secreted gonadotropins may feed back at the level of the pituitary to establish an autoinhibition: both in vivo and in vitro, acute increases in blood or medium concentrations of LH inhibit basal and GnRH-stimulated LH secretion. This effect is gonadotropin-specific as there is no inhibition of GnRH-stimulated LH secretion by FSH.

Prolactin Secretion.   Injection of PRL or implantation of PRL into the median eminence of rats reduces the secretion of PRL from the pituitary. In some of these studies the hypothalamic content of PIF (dopamine) was found to be increased; these results suggested that a short-loop feedback system might regulate pituitary PRL secretion. There is other evidence that PRL can inhibit its own secretion by a direct action on the lactotrophs of the anterior pituitary gland.

Growth Hormone Secretion.   The central nervous system control of pituitary growth hormone secretion is believed to be mediated by a balance between somatostatin and somatocrinin. There is evidence that GH acts at the level of the hypothalamus to stimulate the synthesis and release of SRIF. Somatotropin mediates most of its effects indirectly through the stimulation of somatomedin production and release by the liver. The somatomedins then act on many tissues and organs to enhance growth. There is also evidence that IGF-I acutely stimulates SRIF release by the hypothalamus. IGF-I also exerts a much slower direct inhibitory effect on pituitary GH secretion. These observations suggest that IGF-I participates in a long-loop negative feedback action on SRIF secretion by the hypothalamus, as well as a slower long-loop action at the level of the pituitary.

Thyrotropin Secretion.   TSH secretion is enhanced following thyroidectomy or inhibition of thyroid hormone (T_4/T_3) production by drugs. This enhanced TSH secretion is abolished by the concomitant administration of T_4 or T_3 to an animal. Thyroid hormones also control TRH synthesis by regulating gene expression of the TRH prohormone in the "thyrotropic area" of the hypothalamus. Regulation of TRH production by thyroid hormones occurs primarily at the translational level rather than by post-translational processing [4]. Experimental data support the view that hypothalamic TRH production is regulated by thyroid hormones and that the rise in plasma TSH in hypothyroidism likely is due to increased release of TRH from the median eminence [4]. TSH secretion from isolated pituitaries in culture induced by TRH is also inhibited by thyroid hormones. These results demonstrate control of pituitary TSH secretion by actions at the level of the hypothalamus, as well as the pituitary.

Rhythms of Hypophysiotropin Secretion

During the process of evolution certain physiological processes of animals have become regulated by endogenous rhythms that are closely attuned to the daily periodicities of the light-dark cycle. The term *circadian* (from the Latin for *circa*, about, and *dies*, day) was coined to describe these diurnal rhythms of activity. These endogenous rhythms undoubtedly evolved in response to the daily environmental light cycle; daily exogenous light cues, however, no longer act as the immediate cause of the *biologic rhythm*, but only as a synchronizing mechanism or *Zeitgeber* (time-givers). In the absence of environmental information, the biological rhythm free-runs with its own frequency and can be entrained to a range of frequencies, however limited, that differ from the 24-hour cycle.

The control of biological rhythms is regulated by a so-called *biological clock* whose anatomical site may be the *suprachiasmatic nucleus* of the hypothalamus. Because seasonal changes in animals may be triggered by changes in the length of the day, some mechanism must exist whereby the duration of the daylight period can be measured and translated into changes in pituitary hormone secretion. The mechanisms involved in measurement and translation are unknown, but they must involve neural inputs to hypophys-iotropin-secreting cells (Chap. 20). It is not generally realized that all hormones of the pituitary gland are secreted in an episodic or rhythmic manner. This may relate to the fact that some hormone receptors down-regulate in the presence of continuous hormone secretion. Such an understanding is essential if certain hypophysiotropins are to be used in clinical medicine.

In humans the plasma concentration of cortisol rises in the morning and declines in the afternoon and evening. A similar adrenocortical rhythm, present in many mammalian species, may be associated with a 24-hour variation in secretion rates of CRH and ACTH as the plasma concentration of ACTH and the hypothalamic content of CRH exhibit a similar circadian rhythm. The secretion of GH has been shown to be pulsatile in nature in every species of animal studied, from rat to man. For example, in human male and female subjects at various stages of pubertal development, nonsleep-related bursts of GH secretion occur. Generally, two episodes of GH secretion are observed during a 6-hour sampling period.

Neuropharmacology

Pharmacological methods have been used successfully to determine the particular neural components involved in hypophysiotropin regulation of pituitary hormone secretion. For example, it was demonstrated that reflex ovulation in the rabbit could be blocked by rapid postcoital intravenous injections of Dibenamine, an α-adrenoceptor (see Chap. 14) blocking agent. Infusions of norepinephrine into the third ventricle of the brain resulted in an ovulatory surge of pituitary gonadotropins that was blocked by an α-adrenoceptor blocker and also by pentobarbital (a CNS-acting anesthetic), indicating that norepinephrine was acting within the brain [1].

Many drugs are available that can specifically modify neuronal activity and, in turn, hormonal secretion. The neuronal events are classified as presynaptic, synaptic, and postsynaptic. There are drugs that can modify the presynaptic events by affecting availability of neurotransmitter precursors, synthesis of neurotransmitters, transport of neurotransmitters along the axon, storage of neurotransmitters within secretory vesicles, exocytotic release of neurotransmitters from these vesicles, and inhibition of reuptake of neurotransmitters by presynaptic neurons. There are drugs that specifically interfere with the synaptic event by inhibiting the action of enzymes normally responsible for neurotransmitter inactivation, thereby prolonging the action of neurotransmitters. Drugs can also affect postsynaptic events by blocking neurotransmitter receptors, by mimicking the receptor-mediated actions of the neurotransmitter, and by interfering with cAMP production and degradation within presynaptic or postsynaptic neurons. Increased or decreased release of a pituitary hormone by one of these drugs is interpreted to imply that a particular neurotransmitter is involved somewhere in the hypothalamic pathway of control of the hormone.

MECHANISMS OF HYPOPHYSIOTROPIN ACTION

Attempts to determine the mechanisms of hypophysiotropic hormones' action on pituitary target cells are complicated due to the heterogeneity of the pituitary cell population. Nevertheless, the action of hypophysiotropins directly on hypophysial cells has been demonstrated [22, 46]. Pituitaries or pituitary cell cultures can be studied using a perifusion system (Fig. 6.17) wherein the actions of a hormone or drug on hormone secretion can be monitored. Electrophysiological activities of individual pituitary cells have been monitored. Application of TRH by micropipette to individual dissociated anterior pituitary cells elicited action potentials in previously silent cells and increased the frequency of such potentials in spontaneously active cells (Fig. 6.18). The respondent cells probably

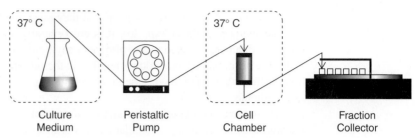

Figure 6.17   Schematic representation of a pituitary cell perifusion system. (From Weiss and Jameson, "Perifused pituitary cells as a marker for studies of gonadotropin biosynthesis and secretion." [51]. Reprinted with permission of the publisher from *Trends in Endocrinology and Metabolism* 4:265–269. ©1993 by Elsevier Science, Inc.)

represent thyrotrophs (or possibly lactotrophs). TRH-induced depolarization of thyrotrophs is Ca^{2+} dependent, which suggests that the hypophysiotropic factor stimulates thyrotropin secretion through a stimulus-secretion coupling mechanism [46].

Further evidence that hypophysiotropins mediate their action on the pituitary by a modulation of membrane action potentials was demonstrated on prolactin-secreting cells of a fish. In some teleost fishes the PRL-secreting cells are segregated to a specific region of the pituitary, making it possible to study a pure population of cells. These cells, as in the mammal, are under an inhibitory hypothalamic dopaminergic control. Isolated cells removed from this inhibitory influence spontaneously depolarize, which results in PRL secretion. Addition of dopamine to these cells inhibits the spontaneous discharge of the action potentials. Dopamine, the putative MIF, has a similar action on cells of the pars intermedia and is inhibitory of MSH secretion (see Chap. 8). Taken together these results provide evidence that the stimulatory and inhibitory effects of hypophysiotropins are mediated through their immediate actions at the level of the plasma membrane.

Methylxanthines and cAMP derivatives stimulate secretion of each of the six anterior pituitary hormones. Thus cAMP is considered to be one intracellular messenger regulating adenohypophysial cell hormone secretion in response to hypophysiotropic factors. Somatostatin, whose action is inhibitory to GH secretion, inhibits pituitary cAMP production, which is accompanied by an inhibition of both GH and TSH secretion. SRIF also inhibits theophylline-induced hormone secretion, which suggests that the hypothalamic hormone mediates its action at the level subsequent to cAMP production. SRIF inhibits both basal and stimulated transduction systems at the membrane level by interacting with an Ri-type receptor coupled to a G_i component (Chap. 4). This interaction results in inhibition of adenylate cyclase, Ca^{2+} channel opening, and probably phosphoinositide turnover. Besides these effects SRIF is also able to stimulate soluble phosphodiesterase, therefore reinforcing its inhibitory effect on cyclase.

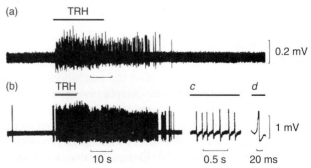

Figure 6.18   TRH-induced action potentials from pituitary thyrotrophs. (From Taraskevich and Douglas [46], with permission.)

Cellular secretions are generally correlated with an elevation in cAMP levels, whereas inhibition of secretion is most often correlated with decreased levels of the cyclic nucleotide. It would be expected that dopamine, the hypophysiotropic PIF and MIF, mediates its inhibitory action on pituitary PRL and MSH secretion through a depression of cAMP production. GnRH stimulates the rapid and specific hydrolysis of phosphoinositides and their conversion to diacylglycerols in enriched gonadotrope cultures. It is likely that the actions of some other hypophysiotropins will be shown to be mediated through a similar pathway (see Chap. 4).

Modulation of Pituitary Hormone Secretion by Thyroid and Steroid Hormones

Thyroid hormones and adrenal and gonadal steroids secreted in response to hypophysial hormones feed back at the level of the pituitary to modulate the action of hypophysiotropins. Thyroid hormones, thyroxine and triiodothyronine, are inhibitory to TSH secretion through actions mainly at the level of the pituitary gland. For example, TRH is stimulatory to TSH release from pituitary glands incubated in vitro, but the release of TSH from pituitaries is prevented by prior incubation of the glands in the presence of T_4 or T_3. The inhibitory effects of these thyroid hormones are, in turn, abolished by concomitant incubation of the glands in the presence of actinomycin or cycloheximide (inhibitors of RNA and protein synthesis, respectively), suggesting that the thyroid hormones stimulate the synthesis of an inhibitor of TRH action.

CRH stimulation of pituitary ACTH secretion is abolished by the synthetic glucocorticoid dexamethasone, both in vivo and in vitro. The negative feedback of adrenal glucocorticoids therefore is mediated, in part, directly at the level of the pituitary. Androgens have an inhibitory action on LH release at the hypothalamic and pituitary levels; their inhibitory effect on FSH release is restricted to the hypothalamus. Progesterone can exert stimulatory and inhibitory effects on gonadotropin secretion at the pituitary and hypothalamic levels. Modulation of hypophysiotropin action can occur by an alteration of hypophysial cell receptor number (and possibly receptor sensitivity). Estradiol increases the sensitivity of FSH- and LH-secreting cells to GnRH by a direct action at the level of the pituitary. The effect of estradiol can be stimulatory or inhibitory, depending on the dose and time of administration of the estrogen. The number of pituitary GnRH receptors is positively correlated with concentrations of estradiol in the serum. Modulation of gonadotroph GnRH receptors may be a necessary component of increased pituitary sensitivity to the hypophysiotropin during the estrous cycle. Estradiol may also increase PRL secretion in humans and in rats, and the steroid is also stimulatory to TSH secretion in rats. Daily injections of estradiol increase the number of pituitary TRH binding sites (see Fig. 19.8). Thyroxine injections in the rat, on the other hand, lead to a progressive decrease in pituitary TRH binding sites. Binding of the TRH to thyrotroph plasma membranes is enhanced by prior treatment with propylthiouracil, a drug that reduces thyroid hormone production by the thyroid (Chap. 13).

PATHOPHYSIOLOGY OF HYPOTHALAMIC DYSFUNCTION ✓

Because each of the pituitary hormones is under stimulatory or inhibitory control by hormones of the hypothalamus, adrenal, thyroidal, and gonadal hypoactivity or hyperactivity may often relate to defects at the level of the hypothalamus, rather than at the pituitary gland [21, 30]. Abnormal pituitary hormone secretion may be related to defects in hypophysiotropic hormone synthesis and secretion or to altered activity of the neuronal inputs to hypophysiotropin neurons [52]. Overproduction or underproduction of dopamine within CNS neurons, for example, is believed responsible for the etiology of schizophrenia and Parkinson's disease, respectively.

An anomalous release of ACTH in response to TRH has been noted in some untreated patients with elevated glucocorticoid levels. TRH also stimulates ACTH release from certain neoplastic pituitary cells, but not from normal pituitary cells in tissue culture. In some cases of these clinical syndromes, a primary abnormality may be intrinsic to the ACTH cells themselves. Neoplastic human ACTH-secreting cells may synthesize receptors for TRH, which are coupled to ACTH release, and allow direct stimulation by TRH.

In 1943 Kallmann first described patients with hypogonadism and anosmia. Patients with the Kallmann syndrome fail to secrete gonadotropic hormones; the disorder is an example of hypogonadotropic hypogonadism. In Kallmann's syndrome there appears to be a failure of migration of GnRH neurons due to deletion of a gene that encodes a protein necessary for controlling normal migration of GnRH neurons (and olfactory neurons). The deleted gene region (referred to as KAL) encodes a protein that is homologous to members of the fibronectin gene family, known to control neural chemotaxis, cell adhesion, and apparently now GnRH/neuronal migration during embryogenesis [9].

GnRH has been used therapeutically to induce ovulation in amenorrheic females. The hormone has also been used to treat oligospermia and hypogonadotropic hypogonadism in males. Highly potent analogs of GnRH have been developed for use in the treatment of hypogonadal function in the male and the female [3, 9]. Although administration of GnRH causes an initial large release of gonadotropins in females, prolonged treatment results in disturbances in gonadotropin secretion, irregular follicular maturation, and a low incidence of ovulation (Chap. 18). A single dose of certain long-acting GnRH analogs is effective in decreasing gonadotropin secretion [8]. These peptides may prove useful as antifertility (contraceptive) agents.

Some tumors may secrete hypothalamic hormones. For example, ectopic secretion of a CRH-like peptide may be responsible for certain cases of Cushing's disease. A number of mechanisms may be invoked to explain the hyperprolactinemia associated with pituitary prolactinomas. First a hypothalamic disorder, involving decreased secretion of PIF or increased secretion of a PRL-releasing factor, could lead to eventual tumor formation. Second, PRL could be produced autonomously by a tumor whose cells, by loss of dopamine receptors or other mechanisms, have become partially or wholly independent of hypothalamic control.

Several neuropeptides classically associated with the hypothalamus have been found in the anterior pituitary. The question arises whether they are locally synthesized and, if so, whether they play a paracrine or autocrine role in pituitary cell functions. Using normal and tumoral human pituitaries, TRH, SRIF, GHRH, and dopamine were found in variable quantities, according to the nature of the tissue. They were all present in normal pituitaries, while stimulatory hormones (TRH and GHRH) were found predominantly in tumoral tissue, implying an imbalance of pathophysiological importance between the stimulatory and inhibitory control of hypophysial hormones (PRL and GH) in pituitary adenomas. Both normal and tumoral pituitaries released TRH and GHRH in large amounts, suggesting their local synthesis. These results indicate that anterior pituitary cells release neuropeptides that are most probably endogenously synthesized and that might play a paracrine or autocrine role on anterior pituitary cell functions [35].

Hypophysiotropins as Diagnostic Agents.   Because synthetic hypophysiotropic hormones are commercially available, one can differentiate hypothalamic dysfunction from defects related to pituitary pathophysiology [50]. Administration of thyrotropin-releasing hormone with subsequent measurement of the TSH response, probably the most widely used of these tests, is used to diagnose subclinical hypothyroidism or hyperthyroidism. Repeated administration of GHRH usually is necessary to determine whether functional gonadotrophs are present. Similarly, GnRH has been administrated to GH-deficient patients to determine whether functional somatotrophs are present [23]. Although a single intravenous dose of somatocrinin may stimulate GH release in some patients with idiopathic GH deficiency, repetitive intermittent administration may be necessary to "prime" the somatotroph before significant GH stimulation occurs.

The specificity of releasing factors to stimulate respective target cells in the anterior pituitary has been shown. There is also convincing evidence that the hypothalamic-releasing factors do not interact at the level of the pituitary gland to enhance, inhibit, or modify the biological actions of each other. These observations are of significance to clinical medicine. It is expected that a single bolus administration of several releasing factors (e.g., GnRH, TRH, CRH, and somatocrinin) will be used to determine pituitary reserve (ability to release appropriate hormones; e.g., FSH, LH, TSH, ACTH, GH). It might be expected that any single or multiple pituitary nonresponse or unexpected response will be due to single or multiple pituitary abnormalities, rather than to an interaction of the secretagogues administered.

Therapy with GHRH. The traditional treatment of GH-deficient children is administration of GH. Because Creutzfeldt-Jakob disease developed in a few young adults who received GH extracted from virus-contaminated human pituitary glands, these biological preparations are no longer available in the United States. Fortunately, the development of techniques for biosynthesis of GH by recombinant-DNA technology has provided an ample supply of human GH for treatment of these children. Clinical trials of a methionyl-GH and pure GH indicate that these preparations are effective in promoting linear growth and are not associated with toxicity. An alternative treatment for GH deficiency is administration of GHRH to stimulate GH release. GH-deficient children have been treated with GHRH-40, GHRH-44, and a 29-amino-acid GHRH analog, with inconsistent results. Despite variations in GHRH preparations, total daily dose, and frequency of administration, a substantial proportion of children showed increased growth velocity during therapy with these GHRHs.

CONCLUSIONS AND SPECULATIONS

The hypothalamus, the coordinating center of the brain, controls endocrine, behavioral, and autonomic nervous system functions. Specifically, it plays an important role in thermoregulation, feeding and drinking behaviors, cardiovascular activity, pituitary gland regulation, and certain types of motivation and learning. The experimental affirmation of the neurovascular hypothesis of Harris [20] was particularly important in establishing the functional role of hypothalamic hypophysiotropic factors in the control of endocrine function. Indeed, the hypothalamus provides the final common neuroendocrine pathway in the control of the peripheral endocrine system. The endocrine hypothalamus is itself regulated by the peripheral endocrine system, as well as by autonomic nervous system afferent inputs. Thus the concept of neuroendocrinology has emerged that emphasizes the reciprocal integrated roles of the nervous and endocrine systems in the control of physiological processes.

The progressive elucidation of the presence and precise distribution of neurohormones within the hypothalamus and other brain centers may provide the exact neuroanatomical-neurohormonal correlates related to normal and abnormal neuroendocrine-physiology. An understanding of the structure of the hypophysiotropins and their subsequent synthesis has provided the clinician with new tools for enhancing pituitary hormone secretion under conditions of hypothalamic dysfunction. Of great interest is the discovery that the hypophysiotropins are not restricted to the hypothalamus, but rather are found throughout the nervous system, the gut, and other peripheral organs. Each of these hypophysiotropins may function in the control of a diverse number of physiological processes. A study of the comparative endocrinology of these peptides reveals that their role in the hypothalamus may indeed be a rather late evolutionary acquisition.

REFERENCES

[1]   Al-Damluji, S. 1993. Adrenergic control of the secretion of anterior pituitary hormones. *Baillière's Clin. Endocrinol. Metab.* 7:355–92.

[2]   Beitins, I. Z., and V. Padmanabhan. 1991. Bioactivity of gonadotropins. *Endocrinol. Metab. Clin. N. Amer.* 20:85–120.

[3]   Blunt, S. M., and W. R. Butt. 1988. Pulsatile GnRH therapy for the induction of ovulation in hypogonadotropic hypogonadism. *Acta Endocrinol. (Copenh.)* 288:58–65.

[4]   Bruhn, T. O., J. H. Taplin, and I. M. D. Jackson. 1991. Hypothyroidism reduces content and increases in vitro release of pro-thyrotropin-releasing hormone peptides from the median eminence. *Neuroendocrinology* 53:511–5.

[5]   Campbell, R. M., and C. G. Scanes. 1992. Evolution of the growth hormone-releasing factor (GRF) family of peptides. *Growth Reg.* 2:175–91.

[6]   Childs, G. V., K. W. Westlund, R. E. Tibolt, and J. M. Lloyd. 1991. Hypothalamic regulatory peptides and their receptors: cytochemical studies of their role in regulation at the adenohypophyseal level. *J. Electron Microscopy Technique.* 19:21–41.

[7]   Chrovsos, G. P. 1992. Regulation and dysregulation of the hypothalamic-pituitary-adrenal axis. The corticotropin-releasing hormone perspective. *Endocrinol. Metab. Clin. N. Amer.* 21:833–58.

[8]   Conn, P. M., and W. F. Crowley. 1991. Gonadotropin-releasing hormone and its analogues. *New Engl. J. Med.* 324:93–103.

[9]   Crowley, W. F. Jr., and J. L. Jameson. 1992. Gonadotropin–releasing hormone deficiency: perspectives from clinical investigation. *Endocr. Rev.* 13:635–40.

[10] De Gennaro Colonna, V., S. G. Cella, V. Locatelli, S. Loche, E. Ghigo, D. Cocchi, and E. E. Muller. 1989. Neuroendocrine control of growth hormone secretion. *Acta Paediatr. Scand.* 349:87–92.

[11] Evans, J. W., and M. B. Nikitovitch-Winer. 1969. Functional reactivation and cytological restoration of pituitary grafts by continuous local intravascular infusion of median eminence extracts. *Neuroendocrinology* 4:83–100.

[12] Foreman, D. 1992. The concept of negative feedback—Moore and Price. *Endocrinology* 131:87–9.

[13] Frohman, L. A., T. R. Downs, and P. Chomczynski. 1992. Regulation of growth hormone secretion. *Front. Neuroendocrinol.* 13:344–405.

[14] Frohman, L. A., and J.-O. Jansson. 1986. Growth hormone releasing hormone. *Endocr. Rev.* 7:223–53.

[15] Guillemin, R. 1992. Somatostatin: the early days. *Metabolism* 41:2–4.

[16] Guillemin, R., P. Brazeau, P. Böhlen, E. Esch. N. Long, and W. B. Wehrenbert. 1982. Growth hormone-releasing factor from a human pancreatic tumor that caused acromegaly. *Science* 218:585–87.

[17] Guillemin, R., and R. Burgus. 1972. The hormones of the hypothalamus. *Sci. Amer.* 227: 24–33.

[18] Halász, B., J. Kiss, and J. Molnar. 1989. Regulation of the gonadotropin-releasing hormone (GnRH) neuronal system: morphological aspects. *J. Steroid Biochem.* 33:663–68.

[19] Halász, B., L. Pupp, and S. Uhlarik. 1962. Hypophysiotropic area in the hypothalamus. *J. Endocrinol.* 25:147–54.

[20] Harris, G. W. 1955. *Neural control of the pituitary gland*. London: Edward Arnold Ltd.

[21] Herman-Bonert, V. S., and G. D. Braunstein. 1991. Gonadotropin secretory abnormalities. *Endocrinol. Metab. Clin. N. Amer.* 20:519–38.

[22] Hsiung, H. M., D. P. Smith, X.-Y. Zhang, T. Bennett, P. R. Rosteck Jr., and M.-H. Lai. 1993. Structure and functional expression of a complementary DNA for porcine growth hormone-releasing hormone receptor. *Neuropeptides* 25:1–10.

[23] Kaplan, S. L. 1993. The newer uses of growth hormone in adults. *Advan. Intern. Med.* 38:287–301.

[24] King, J. A., and R. P. Millar. 1992. Evolution of gonadotropin-releasing hormones. *TEM* 3:339–46.

[25]   Kordon, C., and S. V. Drouva. 1992. Gonadotropin regulation, oestrogens, and the immune system. *Horm. Res.* 37:11–5.

[26]   Lechan, R. M. 1987. Neuroendocrinology of pituitary hormone regulation. *Endocrinol. Metab. Clin. N. Amer.* 16:475–501.

[27]   Liposits, Z. 1993. Ultrastructure of hypothalamic paraventricular neurons. *Crit. Rev. Neurobiol.* 7:89–162.

[28]   Maclean, D. B., and I. M. Jackson. 1988. Molecular biology and regulation of the hypothalamic hormones. *Baillière's Clin. Endocrinol. Metab.* 2:835–68.

[29]   McCarthy, G. F., A. Beaudet, and G. S. Tannenbaum. 1992. Colocalization of somatostatin receptors and growth hormone-releasing factor immunoreactivity in neurons of the rat arcuate nucleus. *Neuroendocrinology* 56:18–24.

[30]   Moghissi, K. S. 1992. Clinical applications of gonadotropin-releasing hormones in reproductive disorders. *Endocrinol. Metab. Clin. N. Amer.* 21:125–40.

[31]   Nikitovitch-Winer, M., and J. W. Everett. 1958. Comparative study of luteotropin secretion by hypophysial autotransplants in the rat. Effects of site and stages of the estrous cycle. *Endocrinology* 62:522–32.

[32]   ———. 1959. Histologic changes in grafts of rat pituitary on the kidney and upon re-transplantation under the diencephalon. *Endocrinology* 65:357–68.

[33]   Palkovits, M. 1977. Neural pathways involved in ACTH regulation. *Ann. New York Acad. Sci.* 297:455–76.

[34]   Paradisi, R., G. Frank, O. Magrini, M. Capelli, S. Venturoli, E. Porcu, and C. Flamigni. 1993. Adeno-pituitary hormones in human hypothalamic hypophysial blood. *J. Clin. Endocrinol. Metab.* 77:523–7.

[35]   Peillon, F., M. Le Dafniet, P. Pagesy, J.-Y. Li, C. Benlot, A.-M. Brandi, and D. Joubert (Bression). 1991. Neuropeptides of anterior pituitary origin. Autocrine or paracrine functions? *Path. Res. Pract.* 187:577–80.

[36]   Porter, J. C., R. S. Mical, I. A. Kamberi, and Y. R. Grazia. 1970. A procedure for the cannulation of a pituitary stalk portal vessel and perfusion of the pars distalis in the rat. *Endocrinology* 87:197–201.

[37]   Porter, J. C., D. D. Nansel, G. A. Gudelsky, M. M. Foreman, N. S. Pilotte, C. R. Parker Jr., G. H. Burrows, G. W. Bates, and J. D. Madden. 1980. Neural control of gonadotropin secretion. *Fed. Proc.* 39:2896–2901.

[38]   Rivier, J., J. Spiess, M. Thorner, and W. Vale. 1982. Characterization of a growth hormone-releasing factor from a human pancreatic islet tumor. *Nature* 300:276–78.

[39]   Robinson, I. C. A. F. 1991. The growth hormone secretory pattern: a response to neuroendocrine signals. *Acta Paediatr. Scand.* 372:70–8.

[40]   Sawchenko, P. E., T. Imaki, E. Potter, K. Kovacs, J. Imaki, and W. Vale. 1993. The functional neuroanatomy of corticotropin-releasing factor. *Ciba Found. Symp.* 172:5–21.

[41]   Schally, A. V., W. Y. Huang, R. C. C. Chang, A. Arimura, T. W. Redding, R. P. Millar, M. W. Hunkapiller, and L. E. Hood. 1980. Isolation and structure of pro-somatostatin: a putative somatostatin precursor from pig hypothalamus. *Proc. Natl. Acad. Sci. USA* 77:4489–93.

[42]   Schwartz, J., and R. Cherny. 1992. Intercellular communication within the anterior pituitary influencing the secretion of hypophysial hormones. *Endocr. Rev.* 13:453–75.

[43]   Sherwood, N. M., D. A. Lovejoy, and I. R. Coe. 1993. Origin of mammalian gonadotropin-releasing hormones. *Endocr. Rev.* 14:241–54.

[44]   Swaab, D. F., M. A. Hoffman, P. J. Lucassen, J. S. Purba, F. C. Raadsheer, and J. A. P. Van De Nes. 1993. Functional neuroanatomy and neuropathology of the human hypothalamus. *Anat. Embryol.* 187:317–30.

[45]   Tannenbaum, G. S. 1988. Somatostatin as a physiological regulator of pulsatile growth hormone secretion. *Horm. Res.* 29:70–74.

[46]   Taraskevich, P. A., and D. W. Douglas. 1977. Action potentials occur in cells of the normal pituitary gland and are stimulated by the hypophysiotropic peptide thyrotropin-releasing hormone. *Proc. Natl. Acad. Sci. USA* 74:4064–67.

[47]   Taylor, A. L., and L. M. Fishman. 1988. Corticotropin-releasing hormone. *New Engl. J. Med.* 319:213–22.

[48] Thorner, M. O. 1993. On the discovery of growth hormone-releasing hormone. *Acta Pae-diatr. Scand.* 388:2–7.

[49] Tse, A., and B. Hille. 1992. GnRH-Induced Ca^{2+} oscillations and rhythmic hyperpolarizations of pituitary gonadotropes. *Science* 255:462–4.

[50] Wade, N. 1978. Guillemin and Schally. *Science* 200:279–82; 411–15; 510–13.

[51] Weiss, J. and J. L. Jameson. 1993. Perifused pituitary cells as a marker for studies of gonadotropin biosynthesis and secretion. *TEM* 4:265–70.

[52] Veldhuis, J. D., R. J. Urban, I. Z. Beitins, R. M. Blizzard, M. L. Jonson, and M. L. Dufau. 1989. Pathophysiological features of the pulsatile secretion of biologically active luteinizing hormone in man. *J. Steroid Biochem.* 33:739–49.

[53] Whitnall, M. H. 1993. Regulation of the hypothalamic corticotropin-releasing hormone neurosecretory system. *Prog. Neurobiol.* 40:573–629.

Neurohypophysial Hormones

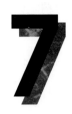

7

*As early as 1895 extracts of pituitaries were discovered to cause a rapid rise in blood pressure when injected into animals [34]. An important advance was made with the subsequent discovery by Howell (1898) that the pressor principle of pituitary extracts resided in the posterior lobe [20]. Dale, an eminent English pharmacologist, was the first to note that an extract of dried bovine pituitary glands caused a contraction of the uterus in addition to an elevation in blood pressure [11]. In 1909 posterior pituitary extracts were first used in clinical obstetrics to induce labor at term. In the years following, it was discovered that posterior lobe extracts caused a rapid flow (release) of milk. **Antidiuresis** as a response to injections of posterior pituitary extracts was demonstrated in 1913. The injections reduced urine flow, increased the osmolality of the urine, and alleviated thirst. Extracts of the neurohypophysis then became established as the clinical method of controlling the polyuria of diabetes insipidus, although the etiology of the syndrome was not yet understood.*

*In the early 1950s the two physiologically active principles of the posterior pituitary, **oxytocin** (OT) and **vasopressin** (AVP), were completely separated so that their individual activities could be studied. Du Vigneaud and his colleagues determined the structures of the oxytocic and antidiuretic principles of the neurohypophysis [23]. European chemists also determined the structures of OT [58] and AVP [1] at about the same time. Among the first peptide hormones to be completely chemically characterized, oxytocin and vasopressin were then synthesized; for this work du Vigneaud was awarded a Nobel Prize. This merging of pure chemistry with physiology provided the foundation for modern endocrinology.*

THE NEUROHYPOPHYSIS

Unlike the adenohypophysis, which derives from an upward evagination of the oral (buccal) epithelium, the posterior pituitary develops from a downward growth of the neural ectoderm. Therefore the neurohypophysis mainly consists of neural endings and associated blood vessels (see Chap. 5). There are only a few cellular elements present within the pars nervosa and they are referred to as pituicytes. Their function is unknown, but they are probably glial cells and may function like the neuroglia of the central nervous system. This paucity of cell bodies was a puzzling observation to the early investigators who ascribed an endocrine role to the pars nervosa. Where or what were the secretory elements of the posterior pituitary?

Lesions within specific areas of the hypothalamus led to degeneration of the pars nervosa and to a disturbance in water balance. These and other observations revealed that the neurons of the pars nervosa originate in two pairs of hypothalamic nuclei. These

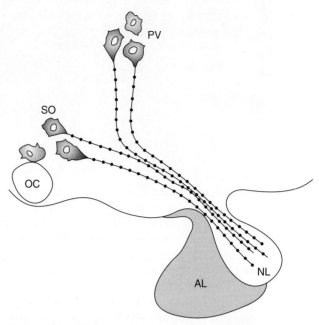

Figure 7.1 Diagram of a sagittal section through the pituitary gland. The relationship of the neurons that compose the supraoptic nuclei (SO) and the paraventricular nuclei (PV) to the hypothalamo-hypophysial tract and the neural lobe (NL), and anterior lobe (AL), is revealed. (From Pickering [38], with permission.)

magnocellular (see Chap. 6) neurons contain a stainable material that allows easy identification of the pathways from the hypothalamic nuclei, through the median eminence, and down the infundibular stalk of the neurohypophysis (Fig. 7.1). The stainable material is composed of granules that are now known to contain the hormones of the neurohypophysis. These large granules are referred to as *neurosecretory granules*; the process of granule formation and release is termed *neurosecretion* [47].

The discovery that the neurohypophysis is the terminal organ of a CNS neurosecretory system, that it is mainly composed of hormone-containing nerve terminals, and that these axonal endings secrete their products into the bloodstream to act as hormones on distant target tissues, was an important landmark in understanding the role of neurons in endocrine function [3]. Thus the discipline of vertebrate neuroendocrinology was established. The concept of neurosecretion in the vertebrate provided information that furthered understanding of the role of the brain in the control of pituitary and other endocrine functions. Neuroendocrinology in the vertebrate began with the study of the neurohypophysis and its hormones.

Anatomically, the vertebrate neurohypophysis is considered to be a storage organ for the products of individual neuronal syntheses. The stored hormones are released into the adjacent vascular network. Such a functional unit is referred to as a *neurohemal organ* and is structurally analogous to the *corpus cardiacum* of some invertebrates. The study of these depot-release structures, the neurohypophysis and corpus cardiacum, and their release of neurohormones has been crucial in understanding brain-endocrine relationships in vertebrates and invertebrates.

SYNTHESIS AND CHEMISTRY

Two nonapeptides, oxytocin (OT) and arginine vasopressin (AVP, also referred to as antidiuretic hormone, ADH), are found within the pars nervosa of most mammalian species. These neurohypophysial hormones are closely related structurally, but they serve quite different physiological roles. Oxytocin, for example, controls milk release from the mammary gland and contraction of the uterus, whereas AVP is concerned with water balance. The neurohypophysial hormones consist of nine amino acids folded into a ring through a disulfide bridge at positions 1 and 6 of the molecule, leaving a terminal tripeptide side chain (Fig. 7.2). AVP differs from OT in possessing a phenylalanine and an arginine at the 3 and 8 positions, respectively, of the molecule and is usually referred to as arginine vasopressin (AVP). Other structurally different neurohypophysial principles are found within the neurohypophysis of nonmammalian vertebrates (Table 7.1).

The neurohypophysial hormones are localized within the axonal endings that make up the pars nervosa. These hormones are, however, synthesized within the cell bodies of the pars nervosa neurons, which are located a long distance away in the hypothalamus. In mammals, birds, and reptiles these cell bodies are found principally within the paired supraoptic nuclei (SON) and paraventricular nuclei (PVN) of the magnocellular neurosecretory system (Fig. 7.1). In other vertebrates this system consists of a single group of neurons in the anterior hypothalamus, the *preoptic nucleus*. In the amphibian, immunocytochemical studies have demonstrated separate hormone-producing neurons within the magnocellular preoptic nucleus, suggesting that the two types of neurosecretory neurons are intermingled. Although there is evidence that individual neurons synthesize only one species of hormone, both types of neurons are found intermingled within each of the hypothalamic nuclei. OT-synthesizing cells predominate in the PVN and AVP-synthesizing cells in the SON. In rats the number of neurosecretory neurons is, however, more than three times greater in the SON than the PVN, and the contribution of OT from the former structure may be several times greater than that from the latter during reflex stimulation of OT release. In humans numerous large- and medium-sized neurons contain AVP mRNA in the PVN, SON, and accessory magnocellular nucleus. Small, lightly labeled AVP neurons are also found in the suprachiasmatic nucleus. Oxytocin mRNA is found in the SON, PVN, accessory magnocellular nucleus and, less frequently, in neurons of the lateral hypothalamus [54]. The relative contribution of oxytocinergic and vasopressinergic neurons within the PVN and SON varies considerably between species; the individual contributions of these two nuclear centers to neurohypophysial hormone secretion,

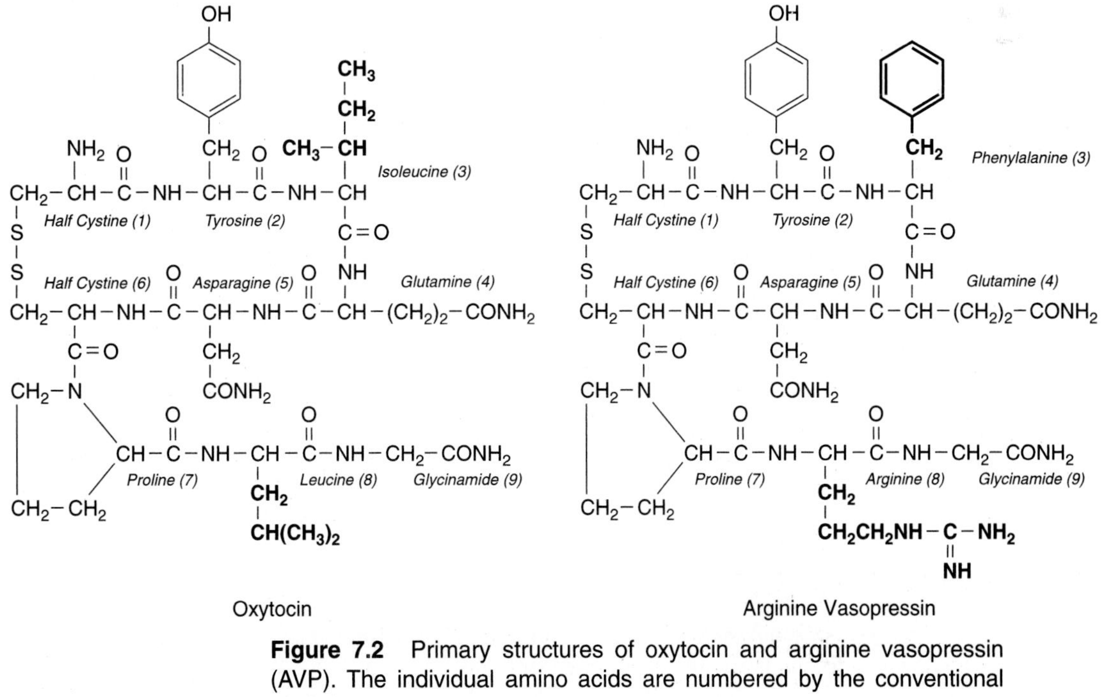

Figure 7.2 Primary structures of oxytocin and arginine vasopressin (AVP). The individual amino acids are numbered by the conventional method.

Gln: glutamine

TABLE 7.1 PRIMARY STRUCTURES OF THE VERTEBRATE NEUROHYPOPHYSIAL HORMONES

Hormone	Positions of amino acid residues	Animal group
Ancestral molecule	1 2 3 4 5 6 7 8 9 Cys–Tyr– X – X – Asn–Cys–Pro– X – Gly–NH$_2$	
Oxytocin	1 2 3 4 5 6 7 8 9 Cys–Tyr–Ile–Gln–Asn–Cys–Pro–Leu–Gly–NH$_2$	Mammals
Arginine vasopressin	1 2 3 4 5 6 7 8 9 Cys–Tyr–Phe–Gln–Asn–Cys–Pro–Arg–Gly–NH$_2$	Mammals except domestic pigs and Macropodidae
Lysine vasopressin (Lysipressin)	1 2 3 4 5 6 7 8 9 Cys–Tyr–Phe–Gln–Asn–Cys–Pro–Lys–Gly–NH$_2$	Placental mammals (Suidae) Marsupials (Macropodidae, Didelphidae)
Phenypressin	1 2 3 4 5 6 7 8 9 Cys–Phe–Phe–Gln–Asn–Cys–Pro–Arg–Gly–NH$_2$	Marsupials (Macropodidae)
Arginine vasotocin	1 2 3 4 5 6 7 8 9 Cys–Tyr–Ile–Gln–Asn–Cys–Pro–Arg–Gly–NH$_2$	Birds, reptiles, amphibians, bony fishes, and cartilaginous fishes
Isotocin	1 2 3 4 5 6 7 8 9 Cys–Tyr–Ile–Ser–Asn–Cys–Pro – Ile – Gly–NH$_2$	Bony fishes (teleosts)
Mesotocin	1 2 3 4 5 6 7 8 9 Cys–Tyr–Ile–Gln–Asn–Cys–Pro – Ile–Gly–NH$_2$	Marsupials, birds, reptiles, amphibians, lung-fishes
Glumitocin	1 2 3 4 5 6 7 8 9 Cys–Tyr–Ile–Ser–Asn–Cys–Pro – Gln–Gly–NH$_2$	Cartilaginous fishes (rays)
Valitocin	1 2 3 4 5 6 7 8 9 Cys–Tyr–Ile–Gln–Asn–Cys–Pro–Val–Gly–NH$_2$	Cartilaginous fishes (spiny dogfish shark)
Aspargtocin	1 2 3 4 5 6 7 8 9 Cys–Tyr–Ile–Asn–Asn–Cys–Pro–Leu–Gly–NH$_2$	Cartilaginous fishes (spiny dogfish shark)
Asvatocin	1 2 3 4 5 6 7 8 9 Cys–Tyr–Ile–Asn–Asn–Cys–Pro–Val–Gly–NH$_2$	Cartilaginous fishes (spotted dogfish shark)
Phasvatocin	1 2 3 4 5 6 7 8 9 Cys–Tyr–Phe–Asn–Asn–Cys–Pro–Val–Gly–NH$_2$	Cartilaginous fishes (spotted dogfish shark)

therefore, remain unresolved. Whether OT or AVP are preferentially secreted from either the SON or PVN in response to a particular physiological need remains to be determined.

Radioisotope studies using [^{35}S]cysteine injected into the third ventricle reveal that incorporation of the radiolabel into protein occurs first within the cell bodies of the neurosecretory neurons. The label is then transported rapidly (2.5 mm/hr) down the axons to terminals within the pars nervosa. Studies revealed that radioactive amino acids injected into the SON appear in the posterior pituitary incorporated into AVP and its precursors within 2 hours of injection. In vitro studies showed that hypothalamo-median eminence tissue, but not neurohypophysial tissue, incorporated [^{35}S]cysteine into AVP. These experimental observations documented the origin of the neurosecretory material of the pars nervosa.

Each of the hormones is found in close association with a larger protein, referred to as a *neurophysin*. There is a specific neurophysin for each hormone, oxytocin-neurophysin (*oxyphysin*) and vasopressin-neurophysin (*pressophysin*). Neurophysins and their associated hormones are derived from the post-translational cleavage of precursor proteins, propressophysin and pro-oxyphysin. Inhibitors of neurophysin formation also repress formation of the associated hormones. In the homozygous state of the Brattleboro strain of rat (which has hereditary diabetes insipidus) there is an absolute lack of AVP secretion, but no comparable defect in OT synthesis and secretion. Pressophysin is also absent from the hypothalamus of these rats, providing further evidence for the common origin of the neurophysin and its associated neurohypophysial hormone. The concept that peptide hormones may arise from the proteolytic cleavage of a precursor *prohormone* (in this case a *proneurophysin*) is now recognized to be of more general significance for the production of most other peptide hormones.

The structural genes for the human preproarginine vasopressin-neurophysin II (prepro-AVP-NPII) and prepro-oxytocin neurophysin-I (prepro-OT-NPI) locus are closely linked. These two loci have been assigned to chromosome 20. Prepro-AVP-NPII consists of a single polypeptide chain containing a secretory signal sequence, the nonapeptide AVP, the hormone carrier protein neurophysin-II (NPII), and another peptide of unknown function. Prepro-OT-neurophysin-I (NPI) consists of the same configuration, except that the AVP moiety is replaced by OT and the neurophysin moiety is NPI instead of NPII. While the prepro AVP and OT genes have been shown to be physically very close, their transcription occurs on opposite DNA strands and is not coupled to the same stimuli. AVP, OT, and their respective neurophysins are cleaved within neurosecretory granules and are reassembled into a hormone-binding protein complex before excretion from the posterior pituitary glands.

The amino acid sequences of the two neurophysins are similar within and between species. This suggests that they have arisen from a common ancestral neurophysin by gene duplication. These two neurophysins have been found in the pituitary of each of the mammals studied. The precursor molecule, with associated proteolytic enzymes, is present within the granules of the neurosecretory cells. These enzymes may be necessary to split the neurophysin from the precursor molecule because cleavage of the precursor occurs inside the granule after it begins migration from the Golgi regions in the hypothalamic perikarya to the axon terminals in the neural lobe. AVP and OT bind noncovalently in a specific manner to neurophysins. Thus the neurophysins are believed to function as transport proteins for the neurohypophysial hormones. Neurophysin is secreted with its hormone into the bloodstream in response to physiologic stimulation. The secreted neurophysins are considered to function only as intraneuronal carrier proteins for the hormones and to lack any systemic hormonal/physiological function.

The early work of Bargmann and Scharrer [3], which used staining techniques for neurosecretory material, established the site of origin of the pars nervosa hormones. It was noted that some axons of the supraopticohypophysial tract project to the external zone of the median eminence and also to the third ventricle. Both AVP and neurophysin are present in granules of axons that are in contact with the hypophysial portal system, and these peptides are secreted into the portal blood. These observations suggest a possible role of AVP in the control of anterior pituitary function. Neurohypophysial hormone secretion into the cerebrospinal fluid may also be important physiologically, for example, in the regulation of cerebrospinal electrolyte composition.

CONTROL OF NEUROHYPOPHYSIAL HORMONE SECRETION

Stimuli received by sensory receptors in the breast or vascular system result in release of OT or AVP, respectively, from the neurohypophysis. Neural afferents to the spinal cord connect with other neural pathways to the neurosecretory cell bodies localized within the PVN and SON. The neurosecretory neurons are in synaptic contact with neurons from these afferent pathways. There may be excitatory (cholinergic) and inhibitory (noradrenergic) connections from the rostral midbrain to the neurosecretory neurons. Destruction of noradrenergic neurons in the rabbit brainstem, for example, elevates plasma AVP, resulting in hypertension. There may also be interneurons that synchronize the activity of the neurosecretory neurons within the hypothalamic nuclei. Release of an excitatory neurotransmitter from afferent neurons onto the neurosecretory neurons results in depolarization of the cells. Action potentials can be recorded from mammalian neurosecretory cells of the SON and PVN. The pattern of firing of OT cells can be distinguished from that of AVP-secreting cells during appropriate stimulation, such as suckling or hemorrhage, respectively [39]. The putative AVP-secreting cells show a rhythmic bursting-type discharge that is increased by high osmotic pressure, whereas OT-producing cells appear to discharge continuously and in a random fashion. This pattern of firing, characteristic of the rat, may not be typical for all species.

Depolarization of neurosecretory cell bodies is propagated along the axons of the hypothalamo-hypophysial tract to the neuron terminals in the pars nervosa. Calcium ions enter the neurosecretory neurons during depolarization, and are required for the secretory process, as neurohypophysial hormone secretion is inhibited in the absence of Ca^{2+}. Neurosecretory granules fuse with the plasmalemma of the cells and are extruded via vesicular exocytosis. The secreted hormone and associated neurophysin enter the bloodstream in the vessels passing out of the neurohypophysis.

A specific facilitatory effect of OT on OT release has been demonstrated for SON- and PVN-neurons in various electrophysiological studies. In addition the morphological finding of oxytocinergic synapses impinging on OT neurons in the SON provides evidence for a facilitatory action of OT on OT release. The stimulatory effect of OT on OT release could be functionally meaningful as a mechanism for enhancement of the burst discharges under conditions of OT demand [13]. Prolactin is also implicated in the control of OT release during suckling (see Chap. 19).

Messenger RNAs of neurohypophysial hormones occur within the axons of magnocellular hypothalamic neurons known to secrete OT and AVP. Brattleboro rats have a genetic mutation that renders them incapable of AVP expression and secretion and thus causes diabetes insipidus. Injection into the hypothalamus of purified mRNAs from normal rat hypothalami or of synthetic copies of the AVP mRNA leads to selective uptake, retrograde transport, and expression of AVP exclusively in the magnocellular neurons. Temporary reversal of their diabetes insipidus can be observed within hours of the injection. Intra-axonal mRNAs may represent an additional category of chemical signals for neurons. These observations suggest that rat hypothalamic magnocellular neurons can take up and translate certain specific exogenous RNAs normally expressed in these neurons. This hypothesis is supported by the finding that degradation of RNA is low in the brain. Oxytocin mRNA is present in secretory vesicles in the hypothalamoneurohypophysial system, suggesting that these mRNAs exist in cellular compartments together with peptide signals known to be secreted. Recent studies with in situ hybridization and electron microscopy indicate a similar situation for AVP mRNA. Axonal uptake, transport, and secretion of mRNA may offer new approaches in regulating interneuronal signaling [21].

PHYSIOLOGICAL ROLES

Control milk
uterine contraction

Oxytocin is involved in the control of milk release and in uterine contraction during labor. Vasopressin, or antidiuretic hormone as its name implies, is important in the homeostatic control of the extracellular fluid volume. The antidiuretic response is of survival value to individuals of both sexes. OT, on the other hand, apparently functions only during specific times in the reproductive cycle of the adult female. No function for OT in the male has been clearly established.

Oxytocin

Oxytocin is an example, along with several others (progesterone and chorionic gonadotropin, Chap. 19), of a hormone that plays only a transitory role, possibly specific to the female, and then, in some cases, only if she becomes pregnant and delivers a child at term.

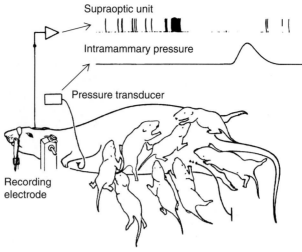

Figure 7.3 Scheme for measuring the electrical activity of hypothalamic neurosecretory neurons associated with reflex release of OT during suckling in the rat. The upper trace (supraoptic unit or SO) shows the action potentials recorded from a cell in the supraoptic nucleus, while the lower trace is a recording of intramammary pressure. Note the burst of potentials that occurs 12 seconds before the increase in pressure. (From Lincoln and Wakerley [26], with permission.)

sensory
nerve
endings
↓
neurohypophysis

Milk Release (Let-Down). OT functions in the control of milk release after parturition. Sensory nerve endings, which are localized to the areolae and nipples of the breasts, are stimulated by suckling (Fig. 7.3), and afferent neural pathways conduct these stimuli to the neurohypophysis [26]. From studies on different animals, the various components of these neural pathways have been traced. The pathways are ipsilateral (same side) to the teat being suckled. Neural impulses conducted along the sensory neurons enter the spinal column and ascend via dorsal, lateral, and ventral spinothalamic tracts to the mesencephalon of the brain. These stimuli are then transmitted via a diencephalic route to the hypothalamus. The neural pathways controlling OT secretion have been determined by electrode stimulation and lesioning experiments [57]. Stimulation of the ventral diencephalon in anesthetized animals results in ejection of milk. On the other hand, lesions in the PVN in lactating animals result in marked diminution in the quantity of milk released from the mammary gland. Electrophysiological recordings from putative oxytocinergic neurons in unanesthetized, freely moving rats established that the electrical activity displayed by these magnocellular neurons, some 10 to 12 seconds before milk ejection, is responsible for OT release under normal physiological conditions.

At parturition dilation of the cervix (vaginal stretching) may also be a stimulus to OT secretion. Cross-circulation experiments have been carried out with pairs of unanesthetized ewes in which the jugular veins had previously been crossed so that each member of a pair received blood only from its partner. Mechanical distension of the vagina in one of the ewes resulted in a milk-ejection response only in the other ewe. Similar results were obtained when the roles were reversed. There is increased uterine activity during mating, and milk ejection during coitus in the human female and other animals has been reported. Auditory and optic sensory stimuli also affect milk let-down in some animals. (Ask any farmer who has milked a cow.)

Ovarian hormones affect the levels of neurohypophysial hormones in the pituitary of the rat. The firing rates of paraventricular neurons are increased during proestrus and estrus and after estrogen treatment in ovariectomized rats. Estrogen treatment also facilitates the activation of paraventricular secretory cell units and the reflex release of OT by genital

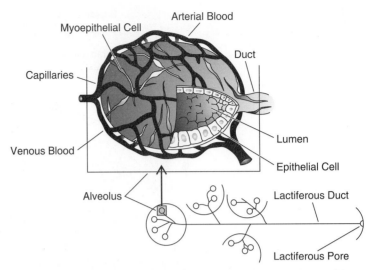

Figure 7.4 Alveolus and mammary gland ductal system. (From Rillema, "Development of the mammary gland and lactation." Reprinted by permission of the publisher from *Trends in Endocrinology and Metabolism* 5:149–54, ©1994 by Elsevier Science Inc.)

tract stimulation. Therefore, ovarian hormones may not only promote the expression of sexual receptivity (see Chap. 18), but may also increase levels of neurohypophysial hormones and facilitate release of these hormones during mating. Because these hormones have potent stimulating effects on uterine and oviduct smooth muscle, they might also enhance the likelihood of fertilization by promoting sperm transport.

The major target organ of OT is the mammary gland of the pregnant female. The alveolar and ductal system of the mammary gland is depicted in Fig. 7.4. OT released from the pars nervosa elicits contraction of cellular musclelike elements [27, 40], myoepithelial cells (Fig. 7.5), which results in increased intramammary pressure and the expression of milk from the alveoli and ducts out through the teats (Fig. 7.6). The effect of OT on milk release from isolated mammary gland tissue in vitro is easily demonstrated [6].

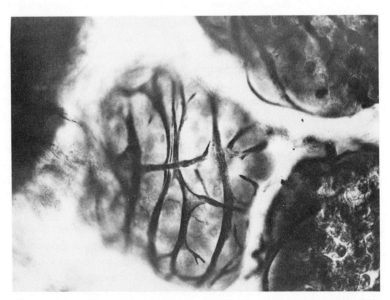

Figure 7.5 Silver-stained section of lactating mammary gland of the goat. A surface view of a contracted alveolus shows a myoepithelial cell with nucleus (N) and branching processes. (From Richardson [40], with permission.)

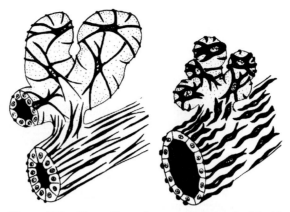

Figure 7.6 Disposition of myoepithelial cells (black) around alveoli and ducts. (Left) Myoepithelial cells relaxed, alveoli full. (Right) Myoepithelial cells contracted, alveoli emptied, ducts widened. (From Linzell [27], by permission of John Wright & Sons.)

High affinity sites that bind [^{3}H]-labeled OT are present in membrane fractions of mammary gland from the lactating rat [53]. OT binding activity is specifically localized by autoradiography to the plasma membrane of myoepithelial cells of mammary tissue (Fig 7.7).

Uterine Contraction. OT has been used for years to induce labor in human females at term. OT contracts the myometrium (uterotropic action), which can be demonstrated in vitro. Whether OT is responsible for initiating labor has been debated. Although OT is found in the maternal circulation throughout pregnancy, OT concentrations in the blood increase only during the final stages of labor, not before. It is suggested that parturition may be triggered not only by an increase in OT secretion per se, but also by an

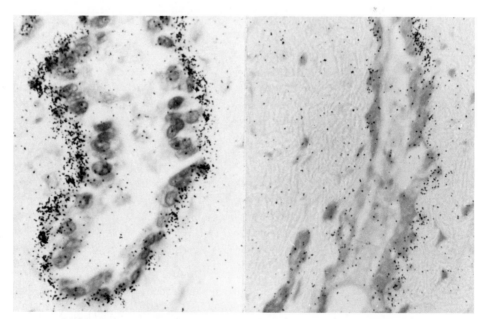

Figure 7.7 Autoradiographic localization of tritium-labeled OT to myoepithelial cells of the rat mammary gland. Radioactivity was accumulated in the regions corresponding to the location of myoepithelial cells in the alveoli (left) and along the ducts (right). (From Soloff et al. [53], with permission.)

increase in the sensitivity of the myometrium of the uterus to the hormone [52]. The response of the myometrium to OT is maximal at or near parturition.

It has been demonstrated that specific binding of [³H]oxytocin to uterine receptors of pregnant rats increases dramatically at term and is maximal during labor [15, 52, 53]. In contrast, there is only a gradual increase in binding of [³H]oxytocin to mammary tissue, but this binding does become maximal during lactation. Changes in the ratio of plasma estradiol to progesterone concentration closely parallel the changes in OT binding: estradiol is elevated and progesterone diminished. Estrogens increase myometrial sensitivity to OT and increase the number of OT receptors in the uterus. Progesterone, on the other hand, suppresses the appearance of OT receptors. Decreased synthesis of progesterone may, therefore, indirectly increase production of OT receptors. Thus it appears that parturition is preceded by a dramatic increase in myometrial OT receptors, which may render the myometrium more sensitive to OT [16]. The meager number of OT receptors before term might make the myometrium insensitive to the circulating hormone. Therefore parturition may be triggered by an increase in myometrial receptor number, as well as an increase in OT levels in the blood during labor. This hypothesis unites many observations and arguments on the role of OT in parturition.

Circulating OT, however, is not essential for the initiation or maintenance of spontaneous labor. Parturition can begin in the absence of circulating OT, and although OT antiserum suppresses lactation it fails to affect parturition. There is no universal agreement as to whether there is an increase in circulating OT levels prior to the onset of labor. OT of pituitary origin therefore may not play a physiological role in parturition. Oxytocin mRNA and peptide in rat uteri are increased more than 150-fold during pregnancy, exceeding that of hypothalamic mRNA (Fig. 7.8) [25]. These observations suggest that the rat uterus itself

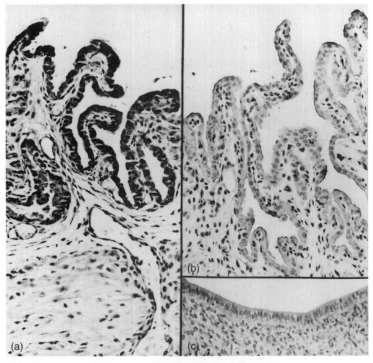

Figure 7.8   Immunocytochemical staining of sections of rat uterus with an antibody to OT. (a) Uterus of 21-day-pregnant rat. (b) Same as (a), but nonimmune serum was used instead of primary antiserum. (c) Uterus, stained with immune serum, of nonpregnant, diestrous female rat. Sections were immunostained with an avidin-biotin complex. (From Lefebvre et al. [25], with permission. *Science* 256:1553–5, 1992. ©1992 by the American Association for the Advancement of Science.)

is the major site of OT gene expression during the later stages of pregnancy. OT therefore may act as a local paracrine or autocrine mediator of parturition, rather than as a circulating hormone. It appears that the uterus contains an intrinsic OT system in which both ligand and receptor are subject to strict regulation. The rise in uterine OT gene expression, in concert with the rise in uterine OT receptors, may represent the "trigger for parturition." Dysregulation of uterine OT gene expression may be an underlying cause of premature or delayed labor. OT gene expression has also been observed in the human uterus [29].

Vascular Smooth Muscle Actions. Neurohypophysial hormones contract or relax vascular smooth muscle [45]. The exact type of response depends on species, vascular bed, and region within a vascular bed. Thus within a single species of animal the neurohypophysial peptides can exert vasoconstrictor actions in one peripheral vascular bed and vasodilator actions in another. There may be two distinct kinds of neurohypophysial hormone receptors, one that subserves contraction and the other that subserves relaxation. There may even be different relative proportions of both receptors that vary in number depending on blood vessel segment and species. In addition OT may act on a distinctly different vascular receptor from that of AVP. For example, OT is highly effective in contracting human umbilical arteries and veins, whereas AVP is relatively inactive. Rat aortic strips, in contrast, are extremely sensitive to the contractile effects of AVP, but are insensitive to OT. Synthesis of neurohypophysial analogs can provide peptides with unique and selective microcirculatory effects that may be clinically useful in the treatment of low vascular flow rates [22].

Effects on Adenohypophysial Function. OT exerts an inhibitory effect on CRH-mediated ACTH secretion when infused into the human male. No effects on other adenohypophysial hormone responses under conditions of submaximal stimulation by hypothalamic-releasing factors could be demonstrated. OT may play a part in the neuroendocrine response to stress in humans [35].

A possible regulatory role of OT in PRL secretion during suckling has been suggested. Although secretion of OT and PRL is not absolutely correlated, it was reported that OT-stimulated release of PRL from dispersed rat pituitary cells in vitro, and immunoneutralization of rats with antiserum specific to OT, significantly reduced PRL release during suckling or after estrogen treatment. Superfusion of rat pituitary cells with OT resulted in a significant PRL-releasing activity. It is likely that OT plays an important role in PRL release, especially during suckling, as reported by several investigators [31].

Maternal Behavior. Intact (nonovariectomized) virgin female rats given OT through lateral ventricular cannulae displayed full maternal behavior toward foster pups [37]. Saline- or AVP-treated animals did not display full maternal behavior. Estrogens also induce maternal behavior, and it was suggested that elevated or recently elevated levels of estrogens may be necessary for the induction of full maternal behavior by OT. Intracerebroventricular (ICV) injected OT in ovariectomized female rats failed to induce maternal behavior, whereas most estrogen-primed animals became fully maternal in response to the hormone.

Ovarian estrogens may promote maternal behavior by increasing OT release or OT binding within the brain, or both. OT levels do rise markedly around the time of parturition. Maternal behavior is significantly reduced following ICV infusion of antibodies to OT. These observations suggest that OT endogenous to the brain may mediate the onset of maternal behavior. OT is widely distributed within neurons of the brain, and cerebral spinal fluid levels of OT rise markedly around the time of parturition. It is possible that OT may be released at many sites within the brain to activate maternal behavior [37].

Mating Behavior. The ventromedial nuclei of the hypothalamus (VMN) are important for the control of feminine mating behavior, and hormone action within these nuclei has been causally related to behavior. Estradiol induces receptors for OT in the VMN and in the area lateral to these nuclei over the course of 1 to 2 days, and progesterone causes, within 30 minutes of its application, a further increase in OT receptor binding and an expansion of the area covered by these receptors lateral to the VMN. The rapid progesterone action appears to be a direct and specific effect of this steroid on membrane receptors, because it was produced in vitro as well as in vivo and was not mimicked by a variety of other steroids. The effect of progesterone occurred in the posterior part of the VMN, where OT infusion facilitated feminine mating behavior; it did not take place in the anterior part of the VMN, where OT infusion had no effect on mating behavior [48, 49].

Human Sexual Response.   Plasma OT levels increase during sexual arousal (self-stimulation) in both women and men and are significantly higher during orgasm/ejaculation than during prior baseline testing [8]. OT is secreted specifically at the time of ejaculation in men. This is preceded by a rise in AVP secretion during arousal, which returns to baseline values by the time of ejaculation. AVP release during arousal may be associated with specific suppression of OT until ejaculation [32]. OT may play a role in the physiology of sexual responses by facilitating contractions of the smooth muscles of the uterus and vagina in women. Likewise, release of OT during sexual responses in men may be related to increased contractility of reproductive smooth muscle tissue. Thus OT may enhance both sperm and egg transport, thereby promoting reproductive success [7].

Control of Feeding Behavior.   Administration of cholecystokinin (CCK) to rats causes a dose-related increase in plasma levels of OT [59]. The effect of CCK on OT secretion was blunted after gastric vagotomy, as was the inhibition of food intake induced by CCK. CCK immunoreactivity has been colocalized in some oxytocinergic neurons. It is possible that multiple vagally-mediated stimuli converge in the hypothalamus to cause secretion of CCK as well as OT. Ablation of the paraventricular nucleus can lead to hyperphagia and obesity in rats. These observations suggest that this hypothalamic nucleus plays an important role in the control of feeding behavior and also that OT and CCK are involved in this regulatory system.

Vasopressin (AVP)

AVP has two major physiological actions: it induces the contraction or relaxation of certain types of smooth muscle, and it promotes the movement of water (and Na^+) across responsive epithelial tissues, notably the distal tubule of the mammalian kidney and the skin and urinary bladder of amphibians. Radioimmunoassay of circulating AVP under varying experimental conditions and pathophysiological states has provided detailed information on the role of AVP in the control of water balance [42].

Osmoregulation.   When body fluid osmolality decreases, AVP levels fall; this causes the excretion of free water via a hypotonic urine. In contrast, when body fluid osmolality rises, AVP is released, stimulating free water retention and excretion of a hypertonic urine [18]. Blood osmolality is important in the control of AVP secretion [42, 43], and injections of small volumes of hypertonic solution into the carotid artery of the dog result in an immediate antidiuresis. Osmoreceptors are localized in the anterior hypothalamus. These osmoreceptors were thought to be near or identical to the magnocellular neurons of the neurohypophysis. It is now believed that the osmoreceptor function is not performed by the neurosecretory cells. An antidiuretic response is evoked only when hypertonic saline is infused in small volumes at sites some distance from the SON. Small lesions in the medial preoptic area of the hypothalamus, which do not involve the neurohypophysis, prevent AVP secretion in response to fluid deprivation. In addition, in the rare clinical syndrome of adipsic hypernatremia, patients have a complete lack of osmotically-mediated AVP secretion, but they secrete AVP in response to hemodynamic (baroreceptor) stimuli. The osmoreceptors in humans would therefore appear to be totally separate from the neurosecretory cells and are apparently not an integral component of the neuronal pathways by which AVP secretion is affected by hemodynamic variables [42].

In summary, the physiologically important osmoreceptor control mechanism is near but neither identical to nor intermixed with the cell bodies of the neurohypophysial neurons (Fig. 7.9A$_1$). Because osmotically mediated AVP release can be totally ablated without altering in any way the hormonal response to hypotension, this excludes the possibility that hemodynamic stimuli are transmitted to the neurohypophysis by way of osmoreceptor neurons (Fig. 7.9A$_1$ and A$_2$). Possibly the AVP-secreting cells of the neurohypophysis are functionally heterogeneous; that is, they are divided into different units that receive afferents from the osmoregulatory or the baroregulatory systems (Fig. 7.9B). If so, one might expect that the function of one unit should have no effect on the other. This is not the case. In addition, electrophysiological recordings from neurosecretory cells in the anterior and lateral hypothalamus revealed firing rates that could be altered by *both* volume and osmotic stimuli. Thus the control system may be organized as depicted (Fig. 7.9C).

In normal individuals the *osmostat* appears to be set so that AVP secretion is suppressed to low or undetectable levels whenever plasma osmolality falls to 280 mOsm/kg or below [43]. Above this concentration AVP secretion rises (Fig. 7.10, left) in direct proportion to the osmolality, affecting maximal antidiursis at a plasma osmolality around 295 mOsm/kg. Changes in plasma osmolality as small as 1% will increase or decrease plasma AVP levels and affect urinary osmolality (Fig. 7.8, right), suggesting that the osmoreceptors are extraordinarily sensitive to changes in blood electrolyte concentration. Osmoreceptors exhibit a specificity for certain solutes. For example, hypertonic saline or sucrose, but not urea or glucose, induces an antidiuretic response. Because well over 90% of the osmotic activity of plasma is normally contributed by Na$^+$ and its anions, the osmoreceptors would be expected to function mainly in the detection of Na$^+$ osmolality changes [42]. Oral saline intake reduces the AVP content of the SON and PVN but is without effect on the AVP content of the median eminence. Salt loading also increases the mRNA content of the neural lobe, suggesting increased synthesis of the hormone [33]. This supports the concept for an independent control of AVP biosynthesis in the median eminence.

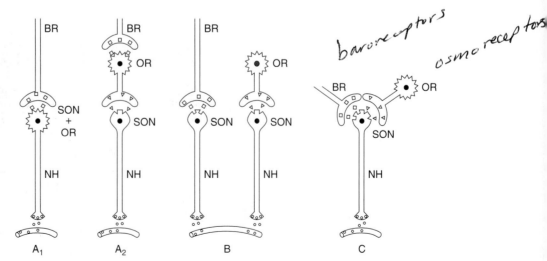

Figure 7.9 Schematic representation of possible modes of organization of the neurohypophysis (NH) and its regulatory afferents from osmoreceptors (OR) and baroreceptors (BR). Supraoptic and paraventricular nuclei are designated as SON. (From Robertson, Athar, and Shelton [42], with permission.)

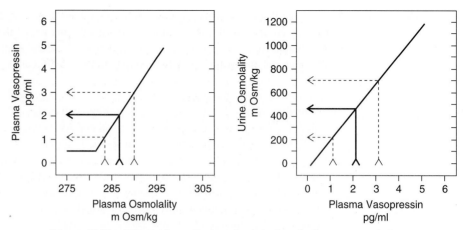

Figure 7.10 Effect of small alterations in basal plasma osmolality on plasma vasopressin and urine osmolality in normal humans. (From Robertson, Shelton, and Athar [43], with permission.)

Blood Volume-Pressure Regulation. Changes in blood volume and pressure affect AVP secretion [9]. Hemodynamic influences are exerted via neural afferents originating in pressure-sensitive receptors (baroreceptors) in the left atrium of the heart, aortic arch, and the carotid sinus ([62], Fig. 7.11). Afferent stimuli in response to changing blood volume or pressure reach the brainstem through the vagal and glossopharyngeal nerves. The central pathways integrating these signals are unidentified, but they may involve a primary synapse in the nucleus tractus solitarius with a secondary relay in the posterior-medial nucleus of the hypothalamus.

Significant increases in plasma AVP (in rats) are not detected until blood volume is reduced by more than 8%. The relationship between AVP and blood volume in humans follows an exponential pattern similar to that of rats. Under more unphysiological conditions, as in excessive hemorrhage, AVP causes maximal antidiuresis and may exert significant pressor effects on certain vascular beds [14]. In humans and other animals there is an exponential relationship between plasma AVP levels and the degree of hypotension produced. Enhanced AVP secretion ensues after a reduction in mean arterial pressure as small as 5%. Volume and Na^+ concentration may also affect AVP secretion through the renin-angiotensin system (see Chap. 15). Angiotensin II, an octapeptide, may act on the

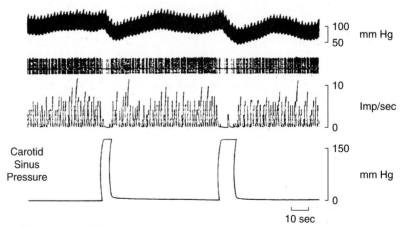

Figure 7.11 Effects of periodically increased pressure in the isolated carotid sinus on the activity of a SON neuron. Upper, middle, and bottom traces show the blood pressure, unit activity, integrated record of the number of spikes per second and carotid sinus pressure. (From Yamashita [62], with permission.)

brain to stimulate AVP secretion. Thus a complex set of factors control AVP secretion and, subsequently, water and electrolyte balance.

Central AVP may play a role in the control of blood pressure and heart rate in both normotensive and hypertensive animals [44]. Administration of AVP into the CNS produces changes in arterial pressure and heart rate that can be reversed by competitive receptor antagonists. AVP is also a potent releasing factor for corticotropin and corticosterone, which in turn act on the cardiovascular system. Central administration of AVP produces cardiovascular responses attributable to stimulation of sympathetic outflow. AVP may, in early stages of hypertension, alter sympathetic outflow via an effect on central neural structures controlling the CNS. Central administration of AVP also causes an increase in heart rate; thus, the peptide appears to override the ability of the baroreceptor reflex to buffer changes in arterial pressure. AVP may therefore participate in baroreceptor reflex resetting in hypertension and alter sympathetic outflow via effects on the baroreceptor reflex system [5].

Adenohypophysial Function.   In the monkey, AVP is present in high concentrations in the portal blood of the anterior pituitary. There is an increase in neurosecretory material in the median eminence of the rat after adrenalectomy. Specifically there is an increase in both neurophysin and AVP, but not OT, in the external zone of the median eminence, and the increase appears to be due to a lack of glucocorticoids.

Vasopressin stimulates the release of ACTH and, subsequently, cortisol from the pituitary and adrenal glands, respectively. This has been described in rats, in humans, in isolated pituitary glands, and in dispersed anterior pituitary cells. The greatest response to AVP occurs when it is coadministered with corticotropin-releasing hormone. In this situation there is synergism between the two releasing factors to cause an augmented release of ACTH. Thus it is now thought that if AVP plays a role in the release of ACTH it is probably through the potentiation of the CRH action.

AVP at physiological concentrations acts specifically on anterior pituitary cells to enhance the release of TSH. The finding that AVP is equipotent with TRH in stimulating TSH release strongly suggests that AVP may indeed be a physiological regulator of TSH secretion. In the hypothalamus, however, AVP may function as a negative auto-feedback agent to regulate signals for TSH release. The fact that centrally administered AVP lowers plasma TSH, but not other hormones, is consistent with observations that hypothalamic-releasing or inhibiting factors, at the appropriate ventricular dose, produce effects that oppose their direct actions on their respective target cells of the adenohypophysis. Others have supported this concept of negative ultrashort-loop feedback for hypothalamic-releasing and inhibiting factors in vitro.

Vasopressin and Behavior.   AVP is said to play a role in behavior (see Chap. 21). Unless the hormone is transported retrogradely from the pars nervosa directly to the brain, one may wonder how this neurohypophysial hormone could play such a role if secreted directly into the peripheral circulation. Circulating peptide hormones at physiological concentrations are not generally considered capable of crossing the "blood-brain barrier." If, on the other hand, this hormone is secreted from neurons within the brain, then it or other neurohypophysial peptides might indeed act as a neurotransmitter or, more likely, as a neuromodulator.

Vasotocin (AVT)

AVT rather than AVP is present in the pituitary gland of nonmammalian vertebrates. Only a few of the many putative roles of this hormone can be discussed here.

Sexual Behavior.   Intracerebroventricular injections of AVT induce sexual activity (amplectic clasping) in male newts (salamanders), a response that was blunted by an

AVT antagonist or by an anti-AVT immune serum. Intracranial implants of certain gonadal steroids in castrated male newts maintained the behavioral response to AVT. Systemic injections of the steroid hormones failed to increase the incidence of sexual behavior. These observations suggest that AVT induces sexual behavior in newts by acting on cells in the brain. In male newts high concentrations of AVT in the cerebrospinal fluid, dorsal preoptic area, ventral infundibular nucleus, and optic tectum are associated with the propensity to exhibit sexual behavior. This is the first direct evidence that the motivational state of an animal to initiate reproduction is regulated, in part, by the concentrations of particular neuropeptides in specific brain areas [64].

Oviposition.   There is evidence, in some reptiles and birds [51] at least, that AVT regulates oviductal muscle contraction. Marine turtles are oviparous reptiles that emerge from the water to construct a nest and deposit a clutch consisting of 100 to 200 eggs. The nesting process can be clearly divided into a series of nine discrete nesting behaviors. Nesting begins when the animal strands (emerges from the water) and proceeds through the production of a body pit (a shallow depression into which the animal positions itself for oviposition); nest construction; digging the egg chamber; depositing the first, middle, and last eggs; covering the nest; and ends when the animal returns to the water. The entire process consumes approximately 1 hour. Circulating levels of AVT were shown to increase dramatically prior to the onset of oviposition and decrease rapidly following its conclusion. The time span of this transient increase is approximately 45 minutes (Fig 7.12). The elevation of systemic AVT coincident with a period of increased oviductal motility indicates a role for AVT in reptilian reproduction analogous to the known reproductive roles of the neurohypophysial peptides in birds and mammals.

Oviposition, the expulsion of the egg from the oviduct, is accompanied by a marked increase in contractions of the oviductal smooth muscle in the hen and generally takes place each day. AVT may play a physiological role in the regulation of oviposition since an increase in plasma levels of AVT and a decrease in AVT content in the neurohypophysis have been demonstrated during egg expulsion from the oviduct. An increase in oviductal contractility may be a stimulus for AVT release during normal oviposition. The mechanisms that initiate an increase in contractions of the oviduct are not known [51].

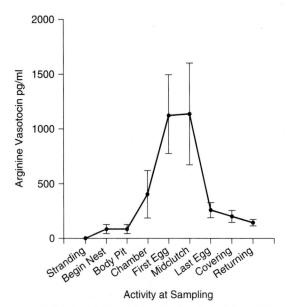

Figure 7.12   Mean serum AVT levels in Olive Ridley sea turtles (*Lepidochelys olivacea*) throughout nesting. (Figure provided by Robert A. Figler, Texas A&M University.)

METABOLISM

A number of enzymes exist in a variety of tissues that can degrade the neurohypophysial hormones in a specific manner. For example, an enzyme capable of inactivating OT appears in human blood during pregnancy. It is produced in the placenta and is referred to as plasma *oxytocinase*. This amino peptidase produces a rupture of the ring of OT by hydrolysis of the hemicystinyl-tyrosyl bond. The colostrum also contains enzymes, apparently produced in the mammary gland, which inactivate neurohypophysial hormones. The kidney, which is also a target organ for neurohypophysial hormones, contains a variety of enzymes that degrade and inactivate these hormones.

MECHANISMS OF HORMONE ACTION

As for other peptide hormones, OT and AVP interact with target tissue cellular membrane receptors. Some of the earliest evidence for a role of cyclic nucleotides in hormone action derived from studies on the mechanism of AVP action.

Oxytocin

Uterine Contraction.   OT interacts not only with myometrial but also with endometrial receptors. OT stimulates the synthesis of $PGF_{2\alpha}$ in the ovine uterus by interacting with the endometrium, which is the principal source of uterine PGs. Estrogens also enhance uterine synthesis of PGs by increasing the activity of PG synthetase in rats. Estrogens also increase the number of endometrial and myometrial OT receptors. Progesterone antagonizes these estrogen effects in rats. Thus estrogen-induced development of endometrial OT receptors would enhance endometrial $PGF_{2\alpha}$ production in the presence of OT. Myometrial contractions, a mechanical event, also induce endometrial $PGF_{2\alpha}$ production; thus OT may affect $PGF_{2\alpha}$ synthesis directly and indirectly.

Prostaglandins of uterine origin are believed to control luteolysis in some species of mammals. OT could induce luteal regression via regulation of uterine synthesis of PGs. The normal course of labor might depend on an early increase in uterine synthesis of PGs to inhibit luteal or placental production of progesterone. Decreased progesterone levels would remove the block to OT-induced uterine contractions, which are maintained up to that time by the steroid hormone (see Chap. 19). The uterotropic actions of OT have now been clarified in some detail. OT exerts its myometrial contractile effect by increasing intracellular levels of Ca^{2+}. OT binding to myometrial receptors inhibits Ca^{2+} extrusion at the sarcolemma by inhibiting a Ca^{2+}-ATPase. OT receptor binding also produces a rapid Ca^{2+} influx (measured with ^{45}Ca) through receptor-mediated Ca^{2+} channel activation. The inhibition of Ca^{2+} extrusion and the concomitant uptake of the cation prolongs the elevation of intracellular Ca^{2+}, thus promoting myometrial contraction. Inositol triphosphate had earlier been shown to release Ca^{2+} from internal stores of myometrial cells. IP_3 causes Ca^{2+} release from SR microsomal fractions. Oxytocin has now been shown to stimulate IP_3 production by human gestational myometrial cells. OT also elevates IP_3 in a dose-dependent manner in the pregnant uterus but is ineffective in the nonpregnant uterus. A model for OT-induced uterine contraction is shown (Fig. 7.13).

Vasopressin

Vasopressin Receptors.   Vasopressin receptors display a diversity in pharmacological, functional, and biological properties. Four subtypes of receptors have been distinguished on a functional and/or pharmacological basis [30]. The renal AVP receptor (V_2-type) that mediates the antidiuretic response was among the first membrane receptors for which a functional coupling with adenylate cyclase was demonstrated. AVP receptors of

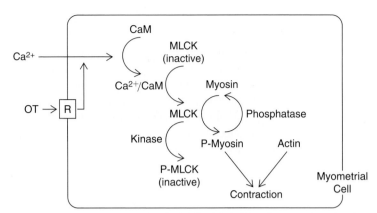

Figure 7.13 Scheme of contraction in uterine smooth muscle [61]. A rise in Ca^{2+}, produced either spontaneously or by an agonist such as OT interacting with its receptor (R), causes Ca^{2+} to bind to calmodulin (Ca^{2+}/CaM). This activates myosin light-chain kinase (MLCK). This kinase then phosphorylates light chains on myosin (P-myosin). This allows actin binding and activates myosin Mg-ATPase, thus contraction can occur with hydrolysis of ATP. P-myosin is dephosphorylated by phosphatases, leading to relaxation. If MLCK is phosphorylated, for example, by Ca^{2+} calmodulin-dependent protein kinase II, then it is much less efficient at phosphorylating myosin, and force falls. Reduction of Ca^{2+} will also promote relaxation (modified from [61]).

the liver (V_{1a}-type) and adenohypophysis (V_{1b}-type) and OT receptors of the uterus and mammary gland act through increased inositol turnover to mobilize intracellular Ca^{2+} [4]. The immediate transmembrane signalling of V_1-vascular AVP receptors involves ligand-receptor complex formation; receptor lateral mobility and internalization, coupling to a G_q protein; activation of phospholipases A_2, C, and D; translocation and activation of protein kinase C; production of inositol 1,4,5-triphosphate and 1,2-diacylglycerol; mobilization of intracellular Ca^{2+}; alteration of intracellular pH with activation of the Na^+/H^+ exchanger; calmodulin activation; and myosin light-chain phosphorylation [55]. The secondary nuclear signal mechanisms triggered by activation of V_1-vascular AVP receptors include tyrosine phosphorylation, induction of gene expression, and protein synthesis [56].

AVP and OT have overlapping pharmacological properties (Table 7.2). More specific agonists are therefore useful in determining whether OT or AVP receptors may be involved in mediating a given biological response. Some examples of agonists available for determining whether responses are mediated by OT or by V_1 or V_2 AVP receptors appear in Table 7.2. Regardless of an AVP receptor's pharmacological properties, it can only be definitively classified based on the cellular second messenger its activation evokes. Although many specific antagonists are available, by themselves they are rarely useful for identifying receptor types. Using antagonists, however, one may distinguish differences among receptors that are not clear from studies using agonists alone. For example, one such study showed that V_{1b} receptors on adenohypophysial cells differ pharmacologically from the V_{1a} receptors on hepatocytes or vascular smooth muscle cells, although they have a similar second-messenger system [46].

The mechanism of action of AVP has been determined from studies on a variety of epithelia—frog skin, toad bladder, and mammalian nephron. The toad bladder, a storage organ for water, is a useful and simple model system and responds to AVP similarly to the distal tubule of the mammalian nephron. The organ is a relatively large sheet of thin epithelium that survives for long periods in vitro. Exposure of isolated toad bladder to AVP results in an increase in Na^+ and water transport from the outer (mucosal or luminal) to the inner (serosal) side. AVP can only affect water permeability if applied to the serosal side of the bladder, and it can only act on the kidney collecting duct when applied to the peritubular (serosal) side. The barrier to water penetration across such membranes is

TABLE 7.2 Relative Potencies of Some Analogs of AVP and OT

AVP: Cys–Tyr–Phe–Gln–Asn–Cys–Pro–Arg–Gly(NH$_2$)

OT: Cys–Tyr–Ile–Gln–Asn–Cys–Pro–Leu–Gly(NH$_2$)

	Activities, U/mg*		
	VP(V$_1$)	AD(V$_2$)	OT[†]
AVP	380	330	60
OT	4	4	490
dDAVP (1-deamino[D-Arg^8]VP)	0.4	1300	3
[Phe^2, Orn^8]OT	121	1.6	5
[Thr^4,Gly^7]OT	<0.01	0.002	860

*Data from [46].

[†]Oxytocic (OT) activities assayed on isolated rat uteri in a medium containing 0.5 mM Mg^{2+}

in the mucosal (luminal) side. This barrier is decreased in the presence of AVP, and water is moved across the cells and leaves at the basal (serosal) margins. In the unstimulated state, the apical membranes of these cells have an extremely low permeability to water; the dramatic increase in permeability occurs within minutes of the addition of AVP to the basolateral side of the epithelium. When AVP is withdrawn, the reversal of permeability also occurs within minutes.

Interaction of AVP with toad bladder serosal plasmalemmal receptors activates adenylate cyclase and intracellular levels of cAMP are elevated [18]. The result is that the mucosal membrane then has an increased permeability to water. Cyclic AMP or its analogs, as well as phosphodiesterase inhibitors (e.g., theophylline), enhance water permeability, thus supporting a role for cAMP as the intracellular messenger of AVP. The actions of AVP on frog skin and the mammalian nephron also involve elevations in cAMP levels.

The site of action of these effects is the membrane of the mucosal surface. Structural changes (intramembranous particle aggregation) occur in this barrier to render the membrane more permeable to water. AVP controls renal water retention by inserting water channels into the normally water-tight apical membranes of the collecting duct. This allows water flow from the tubule lumen along osmotic gradients between the tubular fluid and the surrounding interstitium. AVP also enhances Na$^+$ reabsorption by the collecting duct and, in some animals, increases transepithelial solute transport in the medullary thick ascending limb, thereby increasing osmotic gradients for water reabsorption. In some amphibia dilute urine is stored in a large bladder where it can be reabsorbed in response to AVP secreted when body fluid osmolality rises. Since AVP-responsive properties of toad urinary bladder granular epithelial cells closely resemble those of principal cells of the mammalian collecting duct, the toad bladder is a useful model of ADH-responsive renal epithelia [18].

The cloning of water-selective channels is beginning to reveal the molecular basis of renal water transport. The water-selective channel, aquaporin-1 (CHIP28), is responsible for the constitutively high water permeability in the proximal tubule and the descending thin limb of the loop of Henle. In mammals other mechanisms are needed to regulate the delicate water balance in response to the needs of the organism. This is accomplished in kidney collecting ducts where water resorption is regulated by AVP. Binding of this hormone to its V$_2$ receptor initiates a chain of signalling events that ultimately leads to the transient insertion of water channels in the apical membrane of principal cells and in the inner medullary collecting ducts' cells. The cDNA encoding a second water channel (aquaporin-2, WCH-CD) was cloned, which, on the basis of its exclusive expression in the collecting duct, may be the AVP-regulated water channel [12].

PATHOPHYSIOLOGY

The control of AVP release and regulation of fluid balance occurs primarily in response to alterations in blood tonicity and blood volume so that a relative constancy of these two parameters is maintained. This finely adjusted homeostatic system can be disrupted by disease states that affect neurohypophysial or renal function and by AVP produced independently of normal regulatory influences. The resulting clinical disturbance of body-water balance will be manifest by hypernatremia or hyponatremia and by excessive water loss or retention.

Can't synthesize or release AVP

Diabetes Insipidus. Impairment of the neurohypophysial system to synthesize or release AVP results in a diminished ability of the kidney to conserve water, resulting in pituitary (neurogenic) diabetes insipidus. Failure to synthesize AVP can also occur as a result of disease processes that destroy hypothalamic or posterior pituitary tissue. Diabetes insipidus can also result from traumatic or surgical injury to the hypothalamus.

In the normal individual, plasma osmolality is maintained in a range of 285 to 290 mOsmol/kg with associated plasma AVP levels of 1 to 3μU/ml and urinary AVP levels of 11 to 30 mU/24 hrs [42, 43]. In patients with severe diabetes insipidus, plasma osmolality may rise to more than 330 mOsmol/kg; under this severe osmotic stress, plasma and urinary AVP remain well below the normal range.

A single base deletion in the AVP gene is the cause of diabetes insipidus in the Brattleboro rat. The mRNA produced by the mutated gene encodes a normal AVP but an abnormal NPII moiety, which impairs transport and progression of the AVP-NPII precursor and its retention in the endoplasmic reticulum of the magnocellular neurons where it is produced. Transplantation of vasopressin neurons from normal rat fetuses into the adult Brattleboro rat, which congenitally lacks AVP-producing neurons, alleviates the polydipsia and polyuria that are symptomatic of this genetic defect. Apparently the axons of the grafted fetal neurons make appropriate and functional connections within the brain of the host. The ability of transplanted neurons to correct a CNS deficiency has important theoretical and clinical implications [17].

In *nephrogenic* (AVP-resistant) diabetes insipidus (NDI), there is a defect in the urinary concentration mechanism at the level of the kidney. Pituitary diabetes insipidus can be treated by replacement therapy with AVP, but the hormone is without effect in the nephrogenic disease type. In fact, greater than normal circulating levels of AVP are present in this condition. The antidiuretic response of the kidney to AVP is used clinically to diagnose the specific type of defect responsible for the diuresis. Females may have a subclinical form of the disease or the more severe form that is characteristic in males. A dominant sex-linked inheritance with variable penetrance is suggested. The defect involves a failure to generate intracellular levels of cAMP within distal tubular cells of the kidney in response to AVP. X-linked nephrogenic diabetes insipidus is a rare disorder in which the kidney is insensitive to the antidiuretic hormone, vasopressin. It has been proposed that the kidney-specific V_2 vasopressin receptor, a G protein-coupled receptor, is defective in this disorder as both the disease and the receptor map to chromosome Xq28. As NDI also maps to the Xq28 region, it has been speculated defects in the V_2 vasopressin receptor gene are responsible for this disease [19, 36, 50]. Data suggest that *aquaporin-2* is the AVP-regulated water channel in humans. In NDI patients, mutations have now been identified at the first and last stages of the pathway for AVP-induced antidiuresis. Identification of patients with AVP-resistant diabetes who do not have mutations in either the gene encoding the vasopressin V_2 receptor or the aquaporin-2 gene may help in the identification of further elements essential for AVP-regulated water transport in the kidney [12].

Syndrome of Inappropriate Vasopressin Secretion. The state of continual AVP release without relationship to plasma osmolality or volume is referred to as the syndrome of inappropriate vasopressin secretion [60]. The syndrome is characterized by an inability to excrete a maximally dilute urine, which results in retention of water, an expansion of the extracellular fluid volume, and a resultant dilutional hyponatremia. The most common cause of excessive AVP secretion is malignancy; AVP is secreted from a carcinoma of the lung, and is secreted along with its neurophysin. Although plasma and urinary levels of AVP may be markedly elevated, the amount of hormone in the blood or urine may be similar to that of normal individuals. However, these levels are excessive considering that the hypotonicity should have inhibited AVP secretion.

EVOLUTION OF THE NEUROHYPOPHYSIAL HORMONES

Determination of the structure of the neurohypophysial peptides, present within the pars nervosa of different vertebrate classes, has provided a remarkable understanding of the evolution of the neurohypophysial hormones [2]. This information has also given insight into the structural requirements for neurohypophysial hormone action [22]. From these studies a variety of hormone analogs have been designed for detailed analysis of hormone-receptor interaction.

Neurohypophysial hormones have been characterized in representatives of all vertebrate classes [2]. The neurohypophysis of each vertebrate species contains at least two principles, except in the cyclostomes where only a single peptide, arginine vasotocin (AVT), has been detected so far. In the species studied the same two hormones are usually present in the neurohypophysis of each member of a particular vertebrate group. Only one or two residues differ between the hormones of any two different vertebrate classes. Sequence differences mainly occur at positions 3, 4, and 8 of the nonapeptides (Table 7.1). Structural differences at these positions apparently account for the differing receptor affinities and activities of the neurohypophysial peptides.

Twelve neurohypophysial hormones have been characterized; eight are regarded as oxytocinlike and the remaining four as vasopressinlike. An early gene duplication led to two lines of neurohypophysial principles. Gene mutation following gene duplication may have resulted in one line originating with isotocin, found in bony fishes, which gave rise by further base mutations to the oxytocin-related structures. The other line, originating directly from AVT, gave rise to the vasopressins much later in evolution. Although the uterotropic and antidiuretic roles of neurohypophysial hormones are well documented in mammals, there is no convincing evidence that the neurohypophysial or related peptides subserve these functions in nonmammalian vertebrates, except for the antidiuretic role of AVT in amphibians, reptiles, and birds. Vasotocin is intermediate in structure between OT and AVP and is considered to be phylogenetically the oldest neurohypophysial hormone. AVT was synthesized and found to have properties identical to the naturally occurring amphibian water-balance principle [22]. Chemical analysis of the amphibian neurohypophysis revealed that the natural peptide was AVT. This provided a unique example where a synthetic hormone was prepared before its natural homologue had been identified.

Some members of the piglike mammals (pigs, wart hogs) contain a vasopressin with a lysine rather than arginine at the 8 position of the molecule (Table 7.1). It has been suggested that lysine vasopressin (LVP) arose as a single-step mutation from AVP. AVP and LVP may both be present in individual members of the pig family according to a Hardy-Weinberg distribution. Homozygotes contain one peptide and the heterozygotes contain both, suggesting the gene for vasopressin is present in two allelic forms. Only LVP is present in the domestic pig, which may be the result of the restrictive and selective force of domestication by humans. Both LVP and AVP are present in individual pituitaries of both Australian macropodian peramelids (bandicoot) and American didelphian marsupials (opossums) [2]. The constant presence of two pressor principles within individual pituitaries suggests that these peptides arose by gene duplication. A new neurohypophysial peptide, phenypressin ([Phe^2,Arg^8]-vasopressin) has been found along with LVP in the pituitary of five marsupials, including the red kangaroo and the tammar [2].

Other Neurohypophysial Hormones

Hydrins.   Extended forms of vasotocin, termed hydrins because of their action on the water permeability of frog skin and urinary bladder, are found in the amphibian neurohypophysis, along with vasotocin. In contrast to other AVT-producing vertebrates such as birds or reptiles, some amphibians have evolved provasotocin processing so that an intermediate vasotocinyl-glycine (hydrin 2) peptide is present in the neurohypophysis along with AVT. This peptide stimulates water transport through frog skin and frog bladder epithelia as does AVT, but in contrast to AVT it is virtually devoid of antidiuretic activity on the frog kidney. Because hydrin 2 has been identified in frog neurosecretory granules to be a physiological hormone secreted into the blood, it has been suggested that the differential processing of provasotocin is important to amphibians, allowing formation of two hormones from a single precursor. Water homeostasis in amphibians involves three organs, namely skin, bladder and kidney, and could be under control of both AVT and hydrin 2, the latter acting mainly for external water uptake through the skin [9].

In contrast to vasotocin, hydrins are virtually devoid of oxytocic, pressor, and antidiuretic activities. It has been suggested that in frogs and toads hydrin 2 acts specifically on skin in order to rehydrate animals when bathing in freshwater, whereas vasotocin is mainly active on kidney tubules controlling the recovery of water from urine. The finding of hydrin 2 in isolated frog neurosecretory granules supports the assumption that this peptide is secreted in blood as a hormone. Hydrins are detected neither in birds, such as geese, nor in reptiles, such as vipers [9, 45].

The Caudal Neurosecretory System (Urophysis) and the Urotensins. Within the spinal cord of some teleost and cartilaginous fishes are groups of neurosecretory neurons that possess all the characteristics of a neuroendocrine system, anatomically analogous to the neurohypophysis [5, 24]. This *caudal neurosecretory system* or *urophysis* contains two types of secretory cells based on staining reactions, granule morphology, and response to osmotic or electrophysiological stimuli. Two types of granules have been isolated, and each is associated with its own hormonal-like factor (urotensin I and II). Both aminergic and cholinergic inputs to urophysial secretion are implicated in some species of fishes. The *urotensins* are neuropeptides and, like the neurohypophysial hormones of the pars nervosa, are associated with two or more transport proteins, *urophysins,* which specifically bind either urotensin I or II. There is presently no evidence for the existence of urotensins in nonpiscine vertebrates, although, as noted presently, structurally related peptides are present, and the urotensins have a variety of actions in tetrapods [5, 24].

Extracts of the urophysis are vasoactive in all vertebrate species studied. In general a vasopressor response is observed in poikilothermic vertebrates and a vasodepressor effect observed in homeotherms. There is evidence that these differential effects are produced by two distinct peptides: the vasodepressor factor is referred to as urotensin I, whereas urotensin II is the name given to the vasopressor principle of the urophysis. Both urotensins apparently are present in all fish urophyses thus far examined, suggesting that they are indeed peptidergic hormones of this neurosecretory system. The presence of a third urotensin (III) is based solely on experimental data; urotensin IV appears to be arginine vasotocin (AVT).

Urophysectomy in several teleost species results in ionic imbalance, and exposure of euryhaline teleosts to different salinities results in marked histological and ultrastructural changes in the urophysial cells. In addition, injections of urophysial extracts increase plasma ion levels in fishes. Experimental evidence strongly suggests that urotensin II may act directly on the ion-transporting cells of the urinary bladder involved in teleostean seawater osmoregulation.

Urotensin II, isolated from the urophysis of the teleostean fish *Gillichthys mirabilis,* is reported to be a dodecapeptide with an amino acid sequence somewhat similar to somatostatin. The primary structure of urotensin I has also been determined and found to be strikingly similar to that of a putative corticotropin-releasing hormone of sheep and to sauvagine, a peptide isolated and characterized from frog skin. There is hope that with the elucidation of the structure of urotensin I synthetic analogs may be produced that are of pharmacological value in the clinical treatment of hypertension in humans.

Endothelin.   Originally characterized as a 21-residue vasoconstrictor peptide from endothelial cells, endothelin (ET) is present in the porcine spinal cord and may act as a neuropeptide [28]. Endothelinlike immunoreactivity has now been demonstrated by immunohistochemistry in the paraventricular and supraoptic nuclear neurons and their terminals in the posterior pituitary of the pig and the rat. In situ hybridization demonstrated ET messenger RNA in porcine paraventricular nuclear neurons. ET-like immunoreactive products in the posterior pituitary of the rat were depleted by water deprivation, suggesting a release of ET under physiological conditions. These findings indicate that ET is synthesized in the posterior pituitary system and may be involved in neurosecretory functions [63].

Melanin-Concentrating Hormone (MCH).   This heptadecapeptide is localized to the neurointermediate lobe of teleost fishes (Chap. 8). It is possible that, like the urotensins (see Chap. 21), this peptide plays a unique role in certain teleost fishes. MCH is, however, found within the brain of other vertebrates, including mammals (see Chap. 8).

REFERENCES

[1]   Acher, R., and J. Chavet. 1953. La structure de la vasopressine de boeuf. *Biochem. Biophys. Acta* 12:487.

[2]   ———— . 1988. Structure, processing and evolution of the neurohypophysial hormone-neurophysin precursors. *Biochemie* 70:1197–207.

[3]   Bargmann, W., and E. Scharrer. 1951. The site of origin of the hormones of the posterior pituitary. *Amer. Sci.* 39:255–59.

[4]   Barberis, C., A. Seibold, M. Ishido, W. Rosenthal, and M. Birnbaumer. 1993. Expression cloning of the human V_2 vasopressin receptor. *Reg. Pept.* 45:61–6.

[5]   Bern, H. A., D. Pearson, B. A. Larson, and R. S. Nishioka. 1985. Neurohormones from fish tails: the caudal neurosecretory system. I. "Urophysiology" and the caudal neurosecretory system of fishes. *Rec. Prog. Horm. Res.* 41:533–52.

[6]   Bisset, G. W. 1974. Milk ejection. In *Handbook of physiology,* Section 7. Endocrinology, eds. R. O. Greep and E. B. Astwood. Vol. 4, part 1, pp. 493–520. eds. E. Knobil and W. H. Sawyer. Washington, D.C.: Amer. Physiol. Soc.

[7]   Carmichael, M. S., R. Humbert, J. Dixen, G. Palmisano, W. Greenleaf, and J. M. Davidson. 1987. Plasma oxytocin increases in the human sexual response. *J. Clin. Endocrinol. Metab.* 64:27–31.

[8]   Carter, C. S. 1992. Oxytocin and sexual behavior. *Neurosci. Biobehav. Rev.* 16:131–44.

[9]   Chauvet, J., Y. Rouille, G. Michel, Y. Ouedraogo, and R. Acher. 1991. Adaptive differential processing of neurohypophysial provasotocin in amphibians: occurrence of hydrin 2 (vasotocinyl-glycine) in *Anura* but not in *Urodela. Endocrinology* 313:353–8.

[10] Cowley, A. W. Jr. 1988. Vasopressin and blood pressure regulation. *Clin. Physiol. Biochem.* 6:150–62.

[11]   Dale, H. H. 1906. On some physiological actions of ergot. *J. Physiol.* 34:163–206.

[12]   Deen, P. M. T., M. A. J. Verdijk, N. V. A. M. Knoers, B. Wieringa, L. A. H. Monnens, C. H. van Os, and V. A. van Oost. 1994. Requirement of human renal water channel aquaporin-2 for vasopressin-dependent concentration of urine. *Science* 264:92–4.

[13]   Falke, N. 1989. Oxytocin stimulates oxytocin release from isolated nerve terminals of rat neural lobes. *Neuropeptides* 14:269–74.

[14]   Fox, A. W. 1988. Vascular vasopressin receptors. *Gen. Pharmacol.* 19:639–47.

[15]   Fuchs, A.-R., F. Fuchs, P. Husslein, and M. S. Soloff. 1984. Oxytocin receptors in human uterus during pregnancy and parturition. *Amer. J. Obstet. Gynecol.* 150:734–41.

[16]   Fuchs, A.-R., F. Fuchs, and M. Soloff. 1985. Oxytocin receptors in nonpregnant human uterus. *J. Clin. Endocrinol. Metab.* 60:37–41.

[17]   Gash, D. M., J. R. Sladek, Jr., and C. D. Sladek. 1980. Functional development of grafted vasopressin neurons. *Science* 210:1367–69.

[18]   Harris, H. W. Jr., K. Strange, and M. L. Zeidel. 1991. Current understanding of the cellular biology and molecular structure of the antidiuretic hormone-stimulated water transport pathway. *J. Clin. Invest.* 88:1–8.

[19]   Holtzman, E. J., and D. A. Ausiello. 1994. Nephrogenic diabetes: causes revealed. *Hosp. Pract.* 29:89–104.

[20]   Howell, W. H. 1898. The physiological effects of extracts of the hypophysis cerebri and infundibular body. *J. Exp. Med.* 3:235–58.

[21]   Jirikowski, G. F., P. P. Sanna, D. Maciejewski-Lenior, and F. E. Bloom. 1992. Reversal of diabetes insipidus in Brattleboro rats: intrahypothalamic injection of vasopressin mRNA. *Science* 255:996–8.

[22]   Jost, K., ed. 1987. *Neurohypophysial hormone analogues.* Boca Raton: CRC Press, Inc.

[23]   Katsoyannis, P. G., and V. Du Vigneaud. 1958. Arginine-vasotocin, a synthetic analogue of the posterior pituitary hormones containing the ring of oxytocin and the side chain of vasopressin. *J. Biol. Chem.* 233:1352–54.

[24]   Lederis, K., J. Fryer, J. Rivier, K. L. MacCannell, Y. Kobayashi, N. Woo, and K. L. Wong. 1985. Neurohormones from fish tails II: Actions of urotensins in mammals and fishes. *Rec. Prog. Horm. Res.* 41:533–76.

[25]   Lefebvre, D. L., A. Giaid, H. Bennett, R. Lariviere, and H. H. Zingg. 1992. Oxytocin gene expression in rat uterus. *Science* 256:1553–5.

[26]   Lincoln, D. W., and J. B. Wakerley. 1974. Electrophysiological evidence for the activation of supraoptic neurones during the release of oxytocin. *J. Physiol.* 242:533–54.

[27]   Linzell, J. L. 1961. Recent advances in the physiology of the udder. *Vet. Ann.* 2:44–53.

[28]   Maggi, M., G. Fantoni, A. Peri, S. Rossi, E. Baldi, A. Magini, G. Massi, and M. Serio. 1993. Oxytocin-endothelin interactions in the uterus. *Reg. Pept.* 45:97–101.

[29]   Miller, F. D., R. Chibbar, and B. F. Mitchell. 1993. Synthesis of oxytocin in amnion, chorion and decidua: a potential paracrine role for oxytocin in the onset of human parturition. *Reg. Pept.* 45:247–251.

[30]   Morel, A., S. J. Lolait, and M. J. Brownstein. 1993. Molecular cloning and expression of rat V_{1a} and V_2 arginine vasopressin receptors. *Reg. Pept.* 45:53–9.

[31]   Mori, M., S. Vigh, A. Miyata, T. Yoshihara, S. Oka, and A. Arimura. 1990. Oxytocin is the major prolactin releasing factor in the posterior pituitary. *Endocrinology* 126:1009–13.

[32]   Murphey, M. R., J. R. Seckl, S. Burton, S. A. Checkley, and S. L. Lightman. 1987. Changes in oxytocin and vasopressin secretion during sexual activity in men. *J. Clin. Endocrinol. Metab.* 65:738–41.

[33]   Murphy, D., A. Levy, S. Lightman, and D. Carter. 1989. Vasopressin RNA in the neural lobe of the pituitary: dramatic accumulation in response to salt loading. *Proc. Natl. Acad. Sci. U.S.A.* 86:9002–5.

[34]   Oliver, G., and E. A. Schafer. 1895. On the physiological actions of extracts of the pituitary body and certain other glandular organs. *J. Physiol.* 18:277–79.

[35]   Page, S. R, V. T. Y. Ang, R. Jackson, A. White, S. S. Nussey, and J. S. Jenkins. 1990. The effect of oxytocin infusion on adenohypophyseal function in man. *Clin. Endocrinol.* 32:307–13.

[36] Pan, Y., A. Metzenberg, S. Das, B. Jing, and J. Gitschier. 1992. Mutations in the V_2 vasopressin receptor gene are associated with X-linked nephrogenic diabetes insipidus. *Nature Genetics* 2:103–6.

[37] Pedersen, C. A., and A. J. Prange, Jr. 1985. Oxytocin and mothering behavior in the rat. *Pharmac. Therap.* 28:287–302.

[38] Pickering, B. T. 1978. The neurosecretory neurone: a model system for the study of secretion. *Essays in Biochem.* 14:45–81.

[39] Poulain, D. A., J. B. Wakerley, and R. E. J. Dyball. 1977. Electrophysiological differentiation of oxytocin- and vasopressin-secreting neurones. *Proc. Roy. Soc. London*, B. 196:367–84.

[40] Richardson, K. C. 1949. Contractile tissues in the mammary gland with special reference to myoepithelium in the goat. *Proc. Roy. Soc. London*, B 136:30–45.

[41] Rillema, J. A. 1994. Development of the mammary gland and lactation. *TEM* 5:149–54.

[42] Robertson, G. L., S. Athar, and R. L. Shelton. 1977. Osmotic control of vasopressin function. In *Disturbances in body fluid osmolality*, pp. 125–48. Washington, D.C.: Amer. Physiol. Soc.

[43] Robertson, G. L., R. L. Shelton, and S. Athar. 1976. The osmoregulation of vasopressin. *Kidney Int.* 10:25–37.

[44] Robinson, A. G., and M. D. Fitzsimmons. 1993. Vasopressin homeostasis: coordination of synthesis, storage and release. *Reg. Pept.* 45:225–30.

[45] Rouille, Y., J. Chauvet, and R. Acher. 1991. Heterologue conversion of amphibian hydrin 2 into vasotocin through bovine granule alpha-amidating enzyme. *J. Neuroendocrinol.* 3:15–20.

[46] Sawyer, W. H., and M. Manning. 1989. Experimental uses of neurohypophysial hormone analogs. *TEM* 48–50.

[47] Scharrer, B. 1987. Neurosecretion: beginning a new direction in neuropeptide research. *Annu. Rev. Neurosci.* 19:1–17.

[48] Schumacher, M., H. Coirini, A. E. Johnson, L. M. Flanagan, M. Frank-Furt, D. W. Pfaff, and B. S. McEwen. 1993. The oxytocin receptor: a target for steroid hormones. *Reg. Pept.* 45:115–19

[49] Schumacher, M., H. Coirini, D. W. Pfaff, and B. S. McEwen. 1990. Behavioral effects of progesterone associated with rapid modulation of oxytocin receptors. *Science* 250:691–94.

[50] Seibold, A., W. Rosenthal, D. G. Bichet, and M. Birnbaumer. 1993. The vasopressin type 2 receptor gene. Chromosomal localization and its role in nephrogenic diabetes insipidus. *Reg. Pept.* 45:67–71.

[51] Shimada, K., H. L. Neldon, and T. I. Koike. 1986. Arginine vasotocin (AVT) release in relation to uterine contractibility in the hen. *Gen. Comp. Endocrinol.* 64:362–67.

[52] Soloff, M. S., M. Alexandrova, and M. J. Fernstrom. 1979. Oxytocin receptors: triggers for parturition and lactation. *Science* 204:1313–14.

[53] Soloff, M. S., H. D. Rees, M. Sar, and W. E. Stumpf. 1975. Autoradiographic localization of radioreactivity from [^{3}H]-oxytocin in the rat mammary gland and oviduct. *Endocrinology* 96:1475–77.

[54] Sukhov, R. R., L. C. Walker, N. E. Rance, D. L. Price, and W. Scott Young III. 1993. Vasopressin and oxytocin gene expression in the human hypothalamus. *J. Comp. Neurol.* 337:295–306.

[55] Teitelbaum, I. 1992. Hormone signaling systems in inner medullary collecting ducts. *Amer. J. Physiol.* 263:F985–90.

[56] Thibonnier, M. 1992. Signal transduction of V_1-vascular vasopressin receptors. *Reg. Pept.* 38:1–11.

[57] Tindal, J. S., and G. S. Knaggs. 1971. Determination of the detailed hypothalamic route of the milk-ejection reflex in the guinea pig. *J. Endocrinol.* 50:135–52.

[58] Tuppy, H. 1953. *Biochim. Biophys. Acta* 11:449.

[59] Verbalis, J. G., R. E. Blackborn, B. R. Olson, and E. M. Stricker. 1993. Central oxytocin inhibition of food and salt ingestion: a mechanism for intake regulation of solute homeostasis. *Reg. Pept.* 45:149–54.

[60] Vokes, T. J., and G. L. Robertson. 1988. Disorders of antidiuretic hormone. *Endocrinol. Metab. Clin. N. Amer.* 17:281–99.

[61] Wray, S. 1993. Uterine contraction and physiological mechanisms of modulation. *Amer. J. Physiol.* 264:C1–18.

[62] Yamashita, H. 1977. Effect of baro- and chemoreceptor activation on supraoptic nuclei neurons in the hypothalamus. *Brain Res.* 126:551–56.

[63] Yoshizawa, T., O. Shinmi, A. Giaid, M. Yanagisawa, S. J. Gibson, S. Kimura, Y. Uchiyama, J. M. Polak, T. Masaki, and I. Kanazawa. 1990. Endothelin: a novel peptide in the posterior pituitary system. *Science* 247:462–64.

[64] Zoeller, R. T., and F. L. Moore. 1988. Brain arginine vasotocin concentrations related to sexual behaviors and hydromineral balance in an amphibian. *Horm. Behav.* 422:66–75.

The Melanotropic Hormones

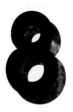

The early studies of Smith and Allen clearly implicated the pituitary gland as the source of a hormone that controlled color changes in amphibians. These color changes were found to be due to the response of certain **chromatophores** (pigment-bearing cells), particularly melanophores (melanin-containing cells), found within the skin. The **melanotropic** substance was specifically localized to the neurointermediate lobe (pars intermedia) of the pituitary [2] This peptide is now referred to as α-**melanocyte-stimulating hormone** (MSH) or α-**melanotropin**. MSH and other structurally related peptides found within the pituitary and the brain are referred to generically as **melanotropins** (Fig. 8.1). There have been some confusing interludes in the story of the melanotropic peptides. It was generally believed that the vertebrate pituitary contains an α-MSH and a β-MSH. Human pituitaries, however, were said to lack an α-MSH but to contain a β-MSH, which consisted of more amino acids than the melanotropins of other mammalian β-MSHs. More confusing was that the pars intermedia of the pituitary gland of the adult human and some other primates is absent or rudimentary in structure, although a fetal zona intermedia is present and may produce a melanotropin. This chapter will review the interesting story of the melanotropins and their newly suggested roles in vertebrate physiology. Several reviews on the melanotropic peptides are now available [11, 18, 19, 20].

humans have only β-MSH

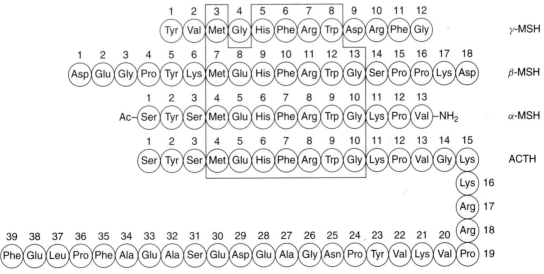

Figure 8.1 Amino acid sequences of bovine γ-, β-, and α-MSH compared to ACTH. (From Sawyer et al. [40], with permission.)

153

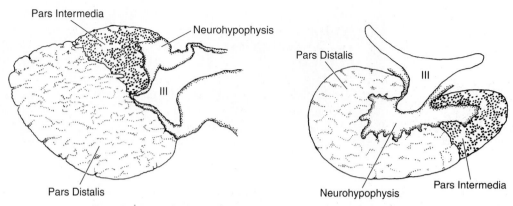

Figure 8.2 Sagittal sections of (left) an amphibian (salamander) pituitary gland and (right) a teleost pituitary gland. The three lobular components of the glands are indicated: neurohypophysis, pars intermedia, and pars distalis. The third ventricle (III) is also indicated.

THE PARS INTERMEDIA

The pars intermedia develops as a result of contact between the infundibulum and the adenohypophysial anlage [25]. In cyclostomes, amphibians, reptiles, and most mammals, the MSH-secreting cells (melanotrophs) form a well-defined pars intermedia or intermediate lobe (Fig. 8.2). Although the pars intermedia of certain mammals is absent (cetaceans, or whales and dolphins), a zona intermedia does exist in the human fetus, though it subsequently becomes rudimentary (see Fig. 5.1). Birds lack a pars intermedia, but it is claimed, on cytological and bioassay evidence, that MSH-secreting cells are present within the pars distalis. In elasmobranchs and teleosts the MSH cells are localized caudally but are contiguous with other cells of the pars distalis (Fig. 8.2). The pars nervosa and the pars intermedia of tetrapods are inseparable from each other; this anatomical unit is often referred to as the neurointermediate lobe.

The size of the pars intermedia is usually positively correlated with whether or not an animal is able to change color in conformity with the coloration of the substratum. The pars intermedia of the lizard, *Anolis carolinensis* (chameleon), is very large, and this reptile has an outstanding ability for color change, being a bright green or dark brown on light or dark backgrounds, respectively. In some mammals, on the other hand, the size of the pars intermedia is said to be correlated with the nature of the environment, large in mammals living in dehydrating conditions [25]. In rats, injection of hypertonic saline or subjection to dehydration results in hypertrophic changes in the cells of the pars intermedia, thus suggesting a role for the pars intermedia in electrolyte regulation.

The pars intermedia is relatively avascular compared to the other components of the pituitary gland and other endocrine tissues. Nevertheless, an extravascular, multibranched transport system penetrates the parenchyma of the pars intermedia and may provide a pathway for the passage of secretory products and regulatory factors to and from the gland. In some species the pars intermedia differs from the pars distalis in that it is penetrated by neurons from the hypothalamus. Neurosecretory and catecholamine-containing neuronal elements may be present; the latter may form a plexus around the secretory cells. These aminergic neurons play a dominant role in the control of melanotroph proliferation and MSH secretion, as will be discussed [15]. Neurons are absent from the neurointermediate lobe of the few lizards that have been studied.

SYNTHESIS AND CHEMISTRY OF MELANOTROPINS

The history of research related to the present understanding of the chemistry and proposed roles of the vertebrate melanotropins began with investigations which established that the pituitary gland contained a number of melanotropic peptides. Indeed, a rather pure MSH (α-MSH) was subsequently isolated from the pituitary of a number of mammalian species. Soon after the discovery of α-MSH, another chemically different MSH, β-melanotropin (β-MSH), was also isolated from the pituitary of these same species.

Human pituitaries were said to lack α-MSH, but to contain a β-MSH that was longer (22 amino acids) than the β-MSHs (18 amino acids) isolated from other mammalian pituitaries. Radioimmunoassays revealed that in normal humans and in those with certain pathological conditions, the plasma concentrations of β-MSH and ACTH were always correlated. It was therefore thought that β-MSH was the principal melanotropic hormone of humans. Subsequently the α-MSHs from a number of mammalian pituitaries were chemically characterized and found to be identical in structure. The structure of α-MSH, however, differs slightly in the few poikilotherms that have been studied. Shark (*Squalus acanthias*) and salmon (*Oncorhynchus keta*) α-MSHs are also tridecapeptides, but the N-terminal serine is unacetylated in these species. In addition, in the dogfish shark the C-terminal amino acid, which is valine in all mammalian α-MSHs, is replaced by methionine.

Eventually it was discovered that pituitaries of a number of species contained a melanotropic peptide that was larger than that of any known pigmentary peptide. The ovine molecule was shown to contain 91 amino acids and was referred to as β-lipotropic hormone, β-LPH (see Fig. 21.4). The complete structure of β-MSH is contained within the 41–58 sequence of this peptide. Further work revealed that the so-called β-MSH of humans is merely a fragment of β-LPH, artifactually formed during extraction of the tissue. Thus the earlier radioimmunoassay measurements of β-MSH in humans were measurements of the β-LPH present within the plasma. The adult human pituitary may therefore produce only two melanotropic peptides, ACTH and β-LPH, and these are probably not involved, under normal conditions, in the control of melanocyte activity. There is no evidence that β-MSH serves any peripheral physiological function other than as a necessary secretory by-product of other hormones derived from the melanotrophs and corticotrophs.

Subsequent to these early studies a corticotropinlike peptide, CLIP, was discovered in the pars intermedia of rat and pig pituitaries. This peptide is composed of the 18–39 amino acid sequence of ACTH. It has been proposed that CLIP and α-MSH are products of the intracellular cleavage of ACTH [31]. No clear function for CLIP has been shown; CLIP may simply be a necessary cleavage product of MSH secretion. Similarly, a larger protein (31,000 MW) has been isolated from both the pars distalis and the pars intermedia (see Chap. 21). As seen in Fig. 8.3 this protein, pro-opiomelanocortin (POMC), contains the sequences of ACTH and β-LPH. In the pars distalis ACTH is released under certain

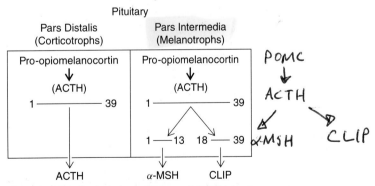

Figure 8.3 Prohormone theory of ACTH and α-MSH biosynthesis. It is unclear whether in the pars intermedia ACTH is first enzymatically released from pro-opiomelanocortin to yield α-MSH and CLIP, or whether the latter two peptides are liberated directly from POMC. (Modified from Lowry and Scott [31].)

physiological conditions to regulate adrenocortical function. In the pars intermedia, on the other hand, enzymes are present within the secretory granules and are responsible for the enzymatic cleavage of POMC to α-MSH. Following cleavage from the precursor protein, post-translational amindation and acetylation of the C-terminus and N-terminus, respectively, of the MSH molecule then occurs.

α-MSH has also been localized to the hypothalamus where it is found within the perikarya of neurons of the arcuate nucleus. These α-MSH-containing cell bodies in the ventral hypothalamus send multiple projections to numerous extrahypothalamic regions of the brain. Destruction of the arcuate nucleus lowers the α-MSH content of extrahypothalamic regions (Chap. 21). Neuronal perikarya of the arcuate region also contain ACTH and β-endorphin, and the reduction in levels of these peptides (including α-MSH) after various treatments suggests that these neuronal peptides are derived from a common precursor, POMC, similar to ACTH and α-MSH in the pituitary gland. A γ-MSH of unknown function is also present within the pituitary gland and hypothalamus as a component of POMC (Fig. 8.1). Thus the precursor protein POMC contains within its primary structure the sequences of five melanotropic peptides: α-MSH, β-MSH, γ-MSH, ACTH, and β-LPH (Fig. 8.4).

The preferential localization of mRNA for the pars intermedia and pars distalis ACTH secretion has been determined by in situ hybridization studies. mRNA for POMC is relatively unaffected by adrenalectomy in the pars intermedia, whereas anterior lobe levels of POMC mRNA are greatly increased. This increase in POMC production is abolished in adrenalectomized animals, however, if the ADX animals are first treated with a synthetic glucocorticoid (dexamethasone). Intermediate lobe levels of POMC mRNA are unaffected by the glucocorticoid (Fig. 8.5). These observations demonstrate the differential control of POMC mRNA synthesis by cells of the pars intermedia and pars distalis [45].

A heptapeptide sequence has been conserved within the structures of α-MSH, β-MSH, and ACTH. The first 13 amino acids of ACTH are identical to those of α-MSH. Unlike the other melanotropins, the N-terminus of α-MSH is acetylated and the C-terminus is amidated. There is a great species heterogeneity in structure of the β-MSHs, which may further support the suggestion that β-MSH serves no functional role other than as a structural component of POMC.

CONTROL OF MSH SECRETION

Disruption of the normal anatomical relationships between the pars intermedia and the hypothalamus results in the release of MSH. The endocrine implications of this observation were first appreciated in the early studies of Etkin [1]. Ectopic transplantation of the entire pituitary gland or the isolated neurointermediate lobe usually leads to hypertrophy of the pars intermedia cells and to an increased (uninhibited) release of MSH. These experiments and others involving hypothalamic lesions or pituitary stalk transection have yielded similar results in a variety of vertebrates. The observations suggest that the hypothalamus exerts an inhibitory control over MSH release.

Dopaminergic Control

There is strong evidence that inhibition of MSH secretion by the hypothalamus is controlled by a catecholamine, most likely dopamine [46]. Catecholamines, such as norepinephrine, epinephrine, and dopamine, are inhibitory to MSH secretion from the isolated neurointermediate lobe of the pituitary [18]. The inhibitory actions of these catecholamines are antagonized by chlorpromazine, a dopaminergic receptor antagonist. Dopaminergic receptor agonists, such as certain ergot alkaloids, on the other hand, are inhibitory to pars intermedia MSH secretion both in vivo and in vitro.

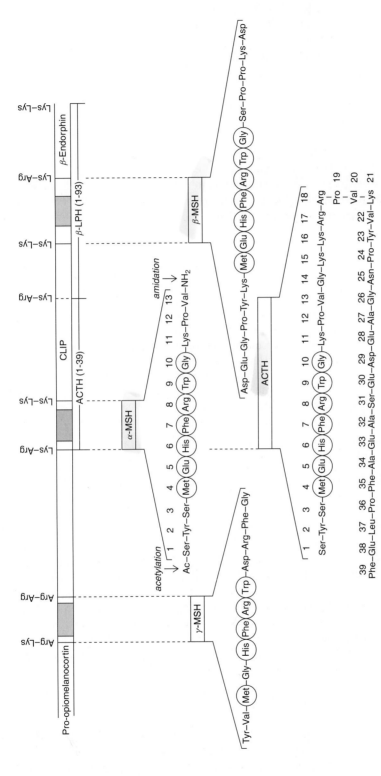

Figure 8.4 Schematic representation of the known, biologically active peptides derived from pro-opiomelanocortin, which is found in the vertebrate pituitary (corticotrophs and melanotrophs) and hypothalamus. (Reprinted with permission from Sawyer et al. [40]. ©1982 by The American Chemical Society.)

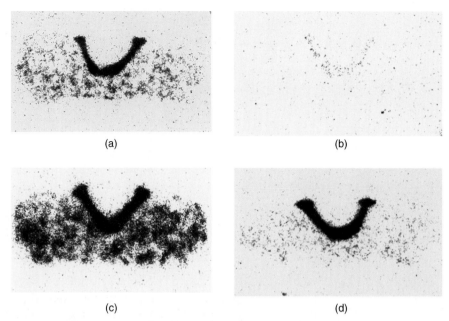

Figure 8.5 Autoradiographs showing hybridization signal in pituitary sections. The intermediate lobe is strongly labeled, whereas a weaker and patchy reaction can be observed in the anterior lobe. (b) Section consecutive to that shown in (a), which has been pretreated with RNAase before prehybridization. No labeling can be observed. (c) Adrenalectomized (ADX) animal. The labeling observed in the anterior lobe is much more intense than that seen in the intact animal. (d) ADX animal treated with dexamethasone (DEX). The intensity of the reaction in the anterior lobe is weaker than that observed in the intact animal. (From Tong et al. [45], with permission. *Molecular and Cellular Neuroscience* 1:78–83, 1990.)

In animals that change color in response to a light- or a dark-colored background, the following model has been proposed from early studies on the frog. The amount of light that is reflected from the background substratum (albedo) to the dorsal aspect of the retina, relative to the amount that reaches the bottom of the retina from the light source overhead, determines whether MSH will be secreted. On a black background very little light is reflected to the upper aspect of the retina compared to the amount reflected from a light substratum. In either case the amount reaching the lower part of the retina remains the same [Fig. 8.6]. The differential stimulation of the two retinal components therefore determines the chromatic response. On a black background animals turn dark colors due to the release of MSH from the pars intermedia, whereas animals become light on a white background due to an inhibition of MSH secretion (Fig. 8.7).

In the absence of any tonic hypothalamic inhibitory input, melanotrophs and lactotrophs exhibit spontaneous electrical activity in vitro and secrete α-MSH and PRL, respectively. They both provide informative model systems for determining the relationship between cellular secretion and membrane bioelectrical activity. For example, hormones that affect MSH or PRL secretion do so by mechanisms that modify the membrane electrical activity of the melanotrophs and lactotrophs [10].

Data obtained from a variety of species suggests the following events may be involved in the control of MSH release from the pars intermedia, at least in animals that change color. Environmental photic cues received by the lateral eyes are relayed via neuronal circuits to the hypothalamus. These neurons of inhibitory or stimulatory nature may terminate and synapse with other neurons within the hypothalamus. Aminergic and peptidergic neurons originating in the postoptic nucleus and preoptic nucleus, respectively,

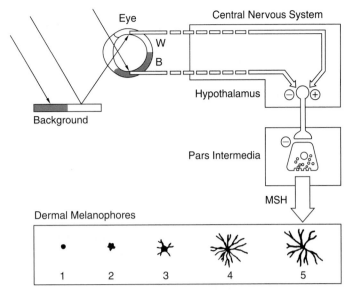

Figure 8.6 The neuroendocrine reflex-regulating pigment dispersion in dermal melanophores of amphibians during the process of background adaptation. (Reprinted with permission from B. G. Jenks, V.-V. Kemenade, and G. J. M. Martens [27]. ©1988 by CRC Press.)

have been shown (in the skate) to course through the basal hypothalamus, as a pair of lateral aminergic fiber tracts and a central neurosecretory tract, to penetrate the pars intermedia. The catecholamine-containing neurons make synaptic contact with the individual melanotrophs. The neurosecretory neurons penetrate only to the pars nervosa–pars intermedia border. Other cholinergic neurons of unknown hypothalamic origin may also penetrate into the pars intermedia of some species.

Dopamine released from the aminergic neurons interacts with dopaminergic receptors possessed by the membranes of the pars intermedia cells. The tonic release of the catecholamine maintains the cells in the hyperpolarized state and is inhibitory to MSH secretion. The cholinergic neurons may antagonize the aminergic neurons by release of

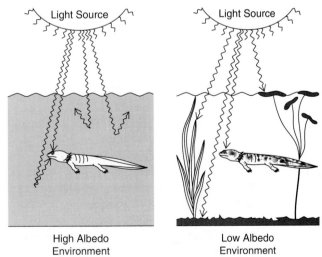

Figure 8.7 Model for the control of MSH secretion and the regulation of integumental coloration. (From Fernandez and Collins [13], with permission.)

acetylcholine at synapses on the aminergic neurons themselves, or by direct synaptic contact with the pars intermedia cells. MSH release would then result from presynaptic inhibition (of dopamine release) or by a direct depolarizing input to the doubly innervated melanotrophs. Release would result if the cholinergic depolarizing input were able to override the aminergic hyperpolarizing inhibitory input. Fine adjustments between the two opposing synaptic events might then modulate the amount of MSH to be secreted.

Control by Other Neurohormones. The pars intermedia melanotrope cells of the pituitary of the South African clawed toad *Xenopus laevis* release α-MSH. Release activity is under complex inhibitory and stimulatory control. In vitro superfusion studies with isolated neurointermediate lobes have indicated that TRH and CRF have stimulatory effects, whereas dopamine, gamma amino butyric acid (GABA) and neuropeptide Y (NPY) inhibit α-MSH release. Superfusion experiments with isolated melanotropes have established that CRF, dopamine, and GABA act directly on melanotropes. Light microscopic immunocytochemistry with an anti-NPY serum has shown that the pars intermedia of *X. laevis* is penetrated by an extensive network of NPY-containing nerve fibers. At the ultrastructural level these fibers appear to form varicosities filled with NPY-containing secretory granules. These varicosities make synaptic contacts not only with melanotropes, but also with folliculo-stellate cells. The latter cells, together with the melanotropes, form the main cell constituents of the pars intermedia. It has been hypothesized that these cells play a role in the control of the endocrine cells' activity within the pars intermedia [46].

In those vertebrates where a direct innervation is absent (e.g., lizards), neurotransmitters released from the median eminence or pars nervosa may be delivered to the pars intermedia by way of vascular or other routes. In the few nonmammalian species studied, serotonin appears to exert a stimulating effect on MSH secretion. Administration of 5-hydroxytryptophan, a precursor of serotonin, is indirectly stimulatory to melanophore dispersion in the skin of some fishes and amphibians. Serotonin stimulates MSH secretion from the isolated neurointermediate lobe of some species, and the frequency of pars intermedia action potentials (depolarizations) is enhanced coincident to MSH secretion. It is possible that in some species (e.g., the lizard *Anolis carolinensis*), where an inhibitory hypothalamic control is lacking and there is minimal autonomous secretion of MSH, serotonin subserves a function as a hypophysiotropin, a so-called MSH-releasing hormone.

PHYSIOLOGICAL ROLES OF MSH

The role of the pars intermedia and MSH in the control of color changes in poikilothermic vertebrates is the one clearly documented physiological function of the hormone and one of the earliest described roles for a vertebrate hormone. Only recently have other putative functions been ascribed to MSH [19].

Melanin Pigmentation of the Skin

The one unquestionable role of MSH is to control melanin pigmentation of the skin of most vertebrate species [17]. In mammals and many other vertebrates melanin-containing pigment cells are found in the basal layers of the epidermis. These *melanocytes* (also referred to as melanophores) use the precursor amino acid tyrosine and, through a number of biochemical events controlled by one or more enzymes, produce a colored polymer called *melanin*. This melanin is incorporated into a subcellular structure referred to as a *premelanosome*. When this organelle becomes fully melanized, it is known as a *melanin granule* or *melanosome*. Brown and black melanins are referred to as *eumelanins*, whereas red or

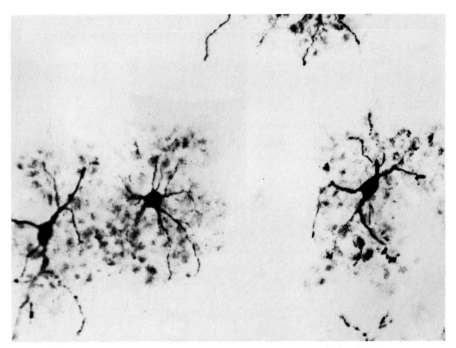

Figure 8.8 Epidermal melanin units of the frog *Rana pipiens*. Melanosomes synthesized by the melanocytes are released into adjacent keratinocytes where they function, at least in humans, as a sunscreen against ultraviolet radiation [24].

lighter colored melanins are known as *pheomelanins*. Mammals with colored pelage patterns produce one or another of these melanins in different anatomical areas of the skin.

The melanin produced within the melanocytes is released into surrounding cells of the skin by a secretory (cytocrine) mechanism that is not fully understood. The functional unit of epidermal pigmentation, made up of a melanocyte and associated epidermal cells, is referred to as an *epidermal melanin unit* [24]. Melanotropins enhance melanin production within melanocytes, and the melanosomes produced migrate into the dendritic processes of the cells where they are released into the surrounding cells of the epidermis (Fig. 8.8). The melanocytes in hair-covered parts of the skin are localized to the hair follicles, and synthesis of melanin by these follicular melanocytes is responsible for pigmentation of the hair; a similar process is responsible for melanin pigmentation of feathers. MSH and steroid hormones may sequentially, or in combination, affect the production of eumelanins and pheomelanins within individual follicular melanocytes, which can lead to hairs containing black, brown, or white bands, a so-called "agouti" pattern. Although MSH affects hair pigmentation in some mammals, the hormonal basis, if any, of melanin pigmentation of feathers is not clearly understood, particularly since birds lack a pars intermedia.

Seasonal alterations in pigment cell melanogenic activity are an important aspect of an animal's ability to conform to yearly change in environmental conditions. An animal, such as the varying hare (*Lepus americanus*), is thus able to change color from a brown summer pelage to a white winter coat. Suntanning in humans also results from enhanced melanin pigmentation of the skin. Ontogenic changes in integumental pigmentation occur as in the development of the nuptial coloration of the skin associated with the sexual activity of such vertebrates as birds. The graying of hair in humans and other mammals is a common phenotypic characteristic of older age, but its physiological significance and etiology is not well understood.

Morphological color changes, which involve alterations in the amount of pigment present within the skin, are generally manifest in response to seasonal changes in background

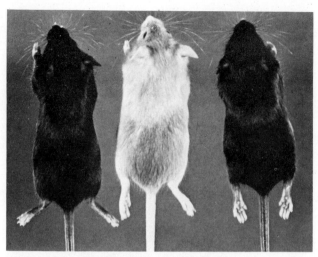

Figure 8.9 Effect of injected α-MSH on melanin pigmentation of the hair of the yellow (C57BL/6JA^y strain) mouse. The yellow control mouse is in the center. (From Geschwind, Huseby, and Nishioka [16], with permission.)

conditions. Rabbits and ptarmigans, for example, develop a white pelage or plumage in conformity with the snow of the winter habitat. During the spring and summer a dark pelage or feather change accompanies the melting of the snows. MSH is implicated in the white-to-brown pelage changes that occur in the short-tailed weasel and the Siberian hamster, in conformity with the winter to spring change [39]. That mammalian melanocytes of some species can respond to MSH is dramatically demonstrated by the response of the yellow mouse to the hormone (Fig. 8.9). Phenotypically this genetic strain of mice is normally yellow in color [16]; the response to MSH is unnatural, but does demonstrate the potential for melanogenic activity in the mammal.

Morphological color changes result from changes in the number and synthetic activity of the integumentary pigment cells. For example, frogs maintained on light- or dark-colored backgrounds for long periods of time become light or dark in color (Fig. 8.10), and the number of melanocytes found in the epidermis of these animals differs dramatically (Fig. 8.11). This morphological color change is controlled by MSH and clearly demonstrates hypertrophy and hyperplasia of melanocytes in response to the hormone [24]. In vitro studies demonstrate that melanotropins are clearly stimulatory to melanoblast cytodifferentiation and proliferation, at least in poikilotherms.

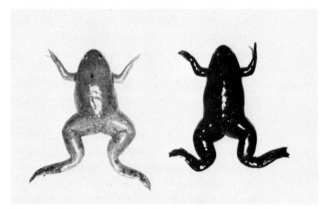

Figure 8.10 Morphological color change. Effect of long-term (9-week) adaptation of frogs, *Xenopus laevis*, to a white (left) or black (right) background [24].

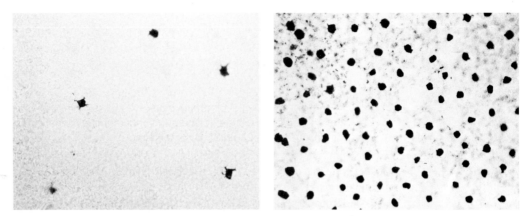

Figure 8.11 Photomicrograph of melanophores in the epidermis of frogs, *Xenopus laevis*, adapted to a white (left) or a black (right) background for a 10-week period.

Because birds lack a pars intermedia, it is possible that certain cells of the pars distalis synthesize and secrete an MSH or some other melanotropin. However, MSH has been shown to be without effect on feather pigmentation in the few species of birds studied. Not much is known about the neuroendocrine control of avian pigmentation. One would like to know, for example, what endocrine or other chemical messengers control winter-to-spring and fall-to-winter plumage color changes, particularly in birds such as ptarmigans.

Because MSH is apparently absent from the pituitary of adult humans, the stimulus for enhanced melanogenic activity during suntanning is not known. Repeated injections of MSH into darkly pigmented individuals, however, increase epidermal pigmentation that is readily visible after a few days. This demonstrates the capability of the human melanocyte system, at least in dark-skinned individuals, to respond to hormonal activation by MSH [18, 22, 23]. Pigmentation of humans is genetically controlled, and radiant energy from the sun may directly activate melanogenic activity within melanocytes. It is also possible that cholecalciferol (hormonal form of vitamin D) or other vitamin D metabolites (see Chap. 9) produced within the skin in response to solar radiation stimulate melanogenesis directly or synergistically in concert with other endogenous hormonal factors. In fact, there is evidence that a melanotropic peptide may be produced within the epidermis of the skin in response to ultraviolet light (UVL) [36].

During pregnancy the areolae of the nipples in human females may become more darkly pigmented. The darkening of the skin is most pronounced in the last trimester and diminishes slowly after parturition. This increased pigmentation has been considered to be due to elevated levels of a melanotropin. It must be pointed out, however, that gonadal steroid levels are also elevated, and steroid hormones are clearly melanogenic in some species. The MSH-like activity of the blood and urine is increased during pregnancy, and indeed, the frog skin bioassay for MSH was originally designed to measure an elevation of the hormone as an index for predicting pregnancy in the human [42]. The source and nature of the MSH-like activity of the blood and urine during pregnancy is unknown. It is interesting to speculate that it might be of fetal origin, as the fetal, but not the adult, pituitary is thought to produce a melanotropin.

Chromatophores and Color Changes

The only known function of MSH in nonmammalian vertebrates is the control of integumental pigmentation [2]. Present evidence implicates α-MSH as the only physiological melanotropin controlling this chromatic behavior. Many poikilothermic vertebrates, for example, fishes, amphibians, and reptiles, rapidly adapt to the color of the background

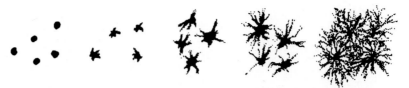

Figure 8.12 A melanophore index is used to evaluate melanosome movements, centrifugal (dispersion) or centripetal (perinuclear aggregation), in response to MSH or other stimuli.

over which they reside. The American anole, *Anolis carolinensis*, can change, chameleon-like, from a bright green to a darker brown in a matter of minutes after moving from a light- to a dark-colored surface. Rapid *physiological color changes* do not involve changes in the amount of pigment in the skin but, rather, changes in the morphology of dermal chromatophores (Fig. 8.12). The chromatophores of poikilotherms are the xanthophores, iridophores, and melanophores. The xanthophores may contain carotenoids and pteridines; these pigments may be yellow, orange, or red, and xanthophores may therefore contain combinations of these pigments. The iridophores contain reflecting crystals of purines and related molecules. These three chromatophore types are often grouped together functionally in a *dermal chromatophore unit* (Fig. 8.13). The individual chromatophores of this functional unit respond to MSH by aggregating or dispersing their pigments; in this way the skin becomes light or dark or even yellow or green in color [1, 44].

A radioimmunoassay for α-MSH has been successfully used to determine pituitary and plasma levels of α-MSH in frogs adapted to various background (albedo) conditions. The results verified what might be expected (although never confirmed before): plasma levels of MSH were elevated in toads on a black background compared to animals main-

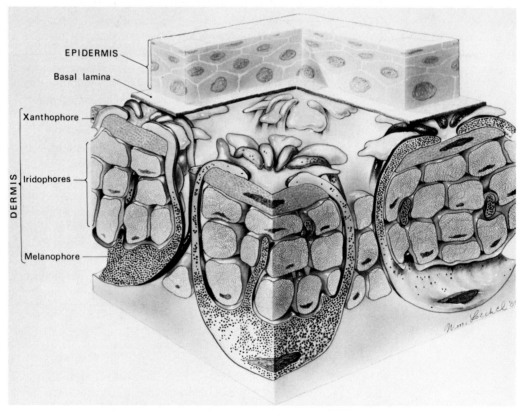

Figure 8.13 Dermal chromatophore unit of the lizard *Anolis carolinensis*. (From Taylor and Hadley [44], with permission.)

tained on a gray or a white background. The inverse relationship was observed for α-MSH levels within the neurointermediate lobe of the pituitary [48].

Other Putative Roles of Melanotropins

Many other physiological roles have been suggested for MSH. A few of these putative functions are discussed, but more information is needed to substantiate them fully.

Fetal Pituitary-Adrenal Axis. The discovery that the pituitary gland produces a family of related hormonal peptides is most interesting. We have seen how α-MSH is derived from a larger (31,000 MW) protein that also contains β-LPH within its structure. Possibly the most exciting recent discovery in endocrinology is that the pituitary and brain contain opiatelike peptides. These peptides interact with so-called opiate receptors of neurons and are believed by some investigators to be the analgesic hormones (endorphins) of humans (Chap. 21). These endorphins (endogenous morphinelike substances) are derived from the β-LHP sequence within POMC. The sequence 61–91 of β-LPH is β-endorphin, and smaller sequences (enkephalins) within this peptide also possess potent analgesic activity. Thus the interesting situation exists where a whole family of hormonal peptides is derived from a common precursor molecule (Fig. 8.4).

Significant alterations in the synthesis of the family tree of hormonal peptides derived from POMC may occur during different stages of development. For example, pituitary α-MSH and CLIP predominate during the fetal life of humans and monkeys but disappear in the adult; the levels of β-endorphin may also be more prominent during fetal life. The presence of these pituitary peptides is suggested to reflect a physiological function in the fetus that is not present in postnatal life. In this regard, then, it is important to discuss current thoughts about the pituitary-adrenal axis in development. The human adrenal cortex possesses a so-called *fetal zone* that is of great size during gestation (see Chap. 15). This steroidogenic zone undergoes rapid involution at parturition, whereas the outer cortical zone hypertrophies to produce the definitive cortical zone. There is evidence that in some animals (e.g., rabbit) the fetal zone is responsive to α-MSH rather than to ACTH and that the definitive cortical zone is responsive to ACTH, but not to α-MSH. Near the time of parturition there is a sharp increase in ACTH production relative to the smaller peptides, such as α-MSH and CLIP.

A key event preceding parturition (at least in sheep) is a surge of cortisol from the fetal adrenal cortex. Infusion of ACTH or cortisol into the ewe will induce premature delivery any time during the second half of pregnancy [30]. It is postulated, therefore, that the increase in ACTH relative to smaller peptides (α-MSH, endorphins) at parturition is responsible for the increasing production of cortisol by the definitive adrenal cortex. Thus the key mechanism in the chain of events controlling parturition may be the switch in pituitary peptide synthesis from α-MSH production in the pars intermedia to ACTH synthesis in the pars distalis [43].

The levels of β-endorphin are also more prominent in fetal than in adult pituitaries; there is, for example, a dramatic increase of β-endorphin in the pituitary of the newborn monkey. Silman and colleagues speculate that because the process of parturition may be a time of intense psychological trauma for the fetus, and the fetus may need to be rendered insensitive to the assault of parturition, "the high levels of plasma β-endorphin present at delivery may serve to protect the infant against a necessary but otherwise intolerable event" [43]. A corticotropin-releasing hormone (CRH) is reported to stimulate ACTH and α-MSH secretion. It was surmised, therefore, that α-MSH may play a role in the physiological response to stress.

Melanotropins and Behavior. Melanotropins have been reported to affect central nervous system activity in laboratory animals and humans (Chap. 21). These effects include arousal, increased motivation, longer attention span, memory retention, and increased learning ability [35]. Immunocytochemical studies have localized melanotropic activity to specific neurons within the brain. The potency of melanotropin action on CNS-related activity is enhanced when administered directly into the ventricles of the brain. It is suggested, therefore, that α-MSH or related melanotropins may function as a neurotransmitter or neuromodulator within the brain (Chap. 21).

Thermoregulation.   Certain lizards (e.g., *Sceloporus jarrovi*) orient themselves so that their dorsal surface is maximally exposed to the early morning sun. During this time they are generally dark in color, compared to later in the day when temperatures are elevated. It can be speculated that this adaptive chromatic response is regulated by MSH and that skin is able to absorb more radiant energy. Experimental verification is needed as it is possible, at least in some species, that skin darkening could be regulated through direct neural innervation of the melanophores.

A melanotropin may be involved in the central control of body temperature and fever. Both α-MSH and ACTH cause dose-related hypothermia when injected into the cerebral ventricles of the rabbit [7]. α-MSH is apparently neither involved in the central mechanisms underlying normal thermoregulation, nor does it act as an endogenous antipyretic in the cat, functions that have been postulated in some other species. α-MSH and ACTH have been immunocytochemically isolated to neurons within areas of the brain (preoptic-anterior hypothalamus) known to be of paramount importance in temperature regulation.

Pregnancy.   In humans pregnancy is the only known physiological state in which MSH is detectable in plasma. The source of this MSH may be the placenta or it may come from a theorized pregnancy-induced pituitary intermediate lobe. The physiological significance of placental MSH is not clear. MSH stimulates the synthesis and secretion of aldosterone and, to a lesser extent, corticosterone from rat adrenals in vitro, acting in synergy with ACTH and angiotensin II, in accord with the increase in the aldosterone production late in pregnancy. In addition, placental MSH may act as a trophic fetal adrenal stimulus. The human placenta contains the POMC-derived peptides ACTH, α-MSH, β-endorphin, and CRH. High concentrations of immunoreactive CRH have been demonstrated recently in maternal plasma during pregnancy.

The development of dopaminergic control of pituitary melanotropes in the rat occurs postnatally. The question arises as to what possible functional significance this event may have for the animal. The completion of tonic inhibitory control over the melanotropes could determine the size of the gland, due to the substantial decrease observed in proliferative rate. Moreover, innervation of the melanotropes would regulate basal serum levels of α-MSH and β-endorphin in the animal. An additional possibility would be the benefits to the fetus of "unregulated" high circulating β-endorphin levels during labor. Previous studies demonstrate that the human fetus has a well-defined pars intermedia, whose constituent cells often migrate into adjoining pituitary regions. It has been shown in humans that fetal and maternal serum α-MSH and β-endorphin levels are elevated. In the pregnant female, however, there is no organized pars intermedia and no difference in the distribution or numbers of α-MSH immunoreactive cells in the pituitary, as compared to nonpregnant females. The most likely source for the material increase is the placenta, as it synthesizes POMC and secretes POMC-derived peptides [32]. It has been shown that the human placenta releases both IR-CRH and POMC peptides in vitro, and their release was independent of glucocorticoid control. Placental CRH may have a dual endocrine (on maternal pituitary) and paracrine (on placental POMC peptide) role. These data add to the existing evidence indicating that the placenta may be part of the maternal and, possibly, fetal hypothalamo-pituitary-adrenal axis during the latter part of pregnancy [32].

Neuroplasticity.   Melanotropic peptides have been shown to alter neurotransmitter synthesis, the electrophysiological parameters of neurotransmission, and excitability in the spinal cord and peripheral nerves, and to affect a number of behavioral responses. These neurotropic actions of MSH/ACTH-related peptides may be required for normal functioning of many neuronal processes. There is hope that these peptides may be used to improve the adaptational abilities of the nervous system and to counteract age-related cognitive disorders [19].

MECHANISM OF MSH ACTION

Studies on the mechanism of action of MSH have used both in vitro and in vivo methods to monitor responses of integumental melanocytes to the hormone. The frog skin and lizard skin assays monitor the mechanical movements of pigment granules within dermal melanophores and other chromatophores. A few in vivo studies have monitored melanin synthesis within epidermal melanocytes in response to MSH. When melanocytes become cancerous, they are referred to as malignant melanoma. Mouse melanoma cells have been successfully grown in tissue culture and, because these relatively undifferentiated cells respond to MSH, the intracellular biochemical parameters of hormone action have been studied in detail.

Melanosome Movements

Melanophores are found within the dermis of the skin of most poikilothermic vertebrates. Like melanocytes, these specialized pigment cells synthesize melanosomes (melanin granules); instead of being secreted into surrounding cells these organelles can be rapidly translocated into the dendritic processes of the cell and back toward the cell center. These movements, centrifugal dispersion and centripetal aggregation, result in the skin becoming dark or light in color, respectively. The responses in the skin can be monitored microscopically by using a so-called melanophore index (Fig. 8.12). These changes in skin color can be objectively monitored in response to MSH or other chemical messengers using photoelectric reflectance methods [42]. The endocrine mechanisms controlling melanosome movements are well detailed, but nevertheless incomplete [20].

MSH induces an outward dispersion of melanosomes into the dendritic processes of melanophores. Melanosome dispersion in response to MSH can be mimicked by methylxanthines (caffeine, theophylline) and by $(Bu)_2$cAMP. MSH increases the concentration of cAMP in frog skins concomitant with melanosome dispersion and darkening of the skins. These results implicate cAMP as the intracellular second messenger of MSH action. Epinephrine and norepinephrine also affect melanosome movements within melanophores. Classical pharmacological studies using a variety of adrenergic agonists and antagonists have established that melanosome dispersion in response to these catecholamines is mediated through melanophore β-adrenergic receptors (Chap. 14). These receptors are distinct from MSH receptors, as demonstrated by the preferential blockade of one receptor while the functional response of the other is maintained. Melanosome dispersion in response to MSH or a catecholamine (acting through β-adrenoceptors) is inhibited or reversed by catecholamines acting through α-adrenoceptors possessed by the melanophores. This antagonism of MSH by α-adrenoceptor stimulation involves a decrease in cAMP formation (see Chap. 14).

The involvement of adrenergic receptors controlling melanophore responses has been demonstrated in teleosts, amphibians, and reptiles. The melanophores of some amphibians lack α-adrenoceptors but possess β-adrenoceptors [1]. Catecholamines, therefore, fail to inhibit MSH action in these species. Stimulation of β-adrenoceptors in all vertebrate tissues studied results in increased cAMP production, and a similar increase of the cyclic nucleotide probably occurs within melanophores. Melatonin, an indoleamine synthesized within the pineal, antagonizes the action of MSH on melanophores. The possible role of the pineal and melatonin in the control of vertebrate pigmentation will be discussed (see Chap. 20).

melanosome
Dispersal ?
_____

— methylxanthines
(caffeine +
theophylline)

— MSH

— prostaglandins

Prostaglandins also disperse melanosomes within fish and amphibian melanophores. As expected, the action of PGs is not inhibited by MSH receptor or β-adrenoceptor blockade. MSH and epinephrine (or isoproterenol), but not PGs, darken lizard (*Anolis*) skins. It has been suggested that some hormones may mediate their effects indirectly by stimulating cellular PG biosynthesis. The failure of some species' melanophores to respond to PGs would argue against such a generalized role for PGs in the control of vertebrate melanophores.

There is a calcium ion requirement for MSH action but not for melanosome movements, per se, because melanosome dispersion proceeds, in the Ca^{2+}-free medium, in response to theophylline or to $(Bu)_2cAMP$ [47]. Calcium is the only cation required for MSH action, as the Na^+ and K^+ of the medium can be replaced by lithium, cesium, or rubidium, other monovalent cations. Epinephrine or isoproterenol, acting through melanophore β-adrenoceptors or PGs, do not require Ca^{2+} for activation of melanophore cAMP production [47]. These results demonstrate a receptor-specific Ca^{2+} requirement for MSH action. It is interesting that ACTH and MSH elevate cAMP levels of cells by receptor mechanisms separate from β-adrenergic receptors, which similarly increase the production of this cyclic nucleotide. Adrenocorticotropin and epinephrine, for example, stimulate lipolysis within adipocytes, but through different receptors. As for MSH, ACTH requires Ca^{2+} for its mechanism of action, whereas epinephrine, acting through β-adrenoceptors of adipose cells, does not.

Both ACTH and MSH, acting as first messengers, stimulate adrenal cortical cells and melanophores, respectively, by interacting with the plasma membrane receptors of these cells. ACTH stimulation of adenylate cyclase, but not the ACTH-receptor interaction, requires Ca^{2+}. Thus there is a Ca^{2+}-dependent step between the binding of ACTH to its receptor and the subsequent activation of adrenal adenylate cyclase. Adrenal cortical cells are more responsive to ACTH as the concentration of Ca^{2+} is increased. It has been suggested that the strength of the signal generated by the interaction of ACTH with its receptor and transmitted to the adenylate cyclase compartment is proportionately increased as the Ca^{2+} concentration is increased. This model for adrenocortical control by ACTH appears to be appropriate as a model for MSH control of melanophores. Because both hormones are related structurally, and presumably evolutionarily, it would seem plausible that they might share a common mechanism of action, as each is capable of stimulating adrenocortical cells and melanophores.

The biochemical events underlying melanophore melanosome dispersion are analogous to those for smooth muscle relaxation: both processes result from increases in cAMP levels as mediated, for example, by catecholamine stimulation of β-adrenoceptors. An increase in cAMP production results in a transport of Ca^{2+} from the cytoplasm to the endoplasmic reticulum and/or mitochondria or out of the smooth muscle cell. Because melanosome dispersion proceeds in the absence of Ca^{2+} and is enhanced under such conditions [20, 47], a similar Ca^{2+} transport mechanism may also be requisite for melanosome dispersion. Such a model would require the presence of extracellular Ca^{2+} for MSH (but not catecholamine or prostaglandin) action, but the cAMP generated would mediate melanosome dispersion by a subsequent sequestering of cytoplasmic Ca^{2+} [47].

Microtubules, microfilaments, and microtrabeculae are abundant in some, but not all, melanophores. There is no clear consensus for a definitive role of these cytoskeletal organelles within melanophores. The general belief is that they provide the intracellular framework for the translocation of pigment organelles within the cell. A hypothetical model for the control of melanophore melanosome movements is shown [40] (Fig. 8.14).

Melanogenesis

The understanding of the α-MSH action mechanisms has traditionally been derived from studies on the integumental chromatophores of frogs, lizards, and fishes. Because of the possible malignancy of melanocytes, it is hoped that the results gleaned from these stud-

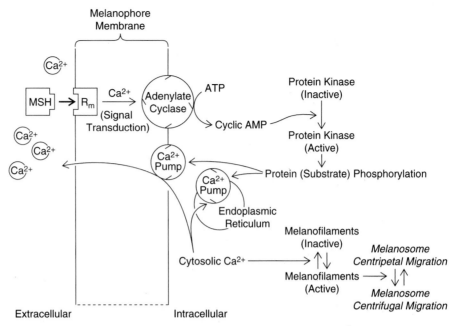

Figure 8.14 Hypothetical model for a role of MSH and Ca^{2+} ions in the control of melanosome movements within melanophores [40].

ies may be extrapolated to mammalian melanocytes. Melanocytes and melanoma cells differ from melanophores in that they are undifferentiated cells. Mouse melanocytes, both normal and abnormal (melanoma), possess MSH receptors and also respond to prostaglandins. These agonists activate adenylate cyclase and elevate intracellular levels of cAMP, which results in enhanced tyrosinase activity and increased melanogenesis. MSH action is blocked by actinomycin D and cycloheximide, thus implicating transcriptional and translational effects of the hormone. Although MSH activates cAMP production, and this cyclic nucleotide activates a cAMP-dependent protein kinase, the mechanism by which this cyclic nucleotide activates nuclear transcriptional processes leading to increased enzyme activity is unknown. A model based on present knowledge of the control of melanogenesis by MSH is shown (Fig. 8.15).

Melanotropin Structure-Function Studies

Numerous analogs of α-MSH and related melanotropins have been synthesized for structure-function studies [26, 41]. The natural melanotropins share a common heptapeptide sequence, -Met-Glu-His-Phe-Arg-Trp-Gly- (Fig. 8.1). Because these peptides (α-MSH, β-MSH, ACTH, β-LPH) possess melanotropic activity, it is believed that this sequence represents the active site of the molecule. Minimal contribution is nevertheless provided by the C-terminal tridecapeptide sequence, -Lys-Pro-Val-NH_2, as well as the N-terminal sequence, Ac-Ser-Tyr-Ser-, in some species. The minimal sequence for biological activity in the frog [26] and lizard skin [5] bioassays is the tetrapeptide sequence His-Phe-Arg-Trp. Insight into the three-dimensional requirements of α-MSH structure related to its biologically active conformation at its receptor has been provided [40].

Melanotropin Receptors

Classical structure-activity studies, derived particularly from frog and lizard skins, reveal that the minimal sequence to stimulate melanosome dispersion is the tetrapeptide sequence, His-Phe-Arg-Trp [5, 26]. Although this sequence is inactive, as might be expected, it apparently represents the minimal natural sequence required for melanotropin receptor

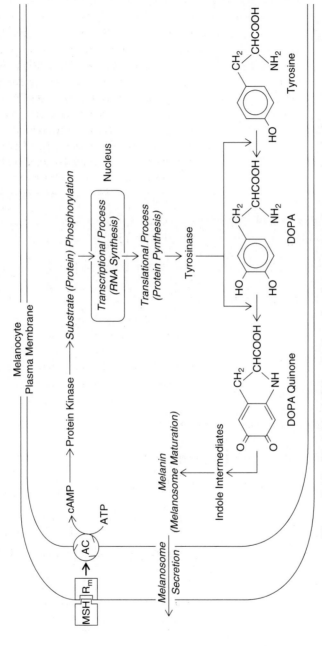

Figure 8.15 Model for MSH activation of melanocyte tyrosinase and melanin synthesis. The substrate for cAMP-dependent protein kinase is unknown. The end result of tyrosinase activation, melanosome formation and release into surrounding keratinocytes, is enhanced skin pigmentation (or follicular melanogenesis in some animals).

binding, receptor signal transduction, and cAMP production leading to melanosome dispersion. In the frog, MSH_{4-12} represents the shortest fragment analog that will give a near equipotent response to the native hormone, MSH. In the lizard, MSH_{4-11} is only slightly less active than MSH. These observations reveal that melanotropin receptors differ between species.

These results also demonstrate that the N-terminal tripeptide sequence is relatively unimportant for receptor activation and cAMP production. The C-terminal valine moiety is also nonessential for the melanotropic activity of α-MSH. The receptors between frogs and lizards differ considerably relative to a need for position 12 (proline) of MSH for activity.

MSH Antagonists. A number of melanotropic peptide antagonists have been designed and their biological actions determined in the frog and lizard bioassays [41]. These peptides differ in their antagonistic activities, pointing out that melanotropin receptors differ between species. Improved efficacy of these antagonists may result in peptides with clinical relevance.

Molecular Biology of Melanocortin Receptors. The receptors for α-MSH and ACTH have been cloned [9, 8, 34, 37]. MSH-R (MC1-R) and ACTH-R (MC2-R) mRNA expression has only been detected in melanocytes and the adrenal cortex, respectively. A neural specific melanocortin receptor that is expressed mainly in the hypothalamus and limbic system has also been described, but it is not found in melanocytes or the adrenal cortex [14, 38]. This melanocortin 3 receptor (MC3-R) is about 43% identical to the α-MSH receptor. This MC3-R is potently activated by γ-MSH peptides. The biological role of γ-MSH is presently unknown but may manifest as yet undefined physiological actions in the brain through this receptor [38].

PATHOPHYSIOLOGY

Because the pituitary of the adult human lacks a pars intermedia, it is not surprising that, unlike most hormones, no pathophysiological states related to overproduction or underproduction of MSH have been described. The discovery that α-MSH is present in the fetal pituitary and may function in the control of fetal growth and development within the uterus should alert the clinician to possible postnatal defects resulting from pars intermedia dysfunction in the fetus. Because α-MSH may function as a neurohormone within the brain, α-MSH may eventually be implicated in the etiology of certain behavioral pathologies.

In Addison's disease destruction of the adrenal cortex results in a subsequent failure of adrenal steroid hormone production. Because of an absence of circulating levels of cortisol, there is a lack of negative feedback inhibition to the hypothalamus and pituitary, which results in enhanced pituitary secretion of ACTH (see Chap. 15). The hyperpigmentation that follows, a cardinal symptom of Addison's disease, is because excessive circulating levels of ACTH or other melanotropic sequences are stimulatory to melanogenesis within epidermal melanocytes. In Cushing's syndrome (of pituitary origin), where excessive amounts of ACTH are secreted, hyperpigmentation is often noted and may be due, again, to elevated circulating levels of POMC-derived melanotropic peptides. Hyperpigmentation may also occur in the *ectopic ACTH syndrome* where excessive amounts of ACTH or other melanotropins are secreted by tumors of nonpituitary origin.

Vitiligo is a malady of the skin where melanocytes in certain areas are absent or fail to become pigmentogenic. Areas of the integument are thus unpigmented. There was hope that melanogenesis within these affected areas might be restored by administration of MSH or related melanotropins. Unfortunately, MSH only increases the pigment in the adjacent normal areas, thus, in effect, accentuating the pigmentary problem.

Biomedical Applications of Melanotropins. A number of unique α-MSH analogs have been synthesized that are superpotent, prolonged acting, and resistant to inactivation by proteolytic enzymes. These peptides provide potential probes for physiological and clinical studies. For example, these analogs can be conjugated to radio-isotopes or fluorescent ligands for the cellular- (receptor-) specific delivery to melanoma (cancer). Melanotropins can also be conjugated to anticancer drugs. Melanotropin analogs, therefore, might be utilized for the localization and chemotherapy of melanoma [21, 23].

It was demonstrated that certain melanotropins can be topically applied and transdermally delivered across the skin of mice and humans in vitro, as determined by bioassay and RIA. Studies are underway to determine whether MSH-related analogues may prove useful as a "tanning hormone" for increasing the pigmentation of light-skinned individuals or possibly even for treating people with certain hypopigmentary disorders. It is hoped this "tanning without the sun" may reduce the incidence of skin cancer. The results of initial studies demonstrated that tanning of human skin by a synthetic melanotropic peptide is feasible [29].

MELANIN-CONCENTRATING HORMONE

In 1931 it was postulated that many lower vertebrates exhibit color changes through dual hormonal control by two antagonistic pituitary melanotropic hormones [3]. *α-Melanotropin* is clearly implicated in regulating darkening of the skin of many animals through stimulation of melanosome dispersion within melanophores. The existence of an antagonist hormone, a *melanin-concentrating hormone* (MCH), in the pituitary gland of teleost fishes was suggested in 1955 [12]. Teleost MCH was then separated from fish pituitary gland extracts in 1958; the highest concentrations of MCH were found in the neurointermediate lobe of the pituitary gland. This hormone induced blanching of the skin (perinuclear aggregation of melanosomes within melanophores) when injected into teleost fishes. MCH was then isolated in pure form from chum salmon pituitaries and was characterized as a cyclic heptadecapeptide [28]. The primary structure of this peptide is shown in Fig. 8.16.

Salmon MCH was effective at concentrations as low as 1 nanoMole, or less, in causing melanosome concentration within teleost melanophores [3, 28]. MCH and several related structural analogs have now been synthesized and characterized for their melanotropic activities in several bioassays [3, 5]. MCH stimulates melanosome concentration within melanophores of all teleost fishes species studied. Melanosome aggregation in response to MCH is reversible, since removal of the peptide from the bathing medium results in a redispersal of the pigment organelles within the chromatophores. The melanosome-aggregating activity of MCH could also be reversed if MSH was added to teleost skin lightened by MCH. These results clearly reveal that in several species of teleosts, melanophores possess receptors responsive to both MSH and MCH. Melanosome aggregation in response to MCH was not blocked by Dibenamine (an α-adrenoceptor antagonist; see Chap. 14), which did block the response to norepinephrine, demonstrating that melanosome-aggregating responses to MCH and NE are mediated through separate receptors [5].

Figure 8.16 Primary structure of melanin-concentrating hormone (MCH).

```
              1      3      5      7      9      11     13     15     17

MCH–1–17   Asp–Thr–Met–Arg–Cys–Met–Val–Gly–Arg–Val–Tyr–Arg–Pro–Cys–Trp–Glu–Val

MCH–1–14   Asp–Thr–Met–Arg–Cys–Met–Val–Gly–Arg–Val–Tyr–Arg–Pro–Cys

MCH–5–17                     Cys–Met–Val–Gly–Arg–Val–Tyr–Arg–Pro–Cys–Trp–Glu–Val

MCH–5–14                     Cys–Met–Val–Gly–Arg–Val–Tyr–Arg–Pro–Cys
```

Figure 8.17   Primary structures of MCH and related fragment analogs.

A most unexpected observation was that MCH, rather than stimulating melanosome aggregation within tetrapod melanophores, instead induced melanosome dispersion. The peptide was about 1/600 as potent as MSH; nevertheless, full melanosome dispersion was effected in melanophores of frogs, toads, and lizards. There are no readily apparent similarities between the primary structures of MCH and α-MSH. To determine the possible structural basis of the opposing actions of MCH, several analogs were synthesized, in addition to the native hormone [5, 33]. These fragment analogs consisted of the central cyclic sequence (MCH$_{5-14}$), as well as the N-terminal (MCH$_{1-14}$) and the C-terminal (MCH$_{5-17}$) extensions of the central sequence of the native peptide (Fig. 8.17). Using skins of the teleost *Synbranchus marmoratus* (an eel) and photoreflectance recordings, it was determined that MCH$_{5-17}$ was at least equipotent to the native hormone, MCH$_{1-17}$. MCH$_{1-14}$ was also quite active, showing about 1/10 the activity of MCH$_{1-17}$. The central cyclic fragment analog, MCH$_{5-14}$, possessed about 1/300 the activity of the parent peptide. Therefore, the potency ranking of the MCH analogs on teleost melanophores was as follows: MCH$_{1-17}$ = MCH$_{5-17}$ > MCH$_{1-14}$ > MCH$_{5-14}$ [33] (Fig. 8.18). The fragment analogs were full agonists, and their melanosome-aggregating actions were reversible when the skins were transferred to physiological saline in the absence of the peptides. It is interesting to note that this fish-skin bioassay is sensitive to MCH at a minimal effective dose of 10^{-12}M. This assay is therefore 10 and 100 times more sensitive, respectively, than are the classical frog and lizard skin assays to MSH.

It was shown that the fragment analog, MCH$_{1-14}$, exhibited MSH-like activity (about 10% of the MCH response) in the frog and lizard skin bioassays. The C-terminal

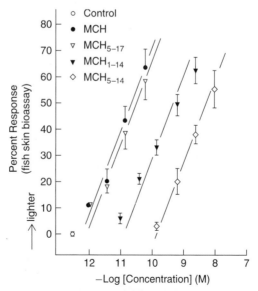

Figure 8.18   In vitro bioassay of MCH and related analogs using skins of the fish *Synbranchus marmoratus* (an eel). (From Castrucci et al. [6], with permission.)

fragment analog, MCH_{5-17}, lacked melanosome-dispersing activity even at the highest concentrations employed ($10^{-5}M$). It appears, therefore, that tetrapod melanophores lack MCH receptors. These results also suggest that one or more amino acids within the N-terminal 1–4 sequence (Asp-Thr-Met-Arg) are required for the MSH-like activity of MCH, but not for the MCH-like activity of the hormone. These observations suggest that MSH and MCH may be evolutionarily related [5, 19].

Mammalian MCH.   Rat hypothalamic MCH is a nonadecapeptide that differs from salmon MCH by an N-terminal extension of two amino acids and four additional substitutions. Rat MCH has the following primary structure: Asp-Phe-Asp-Met-Leu-Arg-Cys-Met-Leu-Gly-Arg-Val-Tyr-Arg-Pro-Cys-Trp-Gln-Val. The sequence of rMCH found by DNA sequencing confirms the sequence deduced from the purified peptide. rMCH is located at the C-terminus of a protein precursor of 165 amino acid residues. Comparison of the amino acid sequence of prepro-MCH and that of the *Aplysia* peptide-A prohormone suggests that these proteins, as well as other precursors, may be evolutionarily related. The human gene for MCH has been isolated and characterized [4].

Both MSH and MCH are present within the brain or the pituitary gland, or both, of several vertebrates [18]. Indeed, MCH has been reported to inhibit corticotropin (ACTH) secretion from the isolated rat pituitary gland and MSH from the fish pituitary gland [3]. This observation suggests that MCH may be a peptidergic neurohormone functioning as a hypophysiotropic factor.

REFERENCES

[1]   Bagnara, J. T., and M. E. Hadley. 1972. *Chromatophores and color change: comparative physiology of animal pigmentation.* Englewood Cliffs, N.J.: Prentice-Hall Publishing Co., Inc.

[2]   Bagnara, J. T., J. D. Taylor, and M. E. Hadley. 1968. The dermal chromatophore unit. *J. Cell Biol.* 38:67–79.

[3]   Baker, B. I. 1993. The role of melanin-concentrating hormone in color change. *Ann. New York Acad. Sci.* 680:279–89.

[4]   Breton, C., M. Schorpp, and J.-L. Nahon. 1993. Isolation and characterization of the human melanin-concentrating hormone gene and a variant gene. *Mol. Brain Res.* 18:297–310.

[5]   Castrucci, A. M. L., M. E. Hadley, T. K. Sawyer, B. C. Wilkes, F. Al-obeidi, D. J. Staples, A. E. De Vaux, O. Dym, F. M. Hintz, J. P. Riehm, K. R. Rao, and V. J. Hruby. 1989. α-Melanotropin: the minimal active sequence in the lizard skin bioassay. *Gen. Comp. Endocrinol.* 73:157–63.

[6]   Castrucci, A. M. L., M. E. Hadley, B. C. Wilkes, V. J. Hruby, and T. K. Sawyer. 1989. Melanotropin structure-activity studies on melanocytes of the teleost fish, *Synbranchus marmoratus. Gen. Comp. Endocrinol.* 4:209–14.

[7]   Catania, A., and J. M. Lipton. 1993. α-Melanocyte stimulating hormone in the modulation of host reactions. *Endocr. Rev.* 14:564–76.

[8]   Cone, R. D., and K. G. Mountjoy. 1993. Molecular genetics of the ACTH and melanocyte stimulating hormone receptors. *TEM* 4:242–7.

[9]   Cone, R. G., K. G. Mountjoy, L. S. Robbins, J. H. Nadeau, K. R. Johnson, L. Roselli-Rehfuss, and M. T. Mortrud. 1993. Cloning and functional characterization of a family of receptors for the melanotropic peptides. *Ann. New York Acad. Sci.* 680:342–63.

[10] Davis, M. D., and M. E. Hadley. 1978. Pars intermedia electrical potentials: changes in spike frequency induced by regulatory factors of melanocyte stimulating hormone (MSH) secretion. *Neuroendocrinology* 26:277–82.

[11] Eberle, A. N. 1988. *The melanotropins. Chemistry, physiology and mechanisms of action.* Basel, Switzerland: Karger.

[12]   Enami, M. 1955. Melanophore-concentrating hormone (MCH) of possible hypothalamic origin in the catfish, *Parasilurus. Science* 121:36–7.

[13]   Fernandez, P. J. Jr., and J. P. Collins. 1988. Effect of environment and ontogeny on color pattern variation in Arizona tiger salamanders (*Ambystoma tigrinum nebulosum* hallowell). *Copeia* 4:928–38.

[14]   Gantz, I., K. Konda, T. Tashiro, H. Shimoto, H. Miwa, G. Munzert, S. J. Watson, J. Delvalle, and T. Yamada. 1993. Molecular cloning of a novel melanocortin receptor. *J. Biol. Chem.* 265:8246–50.

[15]   Gary, K. A., and B. M. Chronwall. 1992. The onset of dopaminergic innervation during ontogeny decreases melanotrope proliferation in the intermediate lobe of the rat pituitary. *Int. J. Devel. Neuroscience* 10:131–142.

[16]   Geschwind, I. I., R. A. Huseby, and R. Nishioka. 1972. The effect of melanocyte-stimulating hormone on coat color in the mouse. *Rec. Prog. Horm. Res.* 28:91–130.

[17]   Hadley, M. E. 1972. The significance of vertebrate integumental pigmentation. *Amer. Zool.* 12:63–76.

[18]   Hadley, M. E. (ed.) 1988a. *The Melanotropic peptides, Vol. I, Source, synthesis, chemistry, secretion, and metabolism.* Boca Raton, Fl.: CRC Press.

[19]   ——— 1988b. *The Melanotropic peptides, Vol. II, Biological roles.* Boca Raton, Fl.: CRC Press.

[20]   ——— 1988c. *The Melanotropic peptides, Vol. III, Mechanisms of action and biomedical applications.* Boca Raton, Fl.: CRC Press.

[21]   Hadley, M. E., and B. V. Dawson. 1988. Biomedical applications of synthetic melanotropins. *Pigment Cell Res.* 1:69–78.

[22]   Hadley, M. E., and N. Levine. 1993. Hormonal control of melanogenesis. In *Pigmentation and pigmentary disorders*, N. Levine, ed. Boca Raton, FL: CRC Press.

[23]   Hadley, M. E., S. D. Sharma, V. J. Hruby, N. Levine, and R. T. Dorr. 1993. Melanotropic peptides for therapeutic and cosmetic tanning of the skin. *Ann. New York Acad. Sci.* 680:626–45.

[24]   Hadley, M. E., and W. C. Quevedo, Jr. 1967. The role of epidermal melanocytes in adaptive color changes in amphibians. *Advan. Biol. Skin* 8:337–59.

[25]   Holmes, R. L., and J. N. Ball. 1974. *The pituitary gland: a comparative account.* Cambridge, England: University Press.

[26]   Hruby, V. J., B. C. Wilkes, M. E. Hadley, F. Al-obeidi, T. K. Sawyer, D. J. Staples, A. E. De Vaux, O. Dym, A. M. L. Castrucci, M. F. Hintz, J. P. Riehm, and K. Ranga Rao. 1987. α-Melanotropin: the minimal active sequence in the frog skin bioassay. *J. Med. Chem.* 30:2126–30.

[27]   Jenks, B. G., V.-V. Kemenade, and G. J. M. Martens. 1988. Proopiomelanocortin in the amphibian pars intermedia: a neuroendocrine model system. In *The Melanotropic peptides,* M. E. Hadley, ed. Boca Raton, Fl.: CRC Press.

[28]   Kawauchi, H., I. Kawazoe, M. Tsubokawa, M. Kishida, and B. I. Baker. 1983. Characterization of melanin concentrating hormone. *Nature* (Lond.) 305:321–3.

[29]   Levine, N., S. N. Sheftel, T. Eytan, R. T. Dorr, M. E. Hadley, J. C. Weinrach, G. A. Ertl, K. Toth, D. L. Mcgee, and V. J. Hruby. 1991. Induction of skin tanning by the subcutaneous administration of a potent synthetic melanotropin. *J. Amer. Med. Assoc.* 266:2730–6.

[30]   Liggins, G. C., R. J. Faerclough, S. A. Grieves, J. Z. Kendal, and B. S. Knox. 1973. The mechanism of initiation of parturition in the ewe. *Rec. Prog. Horm. Res.* 29:111–59.

[31]   Lowry. P. J., and A. P. Scott. 1975. The evolution of vertebrate corticotropin and melanocyte stimulating hormone. *Gen. Comp. Endocrinol.* 26:16–23.

[32]   Margioris, A. N., M. Grino, P. Protos, P. W. Gold, and G. P. Chrousos. 1988. Corticotropin-releasing hormone and oxytocin stimulate the release of placental proopiomelanocortin peptides. *J. Clin. Endocrinol. Metab.* 65:922–6.

[33]   Matsunaga, T. O., A. M. L. Castrucci, M. E. Hadley, and V. J. Hruby. 1989. Melanin concentrating hormone (MCH): synthesis and bioactivity studies of MCH fragment analogues. *Peptides* 10:349–54.

[34]   Mountjoy, K. G., L. S. Robbins, M. T. Mortrud, and R. D. Cone. 1992. The cloning of a family of genes that encode the melanocortin receptors. *Science* 257:1248–51.

[35] O'Donohue, T. L., and D. M. Dorsa. 1982. The opiomelanotropinergic neuronal and endocrine systems. *Peptides* 3:353–95.

[36] Pawelek, J. M., A. K. Chakraborty, M. P. Osber, S. J. Orlow, K. K. Min, K. R. Rosenzweig, and J. L. Bolognia. 1992. Molecular cascades in UV-induced melanogenesis: a central role for melanotropins? *Pigment Cell Res.* 5:348–56.

[37] Robbins, L. S., J. H. Nadeau, K. R. Johnson, M. A. Kelly, L. Roselli-Rehfuss, E. Baack, K. G. Mountjoy, and R. D. Cone. 1993. Pigmentation phenotypes of variant extension locus alleles result from point mutations that alter MSH receptor function. *Cell* 72:827–34.

[38] Roselli-Rehfuss, L., K. G. Mountjoy, L. S. Robbins, M. T. Mort, M. J. Low, J. B. Tatro, M. L. Entwistle, R. B. Simerly, and R. D. Cone. 1993. Identification of a receptor for γ-melanotropin and other proopiomelanocortin peptides in the hypothalamus and limbic system. *Proc. Natl. Acad. Sci. USA* 90:8856–60.

[39] Rust, C. C., and R. K. Meyer. 1969. Hair color, molt, and testis size in male, short-tailed weasels treated with melatonin. *Science* 165:921–22.

[40] Sawyer, T. K., V. J. Hruby, M. E. Hadley, and M. H. Engel. 1983. α-Melanocyte stimulating hormone: chemical nature and mechanism of action. *Amer. Zool.* 23:529–40.

[41] Sawyer, T. K., D. J. Staples, A. M. L. Castrucci, M. E. Hadley, F. A. Al-obeidi, W. L. Cody, and V. J. Hruby. 1990. α-Melanocyte stimulating hormone message and inhibitory sequences: comparative structure-activity studies on melanocytes. *Peptides* 11:351–7.

[42] Schizume, K., A. B. Lerner, and T. B. Fitzpatrick. 1954. In vitro bioassay for the melanocyte stimulating hormone. *Endocrinology* 54:553–60.

[43] Silman, R. E., D. Holland, T. Chard, P. J. Lowry, J. Hope, L. H. Rees, A. Thomas, and P. Nathanielsz. 1979. Adrenocorticotropin-related peptides in adult and fetal sheep pituitary glands. *J. Endocrinol.* 81:19–34.

[44] Taylor, J. D., and M. E. Hadley. 1970. Chromatophores and color change in the lizard *Anolis carolinensis. Z. Zellforsch. Mikroskop. Anat.* 104:282–94.

[45] Tong, Y., J. Couet, J. Simard, and G. Pelletier. 1990. Glucocorticoid regulation of proopiomelanocortin mRNA levels in rat arcuate nucleus. *Mol. Cell. Neurosci.* 1:78–83.

[46] Van Zoest, I. D., P. S. Heijmen, P. M. J. M. Cruijsen, and B. G. Jenks. 1989. Dynamics of background adaptation in *Xenopus laevis*: role of catecholamines and melanophore-stimulating hormone. *Gen. Comp. Endocrinol.* 76:19–28.

[47] Vesley, D. L., and M. E. Hadley. 1979. Ionic requirements for melanophore stimulating hormone (MSH) action on melanophores. *Comp. Biochem. Physiol.* 62A:501–8.

[48] Wilson, J. F., and M. A. Morgan. 1979. α-Melanotropin-like substances in the pituitary and plasma of *Xenopus laevis* in relation to colour change responses. *Gen. Comp. Endocrinol.* 38:172–82.

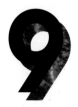

Hormonal Control of Calcium Homeostasis

The calcium ion (Ca^{2+}) is a key element in numerous physiological functions. Derived from the diet or from the structural component of bone, this divalent cation is important in bone growth, and it is readily available to serve in a variety of intracellular and extracellular roles. Ca^{2+} is necessary for normal blood clotting, and, with Na^+ and K^+, it aids in maintaining the transmembrane potential of cells and is involved in mechanisms of cell replication [32]. Ca^{2+} may be necessary for the transduction of signal between hormone receptor and second-messenger formation and action in some cells. Stimulus-secretion and stimulus-contraction coupling also require the participation of Ca^{2+}.

*Three hormones are of prime importance in the control of Ca^{2+} homeostasis, and a number of other hormones also directly or indirectly affect the availability of this cation [15]. **Parathyroid hormone**, or parathormone (PTH), derived from the parathyroid glands, increases circulating levels of Ca^{2+}, whereas **calcitonin** (CT), derived from the parafollicular cells of the mammalian thyroid, lowers the circulating levels of the ion. A metabolite of vitamin D, 1,25-dihydroxyvitamin D_3, also increases serum levels of Ca^{2+}. These three hormones interact to maintain normal plasma Ca^{2+} levels. A recently discovered **PTH-related peptide** (PTHrP) is now also implicated in the control of Ca^{2+} homeostasis. Because of the importance of Ca^{2+} to normal bodily function and because of the complex number of interactions between the hormones regulating Ca^{2+} homeostasis, it is not surprising that a large number of endocrinopathies related to Ca^{2+} homeostasis and bone mineral metabolism have been described.*

CALCIUM AND BONE PHYSIOLOGY

Cytosolic and extracellular fluid concentrations of Ca^{2+} must be maintained within narrow limits despite the wide fluctuations in Ca^{2+} intake. In humans, the Ca^{2+} level of plasma is maintained at about 10 mg/100 ml. Serum Ca^{2+} derived from the diet is delivered to the blood after being actively transported across the intestinal mucosa. Urinary Ca^{2+} loss is partially prevented by active transport of the cation back across the renal tubular epithelium. Bone serves as the immediate source of Ca^{2+} to maintain serum Ca^{2+} homeostasis. Half of the Ca^{2+} present in blood is in the free ionized form and half is bound to albumin. The free ionized form of Ca^{2+} is readily available and important in physiological processes. Three factors can alter the distribution of Ca^{2+} in plasma: albumin concentration, acid-base disturbances, and protein abnormalities. Calcium metabolism consists of relationships between a large skeletal pool, a smaller soft tissue pool, and a much smaller

177

extracellular fluid pool, modified by input from intestinal absorption and loss via renal and fecal excretion. The placenta and the mammary glands represent other routes of Ca^{2+} loss.

To understand the actions of hormones on skeletal formation and resorption, it is necessary to review the cellular processes involved in the mineralization and demineralization of bone. Bone is covered by the periosteum, which consists of connective tissue fibers. A layer of *osteoblasts* within the deeper layer of the fibrous periosteum synthesizes and releases molecules of collagen. The individual collagen molecules become oriented in a specific molecular architecture to form an extracellular matrix around the osteoblasts. Calcium and phosphate ions are stereochemically bound to specific sites on the collagen matrix where they are precipitated as $Ca_{10}(PO_4)_6(OH)_2$, hydroxyapatite. Precipitation of calcium phosphate depends on the product of the concentrations of Ca^{2+} and PO_4^{-3}. Whenever the concentration of $[Ca^{2+}] \times [PO_4^{-3}]$ exceeds the solubility product at the local site of ossification, calcium phosphate precipitates. Precipitation of bone mineral may be enhanced under conditions of local alkalinization resulting from osteoblastic activity. After calcification of the collagen matrix, the embedded cells are referred to as *osteocytes*. Demineralization of bone is effected by large multinucleate cells, *osteoclasts*, which release acid phosphatase and hyaluronic acid. Local decreases in pH caused by the osteoclasts favor the solubilization of hydroxyapatite with the resulting release of Ca^{2+} and PO_4^{-3} from the collagen matrix.

Bone remodeling is the process by which the catabolic effects (bone resorption) of one cell type of bone, osteoclasts, are balanced by the anabolic effects (bone formation) of a second cell type, osteoblasts. Normal bone remodeling proceeds in a highly regulated cycle in which osteoclasts adhere to bone and subsequently remove it by acidification and proteolytic digestion. Once osteoclasts leave the removal site, osteoblasts enter and secrete osteoid (a matrix of collagen and other proteins), which is then calcified into new bone. Osteoclast-mediated resorption is influenced by two processes: activation, in which the resorptive function of mature osteoclasts is increased, and recruitment, in which osteoclast progenitors are stimulated to yield more mature cells [19].

Bone serves as a reservoir for the rapid uptake and release of Ca^{2+} during daily plasma Ca^{2+} fluctuations. A layer of osteoblasts is separated from the underlying layers of osteocytes by a *bone fluid compartment*, a so-called bone-lining cell/osteocyte unit. Calcium stored in the bone fluid compartment is present in a labile, metastable form, which is kept from being transferred to hydroxyapatite crystals.

PARATHORMONE

Historically, parathormone (PTH) was the first of the trio of calcitropic hormones controlling Ca^{2+} homeostasis to be discovered. Because Ca^{2+} is essential in cellular function, PTH is necessary for life. Although other hormones may be required for normal body function, with the exception of aldosterone (Chap. 15), they are not essential for survival.

The Parathyroid Glands

Parathormone is derived from the parathyroids, which in most mammals are embedded on the surface of the thyroid gland. In humans four parathyroid glands are present; they are located on the back side of the thyroid gland, one near each pole of the two lobes of the thyroid gland (Fig. 9.1). The parathyroid glands are derived from the third and fourth pharyngeal pouches, the two superior glands from the fourth and the two inferior glands from the third. Removal of the thyroid gland usually leads to death in animals; it was subsequently discovered, however, that the lethal effects of thyroidectomy could be duplicated solely by removal of the parathyroids, rather than the thyroid itself. In mammals other than humans there may be one or two pairs of parathyroids that may or may not be associated with thyroid tissue. The parathyroids are composed of two cell types, the *chief* cells, which

[handwritten margin note: Parathyroids on Surface of the thyroid gland.]

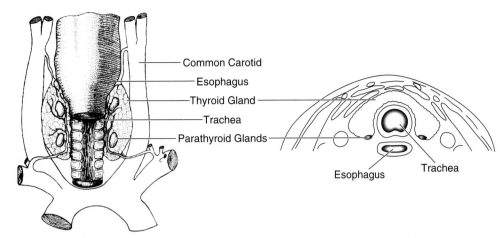

Figure 9.1 Posterior (left) and transverse (right) views of the human thyroid with attached parathyroids.

are the source of PTH, and the *oxyphil* cells, of unknown function. The chief cells are most numerous and in some mammals may be the only cells present. Oxyphil cells in humans appear around puberty and increase in number with age; they contain an eosinophilic granular cytoplasm.

Removal of the parathyroids results in a drop in plasma Ca^{2+} levels, which usually results in tetanic convulsions and death. In 1925 Collip isolated a biologically active fraction from bovine parathyroid glands that could restore Ca^{2+} levels in parathyroidectomized dogs. This active substance of the parathyroid glands was appropriately named parathyroid hormone, or as it is more commonly known, parathormone (PTH).

Synthesis, Chemistry, and Metabolism

Parathormone, a polypeptide 84 amino acids long, is derived from a precursor molecule of 115 amino acid residues. This so-called preproparathyroid hormone (PreProPTH) then undergoes proteolytic cleavages to yield a proPTH of 90 amino acids, from which six residues are then removed to yield the definitive hormonal product. In an in vitro translation system (for the production of protein from messenger RNA), PreProPTH has been biosynthesized and shown to be converted to PTH in the Golgi zone of the chief cells by a trypsin-like protease. The hormone is then packaged into secretory vesicles that migrate to the periphery of the cell where the hormone is secreted by a mechanism of vesicular exocytosis.

The primary structures of human PTH, as well as those of the pig, cow, and other mammals, have been determined (Fig. 9.2). There is extensive sequence homology among the three species of hormone. The 84-amino-acid sequence appears to be the major form of the hormone secreted from the parathyroids. In the peripheral circulation the intact hormone is cleaved into two major fragments, one of which, PTH-(1-34), retains some biological activity. Studies using radiolabeled bovine PTH in calves showed an initial rapid disappearance of most of the hormone, with a half-life of 3 to 4 minutes. In humans, PTH has approximately the same half-life as measured after parathyroidectomy. In the isolated perfused kidney, intact PTH is taken up and cleaved into its N- and C-terminal fragments. The kidney may not be the only site of hormone degradation, and metabolism of the hormone may vary from person to person.

Control of Secretion

The release of PTH from the parathyroid glands is controlled by circulating levels of Ca^{2+}. Parathyroid cells possess recognition sites (receptors) for Ca^{2+}, as incubation of parathyroid slices in a low concentration of Ca^{2+} increases PTH release, and high

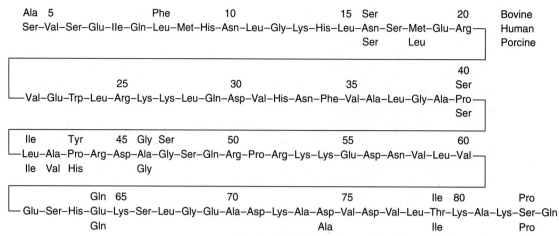

Figure 9.2 Comparative structures of parathormone.

concentrations of the cation decreases PTH release. The Ca^{2+}-sensing receptor has recently been cloned from bovine parathyroid glands (see Fig. 9.13) [4]. Theophylline stimulates PTH release as does $(Bu)_2$ cAMP, thus suggesting that cAMP is involved in the mechanism of PTH release. As discussed later, vitamin D is inhibitory to PTH secretion; its action is on PTH gene expression since short-term incubations with the hormone have no effect on PTH release [49].

Physiological Roles

Parathormone acts on a number of tissues, in most cases elevating, directly or indirectly, plasma levels of Ca^{2+} and decreasing circulating concentrations of PO_4^{-3}.

Bone Mineral Metabolism. A major target tissue of PTH is bone, specifically stromal osteoblast cells of the bone marrow. In response to PTH these cells secrete one or more cytokines (growth regulatory factors) that then stimulate osteoclastic activity leading to the resorption of bone. In this way demineralization of bone results in elevated levels of Ca^{2+}. More specific details of PTH action on bone will be discussed later (see Fig. 9.12).

Renal Reabsorption of Calcium. A major physiological role of PTH is to increase renal tubular reabsorption of Ca^{2+}. Parathyroidectomy, for example, leads to calciuria, which can be corrected immediately by injections of PTH.

Renal Excretion of Phosphate. Parathyroidectomy leads to a decrease in urinary phosphate levels and elevated serum PO_4^{-3} levels (phosphatemia). Injections of PTH, on the other hand, cause a rapid increase in urinary PO_4^{-3} concentration (phosphaturia). Increased renal excretion of PO_4^{-3}, in response to PTH (phosphaturic action of PTH), enhances the ionization of plasma Ca^{2+} through a lowering of the $[Ca^{2+}] \times [PO_4^{-3}]$ solubility product. Other renal effects of PTH include enhanced Mg^{2+} reabsorption and inhibition of exchange of hydrogen ions for Na^+ ions by the tubules. The resulting metabolic acidosis favors removal of Ca^{2+} from plasma proteins and bone, thereby increasing circulating levels of Ca^{2+}.

Intestinal Absorption of Calcium. Parathormone enhances intestinal uptake of Ca^{2+}, but this action may be mediated indirectly through its effect on vitamin D metabolism.

Control of Vitamin D Synthesis. A major role of PTH in Ca^{2+} homeostasis is to stimulate the biosynthesis of 1,25-dihydroxyvitamin D_3 from vitamin D precursors by the kidney. Thus, some of the actions of PTH are mediated indirectly through the action of this steroid hormone.

Other Possible Actions of PTH.   Parathormone increases the mitosis rate of red cell progenitors (reticulocytes) and thymic lymphocytes. Mitotic activity is also increased in regenerating rat liver following partial hepatectomy in response to PTH. The physiological significance, if any, of these observations on the mitogenic actions of PTH is unknown. PTH and related fragments produce vasodilation in coronary and other vascular beds in the dog. The blood-pressure lowering effect of bPTH is not blocked by α- or β-adrenergic, cholinergic, or histaminergic blocking agents, thus suggesting direct effects of the peptide on vascular smooth muscle receptors. This vasodepressor response has been demonstrated in a variety of species.

PARATHORMONE RELATED PEPTIDE (PTHrP)

PTH-related peptide (PTHrP) originally was isolated from human tumor cells or tissues obtained from patients with humoral hypercalcemia of malignancy. PTHrP consists of 139–173 residues, depending upon the species [5, 27]. Both the PTH-like and the non-PTH-like regions of the peptide are highly conserved across species. PTHrP shows a high degree of N-terminal homology with PTH (Fig. 9.3) and appears to interact with the same receptor as PTH in renal and osseous tissues, thereby accounting for its hypercalcemic activity in certain cancer patients. Unique biological actions also have been attributed to peptide sequences in the midportion and C-terminal region of the molecule. Unlike PTH, PTHrP and its mRNA have been detected in a wide variety of normal tissues, prompting considerable interest in potential physiological roles for the peptide. Although no physiological roles have been established unequivocally, the widespread expression of the PTHrP gene and its organizational similarity to that of certain growth factor genes have led to the suggestion that PTHrP may play a paracrine or autocrine role in growth and development.

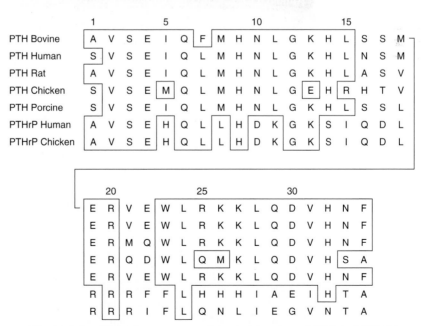

Figure 9.3   Aligned sequences of the 1–34 region of PTH and PTHrP from various species. Conserved human residues are outlined in black. Note the lack of substantial sequence identity between PTH and PTHrP from amino acid residue 14 through the C-terminus. (From Cohen et al., *Journal of Biological Chemistry* 266:1997–2004.)

Both developmental and Ca^{2+} regulatory roles have been suggested as important possibilities in the developing fetus [10, 38].

The lactating rat mammary gland has been shown to contain high levels of PTHrP mRNA that decrease rapidly when suckling is interrupted by removal of pups and reappear within 2 hours of the resumption of suckling or PRL injection. In addition, large quantities of PTHrP or fragments of PTHrP have been found in the milk of a number of species and in the blood of suckling calves. Other recent studies have indicated that mammary gland-derived PTHrP may reach the maternal circulation and influence Ca^{2+} homeostasis in the mother [43]. These findings have aroused considerable interest in the idea that PTHrP might play some role in development of the lactating breast, milk Ca^{2+} transport, maternal or fetal Ca^{2+} homeostasis, or neonatal gut function. PTHrP may play a role in modulating the delivery of milk to the nipple during suckling, and myoepithelial cell-derived PTHrP could contribute to the large pool of PTHrP found in milk. Alternatively, myoepithelial cell-derived PTHrP could act on neighboring secretory epithelial cells in a paracrine fashion to alter growth and differentiation, or affect milk formation [38, 43].

Other roles for PTHrP are now being discovered [10]. For example, there is evidence that the elevated levels of fetal serum Ca^{2+} are due to PTHrP of fetal parathyroid origin. It has been proposed that PTHrP is expressed by fetal tissue during pregnancy for maintenance of the Ca^{2+} gradient across the placenta, which is required for normal skeletal development. In studies with sheep, thyroparathyroidectomy of fetuses in utero results in substantial fetal hypocalcemia. However, serum Ca^{2+} levels were returned to normal upon infusion of a partially purified preparation obtained from cell-culture medium containing PTHrP. PTH infusion was ineffective, suggesting a unique role for PTHrP in fetal physiology [25, 27].

(margin handwritten note: lactating breasts after pregnancy)

CALCITONIN

Although Ca^{2+} is directly inhibitory to PTH release from the parathyroids, this is not the only means of protecting an animal against the elevated Ca^{2+} levels that occur, for example, after a meal. If plasma Ca^{2+} levels are elevated by injecting Ca^{2+} salts, Ca^{2+} concentrations rapidly return to normal. Infusion of a Ca^{2+} chelator, on the other hand, effectively lowers Ca^{2+} levels, which soon return to normal after cessation of the infusion. It was discovered, however, that depressed or elevated Ca^{2+} levels fail to return to normal in thyroidectomized animals. This failure could be partly explained by the absence of PTH, due to the removal of the parathyroids along with the thyroid glands. The solution, however, was not so simple. It was concluded that the thyroid might also produce a hormone whose role is to lower Ca^{2+} levels under conditions where the cation is elevated. Although this hypocalcemic factor, referred to as calcitonin (CT), was initially believed to be derived from the parathyroids, other experimental evidence pointed toward the thyroid [28].

The Parafollicular Cells

The thyroid gland is mainly composed of follicular cells (see Fig. 13.2), which synthesize and store thyroid hormones (Chap. 13). Another cell nestled among the follicular cells of the thyroid is referred to as a C (clear) cell. Immunohistochemical staining techniques reveal that these C cells synthesize and secrete CT. In mammals, including humans, these cells are derived from the ultimobranchial bodies that develop from the most posterior branchial pouch. Cells of the neural crest migrate to the posterior branchial pouch to form the *ultimobranchial glands* early in development. In nonmammalian vertebrates (cartilaginous and bony fishes, amphibians, reptiles, birds) the ultimobranchial glands persist and are the source of CT in the adult animal. In the human fetus the appearance of func-

```
        ┌─S──────────────S─┐
Cys–Gly–Asn–Leu–Ser–Thr–Cys–Met–Leu–Gly–Thr–Tyr–Thr–Gln–Asp–Phe–Asn–
 1    2    3    4    5    6    7    8    9   10   11   12   13   14   15   16   17

      Lys–Phe–His–Thr–Phe–Pro–Gln–Thr–Ala–Ile–Gly–Val–Gly–Ala–Pro–NH₂
       18   19   20   21   22   23   24   25   26   27   28   29   30   31   32
```

Figure 9.4 Primary structure of human calcitonin.

tional activity of parafollicular cells at the onset of skeletal calcification suggests a role for CT in fetal bone growth.

Synthesis, Chemistry, and Metabolism

Calcitonin was purified in 1967 and its amino acid sequence determined in 1968 [7]. Human CT (Fig. 9.4) was isolated from medullary carcinoma of the thyroid and found to be structurally similar to circulating CT. The primary sequence of CT has been determined from a number of species and the peptides are structurally similar (Fig. 9.5). All contain 32 residues, have a 1–7 intrachain disulfide ring, and have a prolinamide carboxyterminal group. As are many peptide hormones, CT is derived from a larger precursor molecule. Analysis of CT from four separate species of salmon reveals that each species produces two forms of the molecule, a salmon I plus a salmon II or salmon III variant of the molecule. These molecular varieties of CT represent *isohormonal* forms of the hormone; that is, the primary structure of these forms varies slightly from one to another. Human and salmon CT share only 16 of 32 amino acids in common. Surprisingly, eel and salmon CT are more potent in mammalian species (particularly well-tested in humans) than are the corresponding human and other mammalian calcitonins. This potency may be due to resistance of the peptides to degradation and may also have to do with greater receptor affinity [34].

A second peptide also related to CT has been discovered. This *calcitonin gene-related peptide* (CGRP) is mainly found in the nervous system. The homology between CGRP and CT reflects their common origin [23]. Human CGRP shares a greater structural homology with salmon than with human CT. Human CT and CGRP exert their actions on separate receptors that are distributed differently throughout the body.

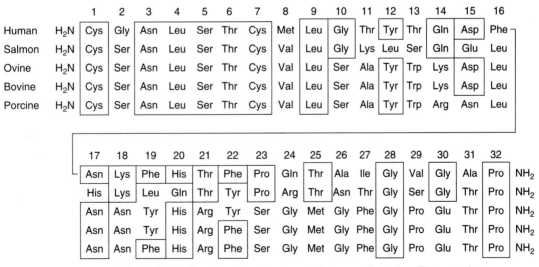

Figure 9.5 Comparative structures of some calcitonins. Three molecular species (isoforms) of salmon CT exist; the structure of salmon I calcitonin is shown, which differs from eel CT at only three residues (eel: 26, Asp; 27, Val; 29, Ala).

Control of Secretion

Perfusion of hypercalcemic blood through the thyroid is a stimulus to CT secretion, and incubation of thyroid tissue in a hypercalcemic medium also results in secretion of the hormone. Is there evidence that elevated levels of Ca^{2+} are also a stimulus to CT secretion in humans? Changes in plasma Ca^{2+} (caused by oral ingestion of Ca^{2+}) within the physiological range are indeed associated with parallel changes in circulating levels of CT in humans. The increase in CT release in response to Ca^{2+} infusion is greater in males than in females, and the basal levels of CT and the response to Ca^{2+} wane with age in both sexes [9]. Animal studies indicate that estrogens and androgens enhance CT secretion, and the progressive decreases in gonadal function may therefore contribute to the age- and sex-related changes in CT secretion in humans [9].

If a very small amount of Ca^{2+} is delivered to the stomach (of the pig) so as not to produce a detectable hypercalcemia, plasma CT still increases severalfold. It was hypothesized that some GI factor in addition to Ca^{2+} might be a CT secretogogue. Gastrin is a potent stimulator of CT secretion, and analogs of gastrin (Chap. 10) exhibit a potency profile similar to their effectiveness in stimulating gastric acid secretion. Cholecystokinin is also effective, due most likely to its partial structural similarity to gastrin. Physiological stimuli that increase gastrin levels in the blood cause a parallel increase in CT secretion. In some patients with Zollinger-Ellison syndrome (hypergastrinemia), there is an elevation in circulating CT.

Because it is composed almost entirely of CT-secreting cells, the ultimobranchial gland of nonmammalian vertebrates is a rich source of CT. Isolated cells from the fish ultimobranchial gland have been used in vitro for studies on CT secretion. Secretin, glucagon, and pentagastrin are stimulatory to CT secretion and, in combination, secretin and pentagastrin or secretion and glucagon have a synergistic effect on CT secretion from isolated teleost ultimobranchial cells. cAMP is the second messenger controlling CT secretion.

Physiological Roles

Bone Mineral Metabolism. Because CT is released from the parafollicular cells in direct relation to the circulating level of Ca^{2+}, it has been suggested that CT functions in the prevention of hypercalcemia [42]. In particular, CT may prevent the postprandial hypercalcemia that results from the absorption of Ca^{2+} from foods during a meal. Calcitonin might also promote mineralization of skeletal bone via Ca^{2+} absorbed from milk in preweanling animals. In addition, CT may protect against Ca^{2+} loss from the skeleton during such periods of Ca^{2+} stress as pregnancy, lactation, and prolonged Ca^{2+} deprivation.

The CT secreted in response to food entering the digestive tract causes the movement of serum Ca^{2+} into the bone mineral compartment. This labile Ca^{2+} then returns to the extracellular compartment as postprandial plasma Ca^{2+} levels decline. By this process Ca^{2+} levels are maintained during periods of fasting. The return of Ca^{2+} to the extracellular fluid would be inhibitory to PTH release, and this might be an effective safeguard against bone resorptive activity during fasting. High circulating levels of CT have been observed during gestation and lactation. At least in ruminants (goats and ewes), CT may protect the maternal skeleton against excessive demineralization.

Calcitonin as a Satiety Hormone. Subcutaneous injections of CT inhibit the 24 hour food intake of rats and rhesus monkeys. Intracerebroventricular injections of CT in the rat are also inhibitory to feeding. In humans, significant reduction in body weight is observed 24 to 36 hours following a single subcutaneous injection of CT. These results suggest that CT may have a physiologically relevant action on the CNS (Chap. 21). It is speculated that CT is involved in the regulation of feeding and appetite, possibly under specialized circumstances such as infancy, lactation, or Ca^{2+}-specific hunger.

Vitamin D Regulation.   Calcitonin directly stimulates vitamin D metabolism and indirectly stimulates it by lowering plasma Ca^{2+} levels, resulting in the release of PTH that activates renal vitamin D synthesis and secretion.

VITAMIN D

Historically, vitamin D is the name applied to two fat-soluble substances, cholecalciferol and ergocalciferol that possess the common ability to prevent or cure rickets. Rickets (osteomalacia in adults) develops from a failure of the bones to ossify properly in the child, and it was originally believed that the disease was due to a lack of sunshine or to some dietary factor. There is some truth in both these early theories. Vitamins are defined as organic dietary constituents necessary for life and development, but that do not act as dietary energy sources. In that respect it has been argued that the term vitamin D is a misnomer because normally the active hormonal form of vitamin D is produced within the body from dietary substrates or endogenous substances [24]. It is now accepted that vitamin D is not a vitamin but rather a precursor of one or more steroidlike hormones produced by specific tissues within the body. These vitamin D metabolites mediate their actions on a number of target tissues, and in the absence of the hormones bones fail to mineralize.

Source, Synthesis, Chemistry, and Metabolism

In 1924 it was discovered that, in animals, prior irradiation of certain dietary foodstuffs was as effective in curing rickets as direct irradiation of the animal itself. Vitamin D_3 (cholecalciferol) is actually produced in the skin of humans by the action of ultraviolet light on a precursor molecule, 7-dehydrocholesterol (an intermediate in the biosynthesis of cholesterol). Actually 7-dehydrocholesterol is first converted to a so-called pre-vitamin D_3, which subsequently equilibrates in the skin to form cholecalciferol through a temperature-dependent thermal isomerization (Fig. 9.6). From the skin, cholecalciferol is transported by a binding protein (transcalciferin) present in the general circulation. Under continuous exposure to the sun, previtamin D_3 also photoisomerizes to lumisterol and

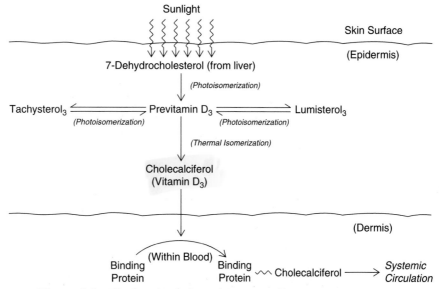

Figure 9.6 Photic stimulation of integumental cholecalciferol (vitamin D_3) formation and subsequent transfer to the general circulation by a cholecalciferol-binding protein.

tachysterol, which are biologically inert. Because transcalciferin has no strong affinity for these isomers, they are not translocated into the circulation but instead remain in the skin. Within the skin these photoisomers are in a quasi-stationary state and may serve as reserve substrates for photoconversion back to previtamin D_3 when the latter substance is converted to vitamin D_3 [17].

Rickets, a vitamin D–deficiency disease, may therefore develop if the skin does not receive adequate irradiation. The disease is now a rarity in most countries because irradiated foods provide an adequate supply of the vitamin. Ergosterol is a provitamin for vitamin D_2 (ergocalciferol), and both differ from 7-dehydrocholesterol and vitamin D_3, respectively, because they possess a double bond between C22 and C23 and a methyl group at the C24 position. Vitamin D_2 is the antirachitic principle of irradiated foodstuffs. Although vitamin D_3 is the normal physiologically relevant antirachitic substrate, vitamin D_2 is equally effective as vitamin D_3 in some species, including humans.

Actually, cholecalciferol is without biological activity at physiological concentrations. Cholecalciferol must first be converted to 25-hydroxyvitamin D_3 (25-OH-D_3, 25-hydroxycholecalciferol) in the liver (Fig. 9.7). The liver appears to be the major site of 25-hydroxylation in mammals. In the chicken, however, the 25-hydroxylase enzyme exists in extrahepatic sites such as the intestine and kidney. Although this steroid is the major circulating metabolite of cholecalciferol, it must undergo one other chemical modification before it can function as a hormone. The 25-OH-D_3 produced in the liver then circulates to the kidney where it is converted by a mitochondrial 1α-hydroxylase to $1\alpha,25$-$(OH)_2D_3$ ($1\alpha,25$-dihydroxycholecalciferol), the hormonal form of cholecalciferol [31]. The exclusive synthesis in the kidney of $1,25$-$(OH)_2D_3$ was demonstrated by the failure of nephrectomized rats given radioactive 25-OH-D_3 to produce radiolabeled $1,25$-$(OH)_2D_3$. Nephrectomized animals do not show physiological responses to 25-OH-D_3, whereas physiological responses on gut and bone, whether the kidneys are present or not, are produced by $1,25$-$(OH)_2D_3$. Chick kidney homogenates, as well as isolated renal mitochondria, convert 25-OH-D_3 to the active hormone. The $1,25$-$(OH)_2D_3$ product was originally detected in chick intestinal chromatin, one of its now recognized sites of action. $1,25$-$(OH)_2D_3$ functions as a hormone in the classical sense because it must be carried by the blood from its site of synthesis to its target cells. Cholecalciferol and its hydroxylated metabolite, 25-OH-D_3, and other hydroxylated metabolites are bound to a plasma protein, originally referred to in the human as transcalciferin or calciferol-binding protein. Although $1\alpha,25$-$(OH)_2D_3$ ($1,25$-$(OH)_2D_3$, for brevity) is the active antirachitic principle, the literature often refers to this hormone simply as vitamin D, or, more recently, as calcitriol.

Another enzyme present in kidney mitochondria and possibly other extrarenal sites, 25-hydroxyvitamin D_3-24 hydroxylase, produces $24,25$-$(OH)_2D_3$ (Fig. 9.6), which is inactive biologically in mammals. A trihydroxylated derivative of vitamin D_3, $1,24,25$-trihydroxyvitamin D_3 ($1,24,25$-$(OH)_3D_3$), has also been isolated from the plasma, but it too is biologically inactive (Fig. 9.7). 25,26-Dihydroxyvitamin D_3 has also been isolated from the blood of humans and some animals receiving pharmacological doses of cholecalciferol. The origin and possible significance of this metabolite is unknown, and the physiological importance, if any, of the other cholecalciferol metabolites is also unclear. Pregnant anephric female rats synthesize $1,25$-$(OH)_2D_3$, and conversion of 25-OH-D_3 to $1,25$-$(OH)_2D_3$ apparently takes place in the fetal placental unit of the rat. The physiological significance, if any, of the placental synthesis of $1,25$-$(OH)_3D_3$ is unknown.

Regulation of Vitamin D Metabolism

If a kidney 1α-hydroxylase is the key enzyme in $1,25$-$(OH)_2D_3$ biosynthesis, it might be expected to be tightly regulated by endocrine or other factors released under conditions of hypocalcemia. Indeed, the production of $1,25$-$(OH)_2D_3$ is markedly stimulated in animals on low Ca^{2+} diets and is suppressed in animals given high Ca^{2+} diets. Thus, there is a strict

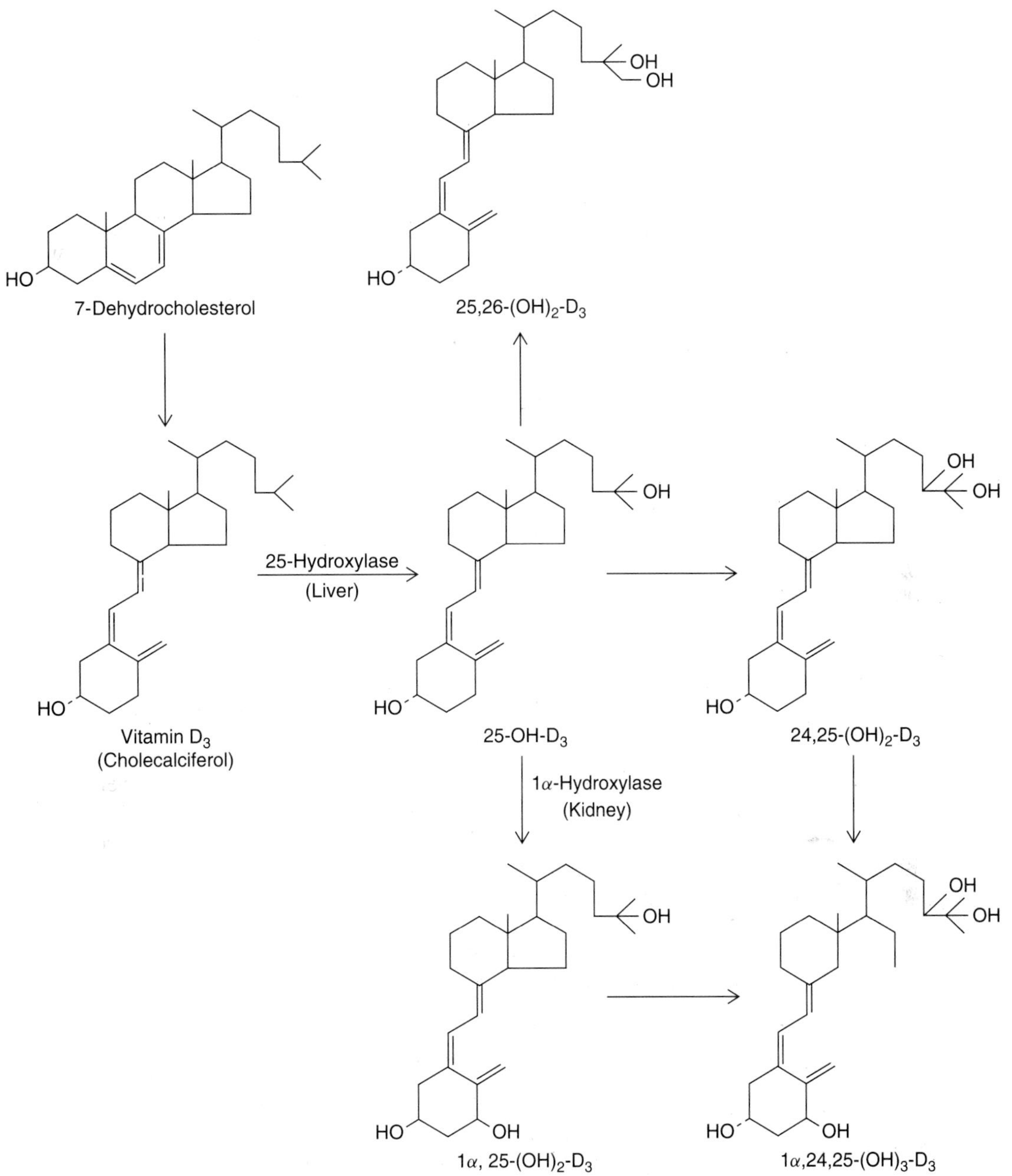

Figure 9.7   Sequential steps in the biosynthesis of vitamin D.

inverse relationship between the serum Ca^{2+} level and the ability of animals to produce $1,25\text{-}(OH)_2D_3$. Conversely, whenever $1,25\text{-}(OH)_2D_3$ synthesis is suppressed, $24,25\text{-}(OH)_2D_3$ synthesis is stimulated. There is no evidence, however, that hepatic 25-OHase activity is regulated by a feedback control mechanism. Removal of the parathyroid glands eliminates the hypocalcemic stimulation of $1,25\text{-}(OH)_2D_3$ production, and $24,25\text{-}(OH)_2D_3$ is produced. Conversely, PTH restores the ability of hypocalcemic animals to make $1,25\text{-}(OH)_2D_3$ and suppresses the production of $24,25\text{-}(OH)_2D_3$. In vitamin D-deficient animals there is an increase in renal 1α-OHase activity, whereas administration of vitamin D causes a dramatic disappearance of this enzyme. A direct effect of PTH on renal tubular production of 1,25-$(OH)_2D_3$ has been demonstrated. Suppression of renal 1α-OHase activity is correlated with increased 24-OHase activity. PTH alters 25-OH-D_3 metabolism through a cAMP-mediated mechanism. The metabolic tendency of the kidney to produce primarily $1,25\text{-}(OH)_2D_3$ or

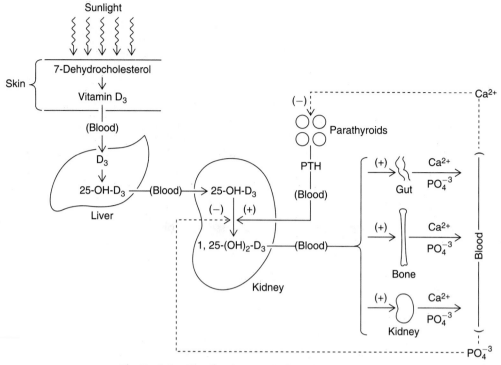

Figure 9.8   Feedback control of vitamin D biosynthesis.

$24,25\text{-}(OH)_2D_3$ is subject to dynamic modulation by the opposing effects of $1,25\text{-}(OH)_2D_3$ and PTH either directly or indirectly.

The feedback mechanism regulating $1,25\text{-}(OH)_2D_3$ production can be summarized as follows (see also Fig. 9.8): Hypocalcemia is stimulatory to PTH secretion from the parathyroids; PTH stimulates renal cortical $1\alpha\text{-OHase}$ activity and $1,25\text{-}(OH)_2D_3$ biosynthesis; $1,25\text{-}(OH)_2D_3$ then stimulates Ca^{2+} absorption from the gut, increases release of Ca^{2+} from the bone, and stimulates Ca^{2+} reabsorption from the kidney. The increasing levels of Ca^{2+} then feed back to inhibit further synthesis of PTH. In the absence of further stimulation of $1\alpha\text{-OHase}$ production, 24-OHase activity is increased and any available $25\text{-}(OH)_2D_3$ is converted to the inactive metabolite, $24,25\text{-}(OH)_2D_3$ (Fig. 9.7). Parathyroid gland cells possess $1,25\text{-}(OH)_2D_3$ receptors, and there is evidence that $1,25\text{-}(OH)_2D_3$ may exert a negative feedback on this gland to inhibit PTH production.

Besides its effect on renal $1,25\text{-}(OH)_2D_3$ production, PTH stimulates renal excretion of phosphate. Low plasma levels of PO_4^{-3} are directly stimulatory to renal $1\alpha\text{-OHase}$ activity and $1,25\text{-}(OH)_2D_3$ production, whereas elevated levels of PO_4^{-3} are inhibitory to production of the hormone. Thyroparathyroidectomized rats maintained on a low phosphate, high Ca^{2+} diet also synthesize $1,25\text{-}(OH)_2D_3$ from 25-OH-D_3. The plasma concentration of PO_4^{-3} may therefore be an important local regulator of renal $1,25\text{-}(OH)_2D_3$ biosynthesis. Although the synthesis of $1,25\text{-}(OH)_2D_3$ can be stimulated directly by low plasma PO_4^{-3} concentration, this hypophosphatemia does not stimulate PTH secretion. Without stimulation by PTH, resorption of Ca^{2+} from bone, renal reabsorption of Ca^{2+}, and renal excretion of PO_4^{-3} is minimal. The net change is predominantly an increase in plasma PO_4^{-3} concentration [21].

Physiological Roles

Intestine. Ca^{2+} absorption from the intestine is the best-documented action of vitamin D. The hormone also causes translocation of PO_4^{-3} across the gut epithelium. Both processes require metabolic energy and are therefore active transport processes.

1,25-$(OH)_2D_3$ stimulates transepithelial Ca^{2+} transport in the intestine by stimulating: Ca^{2+} entry, Ca^{2+} buffering by fixed cellular sites, and Ca^{2+} extrusion at the basolateral pole of the cell. Each of these steps is important, but the major effect of 1,25-$(OH)_2D_3$ is to facilitate intracellular diffusion from mucosa to serosa via a cytosolic Ca^{2+}-binding protein.

Bone.   In the absence of sunlight or a dietary source of vitamin D precursors, rickets (bone demineralization) develops. Although vitamin D is necessary for proper bone growth, it seems a paradox that vitamin D also causes demineralization to provide Ca^{2+}, and possibly PO_4^{-3}, to maintain the critical plasma levels of these ions. The demineralization process may, however, be necessary to provide Ca^{2+} and PO_4^{-3} for accretion of new bone.

Kidney.   There is evidence to suggest that 1,25-$(OH)_2D_3$ stimulates tubular reabsorption of Ca^{2+} in the kidney. In addition, data support a direct role of the hormone on proximal tubular retention of PO_4^{-3}. Because PTH causes phosphaturia and 1,25-$(OH)_2D_3$ production, feedback inhibition of parathyroid PTH release by the steroid might favor PO_4^{-3} retention. A specific 1,25-$(OH)_2D_3$ receptor has been isolated from rat kidney cytosol. A renal Ca^{2+}-binding protein has also been demonstrated and may facilitate tubular uptake of Ca^{2+} by the kidney, as it does in the intestine.

Pregnancy.   A hypophysial factor, probably prolactin, causes a marked suppression of plasma transcalciferin levels. During chronic hyperprolactinemia (pregnancy and lactation) a similar decrease in this binding protein occurs. Androgens, on the other hand, elevate the plasma levels of this protein. It is interesting that PRL, which may regulate the production of transcalciferin, is also regulated in turn by 1,25-$(OH)_2D_3$.

Other Putative Roles.   A number of tissues possess specific 1,25-$(OH)_2D_3$ receptors: skin, mammary gland, placenta, avian shell gland, and such peptide-secreting endocrine tissues as the parathyroids, pituitary, pancreas, and even the brain. The parathyroid glands might be expected to represent a site for 1,25-$(OH)_2D_3$ feedback inhibition of parathormone secretion. Elevated serum levels of 1,25-$(OH)_2D_3$ are known to lead to a decrease in the release of PTH through two different mechanisms. A long feedback loop is established by means of increased serum concentrations of Ca^{2+}, which represent an inhibitory signal for the secretion and production of PTH. In a short feedback loop, 1,25-$(OH)_2D_3$ directly inhibits the synthesis of PTH through an interaction with the preproparathyroid hormone gene [49]. There is evidence that insulin is required for optimal 1,25-$(OH)_2D_3$ production, and PRL and STH also appear to stimulate production of the hormone. These endocrine glands may therefore represent additional sites for negative feedback inhibition by 1,25-$(OH)_2D_3$. Nuclear receptors for 1,25-$(OH)_2D_3$ are also present in cells of the pituitary's pars distalis, and it has been reported that the hormone may regulate PRL production.

The hormone is also known to play essential roles in more basic cellular responses, such as those involved in proliferation and differentiation. Examples include the differentiation and maturation of hematopoietic stem cells, myoblasts, and dermal keratinocytes. In addition, actions on mature B and T cells of the immune system clearly support a physiological role for 1,25-(OH)2D3 in immunoregulation. The hormone also appears to induce a family of catabolic enzymes in all target cells, which metabolize it through a discrete pathway to calcitroic acid. Evidence from autoradiographic studies with [³H]1,25-$(OH)_2D_3$ about its many sites of nuclear binding and multiple actions suggests that the traditional view of vitamin D and Ca^{2+} is too limited and requires modification. It has been proposed that the skin-derived hormone of sunshine, "soltriol" (1,25-$(OH)_2D_3$), is a somatotrophic activator and modulator that affects all vital systems. Regulation of Ca^{2+} homeostasis may be only one of its many actions [39, 40].

Although the role of 1,25-(OH)$_2$D$_3$ in mammals and birds is well documented, the role of the hormone or related metabolites in other vertebrates is less understood. Apparently, teleost fishes synthesize cholecalciferol without the aid of sunlight, and the livers of such animals are a well-known source of precursor metabolites for 1,25-(OH)$_2$D$_3$ production in humans. Frogs and other amphibians are reported to be susceptible to vitamin D deficiency. The availability of Ca^{2+} and PO$_4^{-3}$ in aquatic environments could eliminate the need for vitamin D in some aquatic vertebrates.

HORMONE MECHANISMS OF ACTION IN CALCIUM HOMEOSTASIS

The mechanisms of action of the calcitropic hormones are being very precisely delineated, thus providing a clearer understanding of the molecular basis of disease states related to Ca^{2+} homeostasis.

Parathormone

Because the renal cortex is a major site of PTH action, this tissue has provided the main source of information on the action mechanism of PTH. [^{3}H]-labeled PTH is localized preferentially to the proximal tubule cells of the kidney cortex. Renal cortical membranes bind PTH and respond by increasing the production of cAMP. Human PTH$^{1-34}$ is a full agonist in that it can produce a maximal effect, but has approximately 1/10 the potency of the parent molecule (hPTH 1–84). Deletion of the two amino-terminal residues completely abolishes the activity of PTH, thus demonstrating the importance of the N-terminus for biological activity of the hormone. The mechanism of action of PTH is unique in that interaction of PTH with its receptor results in activation of two different transduction pathways, one leading to cAMP formation and one to IP$_3$/DG production. Different G proteins are involved in these separate pathways (Fig. 9.9).

PTH depends to a remarkable degree on vitamin D for mobilization of Ca^{2+} from bone in vivo. In rats on a vitamin D-deficient, low Ca^{2+} diet, serum Ca^{2+} levels drop to

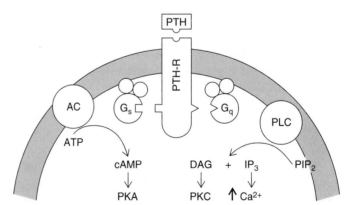

Figure 9.9 Cell surface receptors for PTH are coupled to two classes of G proteins. G$_s$ mediates stimulation of adenylyl cyclase (AC) and the production of cAMP, which in turn activates protein kinase A (PKA). G$_q$ stimulates phospholipase C (PLC) to form the second messengers inositol-(1,4,5)-triphosphate (IP$_3$) and diacylglycerol (DAG) from membrane-bound phosphatidyl-inositol-(4,5)-biphosphate. IP$_3$ increases intracellular calcium (Ca^{2+}) and DAG stimulates protein kinase C (PKC) activity. Each G-protein consists of a unique α chain and a $\beta\gamma$ dimer. (Reprinted by permission of the publisher from W. F. Schwindinger and M. A. Levine, "Albright hereditary osteodystrophy," *The Endocrinologist* 4:17–26. 1994. ©1994 The Endocrine Society.)

very low values in spite of secondary hyperparathyroidism, and there is no histological evidence of enhanced bone resorption. It appears, therefore, that PTH and vitamin D act in concert to effect mobilization of bone mineral. PTH stimulates adenylate cyclase activity in particulate bone cell fractions from vitamin D-deficient and normal rats. The data suggest that the cause of skeletal refractoriness to PTH in vitamin D-deficient animals is not a defective activation of adenylate cyclase. Most likely the vitamin D requirement for PTH action is related to later steps in the biochemical events leading to bone cell activation. In addition, vitamin D may be necessary for recruitment of new (additional) osteoblasts (see Fig. 9.12). Vitamin D appears to be permissive to the actions of PTH, possibly by one or more mechanisms described for steroid hormone actions (see Fig. 4.12).

Calcitonin

The entire 32-amino-acid sequence of CT appears to be required for biological activity. Seven of the nine common residues of the salmon CTs are at the N-terminal end of the molecule and are probably intimately involved in biological activity. Cleavage of the 1—7 disulfide bond in the hormone causes considerable loss of biological activity. The C-terminal prolinamide is also essential for activity. When studied in the rat, piscine (salmon, eel) CTs show markedly enhanced biological activities compared to human and other mammalian CTs. The high biological effectiveness of salmon CT relative to that of mammals may be due to a longer half-life in vivo, due to resistance of the hormone to degradation by plasma or tissue enzymes.

Receptors for CT are present in skeletal tissue, kidney, and testicular Leydig cells. The affinities of several CT analogs for specific receptors in vitro parallel closely the biological activity of those analogs in vivo. Human CT has no greater relative potency when tested against receptors from human tissue than for receptors from rat tissues. Thus in contrast to the marked evolutionary changes in CT structure, there is no evidence suggesting phylogenetic modification in the nature of the CT receptor. CT receptor complementary DNA (cDNA) has been cloned. The receptor has high affinity for CT and is functionally coupled to adenylate cyclase activation. The receptor is homologous to the PTH/PTHrP receptor, suggesting these Ca^{2+} regulatory G protein-coupled receptors are evolutionarily related [22]. The CT receptor may be coupled to different G proteins, Gs, Gi, and possibly Gp (a G protein coupled to PKC) in a cell cycle-dependent fashion. Coupling of the CT receptor to one pathway leads to an opposite biological response from that induced by activation of the other receptor. The basis for cell cycle-regulated coupling of different G proteins to the CT receptor (or subtypes thereof) is unknown. It might be speculated that cell cycle-related changes in phosphorylating and dephosphorylating enzyme activities may affect the particular transduction pathway and the biological responses associated with activation of the receptors. Therefore CT may induce different biological responses in target cells, depending on their position in the cell cycle [6].

PTH-related Peptide

The cDNA encoding a 585-amino acid PTH/PTHrP receptor with seven potential membrane-spanning domains was cloned from a cDNA library. The expressed receptor binds PTH and PTHrP with equal affinity, and both ligands stimulate adenylate cyclase. Striking homology with the CT receptor and lack of homology with other G protein-linked receptors indicate that receptors for these Ca^{2+}-regulating hormones are related and represent a new family of peptide hormone receptors. The surprising structural similarity between the PTH/PTHrP receptor and the CT receptor suggests that these novel receptors may share functional features distinguishing them from other G protein-linked receptors [20]. This family of receptors also includes the rat secretin receptor, which is similar in sequence to both the CT and PTH/PTHrP receptors, with 30% and 42% identity, respectively [22].

Most surprising is the observation that stimulation of placental Ca^{2+} transport requires the 75–85 region of PTHrP and is unresponsive to PTH 1–84. The possibility exists that PTHrP possesses the potential for different biological actions depending on the molecular species present, which may be regulated by tissue-specific processing by target tissues [35]. The term *polyhormone* has been suggested to describe the plural potential of these peptides [25].

Vitamin D

As for steroid hormones, $1,25\text{-}(OH)_2D_3$ interacts with target-tissue nuclear receptors to activate transcriptional and translational processes [13, 14, 30]. In this regard the action of the hormone on the intestine has been well characterized, whereas the effects of $1,25\text{-}(OH)_2D_3$ on bone, kidney, and other tissues is less understood (Fig. 9.10). There is a lag period of some 2 hours before the effects of the hormone can be noted, suggesting that the induction of new proteins is a prerequisite for the actions of the hormone. One of these is a Ca^{2+}-binding (transport) protein (CaBP). This protein may enhance the movement of Ca^{2+} from the brush border into the cytoplasm. An early event in the action of $1,25\text{-}(OH)_2D_3$ in intestinal cells is a rapid, apparently nongenomic, activation of Ca^{2+}-channels (termed transcaltachia), which have recently been linked to PKC activity [46].

The sequence of the avian, rat, and human vitamin D receptor has been deduced from molecular cloning data, revealing that the receptor belongs to a family of related proteins, including several other steroid hormone receptors. The members of this family all have a ligand-binding domain at the carboxy terminus, a DNA-binding domain in the middle, and a less evolutionary conserved amino terminus that may have domains that help select among potentially responsive genes (Fig. 9.11). After binding to the specific ligand, these receptor proteins influence gene expression via association with specific DNA elements known as hormone-responsive elements (HREs). $1,25\text{-}(OH)_2D_3$ exerts its effects through a vitamin D-responsive element (VDRE [13, 14]).

The gene that produces osteocalcin, the major noncollagenous bone protein, is stimulated by vitamin D but inhibited by glucocorticoids. The DNA sequence of the vitamin D-response element, which is within the promoter gene for osteocalcin, was shown to be unresponsive to other steroid hormones. On the other hand, a DNA domain of this pro-

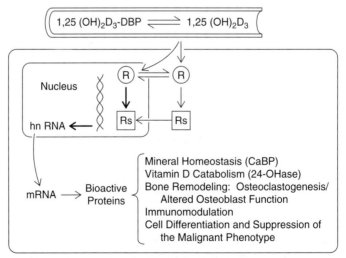

Figure 9.10 Mechanism of action and general functions of $1,25(OH)_2D_3$ in target cells. DBP is the serum vitamin D binding protein, R, unoccupied receptor, and Rs, hormone occupied receptor. (From Haussler et al., [14] with permission. ©1988, Alan R. Liss, Inc. Reprinted by permission of Wiley-Liss, a division of John Wiley and Sons.)

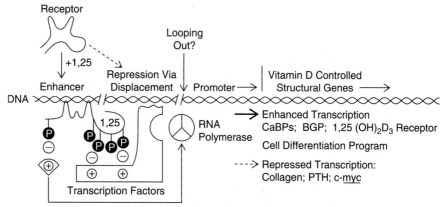

Figure 9.11 Proposed mechanism for 1,25(OH)$_2$D$_3$ receptor molecular action: enhancement of gene expression by transcriptosome formation or repression via displacement of transcription factors. The occupied 1,25(OH)$_2$D$_3$ receptor is postulated to bind to cis enhanced sequences where it becomes phosphorylated on serine residues (the positioning and number of phosphoserines are arbitrary). The resulting patches of negative charge on the receptor are proposed to interact with positive domains in transcription factors and facilitate their activation of RNA polymerase II. Looping out of DNA, which is pictured as a break in the double helix, could occur either between the receptor and the transcription complex, or between transcription factors and RNA polymerase, or both. 1,25(OH)$_2$D$_3$; P, phospho-groups on serine or threonine; CaBP, calcium-binding protein; BGP, bone gamma-carboxygultamic acid (Gla) containing protein; PTH, parathyroid hormone. (From Haussler et al. [13], with permission.)

moter, distinct from the element, controls the potent glucocorticoid repression of vitamin D's induction of osteocalcin. Thus the low circulating serum osteocalcin levels associated with glucocorticoid excess could be explained by a direct influence of the hormone on the osteocalcin gene promoter, resulting in antagonism of the gene [14].

Receptors for 1,25-(OH)$_2$D$_3$ are present in bone, and vitamin D causes a large (100-fold) increase in immunoreactive CaBP in chick bone. 1,25-(OH)$_2$D$_3$ stimulates alkaline phosphatase activity of osteoblastlike bone tumor cells in tissue culture. In view of the postulated role of the enzyme in calcification, these observations suggest a direct involvement of vitamin D in bone mineralization. There is also evidence that the action of vitamin D on the kidney may involve synthesis of a Ca^{2+}-binding protein; a vitamin D-dependent CaBP has been localized immunohistochemically in distal tubules of avian and mammalian kidneys. Autoradiographic studies with 1,25-(OH)$_2$D$_3$ also reveal that the hormone is preferentially localized to cells of the distal tubules.

HORMONE INTEGRATION IN CALCIUM HOMEOSTASIS

Isolated bone cell populations of osteoblasts and osteoclasts have been obtained and the effects of PTH, CT, and vitamin D on these cells studied. CT inhibits the actions of the two hormones on osteoclasts but not on osteoblasts. PTH, but not vitamin D, mediates its effects through cAMP production. Although vitamin D and PTH activate similar cellular processes, they do so through separate receptors, plasma membrane, and cytosolic, respectively. The actions of PTH and vitamin D elevate serum Ca^{2+} levels by enhancing the bone-resorbing activities of the osteoclasts, while inhibiting concomitantly the bone-building activities of the osteoblasts. CT mediates its serum Ca^{2+}-lowering effect by preferentially inhibiting osteoclastic (bone-resorbing) activity without disturbing the mineralization (bone-building) activity of osteoblasts. The fact that both PTH and CT increase cAMP production in bone has been explained by the PTH effect taking place in osteoblasts and the CT effect in osteoclasts.

The multinucleate osteoclast has long been recognized as the principal cell involved in bone resorption; its characteristic resorbing apparatus consists of a ruffled border. CT inhibits bone resorption by altering the morphology and activity of the osteoclast. CT-treated osteoclasts separate from bone surface, lose their ruffled borders, and demonstrate decreased release of lysosomal enzymes.

Strong evidence indicates that the osteoblast is the main target cell for PTH action, regulating indirectly, via cell-cell communication, osteoclastic bone resorption. Precursor cells, possibly of mesenchymal origin, give rise to cells that can differentiate under the influence of the vitamin D hormone ($1\alpha,25$-$(OH)_2D_3$) to a mature phenotype, the osteocyte, which synthesizes and secretes a number of matrix proteins, including collagen and osteocalcin. Some precursor cells follow another path of differentiation to become mature osteoblasts. Osteoclasts also derive from precursor cells, possibly from immature hematopoietic cells, which fuse to become multinucleate osteoclasts. Under the influence of either parathormone (PTH) or vitamin D hormone, or cytokines such as interleukin-1 (IL-1) and tumor necrosis factor (TNF), osteoblasts secrete one or more "osteoclast differentiation-inducing" factors such as interleukin-6 (IL-6). These cytokines stimulate osteoclastogenesis. They also stimulate osteoclasts to undergo morphological (shape) changes and to secrete hydrogen ions and acid proteases of lysosomal origin. Under these acidic conditions proteolysis of osteocyte matrix proteins takes place. This results in the release of Ca^{2+} and PO_4^{-3} to enter the general circulation. Calcitonin is inhibitory to osteoclastogenesis and osteoclastic activity and therefore prevents bone demineralization. Estrogens such as estradiol (E_2) are inhibitory to cytokine release by their actions on osteoblasts and possibly osteoclasts as well. E_2 is also inhibitory to the release of IL-1 and TNF from peripheral blood monocytes.

In the absence of estrogens, in postmenopausal women, the enhanced secretion of cytokines by osteoblasts and the resulting increased osteoclastic activity result in osteoporosis. Under other pathological states (e.g., Paget's disease) the actions of other cytokines, such as tumor necrosis factor (TNF) and interleukin-1 (IL-1), may also increase osteoclastic activity by their stimulation of osteoblasts. An even more complex cytokine circuitry than depicted here is undoubtedly involved in the reciprocal regulatory interactions between osteoblasts, osteoclasts, and osteocytes, (Fig. 9.12) [19, 29, 41].

PATHOPHYSIOLOGY

Decreased or increased production of PTH leads to hypocalcemic or hypercalcemic states, respectively. Because an important role of PTH is to enhance production of $1,25$-$(OH)_2D_3$, the etiology of either calcemic state is most directly related to decreased or increased levels of this steroid hormone. Calcium ions play a critical role in nerve and muscle excitability. Alterations in extracellular Ca^{2+} concentrations may therefore affect neural transmission and contractility of cardiac and skeletal muscle, thus leading to serious clinical problems.

Hypoparathyroidism

Hypoparathyroid patients display hypocalcemia as their major clinical symptom. This hypocalcemia is caused, in part, by a partial deficiency of $1,25$-$(OH)_2D_3$. The hyperphosphatemia resulting from PTH deficiency might also suppress $1,25$-$(OH)_2D_3$ production. Restoration of normocalcemia may be attained by treatment with $1,25$-$(OH)_2D_3$ or related metabolites. Tetany and convulsions are the most serious complications of the

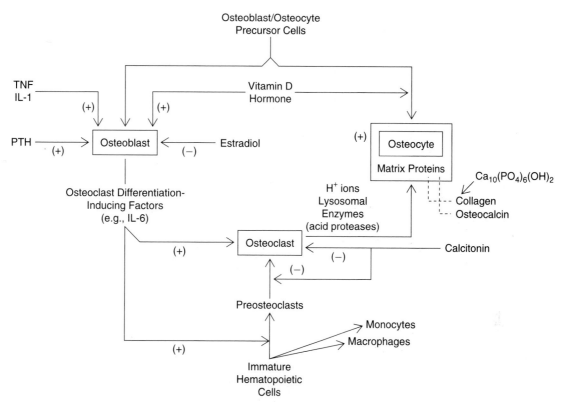

Figure 9.12 Generalized model of the role of hormones controlling bone mineralization and demineralization.

hypoparathyroid state. Latent tetany may be detected by tapping over the facial nerves, which results in a contraction of the facial muscles (Chvostek's sign), or by producing carpal (wrist) spasm (Trousseau's sign) following occlusion of arterial blood supply to the forearm, as often happens when applying a sphygmomanometer to the arm. In some disorders, although Ca^{2+} levels are depressed, suggestive of PTH deficiency, the levels of the hormone may actually be increased above normal. The defect responsible in one type of *pseudohypoparathyroidism* is related to a failure to generate cAMP. The pathology may be specifically related to a defect in a receptor-cyclase coupling protein necessary for transduction of signal between PTH receptor and adenylate cyclase.

Hyperparathyroidism

Patients with primary hyperparathyroidism have moderate to severe hypercalcemia and elevated plasma $1,25\text{-}(OH)_2D_3$ levels. The pathology of primary hyperparathyroidism may involve *neoplasia* or *hyperplasia*. Primary hyperparathyroidism usually results from a benign adenoma of one of the parathyroids. Hyperparathyroidism due to primary hyperplasia, on the other hand, involves overactivity of all the parathyroid glands usually due to an unknown (idiopathic) etiology. Secondary hyperparathyroidism often results from a peripheral defect of PTH action; the resulting hypocalcemia is the stimulus to enhanced parathyroid chief cell activity. Secondary hyperparathyroidism is a frequent consequence of chronic renal failure [12]. Retention of phosphate depresses serum Ca^{2+} levels, and reduced synthesis of $1,25\text{-}(OH)_2D_3$ by the kidney impairs intestinal Ca^{2+} absorption. Excessive levels of PTH are then secreted in response to lowered levels of Ca^{2+}.

The structure of the Ca^{2+}-sensing receptor has been cloned and biologically characterized (Fig. 9.13) [4]. Defects in this receptor that cause "familial hypocalciuric hypercalcemia and neonatal severe hyperparathyroidism" have now been described [33]. Defective Ca^{2+}-sensing receptors cause chief (PTH) cell hypertrophy and hyperplasia; the

neoplasia
hyperplasia

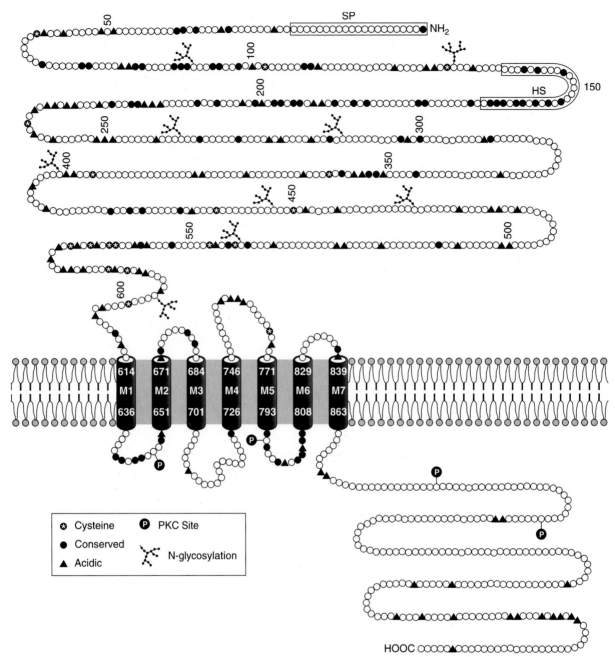

Figure 9.13 Proposed structural model for the predicted BoPCaR1 Ca²⁺-sensing receptor protein. The large N-terminal domain is located extracellularly and contains nine potential N-linked glycosylation sites (shown as branched chains). Amino acids are indicated at intervals of 50 in the N-terminal domain. Amino acid segments forming each of the seven putative membrane-spanning helices are numbered. Potential phosphorylation sites for PKC are shown. Symbols represent individual amino acids. The hydrophilic signal protein (SP) and hydrophobic A-segment (HS) are indicated. (With permission from Edward M. Brown et al., *Nature Lond.* 366:575–80, 1993.)

resulting hyperparathyroidism causes excessive bone resorption and elevated serum Ca²⁺ levels (hypercalcemia) and excessive renal tubular Ca²⁺ reabsorption causes decreased urinary Ca²⁺ concentrations (hypocalciuria).

Malignant Hypercalcemia

One mechanism considered responsible for the hypercalcemia that frequently accompanies malignancy is secretion of a circulating factor that alters Ca^{2+} metabolism by the tumor (see earlier discussion). The structure of a tumor-secreted peptide was recently determined and found to be partially homologous to PTH. The amino-terminal 1–34 region of the factor was synthesized and evaluated biologically. In vivo it produced hypercalcemia, acted on bone and kidney, and stimulated $1,25\text{-}(OH)_2D_3$ formation. In vitro it interacted with PTH receptors and, in some systems, was more potent than PTH. These observations support a long-standing hypothesis regarding pathogenesis of malignancy-associated hypercalcemia [18].

An immunometric assay that measures intact PTH is replacing the traditional RIA, because it provides for the differential diagnosis of hypercalcemic disorders [37]. These assays take advantage of saturation kinetics, rather than competitive binding [50], and use two affinity-purified antisera (or monoclonal antibodies), both of which can simultaneously bind to the ligand with little, if any, steric interference. One of the antisera also binds to a solid-phase matrix, and the other is labeled with radioiodine or with a chemiluminescent compound. Immunoradiometric and immunochemiluminometric assays for iPTH measure intact hormone by "capturing" iPTH with immobilized affinity-purified antisera by epitopes with PTH's middle and carboxyl-terminal sequence and reacting the serum iPTH with soluble, labeled, affinity-purified amino-terminal antisera. The concentration of hormone is determined by quantifying the amount of labeled amino-terminal antisera bound to the solid phase by gamma-counting or with a luminometer (Fig. 9.14 and Fig. 9.15) [37].

Osteomalacia

This disorder is characterized by a failure of normal mineralization of bone in the adult. (In children the disease is referred to as rickets.) This undermineralization of cartilage and bone results in retardation of growth and in development of characteristic skeletal deformities. Rickets and adult osteomalacia encompass a group of diseases that have similar skeletal defects but diverse causes. Osteomalacia is classified as vitamin D-responsive or vitamin D-resistant. The vitamin D-responsive disorders may be due to a deficiency in dietary intake of vitamin D precursors (vitamin D-deficiency rickets), inadequate exposure to sunlight, or intestinal malabsorption of Ca^{2+}. The vitamin D-resistant disorders result from diverse etiologies, such as familial or acquired renal-tubular phosphate wasting, defective collagen matrix formation, and specific hereditary defects in the metabolic transformation of vitamin D to its active form, probably due to failure of 1α-hydroxylation. Several unusual forms of vitamin D-resistant rickets have been described, which involve end-organ hyposensitivity (pseudovitamin D deficiency) to biologically active vitamin D [31]. Hypocalcemic vitamin D-resistant rickets is a human genetic disease resulting from target organ resistance to the action of $1,25\text{-}(OH)_2D_3$. Two families with affected children homozygous for this autosomal recessive disorder were studied for abnormalities in the intracellular vitamin D receptor (VDR) and its gene. Although the receptor displayed normal binding of $1,25\text{-}(OH)_2D_3$, VDR from affected family members had a decreased affinity for DNA. Genomic DNA isolated from these families was subjected to oligonucleotide-primed DNA amplification, and each of the exons encoding the receptor protein was sequenced for a genetic mutation. In each family, a different single nucleotide mutation was found in the DNA-binding domain of the protein [26] (Fig. 9.16).

Paget's Disease

This focal disorder, which is often familial and is fairly common in England and certain Northern European countries, is characterized by the presence of excessive numbers of osteoclasts, which leads to structurally weakened bone tissue [3]. Although susceptibility

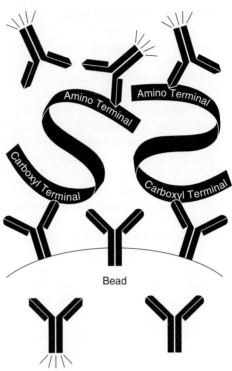

Figure 9.14 A schematic illustration of an immunoradiometric assay for iPTH. (Reprinted by permission of the publisher from "Advances in techniques for measurement of parathyroid hormone. Current applications in clinical medicine and directions for future research," Segre, *Trends in Endocrinology and Metabolism* 1:243–247, 1990. ©1990 by Elsevier Science Inc.)

to Paget's disease is believed to be transmitted by a simple autosomal Mendelian dominant gene, the etiology remains elusive. Osteoclasts from Pagetic bone may be enlarged and contain greatly increased numbers of nuclei. Viruslike inclusions have been noted in the nuclei of some Pagetic osteoclasts. Certain individuals may be born with the genetic susceptibility to osteoclastic invasion by a virus organism. The expression of the abnormality is, however, usually only manifested later in life. Calcitonin is a powerful pain suppressant, stimulating the secretion of the natural opiate, β-endorphin, and reducing the evoked potentials in central pain pathways. Because CT inhibits bone resorption and relieves pain, it is now widely used in the treatment of bone disease (e.g., Paget's disease). Worldwide sales of CT approach $1 billion a year, ranking it second only to insulin as a peptide used in clinical medicine [7].

Osteoporosis

This disease is manifested as a decrease in bone density, with demineralization being attributable to several possible etiologies [47].

Postmenopausal (Type I) Osteoporosis.   In the United States nearly 1.2 million women begin menopause each year. During her expected remaining lifetime of about 30 years, the average woman will lose approximately 30%–50% of her bone mass. After age 65, the incidence of spine and hip fractures rises almost exponentially [47].

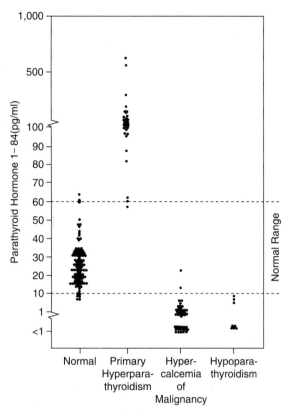

Figure 9.15 Intact iPTH measured by an immuno-radiometric assay in sera of normal subjects, and patients with hyperparathyroidism, hypercalcemia of malignancy, and hypoparathyroidism. (Reprinted by permission of the publisher from "Advances in techniques for measurement of parathyroid hormone. Current applications in clinical medicine and directions for future research," Segre, *Trends in Endocrinology and Metabolism* 1:243–247, 1990. ©1990 by Elsevier Science Inc.)

The pathogenesis of osteoporosis that occurs after menopause is related to a decrease in gonadal steroids (Chap. 19). Common sites of fracture among postmenopausal females are the vertebrae, forearm, and hip. The incidence of such fractures among males of similar age is much less, whereas in younger adults there is little difference in incidence between the sexes. On this basis the prevention of such fractures might be realized if estrogen treatment is continued after menopause. Virtually all the available evidence indicates that the use of estrogens lowers the risk of postmenopausal fractures, and therefore some women may benefit from long-term estrogen use (see also Chap. 19). Postmenopausal osteoporosis appears not to be associated with (or be) the result of CT deficiency [44]. CT alone or in combination with 1,25-$(OH)_2D_3$ is effective in enhancing the bone mineral content of postmenopausal and elderly osteoporotic patients [11]. Three years of 1,25-$(OH)_2D_3$ therapy in women with postmenopausal osteoporosis significantly reduced the incidence of new vertebral fractures, as compared with Ca^{2+} gluconate supplementation. When administered in a dose of 0.25 μg twice a day, 1,25-$(OH)_2D_3$ had no important side effects. The results suggest that 1,25-$(OH)_2D_3$ may be an important therapeutic option in the treatment of women with postmenopausal osteoporosis [45].

The role of estradiol in bone physiology and its relationship to postmenopausal osteoporosis is depicted in Fig. 9.12.

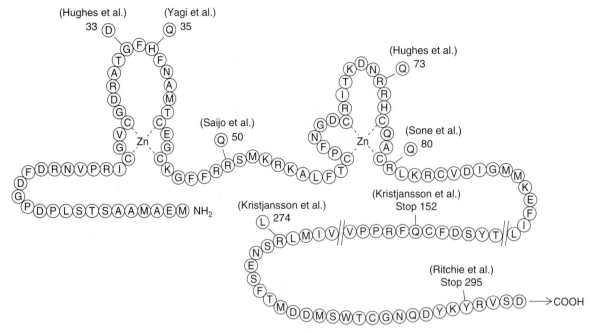

Figure 9.16 Natural mutations in the VDR from patients with hereditary hypothalamic vitamin-D-resistant rickets. The amino acid residues are indicated in the diagram by the single letter abbreviations: A, Ala; C, Cys; D, Asp; E, Glu; F, Phe; G, Gly; H, His; I, Ile; K, Lys; L, Leu; M, Met; N, Asn; P, Pro; Q, Gln; R, Arg; S, Ser; T, Thr; V, Val; W, Trp; and Y, Tyr. (From Macdonald, Dowd, and Huassler, "New insights into the structure and functions of the vitamin D receptor," in Seminars in Nephrology, 14:101–118, 1994. Used by permission.)

Senile (Type II) Osteoporosis.   In elderly people with osteoporosis there is not only reduced 1,25-$(OH)_2D_3$ secretion, but also PTH plasma levels are diminished. Whether these phenomena are specific characteristics of osteoporosis or are just endocrine changes common to all aging persons is unclear. Deficiency of vitamin D is uncommon in the general population of the North American continent because of the availability of sunlight, vitamin D-fortified milk, and over-the-counter preparations containing the vitamin. There are elderly individuals who are, however, at risk of developing a deficiency of the vitamin because of lack of exposure to sunlight and failure to ingest milk or vitamin supplements containing vitamin D. Vitamin D deficiency is a real risk in old age. It may be preceded by a period of active bone disease, which can be mistaken clinically for osteoporosis. If aging patients are to be maintained in an optimal state of health, "it is important to evaluate their exposure to sunlight and their vitamin D intake, and recommend vitamin D prophylaxis to patients at risk" [1].

Winter decreases 1,25-$(OH)_2D_3$ and increases PTH plasma levels; these changes are well documented. It has been postulated that these hormonal changes in the winter could have deleterious effects on the skeleton because 1,25-$(OH)_2D_3$ is required to maintain Ca^{2+} absorption, and PTH is a potent stimulator of bone resorption. Serum PTH and plasma 25-hydroxyvitamin D levels vary inversely with one another, and the concentration of each changes with the season in the temperate zone. There is indirect evidence that seasonal increases in PTH may affect bone mass adversely. Patients with hip fractures have been shown to have wintertime increases in PTH and lower levels of 1,25$(OH)_2D_3$ than controls. At latitude 42°, healthy postmenopausal women with vitamin D intake of 100 IU daily can significantly reduce late wintertime bone loss and improve net bone density of the spine over one year by increasing their intake of vitamin D to 500 IU daily [8].

Pharmacology

Pharmaceutical Preparations of Vitamin D. The oral administration of $1,25\text{-}(OH)_2D_3$, although effective in the treatment of some vitamin D-deficiency syndromes, may cause hypercalcemia due to the high transient local concentrations of the hormone in the serum. A novel alternative method of providing vitamin D to the patient may be through the topical application of $1,25\text{-}(OH)_2\text{-}7$-dehydrocholesterol, combined with phototherapy. Cutaneous generation of $1,25\text{-}(OH)_2D_3$ results (see Fig. 9.6), which may provide a more prolonged release and sustained stimulation of intestinal Ca^{2+} absorption [16, 17].

A number of plant species throughout the world cause severe calcinosis in domestic animals when ingested as part of their forage. A calcinogenic factor extracted from the leaves of *Solanum malacoxylon* has been found to be $1,25\text{-}(OH)_2D_3$ glycoside. After ingestion, endogenous glycosidases or intestinal microbes hydrolyze the glycoside to the hormonally active form. The reason for the existence of such a calcinogenic factor is unclear, but it and other related substances may function in mineral metabolism in plants [48]. The controlled administration of powdered leaves of *S. malacoxylon* has been used therapeutically in both humans and farm animals and improves eggshell quality when given to hens [2].

Dietary Calcium and Osteoporosis. It has been reported that, contrary to popular belief, Ca^{2+} intake in adulthood may have nothing to do with osteoporosis. Studies call into question the dietary recommendations of a 1984 National Institutes of Health consensus panel on osteoporosis, yet they are consistent with a large body of evidence indicating no relationship between Ca^{2+} intake and bone density within populations. A high Ca^{2+} intake can lead to kidney stones in susceptible people, and Ca^{2+} supplements may cut off vitamin D production, which is necessary for the cellular activation of bone cells (but see [36]).

REFERENCES

[1] Barzel, U. S. 1993. Vitamin D deficiency: A risk factor for osteomalacia in the aged. *J. Amer. Geriatrics Soc.* 35:598–601.

[2] Boland, R. L. 1986. Plants as a source of vitamin D_3 metabolites. *Nutr. Rev.* 44:1–8.

[3] Bone, H. G., and M. Kleerekoper. 1992. Clinical Review 39. Paget's disease of bone. *J. Clin. Endocrinol. Metab.* 75:1179–82.

[4] Brown, E. M., G. Gamba, D. Riccardi, M. Lombardi, R. Butters, O. Kifor, A. Sun, M. A. Hediger, J. Lytton, and S. C. Hebert. 1993. Cloning and characterization of an extracellular Ca^{2+}-sensing receptor from bovine parathyroid. *Nature Lond.* 366:575–80.

[5] Burtis, W. J. 1992. Parathyroid hormone-related protein: structure, function, and measurement. *Clin. Chem.* 38:2171–83.

[6] Chakraborty, M., D. Chatterjee, S. Kellokumpu, H. Rasmussen, and R. Baron. 1991. Cell cycle-dependent coupling of the calcitonin receptor to different G proteins. *Science* 251:1078–82.

[7] Copp, D. H. 1992. Remembrance: Calcitonin: discovery and early development. *Endocrinology* 131:1007–8.

[8] Dawson-Hughes, B., G. F. Dallal, E. A. Krall, S. Harris, L. J. Sokoll, and G. Falconer. 1991. Effect of vitamin D supplementation on wintertime and overall bone loss in healthy postmenopausal women. *Ann. Int. Med.* 115:505–12. [14]

[9] Deftos, L. J., M. H. Weisman, G. W. Williams, D. B. Karpe, A. M. Frumar, B. J. Davidson, J. G. Parthemore, and H. L. Judd. 1980. Influence of age and sex on plasma calcitonin in human beings. *New Engl. J. Med.* 302:1351–53.

[10] De Papp, A. E., and A. F. Stewart. 1993. Parathyroid hormone-related protein. A peptide of diverse physiologic functions. *TEM* 4:181–7.

[11] Ettinger, B. 1988. Estrogen replacement therapy symposium. *Obstet. Gynecol.* 72:15–5, 125–7, 315–6.

[12] Feinfeld, D. A., and L. M. Sherwood. 1988. Parathyroid hormone and $1,25(OH)_2D_3$ in chronic renal failure. *Kidney Int.* 33:1049–58.

[13] Haussler, M. R., D. J. Mangelsdorf, B. S. Komm, C. M. Terpening, K. Yamaoka, E. A. Allegretto, A. R. Baker, J. Shine, D. P. McDonnell, M. Hughes, N. L. Weigel, B. W. O'Malley, and J. W. Pike. 1988. Molecular biology of the vitamin D hormone. *Rec. Prog. Horm. Res.* 44:263–305.

[14] Haussler, M. R., D. J. Mangelsdorf, K. Yamaoka, E. A. Allegretto, B. S. Komm, C. M. Terpening, D. P. McDonnell, J. W. Pike, and B. W. O'Malley. 1988. Molecular characterization and actions of the vitamin D hormone receptor. *Steroid Horm. Action* 247–62.

[15] Hohmann, E. L., R. P. Elde, J. A. Rysavy, S. Einzig, and R. L. Gebhard. 1986. Innervation of periosteum and bone by sympathetic vasoactive intestinal peptide-containing nerve fibers. *Science* 232:868–71.

[16] Holick, M. F., J. A. MacLaughlin, and S. H. Doppelt. 1981. Regulation of cutaneous previtamin D_3 photosynthesis in man: skin pigment is not an essential regulator. *Science* 211:590–93.

[17] Holick, M. F., M. Uskokovic, J. W. Henley, J. MacLaughlin, S. A. Hollick, and J. T. Potts, Jr. 1980. The photoproduction of $1\alpha,25$-dihydroxyvitamin D_3 in the skin. *New Engl. J. Med.* 303:349–54.

[18] Horiuchi, N., M. P. Caulfield, J. E. Fisher, M. E. Goldman, R. L. McKee, J. E. Reagan, J. J. Levy, R. F. Nutt, S. B. Rodan, T. L. Schofield, T. L. Clemens, and M. Rosenblatt. 1987. Similarity of synthetic peptide from human tumor to parathyroid hormone in vivo and in vitro. *Science.* 238:1566–70.

[19] Horowitz, M. C. 1993. Cytokines and estrogen in bone: Anti-osteoporotic effects. *Science* 260:626–7.

[20] Juppner, H., A.-B. Abou-Samra, M. Freeman, X. F. Kong, E. Schipani, J. Rochards, L. F. Kolakowski, Jr., J. Hock, J. T. Potts, Jr., H. M. Kronenberg, and G. V. Segre. 1991. A G protein-linked receptor for parathyroid hormone and parathyroid hormone-related peptide. *Science* 254:1024–6.

[21] Klee, G. G., P. C. Kao, and H. Heath III. 1988. Hypercalcemia. *Endocrinol. Metab. Clinics N. Amer.* 17:573–600.

[22] Lin, H. Y., T. J. Harris, M. S. Flannery, A. Aruffo, E. H. Kaji, A. Gorn, L. F. Kolakowski, Jr., H. F. Lodish, and S. R. Goldring. 1991. Expression cloning of an adenylate cyclase-coupled calcitonin receptor. *Science* 254:1022–4.

[23] Lips, C. J. M., P. H. Steenbergh, J. W. M. Hoppener, R. A. L. Bovenberg, J. van der Sluys Veer, and H. S. Jansz. 1988. Evolutionary pathways of the calcitonin genes. *Mol. Cell. Endocrinol.* 57:1–6.

[24] Loomis, W. F. 1970. Rickets. *Sci. Amer.* 233:77–91.

[25] Mallette, L. W. 1991. The parathyroid polyhormones: new concepts in the spectrum of peptide hormone action. *Endocr. Rev.* 12:110–7.

[26] Marx, S. J., and J. Barsony. 1988. Tissue-selective 1,25-dihydroxyvitamin D_2 resistance: novel applications of calciferols. *Bone Miner.* 3:481–87.

[27] McKee, R. L. and M. P. Caulfield. 1989. Synthetic peptides as tools for investigating the pathogenicity of disease: humoral hypercalcemia of malignancy. *Peptide Res.* 2:161–6.

[28] Munson, P. L., and P. F. Hirsch. 1966. Thyrocalcitonin: newly recognized thyroid hormone concerned with metabolism of bone. *Clin. Orthoped.* 49:209–32.

[29] Oursler, M. J., J. P. Landers, B. L. Riggs, and T. C. Spelsberg. 1993. Oestrogen effects on osteoblasts and osteoclasts. *Ann. Med.* 25:362–71.

[30] Ozono, K., T. Sone, and J. W. Pike. 1991. The genomic mechanism of action of 1,25–dihydroxyvitamin D_3. *Bone Miner.* 6:1021–7.

[31] Pike, J. W. 1991. Vitamin D_3 receptors: structure and function in transcription. *Annu. Rev. Nutr.* 11:189–216.

[32] Poenie, M., J. Alderton, R. Steinhardt, and R. Tsien. 1986. Calcium rises abruptly and briefly throughout the cell at the onset of anaphase. *Science* 233:886–89.

[33] Pollak, M. R., E. M. Brown, Y.-H. W. Chou, S. C. Hebert, S. J. Marx, B. Steinmann, T. Levi, C. E. Seidman, and J. G. Seidman. 1993. Mutations in the human Ca^{2+}-sensing receptor gene cause familial hypocalciuric hypercalcemia and neonatal severe hyperparathyroidism. *Cell* 75:1297–303.

[34] Potts, J. T. Jr. 1992. Chemistry of the calcitonins. *Bone and Mineral* 16:169–73.

[35] Ratcliffe, W. A. 1992. Role of parathormone-related protein in lactation. *Clin. Endocrinol* 37:402–4.

[36] Reid, I. R., R. W. Ames, M. C. Evans, G. D. Gable, and S. J. Sharpe. 1993. Effect of calcium supplementation on bone loss in post-menopausal women. *New Engl. J. Med.* 328:460–4.

[37] Segre, G. V. 1990. Advances in techniques for measurement of parathyroid hormone. Current applications in clinical medicine and directions for future research. *TEM* 1:243–7.

[38] Sietz, P. K., K. M. Cooper, K. L. Ives, J. Ishizuka, C. M. Townsend, Jr., S. Rajarman, and C. W. Cooper. 1993. Parathyroid hormone-related peptide production and action in a myoepithelial cell line derived from normal human breast. *Endocrinology* 133:1116–24.

[39] Stumpf, W. E. 1988. Vitamin D-soltriol the heliogenic steroid hormone: somatotrophic activator and modulator. Discoveries from histochemical studies lead to new concepts. *Histochemistry* 89:209–19.

[40] Stumpf, W. E. 1989. The endocrinology of sunlight and darkness: complementary roles of vitamin D and pineal hormones. *Naturwissenschaften* 75:247–51.

[41] Suda, T., N. Takahashi, and J. Martin. 1992. Modulation of osteoclast differentiation. *Endocr. Rev.* 13:66–80.

[42] Talmage, R. V., S. A. Grubb, H. Norimatsu, and C. J. VanderWiel. 1980. Evidence for an important physiological role for calcitonin. *Proc. Natl. Acad. Sci. USA* 77:609–13.

[43] Thiede, M. A., and G. A. Rodan. 1988. Expression of a calcium-mobilizing parathyroid hormone-like peptide in lactating mammary tissue. *Science* 242:278–80.

[44] Tiegs, R. D., J. J. Body, H. W. Wahner, J. Barta, B. L. Riggs, and H. Heath. 1985. Calcitonin secretion in postmenopausal women. *New Engl. J. Med.* 312:1097–1100.

[45] Tilyard, M. W., G. F. S. Spears, J. Thomson, and S. Dovey. 1992. Treatment of post-menopausal osteoporosis with calcitrol or calcium. *New Engl. J. Med.* 326:357–62.

[46] Walters, M. R. 1992. Newly identified actions of the Vitamin D endocrine system. *Endocr. Rev.* 13:719–64.

[47] Wasnich, R. D., P. D. Ross, and J. W. Davis. 1991. Osteoporosis. Current practice and future perspectives. *TEM* 2:59–62.

[48] Wasserman, R. H., J. D. Henion, M. R. Haussler, and T. A. McCain. 1976. Calcinogenic factor in *Solanum malacoxylon*; evidence that it is 1,25-dihydroxyvitamin D_3-glycoside. *Science* 194:853–54.

[49] Watson, P. H., and D. A. Hanley. 1993. Parathyroid hormone: regulation of synthesis and secretion. *Clin. Invest. Med.* 16:58–77.

[50] Wood, P. J. 1992. The measurement of parathyroid hormone. *Ann. Clin. Biochem.* 29:11–21.

10

Gastrointestinal Hormones

*The first hormone to be discovered was **secretin**, a chemical messenger released from the epithelium of the small intestine in response to acid released from the stomach [2]. The gut is the source of many hormones; in fact, the gastrointestinal mucosa may be considered the largest endocrine organ. Elucidation of the chemical nature of the gut hormones has been difficult because the endocrine-secreting cells are distributed individually throughout the gut epithelium. Thus an easy source of the hormones is not readily available for chemical identification. Their specific cellular distribution has, however, been determined precisely in a number of animal species by immunocytochemical methods.*

Of the known gastrointestinal (GI) peptides, four clearly function as hormones: gastrin, secretin, cholecystokinin (CCK), and gastric inhibitory peptide (GIP). Other candidate hormones will probably derive full hormonal status after further studies. One of the major problems confronting the endocrinologist is to determine whether the experimentally determined biological effects of the hormones are indeed indicative of such a physiological function. Many GI hormones fall into families of related hormones that share overlapping structures. Thus members of the same hormonal family evoke similar target tissue responses, which confuses any issue relating to their individual putative physiological roles.

The actions of the GI hormones are primarily concerned with the digestion and movement of food products along the GI tract. They release the enzymes necessary to split specific food substrates, such as proteins, carbohydrates, and fats, into their simpler components, amino acids, sugars, and fatty acids (FFAs), respectively. The GI hormones also enhance the activity of enzymes by stimulating the secretion of acid, which provides the pH optimum for enzymatic action. Stimulation of bile salts secretion provides the medium in which fat globules can become emulsified, thus increasing the surface area for enzyme activity. Thus a major role of the GI hormones is to facilitate the conversion of food substrates into molecular forms that can then gain access into the bloodstream. A number of reviews on the endocrinology of GI function are available [13, 32, 42].

GASTROINTESTINAL TRACT STRUCTURE AND FUNCTION

In order to appreciate the roles and actions of hormones on digestive processes it is necessary to review briefly the structure and function of the GI tract. Food enters the mouth, is mixed with saliva, passes down the esophagus, and enters the stomach through the lower esophageal sphincter. The emulsified, partly digested food is then released as a bolus of chyme through the pyloric sphincter into the duodenum, the initial segment of the small intestine (small bowel). The food continues through the jejunal (jejunum) and ileal (ileum) segments of the small intestine to enter the large intestine (colon), where the undigested components of the food making up the stool are dehydrated before defecation from the anus.

Food is propelled distally along the GI tract because of peristaltic contractions of the gut. Peristalsis results from the rhythmic contractions and relaxations of the longitudinal and circular layers of muscle that comprise part of the gut wall. Muscle contraction and relaxation are controlled by neurons of the parasympathetic and sympathetic components of the autonomic nervous system. These *extrinsic nerve fibers* innervate *intrinsic neurons* of the *myenteric plexus of Auerbach*, which are found between the circular and longitudinal muscle layers. Other intrinsic neurons of the gut form the *submucosal plexus of Meissner*, which regulates the activity of muscles responsible for movements of the villi.

The pancreas plays an important role in GI function. The islets of Langerhans (the endocrine pancreas) are the source of insulin and glucagon, two hormones important in the control of carbohydrate metabolism (Chap. 11). The exocrine pancreas is composed of the *acinar cells* that are the source of a variety of enzymes essential to digestion of foodstuffs arriving in the small intestine [1]. The pancreatic duct provides an exit for the release and delivery of these enzymes to the small intestine. Certain ductule cells lining this excretory passageway provide water and electrolytes (i.e., bicarbonate ion), which are also important to digestive processes.

The gallbladder is a pear-shaped hollow organ that serves as a reservoir for bile salts excreted by the liver. Contraction of the smooth muscles of the walls of the gallbladder discharges the *bile salts* into the common bile duct, which then connects with the pancreatic duct leading to the opening into the small intestine. The bile salts are necessary for emulsification of fats within the intestine.

In the mouth, starch is acted on by ptyalin, an α-amylase present within the saliva. The saliva is secreted from the salivary (parotid, sublingual, submaxillary) glands. Because the optimal pH for α-amylase activity is 6.7, the action of the enzyme is subsequently inhibited by the acidic environment of the stomach. In the small intestine an α-amylase secreted by the *exocrine pancreas* acts on the various polysaccharides present in the partly digested food. Other enzymes localized within the luminal surface of the mucosa further hydrolyze sugars to glucose. Glucose and other hexoses and pentoses are rapidly absorbed across the wall of the duodenum and ileum to enter the bloodstream.

Protein digestion begins in the stomach where enzymes, the pepsins, cleave particular peptide linkages. The pepsins are released from the chief cells of the body of the stomach as precursor (proenzyme) molecules, pepsinogens, which are activated by gastric hydrochloric acid released from *parietal* or *oxyntic* (from the Greek for to make sour or acid) cells of the gastric glands. The actions of the pepsins are terminated in the alkaline pancreatic juice of the duodenum. In the small intestine the shorter peptides are formed by the action of protein-splitting enzymes, trypsin and chymotrypsin, released from the pancreas. Other enzymes, pancreatic carboxypeptidases, intestinal amino-peptidases, and dipeptidases, split the smaller peptides to free amino acids. These amino acids are actively transported across the intestinal lumen and enter the bloodstream.

The digestion of fats begins in the intestine. Free fatty acids are liberated by the enzymatic actions of *pancreatic lipase* on dietary triglycerides. This enzyme acts on fats that have been emulsified by the detergent action of bile salts released into the intestinal lumen following contraction of the gallbladder. Small micelles consisting of lipids and bile salts provide the reactive surface for lipase activity. The FFAs and monoglycerides within the micelles are released by enzymatic action to enter the mucosal cells by passive diffusion; they may then pass directly into the portal blood or they may become re-esterified to triglycerides within the mucosal cells and then enter into the lymphatics.

SOURCE AND CHEMISTRY OF THE GASTROINTESTINAL HORMONES

The GI hormones are synthesized within a system of clear cells (enterochromaffin, argyrophil, or argentaffin cells), so called because they are selectively stained by certain silver salts. These clear cells, scattered within the GI tract mucosa from the stomach through the colon, are often referred to as the diffuse or dispersed endocrine system, or, along with the pancreatic hormones, as the gastroenteropancreatic hormones [27]. This diffuse distribution of enterochromaffin-like (ECL) cells prevents the endocrinologist from surgically removing the source of any one hormone as is done for many other endocrine glands. It is suggested that the distribution of ECL cells throughout extensive areas of mucosa "ensures that hormone release is regulated by an integrated sampling of mixed luminal contents rather than by a specific stimulus that might exist transiently at only one point" [14]. One surface of each of the ECL cells often reaches the lumen, thus providing a receptive surface for metabolite recognition.

The ECL cells of the gut and pancreas have been classified as deriving from certain cell types, designated, for example, as D (somatostain), G (gastrin), or S (secretin). A tenet of neuroendocrinology has been the "one hormone, one cell" concept. However, in the gut and elsewhere, a peptide hormone (e.g., substance P) and the biogenic amine, serotonin (5-HT), are often found within the same cell. The physiological significance of two biologically active moieties within the same cell is unclear.

Based on their homology of structure, the gut hormones can be conveniently grouped into two families. The *gastrin family* comprises the gastrins and the cholecystokinins. The *secretin family* consists of secretin, glucagon, vasoactive intestinal polypeptide (VIP), and gastric inhibitory peptide (GIP). There may be molecular heterogeneity (isoforms) of a particular hormone; the hormone may exist in a number of molecular forms of variable length with differing biological potencies. Only one of these peptides is generally considered to be the physiological messenger, and it usually constitutes the principal form stored within the secretory granules of the cell. Molecular forms larger than the principal form may be viewed as biosynthetic precursors (prohormones), which may escape and be detected in the circulation. Molecular forms smaller than the principal form probably represent postsecretory degradation products.

The Gastrin Family of Hormones

The C-terminal five-amino-acid sequences of gastrin and CCK are identical (Fig. 10.1). Because the biologically active site of these peptides is this pentapeptide sequence, the overlapping actions of one hormone on the physiologically relevant target tissues of the other hormone are explained. The minimal active fragment of these peptides is actually the C-terminal tetrapeptide. Pentagastrin, which exhibits full agonistic activity, is often used in physiological and clinical studies where the actions of gastrin are to be deter-

```
                    1    2    3    4    5    6    7    8    9   10   11  12   13  14   15   16   17
Gastrin (G-17)   (pyro)Glu–Gly–Pro–Trp–Leu–Glu–Glu–Glu–Glu–Glu–Ala–Tyr–Gly–Trp–Met–Asp–Phe–NH2
                                                                        |
                                                                      SO3H

Cholecystokinin    Lys–Ala–Pro–Ser–Gly–Arg–Val–Ser–Met–Ile–Lys–Asn–Leu–Gln–Ser–Leu–Asp–
                      Pro–Ser–His–Arg–Ile–Ser–Asp–Arg–Asp–Tyr–Met–Gly–Trp–Met–Asp–Phe–NH2
                                                                |
                                                              SO3H
                    18   19   20   21  22  23   24  25   26  27   28   29   30   31   32   33
```

Figure 10.1 Amino acid sequences of human G-17 gastrin and cholecystokinin (CCK). Identical C-terminal pentapeptide sequences are indicated.

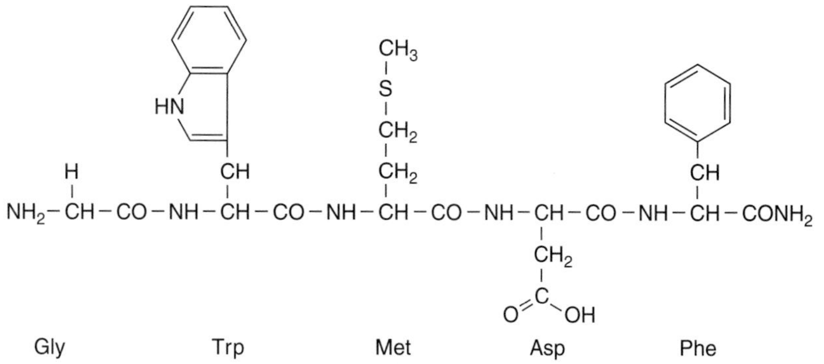

Figure 10.2　Structure of pentagastrin.

mined (Fig. 10.2). The NH_2-terminal component of gastrin and CCK influences the potency of the hormones, and may also be responsible in part for providing target cell specificity. Note that there are sulfated tyrosyl residues at the 6 and 7 (numbering from the C-terminal end) positions of gastrin and CCK, respectively. Approximately half the gastrin isolated from the gastric mucosa is sulfated on tyrosine. In the case of CCK where tyrosine is always sulfated, however, the sulfated form of the hormone is about 160-fold more potent than the nonsulfated form in binding to CCK_A receptors on pancreatic acini and in promoting gallbladder contraction [15]. CCK_B receptors are less specific and sulfation is not required for receptor activation. The CCK_B receptor is, in fact, the gastrin receptor through which acid secretion is stimulated.

Gastrin circulates in most mammalian species in at least three molecular forms (Table 10.1). A macromolecular form of gastrin called big-big gastrin (component I) apparently does not circulate, but could exist as an early intracellular biosynthetic precursor for one or more of the gastrins. It is believed that component I serves as a *preprogastrin* for gastrin-34 (big gastrin, component II), which may in some cells function as a hormone or as a progastrin. Component III, gastrin-17, may be the physiologically relevant form of the hormone secreted by some cells, and component IV (minigastrin, gastrin-14) is considered to be an extracellular degradation product of component III.

TABLE 10.1　Amino Acid Sequences of Human Gastrin Components

Component[a]	Sequence
I Gastrin 　(big-big gastrin)	Preprogastrin (95 amino acid residues)
II Gastrin$_{34}$ 　(big gastrin)	(pyro)Glu–Leu–Gly–Pro–Gln–Gly–His–Pro–Ser–Leu–Val–Ala–Asp–Pro–Ser–Lys–Lys– Gln–Gly–Pro–Trp–Leu–Glu–Glu–Glu–Glu–Glu–Ala–Tyr–Gly–Trp–Met–Asp–Phe–NH_2 　　　　　　　　　　　　　　　　　　　　　　　　　　　$\mid$ 　　　　　　　　　　　　　　　　　　　　　　　　　SO_3H
III Gastrin$_{17}$ 　(little gastrin)	(pyro)Glu–Gly–Pro–Trp–Leu–Glu–Glu–Glu–Glu–Glu–Ala–Tyr–Gly–Trp–Met–Asp–Phe–NH_2 　　　　　　　　　　　　　　　　　　　　　　　　$\mid$ 　　　　　　　　　　　　　　　　　　　　　　SO_3H
IV Gastrin$_{14}$ 　(mini-gastrin)	Trp–Leu–Glu–Glu–Glu–Glu–Glu–Ala–Tyr–Gly–Trp–Met–Asp–Phe–NH_2 　　　　　　　　　　　　　　　　　　　$\mid$ 　　　　　　　　　　　　　　　　SO_3H

[a]Gastrin-34, G-17, and G-14 also exist without a sulfate ester at their tyrosyl residue.

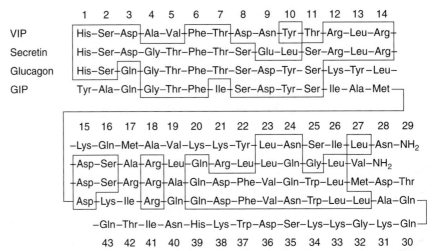

Figure 10.3 Amino acid sequences of porcine peptides of the secretin family. Boxed areas indicate identical amino acid sequences between peptides.

The Secretin Family of Hormones

Secretin is similar to glucagon in structure: 14 of the 27 amino acids of secretin are similar to those found in glucagon, which is 29 amino acids long. The structures of GIP and VIP possess many amino acids in common with those found in glucagon and secretin (Fig. 10.3). A glucagonlike peptide is also found in the small intestine; this *enteroglucagon* (glucagonlike peptide 1, GLP-1) regulates, in concert with other hormones, pancreatic insulin secretion. Most of the entire sequences of each of the peptides is required for their biological actions on their respective target tissues. The hormones of the secretin family lack a well-defined function site where, as in the melanotropins, a particular amino acid sequence has been conserved within the individual peptides (see Fig. 8.1).

Other Candidate Hormones

The other putative hormones of the GI tract are motilin, somatostatin, substance P, neurotensin, and gastrin-releasing peptide. The formulae of some of these peptides are provided; they bear no structural similarity to each other or to the other GI hormones (Table 10.2). These peptides are variably localized to immunocytochemically characterized cells of the GI mucosa. Other physiologically active peptides are also present within the GI tract and, in time, may also obtain hormone status. These include bulbogastrone, urogastrone, villikinin, calcitonin gene-related peptide, and one or more endorphins.

TABLE 10.2 Candidate Hormones of the Gut

Hormone	
Substance P	Arg–Pro–Lys–Pro–Gln–Gln–Phe–Phe–Gly–Leu–Met–NH$_2$
Somatostatin	Ala–Gly–Cys–Lys–Asn–Phe–Phe–Trp–Lys–Thr–Phe–Thr–Ser–Cys
Motilin	Phe–Val–Pro–Ile–Phe–Thr–Tyr–Gly–Glu–Leu–Glu–Arg–Met–Glu–Gly–Lys–Glu–Arg–Asn–Lys–Gly–Glu
Neurotensin	(pyro)Glu–Leu–Tyr–Glu–Asn–Lys–Pro–Arg–Arg–Pro–Tyr–Ile–Leu

PHYSIOLOGICAL ROLES OF THE GASTROINTESTINAL HORMONES

A major role of the GI hormones is to stimulate the secretion of enzymes necessary to degrade complex food substrates into their simpler molecular components so that these smaller molecules can cross the luminal mucosal cells into the bloodstream. GI hormones also stimulate the secretion of acid or base to provide the optimal pH conditions for enzyme activity. By their actions on smooth muscle, the GI hormones move the food distally down the GI tract to the colon. They stimulate release of hormones from the pancreatic islets, which then aid in cellular utilization of metabolic substrates after reaching the bloodstream. The GI hormones may even provide satiety signals to the brain to affect eating behavior (see Chap. 21).

Each of the GI hormones has a number of known biological actions of questionable physiological significance. Because many of the hormones are related in structure, they can exhibit overlapping actions when studied experimentally. Gastrin and CCK are partially similar in structure; they both stimulate gastric acid and pancreatic enzyme secretion. It is likely, however, that each hormone is delivered by specific circulatory routes to its own target tissues. This would then provide the mechanism for the necessary specificity of its actions. The release of each of the GI hormones is in response to chemical stimuli, such as hydrogen ions, certain amino acids, FFAs, and sugars. It is believed that nutrient receptors are present on the surface of the hormone-secreting cells, which are in open communication with the lumen of the GI tract (Fig. 10.4).

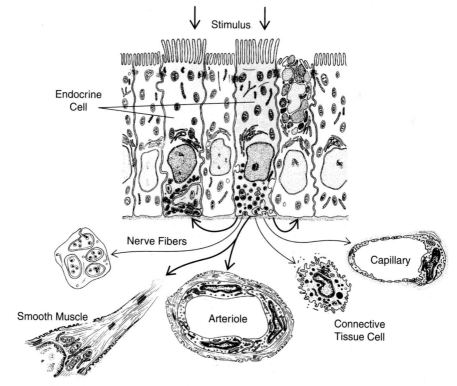

Figure 10.4 Schematic drawing indicating the possible actions of enteroendocrine cells. The stimulus from the intestinal lumen acts on the receptors of the brush-border membrane, resulting in a release of hormones by exocytosis. The peptide hormones may exert their effect on the following: (a) adjacent epithelial cells, nerve fibers, nerve cells, smooth muscle, and connective tissue cells of the lamina propria; (b) cells of the whole organism following delivery to the systematic circulation. Method (a) is described as paracrine; method (b) is referred to as endocrine. (From Grube and Forssmann [14], with permission.)

Gastrin

Although the existence of an antral hormone controlling gastric acid secretion was postulated as early as 1905, the hormone gastrin was not isolated until 1964. The antral mucosa of the stomach is the richest source of gastrin in all investigated species, although the peptide is also present in G cells of the duodenal mucosa, particularly in humans. In the antrum and small intestine the apical pole of the cell, which possesses numerous villi, is in contact with the lumen. Gastrin is present in the gastric juice, which has aroused speculation that gastrin might be released from the luminal surface (as a lumone), as well as from the basal surface. Electrical stimulation of the vagus nerve of the cat causes a minor increase in circulating gastrin, whereas a much greater amount can be detected in the gastric juice.

Food is the primary physiological stimulus of gastrin secretion. Peptide fragments, amino acids, and to a lesser extent FFAs are stimulatory to gastrin secretion, but sugars are without such an effect. Gastrin secretion is under autonomic nervous system control [4]. For example, in some species the vagus nerve stimulates gastrin secretion in anticipation of the ingestion of food or through activation of local neural reflexes following distension of the stomach after food intake. Somatostatin- and VIP-secreting cells are found in close association with antral gastrin-secreting cells and may function in an inhibitory role by a paracrine mechanism.

One physiological function of gastrin is to stimulate hydrochloric acid and pepsinogen secretion within the fundus of the stomach; the activated enzyme then initiates the digestion of proteins. The known targets for gastrin mediating these responses are (a) histamine-releasing ECL cells, and (b) acid-secreting parietal cells [24]. Both cell types have been shown to possess a gastrin-CCK_B receptor. (The CCK_B receptor is a CCK receptor subtype mainly found in the brain, and possesses pharmacologic characteristics similar to those of the gastrin receptor.) Gastrin may also stimulate acid secretion indirectly and gastrin receptors are present on cells other than parietal cells. More recent evidence suggests that gastrin (and agents used to treat ulcers) may act on ECL cells in the lamina propria and not on parietal cells as previously thought. The actions of gastrin may be indirectly transmitted to the epithelial (parietal) cells via the ECL cells [24]. Gastrin does not stimulate pepsinogen secretion directly, but rather indirectly, through release of HCl. In other words, hydrogen ions from the acid are stimulatory to pepsinogen secretion from the chief cells (Fig. 10.5).

The gastrin present within the antrum is the small (G-17) form of the molecule. The cell responsible for gastrin production in the duodenum contains the larger (G-34) form of the peptide. It is only in humans, where high concentrations of duodenal gastrin occur, that a significant proportion of G-34 appears in the circulation. These two cells, therefore, contain different molecular forms of the peptide, which supports the observation that the two cells are ultrastructurally distinguishable. It is possible that these two circulating forms of

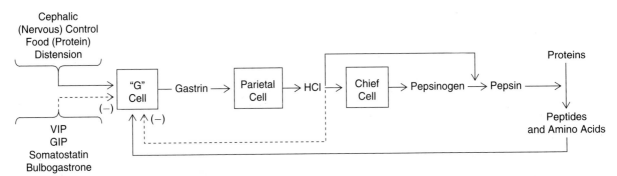

Figure 10.5 Neuroendocrine integration of gastric acid secretion. (Also see Fig. 10.14.)

gastrin have selective actions on different target cells. It is also possible that a particular molecular form of gastrin may be less susceptible to enzyme degradation.

Starvation or total parenteral (venous) nutrition dramatically reduces the levels of both antral and serum gastrin. This suggests that hormone secretion is acutely dependent on the presence of food in the gut. If rats are fed totally by vein, tissue sensitivity to the trophic action of gastrin becomes diminished. This loss of sensitivity can be prevented by the concomitant infusion of pentagastrin. The pancreatic and colonic mucosa, as well as the duodenal and oxyntic gland mucosa, undergo atrophy in the antrectomized rat, but these deleterious effects can be reversed by supplying gastrin exogenously. These observations suggest that gastrin is an important regulator of gastromucosal cellular growth [5].

The following additional biological effects are ascribed to gastrin: stimulation of lower esophageal sphincter pressure; relaxation of the pyloric sphincter; stimulation of pancreatic enzyme secretion; enhancement of motor activity in the intestine; and moderate stimulation of pancreatic bicarbonate and water secretion.

Secretin

Secretin is one of many peptide hormones of the small intestine. The tissue concentration of secretin diminishes from duodenum to ileum. Secretinlike immunoreactivity is localized to the granular S cells, which are present between the crypts and villi of the mucosa of the small intestine, where maximum concentrations of the hormone have also been extracted. Acidification of the duodenal mucosa, resulting from HCl arriving in the duodenum from the stomach, is the normal stimulus for secretin secretion. At a pH above 4.5, secretin is not released in sufficient amounts to stimulate pancreatic bicarbonate secretion and continued release of secretin is pH dependent. Nevertheless, it has been difficult to demonstrate increases in plasma secretin levels after a meal. Because a secretin response (increased pancreatic secretion of water and bicarbonate) is observed in humans and dogs after ingestion of meat, a small amount of secretin (insufficiently large to be detected by radioimmunoassay) may be released from the duodenum and may interact with CCK to stimulate bicarbonate secretion. There is an endocrine closed-loop type of relationship governing secretin and HCO_3^- release. Secretin stimulates pancreatic secretion of HCO_3^- into the duodenum; the HCO_3^- neutralizes the H^+ from the stomach, which raises the pH, hence decreasing the release of secretin, which removes any further stimulus to bicarbonate secretion (Fig. 10.6).

The clearly defined roles of secretin are to stimulate pancreatic bicarbonate secretion and to potentiate CCK-stimulated pancreatic enzyme secretion. The numerous other physiological actions of secretin may only be pharmacological in nature and may relate to similarities in structure to glucagon, VIP, and GIP, the other members of the secretin family of hormones.

Cholecystokinin (CCK)

The presence of a hormone in the duodenal mucosa that is liberated by food (particularly lipids) and causes contraction and emptying of the gallbladder was discovered by Ivy and

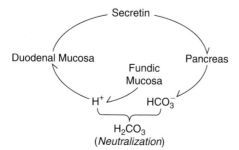

Figure 10.6 Homeostatic closed-loop endocrine mechanism of small intestine pH control.

Oldberg in 1928 and named *cholecystokinin* (CCK). Another hormone from the same source that stimulated the release of pancreatic enzymes and also contracted the gallbladder was named *pancreozymin* (PZ). It was subsequently established that CCK and PZ were the same hormone. CCK is a polypeptide hormone of 33-amino-acid residues, but the peptide also exists in a number of other forms. The carboxyterminal five amino acids of CCK are identical to those in gastrin (Fig. 10.1). The seventh amino acid from the carboxyterminus is sulfated, which is necessary for the normal physiological activity of the molecule. All C-terminal forms of CCK that exceed seven residues are virtually equipotent in stimulating pancreatic enzyme secretion and gall bladder contraction [15].

The physiological significance of the tissue-specific distribution of CCK variants may be related to the fact that small forms of CCK, such as the octapeptide (CCK-8), are efficiently cleared by the liver and thus could not subserve an effective endocrine role in the GI tract, while larger forms more readily survive hepatic transit. This constraint is not present in the CNS, and the majority of C-terminal CCK-like immunoreactivity in the brain comprises CCK-8. It may also be that using shorter forms as central neurotransmitters or neuromodulators promotes delivery to target receptors and subsequent rapid deactivation.

CCK is immunocytochemically localized to the I cells of the duodenal, jejunal, and ileal mucosa. CCK is released by L-isomers of amino acids, hydrochloric acid, and certain fatty acids. Entry of high levels of hydrogen ion into the duodenum results in gallbladder contraction, a specific biological response attributed to circulating CCK. CCK plays a major role in gallbladder regulation, although other neural or hormonal factors may also participate. CCK in physiological concentrations has been shown to correlate with postprandial gallbladder contraction in humans [20].

The other recognized physiological roles of CCK are stimulation of pancreatic enzyme secretion, inhibition of gastric emptying, and potentiation of secretin-induced pancreatic bicarbonate secretion. CCK also appears to be a physiological regulator of the growth of the exocrine pancreas. Although the peptide shares structural similarity with gastrin, which has a trophic growth effect on the GI mucosa, CCK is without such an effect, its trophic actions being specific to the acinar cells of the pancreas.

CCK, or related peptide, may also function as a satiety hormone (Chap. 21) [8, 28]. A CCK-related peptide is also present within the brain where it may subserve a number of physiological functions as a neuroregulator [12]. Bulimia nervosa is a prevalent disorder of unknown cause, characterized by recurrent episodes of uncontrollable eating. Since CCK induces satiety and reduces food intake in laboratory animals and humans, it has been hypothesized that abnormalities in CCK secretion and satiety may occur in patients with bulimia and contribute to their disturbed eating patterns [9]. Individuals with bulimia may not have normal satiety and may have an impaired secretion of CCK in response to a meal. Abnormally low plasma CCK secretion in response to a mixed-liquid meal in patients with bulimia nervosa has been noted. These patients had lower peak levels of CCK immediately after a meal and also had a low total integrated secretion of the hormone. An impaired satiety response to food was also noted. Impaired satiety after a normal-sized meal is consistent with the histories provided by patients with bulimia (Fig. 10.7).

Disturbances in appetite and food intake are often associated with certain states of depression. Patients with melancholic depression frequently have anorexia, whereas atypically depressed patients have hyperphagia. Similarly, it has been proposed that in the anorexia of aging, elevated CCK levels or increased sensitivity to CCK may contribute to decreased appetite by inducing early satiety [9]. There is great hope that CCK or a related analog acting as a "satiety hormone" might prove useful for the control of obesity [26, 29].

Gastric Inhibitory Peptide (GIP)

As early as 1886 it was demonstrated that the presence of fats in a meal inhibited gastric emptying in humans. Fat ingestion was later shown to inhibit gastric acid secretion. Crude

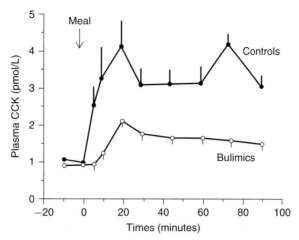

Figure 10.7   Plasma cholecystokinin (CCK) responses to a meal in normal subjects and patients with bulimia. After an overnight fast, 14 patients with bulimia and 10 age- and sex-matched normal volunteers were fed a 400-ml mixed liquid meal. Plasma was collected and extracted at the indicated times and assayed for CCK bioactivity, expressed as cholecystokinin-8 equivalents. Values are means ± SEM. The arrow indicates the beginning of the meal. (From Geracioti and Liddle [9]. Reprinted by permission of the *New England Journal of Medicine*, 319:683–9, 1988.)

intestinal extracts duplicated the actions of fat on gastric acid secretion and motility. The active principle was referred to as *enterogastrone*. Although a number of gut hormones exhibit enterogastronelike activity, only one, gastric inhibitory peptide (GIP), is considered to play such a physiological role. This 43-amino-acid peptide, which bears structural similarity to other members of the secretin family of hormones (Fig. 10.3), is localized to certain K cells of the duodenum and jejunum of humans and dogs.

In addition to its inhibitory effects on gastric acid secretion, GIP is insulinotropic, potentiating insulin release in response to an intravenous infusion of glucose, a response that in humans improves glucose tolerance. GIP has therefore been referred to as the *glucose-dependent insulinotropic peptide*. Oral glucose ingestion in humans produces a sustained increase in serum GIP levels capable of stimulating insulin release. Indeed, glucose ingestion induces a greater insulin release than intravenous administration of the same amount of glucose. The insulinotropic action of GIP appears to be specifically dependent on concomitant glucose administration as fat ingestion increases serum GIP levels but not serum insulin concentrations. Like glucagon and VIP, GIP is a potent stimulator of intestinal juice secretion from the duodenal glands of Brunner (Brunner's glands, located in the vicinity of the pyloric sphincter).

Besides these well-described effects on gastric secretion and pancreatic β cells, GIP also has direct metabolic effects on other tissues and organs, such as adipose tissue, liver, muscle, GI tract, and brain. In adipose tissue it activates lipoprotein lipase; it also inhibits glucagon-induced lipolysis and potentiates the effect of insulin on incorporation of fatty acids into triglycerides. It may play a role in the development of obesity because in obese animals adipose tissue is hypersensitive to some of these actions. It may increase glucose use in peripheral tissues such as muscle. GIP also has an effect on the volume and/or electrolyte composition of intestinal secretion and saliva. The relationship of GIP with insulin is integrated, and the presence of both insulin and GIP is sometimes necessary for the greater efficiency of both hormones. GIP can be considered to be a true metabolic hormone with most of its functions, like insulin, tending to increase anabolism [3].

Vasoactive Intestinal Peptide (VIP)

This peptide, first isolated from the pig intestine, contains 28 amino acid residues and is structurally related to secretin, glucagon, and GIP. Like other members of the secretin family the entire primary structure of VIP is important for biological activity. The structure of VIP is relatively well conserved throughout the animal kingdom. The amino acid sequence of human VIP is identical to that of pigs, cows, and rats, but is slightly different in guinea pigs and chickens. Immunohistochemical studies reveal that the peptide is diffusely distributed throughout the entire length of the mammalian and avian intestinal tract (esophagus through the colon). VIP was named for its potent vasodilator and hypotensive effects [10, 11]. It relaxes a variety of smooth muscles and antagonizes the effects of smooth muscle constrictor agents. VIP inhibits histamine and pentagastrin-stimulated gastric acid secretion. Electrolyte and water secretion by the pancreas are stimulated and bile flow is increased. VIP stimulates lipolysis, glycogenolysis, and insulin secretion, but because these actions are shared by some other members of the secretin family of hormones, these observed effects of VIP may be pharmacological rather than physiological in nature. In addition, the presence of this peptide in nerve cells (Chap. 21) and the absence of a meal-induced change in VIP plasma concentrations further argue against its role as a humoral gastroenteropancreatic hormone. The selective localization of VIP within neurons in the CNS and autonomic nervous system, especially in the superior and inferior mesenteric ganglia, the submucosal (Meissner's) and myenteric (Auerbach's) plexuses of the intestinal wall, the cerebrovascular nerves, and nerves in the female and male genito-urinary tracts, suggests that its role may be restricted to that of a neurohormone acting by a neurocrine or paracrine mechanism in a variety of organs including the GI tract (Fig. 10.8).

There is strong evidence that in humans and other species, the descending relaxation component of the peristaltic reflex is mediated by VIP. This transmitter is released during descending relaxation only, and its neutralization with VIP antiserum or blockade of its effect with VIP antagonists inhibits descending relaxation. Although VIP appears to be the only relaxant transmitter acting at neuromuscular junctions, its release is modulated by two other types of myenteric neurons, somatostatin neurons and opioid neurons [22].

Substance P (SP)

Stimulation of the abdominal vagal nerve releases a substance whose actions on smooth muscle motor activity are not blocked by atropine. This substance, therefore, is not acetylcholine (Chap. 14). This peptide consists of 11 amino acid residues (Table 10.2) and is called substance P (SP) in reference to an early preparation of active gut extract. This was the first neuropeptide to be found in both the brain and gut. SP is found localized within nerve fibers in all areas of the gut wall, including the two muscle layers (the myenteric and submucosal plexuses) the mucosa, and the submucosa. Substance P is also distributed widely but selectively within the brain and spinal column; it is structurally related to a number of peptides present within the skin of anuran amphibians (see Fig. 10.17). Substance P is a member of a family of structurally related peptides (neurokinin A, neurokinin B), called tachykinins, that are involved in the regulation of many biologic processes. Diversity in the generation of tachykinin peptides arises due to encoding these peptides from multiple genes as well as by mechanisms of alternative mRNA processing and differential posttranslational processing. These peptides are neurotransmitters and/or neuromodulator substances, and they bring about their actions mainly by activating three primary types of neurokinin receptors, NK-1, NK-2, and NK-3 [17].

The peripheral action site of SP outside the CNS seems to be mainly on smooth muscle. SP lowers arterial blood pressure and is recognized as one of the most potent vasodilators. Almost all peripheral tissues contain SP-positive nerves, often in close association with blood vessels and secretory cells. The high potency of SP, together with its

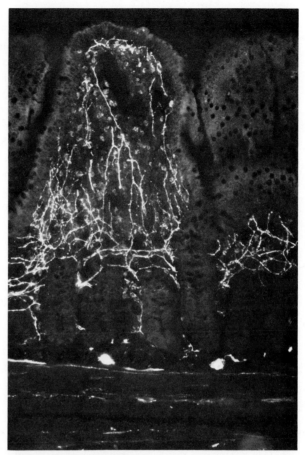

Figure 10.8 Immunoreactive VIP nerve plexus in small intestine of the rat. (Reprinted with permission from T. Hökfelt, R. Elde, O. Johansson, A. Ljungdahl, M. Schulzberg, K. Fuxe, M. Goldstein, G. Nilsson, B. Pernow, L. Terenius, D. Ganten, S.L. Jeffcoate, J. Rehfeld, and S. I. Said. 1978. "Distribution of peptide-containing neurons." In *Psychopharmacology: a generation of progress*. M. A. Lipton, A. DiMascio and K. F. Killam [eds.]. pp. 39–66. New York: Raven Press.)

presence in intrinsic nerves in the gut, suggest that SP may function as a physiological modulator of smooth muscle activity in gut tissue. Intestinal peristalsis changes from bidirectional to unidirectional shortly after birth, concomitant with the appearance in the myenteric plexa of peptidergic nerve fibers. A role for SP in the regulation of intestinal peristalsis has been suggested, and SP may be involved in the postnatal induction of propulsive motility. Intraventricular injections of SP have marked antidipsogenic effect without depressing food intake or producing other behavioral modifications. It has been suggested that because SP is found in the brain, it may be a natural satiator of thirst.

Somatostatin

This tetradecapeptide (Table 10.2), referred to as somatostatin to describe its role as a somatotropin release-inhibiting hormone, is also localized to specialized D cells of the GI mucosa. Highest concentrations are localized to the gastric antrum with progressively decreasing levels found within the small intestine and colon. Somatostatin-producing cells of the stomach have long cytoplasmic processes that terminate on other cell types (Fig. 10.9), including the gastrin-producing and hydrochloric acid-producing cells [19].

The release of gastrin and hydrochloric acid, respectively, from these cells is tonically inhibited by somatostatin. Somatostatin is also localized to D cells of the pancreatic islets and may regulate glucagon and insulin secretion (Chap. 1). The observation that long processes may emanate from other endocrine cells of the gut epithelium suggests that other GI hormones may function by a paracrine mode of control [19].

There are two naturally occurring bioactive forms of somatostatin (Fig. 6.6 and Fig. 6.7), the tetradecapeptide somatostatin-14 (S14) and the N-terminally extended form somatostatin-28 (S28). S14 is the predominant somatostatin present in the D cells of the pancreatic islets and the gastric antrum, while S28 is the predominant form in the epithelial D cells of the duodenal, jejunal, ileal, and colonic mucosa. After a mixed meal, somatostatinlike immunoreactivity (SLI) increases in the peripheral circulation. Changes in peripheral SLI have been shown to arise mainly from gut somatostatin, and, indeed, in humans the postprandial rise in SLI consists predominantly of S28.

Gastrin-releasing Peptide (GRP)

Bombesin is a tetradecapeptide originally isolated from frog (*Bombina*) skin. Bombesin-like immunoreactivity was subsequently localized to both the mammalian brain and GI tract. A 27-amino-acid gastrin-releasing peptide (GRP) was isolated from the porcine gut

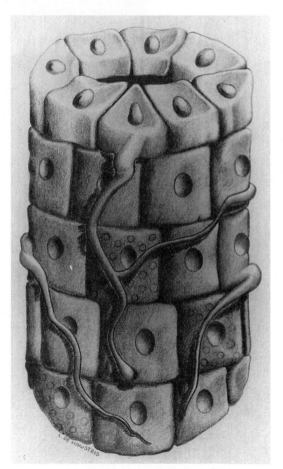

Figure 10.9 Schematic drawing showing a three-dimensional arrangement of the somatostatin cells and their processes in an antral gland. (From Larsson et al. [19], with permission. *Science* 205:1393–94, 1979. ©1979 by the American Association for the Advancement of Science.)

```
                         1    2    3    4    5    6    7    8    9   10   11   12   13   14
Bombesin              pGlu–Gln–Arg–Leu–Gly–Asn–Gln–Trp–Ala–Val–Gly–His–Leu–Met–NH₂


                              1    2    3    4    5    6    7    8    9   10   11   12   13
Gastrin-Releasing Peptide   Ala–Pro–Val–Ser–Val–Gly–Gly–Gly–Thr–Val–Leu–Ala–Lys–


                             14   15   16   17   18   19   20   21   22   23   24   25   26   27
                            Met–Tyr–Pro–Arg–Gly–Asn–His–Trp–Ala–Val–Gly–His–Leu–Met–NH₂
```

Figure 10.10 Primary structures of bombesin and porcine gastrin-releasing peptide (GRP).

that has a C-terminal decapeptide sequence identical to the C-terminal decapeptide of frog skin bombesin, except for a Gln/His interchange at position 20 (Fig. 10.10). The C-terminal octapeptide fragment of GRP retains full biological activity, as does the C-terminal bombesin octapeptide, suggesting that the previously demonstrated effects of bombesin in the mammal are mediated through a GRP receptor. Because GRP and bombesin are structurally related and exhibit similar biological activities, it is likely that GRP is the mammalian equivalent of bombesin.

GRP is present in nerve fibers in the antral mucosa. Bombesin produces atropine-resistant stimulation of gastrin release from isolated rat stomach. This stimulation of gastrin release is not accompanied by a reciprocal decrease in somatostatin release; therefore it clearly differs from the pattern produced by cholinergic stimulation of gastrin secretion. Electrical stimulation of the vagus nerve causes release of immunoreactive GRP from the stomach of anesthetized pigs or sheep. GRP can therefore be added to the growing list of peptides (substance P, neurotensin, CCK, VIP, somatostatin, endorphins) that are present in ECL cells and in central and peripheral neurons.

Motilin

Motilin is a candidate peptide hormone containing 22 amino acid residues, which bears no structural similarity to any other known GI hormone [6]. The peptide is present in highest concentration in the duodenum, where it is present in enteroendocrine cells of the duodenal mucosa, and in lesser amounts throughout the small intestine. The peptide was named for its ability to stimulate gastric motor activity. The potent actions of motilin on GI motility and emptying of chyme into the small intestine suggest possible physiological roles for the peptide. Motilin regulates contractions that occur in 2-hour cycles after meals and that serve to empty the intestine of residual contents. The start of each cycle, which begins in the stomach and travels caudally throughout the intestine, coincides with a peak of circulating motilin. Infusion of motilin can initiate a premature cycle, whereas infusion of motilin antiserum disrupts the phase of maximal contraction. The stimulus for secretion of motilin remains unclear but may be in response to duodenal alkalinization.

Other Putative GI Hormones

A number of other biologically active peptides are also distributed throughout the GI mucosa. They too, in a sense, can be considered candidate hormones. Considering the size of the GI tract, it is not surprising that a number of hormones are distributed throughout this complex organ.

Bulbogastrone. Acidification of the duodenal bulb (area of duodenum just beyond the pylorus) inhibits the gastric acid secretion response to a test meal in certain experimental animals. This secretory response derives specifically from the duodenal bulb because acid perfusion of the postbulbar duodenum has much less effect on gastric-acid secretion. Acidification of bulbar pouches reduces acid secretion from vagally innervated and vagally denervated gastric pouches, suggesting that inhibition of gastric-acid secretion is not mediated by a vagal pathway. Intramural (within the intestinal wall) reflex routes are also not involved, as transection of the pylorus does not abolish the inhibition of acid secretion stimulated by duodenal acidification. The existence of a humoral agent mediating inhibition of gastric secretion is further supported by the observation that extracts of the duodenal bulb inhibit acid secretion. These extracts do not exhibit activities of the other GI hormones because relatively large doses of secretin and CCK are required to inhibit gastric-acid secretin; secretion and CCK may therefore be ruled out as the humoral messengers involved in the response. Bulbogastrone, the name given to this hypothetical factor, interferes with the stimulatory action of gastrin, but not acetylcholine, on the oxyntic glands. Thus bulbogastrone, along with secretin, somatostatin, and GIP, may provide an additional mechanism of regulating gastric acid secretion (Fig. 10.5). The chemical nature and cellular localization of this putative humoral factor is undetermined.

Urogastrone.   Pregnancy causes an improvement in the symptoms of duodenal ulceration. Extracts of urine from pregnant and nonpregnant women, as well as those from men, afford protection against experimentally induced ulceration in dogs. These extracts cause inhibition of gastric acid secretion and also promote fibroblastic proliferation and epithelialization of the mucosa. Purification of urine led to the isolation of two fractions, the *beta* and *gamma* urogastrones, which had different physical properties but the same biological potency. The structure of β-urogastrone consists of a single polypeptide chain of 53 residues with three internal disulfide bonds, whereas γ-urogastrone lacks the C-terminal arginine residue. Although urogastrone is structurally different from other known GI peptides, it is strikingly similar to mouse epidermal growth factor, EGF (Fig. 10.11). Mouse EGF (see Fig. 12.17) is a powerful epithelial mitogen, and urogastrone is equipotent in activity; both peptides are also equally potent in suppressing gastric acid secretion in a number of animals. Urogastrone is considered the human hormonal equivalent of mEGF.

Immunochemical studies have localized urogastronelike activity to the submaxillary glands, to Brunner's glands of the small intestine, and to saliva and gastric juice. Studies in ulcer patients confirmed the ability of urogastrone to suppress basal gastric acid secretion, and acid secretion in response to pentagastrin could also be partially blocked. The action of the peptide was specific as salivary, pancreatic, and bile secretions were not affected similarly by any doses of the peptide. Mouse EGF has a trophic effect on the oxyntic gland mucosa, but, unlike the effects of gastrin, has no such trophic effects on duodenal or colonic mucosa. Secretin inhibits the trophic effects of pentagastrin on the oxyntic mucosa, but not that of mEGF; the trophic action of mEGF is thus not mediated through increased serum gastrin levels. EGF appears to play an important role in the development of the neonatal intestinal epithelium. Administration of EGF in mature animals with a normal intestinal tract results in increased mucosal DNA content and proliferative activity and increased substrate absorption from the intestine. Continuous intravenous infusion of EGF reduces mucosal atrophy and maintains disaccharidase activity during parenteral alimentation. Numerous other studies have supported the concept that EGF is an important trophic hormone of the intestinal mucosa [5].

Glucagonlike Peptide 1.   The structure and biological actions of pancreatic glucagon are well documented (Chap. 11). In addition glucagonlike substances are present within the GI mucosa. Glucagonlike peptide 1 (GLP-1) is an intestinal peptide encoded in the proglucagon gene. Its primary structure is highly conserved from ancient species to humans. The proglucagon gene is expressed in the intestinal L cells, pancreatic α cells, and some neurons in the brainstem. The majority of L cells are located in the distal jejunum and ileum. The L-cell number increases from the proximal colon to the rectum [7]. GLP-1 is released into the circulation after oral ingestion of nutrients. GLP-1 is released rapidly (15 minutes) after the oral ingestion of glucose, fat, and amino acids, and after mixed meals. The nutrient-dependent signal responsible for triggering GLP-1 release

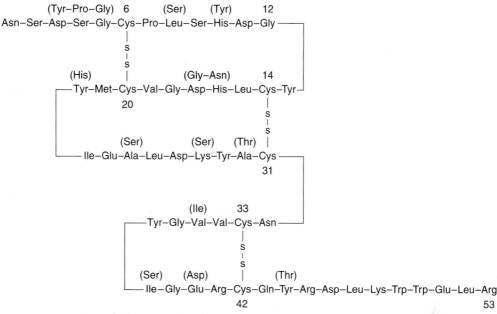

Figure 10.11   Amino acid sequence of human β-urogastrone. Positional amino acid differences between β-urogastrone and mouse EGF are shown in parentheses.

is still unknown, but there is some evidence that neural and probably hormonal (for example, GIP) factors are involved. GLP-1 stimulates insulin secretion in the presence of elevated glucose levels; it stimulates proinsulin gene expression and inhibits glucagon secretion. It lowers glucose levels in non-insulin-dependent diabetes mellitus when administered in pharmacalogical doses.

Villikinin.   Villi are a characteristic cellular feature of the mucosa of the small intestine. The fingerlike villi exhibit a number of peculiar movements, such as contraction and relaxation and a pendular swaying, and each villus moves independently of its neighbors. It is believed that lymph flow within these structures is hastened by their movements. Villous movement is affected by mechanical and chemical stimuli, nervous stimulation, and extracts of intestinal mucosa. Villous motility of an isolated jejunal loop transplanted into the carotid-jugular circulation was shown to be stimulated by intraduodenal administration of HCl. This observation suggested that villous activity might be regulated by a humoral factor. In cross-circulation experiments involving carotid-jugular anastomoses between two animals, administration of HCl into the stomach of one animal caused a substantial increase in villar activity in both animals. Other experiments provide evidence that acid chyme releases a substance that enters the bloodstream to stimulate villous movement. A substance that stimulates villous motility was extracted from the intestinal mucosa and named villikinin to describe its physiological action. Villikinin activity is found only in mucosa of the small intestine, with highest concentrations occurring in the duodenal mucosa of a number of mammalian species, including humans. Villikinin activity increases in human urine after a meal and after intraduodenal acid administration. The substance does not exhibit actions characteristic of the other GI hormones, therefore ruling any of them out as the putative humoral messenger. Villikinin appears to be a polypeptide, but little is known about its chemistry.

Enkephalins.   Endorphins, so-called opiate peptides, which include the enkephalins and β-endorphin, play important roles in CNS function (Chap. 21). Enkephalins have been demonstrated in the ECL cells and nerves of the digestive tract [23]. Opiate drugs, well known for their powerful actions on the GI tract, exhibit pronounced effects on GI motility and secretion. The opiate peptides also profoundly affect activity of the GI tract, by mechanisms identical to opiate drugs. They act as presynaptic or postsynaptic inhibitors and suppress the firing of most neurons tested. For example, opiate peptides specifically inhibit electrically induced contractions of the ileal smooth muscle by inhibiting neurotransmitter (acetylcholine) release. Opiate peptides are potent inhibitors of bicarbonate and protein secretion from the pancreas, suggesting that they affect the secretory mechanisms common to CCK and secretin on pancreatic secretion.

Enkephalins stimulate gastric acid secretion in dogs and also enhance histamine-stimulated acid secretion by isolated rat parietal cells. There are opioid receptors in the gastric muscle layers and in the mucosa. Naloxone and other opiate receptor antagonists inhibit acid secretory responses to food in humans. Large doses of naloxone also inhibit feeding-induced acid secretion in humans. These results suggest that endogenous opioid peptides have some physiological stimulatory role in the regulation of acid secretion in the stomach. However, morphine and some opioid peptides inhibit acid secretion. Both stimulatory and inhibitory opiate receptors may exist in the stomach. The major roles of endorphins in the GI tract may be to act as neurotransmitters and neuromodulators of autonomic nervous system actions on GI motility and secretion.

Neurotensin.   The tridecapeptide neurotensin (NT) was discovered and isolated from the bovine hypothalamus and subsequently found by radioimmunoassay also to be present in the GI tract (Table 10.2). Neurotensin (or a neurotensinlike peptide) is present in the discrete (N) cells rather specifically localized in the ileal mucosa of various birds and mammals. The NT-immunoreactive cells are situated in the upper two-thirds of the villi and appear to communicate with the intestinal lumen by means of microvilli. The morphological features of the NT-containing cells, which have microvilli and secretory granules located at the vascular pole, suggest that they may be sensitive to nutrient or other changes in the gut lumen. This sensitivity may provide the stimulus for the release of the peptide into the circulation.

Peptide YY and Neuropeptide Y.   Peptide YY (PYY), neuropeptide Y (NPY), and pancreatic polypeptide (PP) are three members of a family of regulatory peptides that exhibit considerable sequence homology [18]. In pigs there are 18 sequence identities (50% homology) between PP and PYY or NPY and 25 sequence identities (70% homology) between PYY and NPY. PYY and NPY are evolutionarily highly conserved peptides, with very similar sequences in most mammalian species.

PYY is localized in endocrine cells of the intestinal mucosa from various species. PYY-immunoreactive cells are numerous in the terminal ileum, colon, and rectum, whereas only a few such cells are found in the duodenum and jejunum. PYY cells extend from the basal lamina to the gut lumen. PYY is an intestinal hormone released into the blood in response to a meal or after intestinal perfusion with oleic acid. In contrast to PYY, NPY is strictly a neuropeptide. NPY nerve fibers are found throughout the intestinal tract, with the largest number in the upper small intestine. In the small intestine the occurrence of NPY-containing nerve cell bodies in the submucosal and myenteric ganglia indicates an intrinsic origin of NPY fibers. The distribution of NPY fibers in all layers of the gut wall suggests multiple functions of NPY, including a role in the regulation of intramural neuronal activities, smooth muscle tone, local blood flow, and epithelial transport. PYY and NPY have potent antisecretory effects in the small intestine. There is evidence that the hormone PPY and the neurotransmitter NPY are involved in the regulation of fluid and electrolyte secretion, motility, and blood flow in the intestine. There is evidence for a preferential localization of PYY-preferring receptors negatively coupled to adenylate cyclase and cAMP production in small intestinal crypt cells. Because PYY and NPY are the most potent physiological agents thus far identified as inhibitors of intestinal electrolyte secretion, the cryptic PYY receptor represents a promising target for antidiarrheal drugs [40, 41].

AUTONOMIC NERVOUS SYSTEM CONTROL OF GI FUNCTION

Although hormones play a dominant role in the control of GI function, the autonomic nervous system subserves a similar function [22]. "Acting singly and in concert, neural and hormonal mechanisms control the transverse flow of materials across the mucosa and the axial flow of digesta within the lumen" [21]. In addition, "The overlap of neural and endocrine segments, and the continuously changing character and location of intraluminal stimuli, engender the simultaneous release of several hormones whose interplay on digestive target tissues may be augmentary or inhibitory. The infusion of their effects determines the orderly progress and digestion of food."

The initial phase of neural control of GI function is regulated centrally by the anticipation of food, the so-called cephalic phase [30]. Subsequently, local neural and hormonal mechanisms are activated within the GI tract by mechanical and chemical stimuli derived from ingested foods. The stomach and small intestine are richly innervated by intrinsic and extrinsic nerves [36]. The intrinsic nerves comprise various plexuses that lie between the longitudinal and circular smooth muscle layers of the gut (Auerbach's plexus) and beneath the submucosal muscle layer (Meissner's plexus). These plexuses are innervated by extrinsic nerves derived mainly from the vagus nerve. Axons from neurons within the plexuses synapse with muscle fibers and glandular elements of the gut. Parasympathetic cholinergic (acetylcholine) and sympathetic adrenergic (norepinephrine) neurons affect smooth muscle motor activity and mucosal glandular secretion. Acetylcholine, for example, is a potent stimulus to gastric acid secretion. The intrinsic neurons of the gut contain a number of neurohormones such as VIP, substance P, somatostatin, NPY, and one or more endorphins.

GASTROINTESTINAL HORMONE MECHANISMS OF ACTION

Like other peptide hormones, the GI hormones interact with cell membrane receptors to stimulate or inhibit second-messenger production. Members of the secretin family of hormones (secretin, glucagon, VIP, and GIP) activate adenylate cyclase, which results in an elevation of intracellular levels of target tissue cAMP. Several models of GI hormone action mechanisms are provided.

Gastric Acid Secretion

The regulation of gastric acid secretion by the parietal cell involves complex interactions between a number of humoral or neurohormonal factors [3, 22, 31, 34, 37, 44]. Stimulation of GI secretions (e.g., HCl, pepsinogen, secretion from Brunner's glands) is, as for most secretory processes, regulated by intracellular increases in cAMP. Although gastrin is a potent secretogogue of gastric acid secretion, acetylcholine and histamine are also stimulatory to HCl secretion. The cholinergic neural pathways involved in gastrin and HCl secretion are unresolved. Histamine (see Fig. 6.12) is present in large amounts in the oxyntic mucosa of humans and other mammals. In addition to gastrin and acetylcholine receptors, parietal cells possess histamine (H_2) receptors. The actions of histamine are mediated through cAMP. Although gastrin and acetylcholine also stimulate parietal cell HCl secretion and potentiate the actions of each other and histamine, their actions do not involve cAMP, but rather an activation of phospholipase C and the production of inositol triphosphate and diacylglycerol as second messengers. Somatostatin and prostaglandins of the E series are inhibitory to HCl secretion by a mechanism involving inhibition of

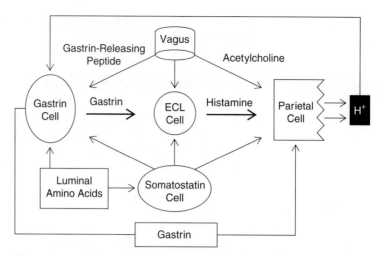

Figure 10.12 This diagram represents the interaction of the gastrin, enterochromaffinlike (ECL), parietal, and somatostatin cells. Both antral and fundic somatostatin cells appear to exert inhibitory influences on gastrin, ECL, and parietal cells, respectively. Neurotransmitter substances from either the vagus or the intrinsic gastric neural system are responsible for modulation of each of the cells and their secretory activity. Luminal amino acids stimulate gastrin release, whereas luminal protons inhibit gastrin release. Systemic secretion of gastrin primarily drives ECL cells to secrete histamine but may play some part in parietal cell secretion, although a trophic regulatory effect is more likely. The ECL cells release histamine, which presumably functions in a paracrine fashion to stimulate parietal cell secretion. (Reprinted by permission of the publisher from "A new look at an old hormone: Gastrin," Modlin and Tang. *Trends in Endocrinology and Metabolism* 4:51–57. ©1993 by Elsevier Science Inc.)

adenylate cyclase activation [25]. A hypothetical model depicting the control of parietal cell HCl secretion is provided (Fig. 10.12).

Exocrine Pancreatic Secretion

Pancreatic acinar cells possess two distinct classes of receptors coupled to the production of different second messengers. Secretin (and VIP in some species) elevates pancreatic cAMP levels and stimulates amylase secretion. Cholecystokinin (and related structures) also stimulates pancreatic amylase secretion and appears to do so by mobilizing cellular Ca^{2+}. Secretogogues that increase Ca^{2+} efflux and cAMP also cause depolarization of acinar cells. Acinar cells within the same acinus are electrically coupled; this coupling may provide a mechanism for amplifying the response of acinar cells to low concentrations of secretogogues. The result may be the potentiation of the CCK action by secretin on acinar enzyme secretion, because the action mechanism of each secretogogue is different and not funneled through the same transduction/second-messenger system. Synergism between CCK and secretin probably reflects their coupling to different signal transduction pathways: adenylate cyclase in the case of secretin, and phospholipase C, phosphoinositide turnover, and Ca^{2+} mobilization in the case of CCK (Fig. 10.13).

Trophic Actions of GI Hormones

The GI mucosa is sensitive to the trophic effects of several peptides. Although gastrin increases RNA, DNA, and protein synthesis in the stomach and duodenum, it does not appear to be trophic to the jejunoileum. The mucosal gastrin receptor has been character-

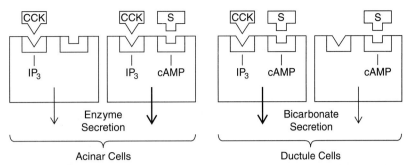

Figure 10.13 Hypothetical model for the synergistic actions of CCK and secretin (S) and second messengers on pancreatic enzyme and bicarbonate secretion.

ized. Specific gastrin binding is present in the oxyntic gland and duodenal mucosa, but is absent from the antral mucosa, liver, spleen, and kidney. Fasting decreases the circulating level of gastrin and the number of gastrin binding sites, whereas refeeding increases the plasma gastrin levels and restores the receptor number to normal. Treatment of fasted animals with pentagastrin prevents the decrease in receptor number. Thus gastric mucosal receptors are autoregulated, that is, their number is influenced by the availability of gastrin; they exhibit up-regulation in response to the hormone (Chap. 4).

Gastrin stimulates RNA, DNA, and protein synthesis along the entire length of the gut, with the exception of the esophagus and antrum. The pancreas is also a target for the trophic action of gastrin. These trophic effects are direct actions of gastrin and are not mediated through the action of another hormone. These observations suggest that increased food intake increases circulating levels of gastrin, which then increase gastrointestinal receptor numbers. This allows an enhanced trophic response to the hormone, which enables the GI tract to better use the increased metabolic substrates available.

EGF appears to play an important role in the development of neonatal intestinal epithelium. Administration of EGF in mature animals with normal intestines results in increased mucosal DNA content and proliferative activity, and increased substrate absorption from the intestine. Continuous intravenous infusion of EGF reduces mucosal atrophy and maintains disaccharidase activity during parenteral alimentation. Numerous other studies support the concept that EGF is an important trophic hormone of the intestinal mucosa [5, 33].

SUMMARY OF THE NEUROENDOCRINE CONTROL OF GI FUNCTION

At the close of the nineteenth century the digestive system was assumed to be solely under nervous control. The discovery of secretin introduced the concept of hormones in the control of GI functions. In recent years a complex system of regulation of these functions has been revealed. In addition to the generally accepted influence of the autonomic nervous system (sympathetic and parasympathetic) and of hormones (peptides), a system of peptide-containing nerves and local-acting peptide-releasing cells has been found to be important. Therefore, regulatory peptides can exert a general humoral control via the blood supply, a local paracrine action, or a neurotransmitter/neuromodulator action when released from nerves [4].

Food is taken into the mouth where ptyalin (salivary α-amylase) initiates digestion of starch. Food in the mouth is responsible for a reflex (cephalic) stimulation of gastric acid secretion. The food then transverses the esophagus to enter into the stomach through the gastroesophageal junction. Local reflex stimuli, resulting from distension of the stomach and from partially digested food products, particularly peptides and amino acids, are stimulatory to gastric acid secretion. Gastrin is the major humoral stimulus to hydrochloric acid secretion from the parietal cells of the gastric mucosa. Gastrin is also indirectly stimulatory to pepsinogen secretion from the chief cells of the mucosa of the body of the stomach. The pepsinogen is acted upon by HCl and split into the active enzyme pepsin. Increased gastric acid secretion then becomes inhibitory to further gastrin secretion. Gastrin and local reflex stimulation may then relax the pyloric sphincter and allow a bolus of food (chyme) to enter the first segment of the small intestine, the duodenum. The acid present in the chyme is stimulatory to secretin release from cells present within the duodenal mucosa. This bloodborne messenger then travels to the exocrine pancreas to cause water and bicarbonate release. These secretory products neutralize the acid present within the small intestine. Fats and proteins in the chyme stimulate the secretion of CCK from cells within the duodenal, jejunal, and ileal mucosa. CCK is carried by the blood to the exocrine pancreas and stimulates the acinar cells to release pancreatic enzymes: α-amylase, trypsin, chymotrypsin, and pancreatic lipase. Proteases split proteins and partially degraded proteins into their constituent amino acids. CCK also contracts the gallbladder, thus releasing bile salts into the intestinal lumen. These salts emulsify the fats into smaller globules and the fats are enzymatically degraded by pancreatic lipase into FFAs and monoglycerides. Starch and its partially degraded components, oligopolysaccharides, are further degraded by pancreatic α-amylase into glucose. Glucose is stimulatory to GIP secretion and possibly GLP-1 secretion from cells of the intestinal mucosa. These humoral messengers may then stimulate the release of insulin from beta cells of the pancreatic islets. By the action of insulin on the liver, the glucose now within the portal vein is taken up into the liver cells where it may be formed into starch and stored (Fig. 10.14).

GIP and possibly other hormones (bulbogastrone) of the small intestine, released in response to gastric acid, glucose, fats, and protein products, may provide feedback to the stomach to inhibit further secretion of gastric acid. Certain intrinsic neurons and other neuronlike cells within the intestinal lining contain peptide hormones such as somatostatin, VIP, substance P, and others. These neuropeptides, acting by neurocrine or paracrine mechanisms, control local secretory events and smooth muscle activity. The autonomic nervous system, particularly through its cholinergic component, plays an equally important augmentary role in the movement and digestion of foods within the GI tract [4].

PATHOPHYSIOLOGY

There are two well-documented examples of direct involvement by GI hormones in abnormal clinical conditions [35]. Most endocrine tumors of the GI system originate in the pancreatic islets. Although these tumors secrete hormones that are normally produced there (e.g., glucagon and insulin), these tumors may also secrete VIP or gastrin. Vasoactive intestinal peptide stimulates intestinal water secretion, and tumors consisting of VIP-secreting cells (VIPomas) are responsible for *pancreatic cholera* or the *watery diarrhea syndrome* (or syndrome of profuse watery diarrhea). Patients with the Zollinger-Ellison syndrome (gastrinoma) have high circulating gastrin levels (hypergastrinemia) of tumor origin. The overproduction of gastric acid usually results in severe duodenal ulcer formation. Two different types of the Zollinger-Ellison syndrome may exist, type I due to a hyperplasia of the antral G cells and type II due to gastrinoma of the pancreatic islets.

Regulation of the lower esophageal sphincter (LES), which is important in preventing the reflux of gastric contents, may be regulated by one or more GI hormones. Gastrin and motilin can contract the LES, whereas VIP is particularly potent as an inhibitor of LES tone. *Achalasia* is a condition where food accumulates in the esophagus because the gastroesophageal junction fails to relax. There is evidence that the smooth muscle of this junction is hypersensitive to normal circulating levels of gastrin, which could account for the prolonged contraction characteristic of this condition. Gastroesophageal reflux, on the

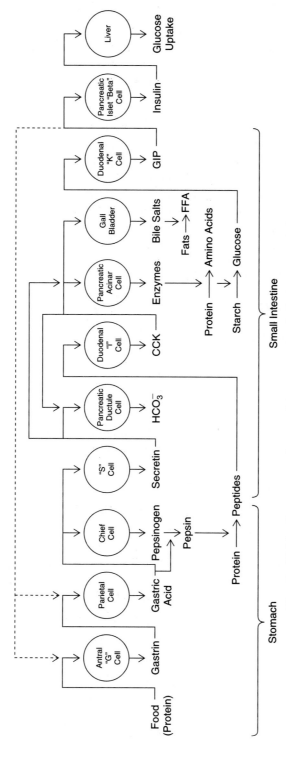

Figure 10.14 Summary scheme of hormone-metabolite control of GI function. Solid lines indicate stimulatory influences, dashed lines represent inhibitory stimuli.

other hand, is due to abnormal relaxation of the sphincter, and it is claimed that in some patients with this condition gastrin levels are low. The available data, however, are controversial.

GIP-containing cells are reported to be most numerous in duodenal samples from patients with low gastric secretory activity and less numerous in patients with duodenal ulcer disease. These observations correlate well with the proposed role of this hormone in the inhibition of gastric acid secretion.

Pernicious anemia is the result of an autoimmune process in which the gastric fundus undergoes atrophy and parietal cells are destroyed. As a result of ablation of the parietal cell mass, varying degrees of hypochlorhydria result. During this process, unregulated hypergastrinemia appears to reflect the lack of an acid feedback effect on the G cell and culminates in a profound trophic effect, predominantly evident in ECL (enterochromaffinlike) cell hyperplasia. Under physiologic conditions, ECL cells multiply by self-replication, and replication is greatly increased under the influence of gastrin. Consequent to sustained elevation of circulating gastrin levels, ECL cells initially undergo hyperplasia, followed by development of micronodules and finally carcinoids [25].

A number of GI hormones have proven useful in clinical practice [26, 28]. Gastrin is used for testing the potential for gastric acid secretion. Pentagastrin, which is commercially inexpensive, is usually used in these studies. CCK is used in the evaluation of gallbladder function; this hormone is also used to test for pancreatic exocrine function. Secretin has been used in the treatment of duodenal ulcer because it is inhibitory to gastric acid secretion and stimulatory to pancreatic bicarbonate-ion secretion. Secretin and glucagon stimulate tumor gastrin release (in contrast to their inhibitory effects on antral release of the hormone) and are used in the diagnosis of the Zollinger-Ellison syndrome.

EVOLUTIONARY RELATIONSHIPS OF THE GUT HORMONES

The gut hormones are localized to specific cells distributed throughout the GI tract. Most interesting, however, is that many of the gut hormones are also found in a variety of other tissues, including in the pancreas, pituitary, in neurons of the central and peripheral nervous systems, and in the skin of some vertebrates [32]. Within each of these tissues they regulate specific functions. In the hypothalamus of the brain, somatostatin regulates pituitary release of growth hormone (somatotropin); in the pancreas this peptide may regulate insulin and glucagon secretion, and in the antrum of the stomach somatostatin controls gastrin secretion.

The skin of anuran amphibians contains a number of biologically active peptides. Two of these peptides, cerulein and phyllocerulein, from related species of frogs (Fig. 10.15), contain the C-terminal pentapeptide sequence found in gastrin and CCK [8]. A peptide containing the C-terminal octapeptide of CCK has been found within the brain of sheep. These structurally related peptides would be expected to have been derived from a common ancestral molecule by gene duplication and divergence. A CCK-related peptide has been found in the brain and gut of cyclostomes and representatives of the agnathans, the oldest of the vertebrates. Immunoreactive gastrin has even been discovered in gut extracts of certain molluscan species and also in ganglia of an insect. Other hormones of the gut and brain are also related to peptides found in the skin of amphibians and in glands of mollusks.

Gastrin, CCK, and cerulein have been proposed as originating from a common ancestor over an evolutionary period. An evaluation of the evolutionary tree at a point near the stem of the vertebrate branch has revealed the existence of a novel neuropeptide, cionin, in the prochordate *Ciona intestinalis*, which is a possible common ancestor for both CCK and gastrin (Fig. 10.16). Evidence thus exists that a common C-terminal pentapeptide has been preserved over a long period of evolution.

$$SO_3H$$
$$|$$
Gastrin(17)   (pyro)Glu–Gly–Pro–Trp–Leu–Glu–Glu–Glu–Glu–Glu–Ala–Tyr–Gly–Trp–Met–Asp–Phe–NH$_2$

$$SO_3H$$
$$|$$
CCK(17-33)   –Asp–Pro–Ser–His–Arg–Ile–Ser–Asp–Arg–Asp–Tyr–Met–Gly–Trp–Met–Asp–Phe–NH$_2$

$$SO_3H$$
$$|$$
Cerulein   (pyro)Glu–Gln–Asp–Tyr–Thr–Gly–Trp–Met–Asp–Phe–NH$_2$

$$SO_3H$$
$$|$$
Phyllocerulein   (pyro)Glu–Glu–Tyr–Thr–Gly–Trp–Met–Asp–Phe–NH$_2$

Figure 10.15 CCK-gastrin family of peptides.

It appears that CCK is the ancestral peptide in this family, since fish and amphibians have CCK-like peptides but not gastrinlike peptides. It has been shown by immunological methods that gastrinlike peptides can first be detected in reptiles, thus suggesting that gastrin evolved at the level of the divergence of amphibians and reptiles in vertebrate phylogeny. Using receptor-binding and biological methods, the presence of gastrin in the chicken has been demonstrated. This suggests that once established, gastrin was conserved and probably did not arise separately in reptilian and mammalian lines [39].

Members of the secretin family of peptides are similar in structure, again suggesting that they are related by a common ancestry. The genes that coded for the ancestral member of this group of peptides probably underwent duplication, thus producing one or more daughter genes. These genes, through independent mutations, diverged to yield distinct, but related, peptide hormones (see Fig. 21.15).

Substance P is structurally similar to certain peptides found in frog skin (Fig. 10.17). These substances are referred to as *tachykinins* (from the Greek, *takus* for fast) because of their rapid actions on smooth muscle. Physalaemin is found in the skin of the South American frog, *Physalaemus bigilonigerus*, and other species of this genus. The shorter peptide, phyllomedusin, is found in the skin of the Amazonian hylid frog, *Phyllomedusa bicolor*, and several related species. Eledoisin, a peptide similar in structure to SP and other tachykinins, is found in the posterior salivary glands of the Mediterranean octopus of the genus *Eledone*.

$$SO_3 \ SO_3$$
$$| \quad |$$
Cionin   Asn–Tyr–Tyr–Gly–Trp–Met–Asp–Phe–NH$_2$

$$SO_3$$
$$|$$
CCK   Asp–Tyr–Met–Gly–Trp–Met–Asp–Phe–NH$_2$

$$(SO_3)$$
$$|$$
Gastrin   –Glu–Ala–Tyr–Gly–Trp–Met–Asp–Phe–NH$_2$

Figure 10.16 Structure of cionin isolated form the protochordate *Ciona intestinalis* compared to the C-terminal sequences of gastrin and CCK. Note that cionin is a perfect hybrid of gastrin and CCK with sulfated Tyr in both positions 6 and 7 from the C-terminus. Modified from Johnson and Rehfeld [16].

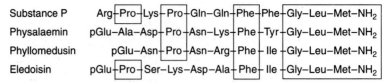

Substance P		Arg	Pro	Lys	Pro	Gln–Gln	Phe	Phe	Gly–Leu–Met–NH$_2$
Physalaemin		pGlu–Ala–Asp	Pro	Asn–Lys			Phe	Tyr	Gly–Leu–Met–NH$_2$
Phyllomedusin		pGlu–Asn	Pro	Asn–Arg			Phe	Ile	Gly–Leu–Met–NH$_2$
Eledoisin		pGlu	Pro	Ser–Lys–Asp–Ala			Phe	Ile	Gly–Leu–Met–NH$_2$

Figure 10.17 Comparative primary structures of peptides related to substance P. Amino acid residues within the peptides located at identical positions to substance P are enclosed.

A most amazing discovery relative to gastric acid secretion has been made in frogs, the implications of which have relevance to clinical medicine [38]. In the frog *Rheobatrachus silus*, the female broods its young (tadpoles) in its stomach. Apparently the young secrete a substance that inhibits gastric acid secretion. This substance has been identified as prostaglandin E$_2$. Inhibition of acid secretion presumably commences when the eggs or early stage larvae are swallowed and lasts until the young emerge from the mother's mouth as frogs (Fig. 10.18). Thus this species of frog has apparently evolved a unique hormonal control of the environment in which the young develop. Prostaglandins are known to inhibit gastric acid secretion and also to stimulate gastric-mucin secretion to form a protective barrier. It is known that nonsteroidal anti-inflammatory drugs inhibit the synthesis of prostaglandins. These drugs, therefore, can induce peptic ulcers by removing the normal protective covering of the mucosal surface normally protected by prostaglandins [38, 43].

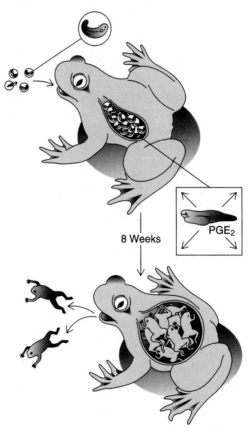

Figure 10.18 Role of a prostaglandin in protecting growth of tadpoles within the stomach of a female frog. (Adapted from "No frogs in Berlin," Nancy Lou Makris, and used by permission. *Hospital Practice* 19(2):33–46, 1984.)

REFERENCES

[1] Adelson, J. W., and P. E. Miller. 1985. Pancreatic secretion by nonparallel exocytosis: potential resolution of a long controversy. *Science* 228:993–96.

[2] Bayliss, W. M., and E. H. Starling. 1902. The mechanism of pancreatic secretion. *J. Physiol.* 28:325–53.

[3] Beck, B. 1988. Gastric inhibitory polypeptide: a gut hormone with anabolic functions. *J. Mol. Endocrinol.* 2:169–74.

[4] Beck, K. 1989. Autonomic control of secretion of gastric acid and pepsin. *J. Auton. Pharmac.* 9:419–28.

[5] Bragg, L. E., J. S. Thompson, and L. F. Rikkers. 1991. Influence of nutrient delivery on gut structure and function. *Nutrition* 7:237–43.

[6] Daikh, D. I., J. O. Douglass, and J. P. Adelman. 1989. Structure and expression of the human motilin gene. *DNA* 8:615–21.

[7] Fehmann, H.-C., and B. Goke. 1993. International symposium on glucagonlike peptide 1, Copenhagen, Denmark, 17–19 May, 1993. *TEM* 4:253–4.

[8] Garlicki, J., P. K. Konturek, J. Majka, N. Kwiecien, and S. J. Konturek. 1990. Cholecystokinin receptors and vagal nerves in control of food intake in rats. *Amer. J. Physiol.* 258:E40–45.

[9] Geracioti, T. D., Jr., and R. A. Liddle. 1988. Impaired cholecystokinin secretion in bulimia nervosa. *New Engl. J. Med.* 319:683–88.

[10] Grider, J. R. 1989. Identification of neurotransmitters regulating intestinal peristaltic reflex in humans. *Gastroenterology* 97:1414–9.

[11] Grider, J. R., and J. R. Rivier. 1990. Vasoactive intestinal peptide (VIP) as transmitter of inhibitory motor neurons of the gut: evidence from the use of selective VIP antagonists and VIP antiserum. *J. Pharmacol. Exper. Ther.* 253:738–42.

[12] Greenstein, R. J., L. Isola, and J. Gordon. 1990. Differential cholecystokinin gene expression in brain and gut of the fasted rat. *Amer. J. Med. Sci.* 299:32–37.

[13] Grossman, M. I. 1979. Neural and hormonal regulation of gastrointestinal function: an overview. *Annu. Rev. Physiol.* 41:27–33.

[14] Grube, D., and W. G. Forssmann. 1979. Morphology and function of the entero-endocrine cells. *Horm. Metab. Res.* 11:589–606.

[15] Huang, S. C., D. H. Yu, S. A. Want, S. Mantey, J. D. Gardner, and R. T. Jenson. 1989. Importance of sulfation of gastrin or cholecystokinin (CCK) on affinity for gastrin and CCK receptors. *Peptides* 10:785–89.

[16] Johnsen, A. H. and J. F. Rehfeld. 1993. Phylogeny of gastrin. In *Gastrin,* ed. J. W. Walsh, pp. 15–27. New York: Raven Press, Ltd.

[17] Krause, J. E., Y. Takeda, and A. D. Hershey. 1992. Structure, functions, and mechanisms of substance P receptor action. *J. Invest. Dermatol.* 98:2S–7S.

[18] Laburthe, M. 1990. Peptide YY and neuropeptide Y in the gut. Availability, biological actions, and receptors. *TEM* 25:168–74.

[19] Larsson, L. I., N. Goltermann, L. De Magistris, J. F. Rehfeld, and T. W. Schwartz. 1979. Somatostatin cell processes or pathways for paracrine secretion. *Science* 205:1393–94.

[20] Liddle, R. A., I. D. Goldfine, M. S. Rosen, R. A. Taplitz, and J. A. Williams. 1985. Cholecystokinin bioactivity in human plasma. *J. Clin. Invest.* 75:1144–52.

[21] Makhlouf, G. M. 1974. The neuroendocrine design of the gut. *Gastroenterology* 67:159–84.

[22] Makhlouf, G. M. 1990. Neural and hormonal regulation of function in the gut. *Hosp. Pract.* 25:79–98.

[23] Manara, L., and A. Bianchetti. 1985. The central and peripheral influences of opioids on gastrointestinal propulsion. *Annu. Rev. Pharmacol. & Toxicol.* 25:249–73.

[24] Mezey, E., and M. Palkovits. 1992. Localization of targets for anti-ulcer drugs in cells of the immune system. *Science* 258:1662–1665.

[25] Modlin, I. M. and L. H. Tang. 1993. A new look at an old hormone: Gastrin. *TEM* 4:51–7.

[26] Morely, J. E. 1989. An approach to the development of drugs for appetite disorders. *Neuropsychobiology* 21:22–30.

[27] Pearse, A. G. E. 1981. The diffuse neuroendocrine system: falsification and verification of a concept. In *Cellular basis of chemical messengers in the digestive system,* eds. M. I. Grossman, M. A. B. Brazier, and J. Lechago, pp. 13–19. New York: Academic Press, Inc.

[28] Peikin, S. R. 1989. Role of cholecystokinin in the control of food intake. *Gastroenterol. Clin. N. Amer.* 18:757–75.

[29] Powers, M. A., and T. N. Pappas. 1989. Physiologic approaches to the control of obesity. *Ann. Surg.* 209:255–60.

[30] Raybould, H. E., E. Kolve, and Y. Tache. 1988. Central nervous system action of calcitonin gene–related peptide to inhibit gastric emptying in the conscious rat. *Peptides* 9:735–37.

[31] Saffouri, B., et al. 1980. Gastrin and somatostatin secretion by perfused rat stomach: functional linkage of antral peptides. *Amer. J. Physiol.* 238:G495–501.

[32] Said, S. I. 1980. Peptides common to the nervous system and the gastrointestinal tract. *Front. Neuroendocrinol.* 6:293–331.

[33] Sakamoto, T., J. S. Swierczek, W. D. Ogden, and J. C. Thompson. 1985. Cytoprotective effect of pentagastrin and epidermal growth factor on stress ulcer formation. *Ann. Surg.* 201:290–95.

[34] Schubert, M. L., et al. 1987. Paracrine regulation of gastric acid secretion by fundic somatostatin. *Amer. J. Physiol.* 252:G485–90.

[35] Silen, M. L., and J. D. Gardner. 1993. Gastrointestinal peptides and cancer. *TEM* 4:131–5.

[36] Sternini, C. 1988. Structural and chemical organization of the myenteric plexus. *Annu. Rev. Physiol.* 50:81–93.

[37] Tache, Y. 1988. CNS peptides and regulation of gastric acid secretion. *Annu. Rev. Physiol.* 50:19–39.

[38] Tyler, M. J., D. J. C. Shearman, R. Franco, P. O'Brien, R. F. Seamark, and R. Kelly. 1983. Inhibition of gastric acid secretion in the gastric brooding frog, *Rheobatrachus silus. Science* 220:609–10.

[39] Vigna, S. R. 1986. Evolution of hormone and receptor diversity: cholecystokinin and gastrin. *Amer. Zool.* 26:1033–40.

[40] Voisin, T., C. Rouyer-Fessard, and M. Laburthe. 1990. Distribution of common peptide YY-neuropeptide Y receptor along rat intestinal villus-crypt axis. *Amer. J. Physiol.* 258:G753–9.

[41] Wahlestedt, C., and D. J. Reis. 1993. Neuropeptide Y-related peptides and their receptors—are the receptors potentially therapeutic drug targets? *Annu. Rev. Pharmacol. Toxicol.* 32:309–52.

[42] Walsh, J. H. 1988. Peptides as regulators of gastric acid secretion. *Annu. Rev. Physiol.* 50:41–63.

[43] Weissmann, G. 1984. No frogs in Berlin. *Hosp. Pract.* 19(2):33–46.

[44] Wolfe, M. M., and A. H. Soll. 1988. The physiology of gastric acid secretion. *New Engl. J. Med.* 319:1707–15.

Pancreatic Hormones and Metabolic Regulation

11

In 1889 Von Mering and Minkowski noted that total pancreatectomy in dogs resulted in severe and fatal diabetes [36]. Subsequent experimenters using a variety of animal species also observed that polyuria and glycosuria (characteristic symptoms of diabetes mellitus) and death always followed removal of the pancreas. It was then noted that after ligation of the pancreatic ducts in rabbits the acinar component of the gland atrophied, but the islets remained normal; the animals did not become hyperglycemic as they did after total pancreatectomy. From these and other observations, it was concluded that the islets of Langerhans, rather than the pancreatic acinar cells, are essential in the control of carbohydrate metabolism.

Two mechanisms of control were suggested: the blood was modified while passing through the islet tissue or the islets produced an internal secretion. Extracts from the ligated pancreases of dogs, which consisted mainly of islet tissue, were shown to reduce blood sugar levels of diabetic dogs. Banting and Best [2, 5] provided convincing evidence that, indeed, the pancreatic islets produced an internal secretion, a hormone, which was responsible for the control of blood glucose levels. In 1926 insulin was obtained in crystalline form and in 1954 Sanger determined the primary structure of this hormone, and received a Nobel Prize for his discovery [43]. The physiological roles and chemistry of the other major pancreatic hormone concerned with carbohydrate metabolism, glucagon, also have been elucidated. More recently it has been discovered that the pancreas is the source of other hormones (e.g., somatostatin and pancreatic polypeptide) also concerned with nutrient homeostasis.

The endocrine roles of the pancreas are to maintain a constant blood glucose level and to facilitate cellular storage of foodstuffs following a meal, and to provide for the mobilization of these depot metabolic substrates during periods of fasting. The underproduction or overproduction of insulin or glucagon can therefore profoundly affect the storage and use of carbohydrates, fats, and proteins within the liver, adipose tissue, and muscle, thus severely affecting cellular metabolic processes. Of all the described endocrinopathies, diabetes mellitus is by far the most common.

THE ENDOCRINE PANCREAS

The endocrine pancreas, which consists of islets of tissue (Fig. 11.1) dispersed among the much larger mass of the exocrine pancreas, was first described by Langerhans in 1869 in his doctoral dissertation. There are approximately 1 to 2 million islets in a

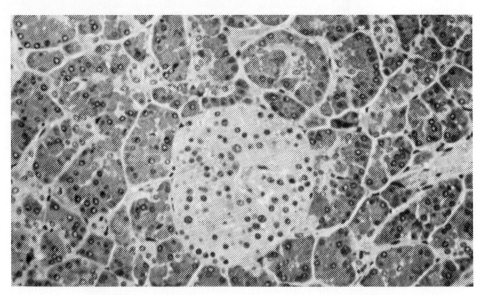

Figure 11.1 Photomicrograph of a human pancreatic islet.

normal human pancreas, but they represent only about 1% to 2% of pancreatic tissue. Two main cell types can be visualized by histological methods; the α cells are the source of glucagon and the more prevalent β cells are the source of insulin. The following cells are present in much smaller numbers: D cells, the source of pancreatic somatostatin (SRIF), and F cells, the source of pancreatic polypeptide (PP). Several lines of evidence point to the β cell as the source of insulin. Fluorescent-labeled antibodies to insulin localize to the β cells, and alloxan, a drug that specifically destroys the β cells, causes diabetes mellitus. In addition, stimuli that excessively increase insulin secretion cause β-cell degranulation.

In humans the pancreas develops during the fifth week of gestation from two diverticula of the duodenum close to the hepatic diverticulum [13, 44]. The two primordia then fuse and the duct of the ventral diverticulum becomes the main pancreatic duct leading to the opening into the duodenum. Initially, each primordium consists of a network of anastomosing tubules lined by a single layer of cells. These cells differentiate into the individual acini that constitute the functional units of pancreatic enzyme secretion. It is believed that the islet cells derive from the embryonic pancreatic ducts, which are endodermal in origin [31].

Although much information has accumulated relative to the endocrine role of the pancreatic islets, it is not clear why the pancreatic cells are disseminated as discrete clusters within the exocrine gland in most higher vertebrates. There is evidence, however, that the *peri-insular acini* differ from the remaining exocrine pancreas, both in their cytological features and secretory activity. There is also evidence for the preferential release of certain enzymes from the exocrine pancreas in response to certain intragastroduodenal nutrients. Therefore, the coordination of particular exocrine gland enzyme secretions may be regulated by hormones deriving from the pancreatic islets. Acinar amylase mRNA levels progressively decrease in rats rendered diabetic. Insulin reverses this effect in the pancreatic acinar cells by inducing a selective increase in amylase mRNA synthesis [29, 35]. Through a paracrine action on amylase production within adjacent acinar cells, insulin may indirectly control the degradation of starch within the gut and thus control the availability of glucose for absorption into the animal.

Glucose homeostasis involves a push-pull system that controls glucose flux into and out of the extracellular space. By their actions on the liver, adipose tissue, and muscle, insulin and glucagon maintain a balance of glucose production and utilization that requires "a coordinated relationship of the glucagon-producing α (A) cells and the insulin-secret-

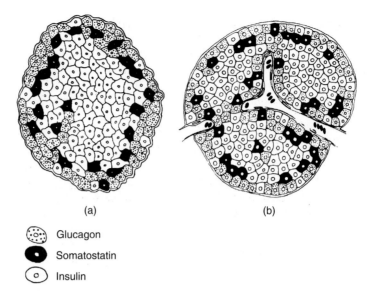

(a)   (b)

Glucagon

Somatostatin

Insulin

Figure 11.2 (a) Schematic representation of the number and distribution of insulin-, glucagon-, and somatostatin-containing cells in the normal rat islet. Note the characteristic position of most glucagon- and somatostatin-containing cells at the periphery of the islet, surrounding the centrally located insulin-containing cells. (b) Schematic representation of the number and distribution of insulin, glucagon- and somatostatin-containing cells in the normal human islet. This pattern divides the total islet mass into smaller subunits, each of which contains a center formed mainly of insulin cells and surrounded by glucagon and somatostatin cells. Cell types for which a definite function and morphology have not been determined are intentionally omitted. (From Unger et al. [52], with permission of Academic Press, Inc., New York.)

ing β (B) cells under the guidance of a perceptive glucose sensor" [52]. The individual insulin cells, glucagon cells, and somatostatin cells are believed to be arranged within the pancreas in such a manner as to accomplish that feat. In humans and rats the generalized arrangement of the cellular subtypes of the pancreatic islets is shown (Fig. 11.2). Endocrine cells are arranged as cords among the capillary channels within the islets [52]. Gap junctions have been demonstrated between β cells, as well as between α and β cells. These plasma membrane specializations are known to permit electrical conductivity between cells, as well as the passage of low molecular weight substances from one cell to another. There is evidence that depolarization of one islet cell may lead to the concomitant depolarization of other islet cells. Thus it is possible that hormone secretion from the pancreatic islets may involve the functional integration of a number of secretory units. It may be significant that the α and D cells contact other cell types, whereas the β cells mainly contact other β cells. The peripheral tricellular zone of the islets is innervated by autonomic afferent nerves and is particularly well vascularized.

INTERMEDIARY METABOLISM

In order to appreciate fully the physiological roles of the pancreatic hormones and the consequences of their underproduction or overproduction, one should review the general outline of carbohydrate metabolism and the relationships of lipid and protein metabolism to glucose production. The consequences of an excess or deficiency of insulin, for example, are hypoglycemia or hyperglycemia, respectively, which result from metabolic defects in glucose metabolism.

As discussed earlier (Chap. 10), the gastrointestinal hormones promote the movement of foodstuffs through the GI tract and provide the chemical environment and enzymes necessary for their degradation into less complex metabolic substrates. These molecular products (e.g., monosaccharides, free fatty acids, and amino acids) then traverse the luminal lining of the gut and enter the hepatic portal vein and/or the lymphatic system. Most venous outflow of the abdominal GI organs passes through the liver before reaching the hepatic veins to be carried to other parts of the body.

The normal fasting level of glucose in the peripheral venous blood of humans is 60 to 80 mg/dl. The movement of glucose into hepatic cells is by facilitated diffusion in response to insulin. Once within the hepatocyte, glucose may move in a pathway toward glycogen formation (glycogenesis), or it may be catabolized through the glycolytic (Embden-Meyerhoff) pathway to pyruvic acid. An alternate pathway for glucose catabolism prominent in certain cells (e.g., adrenal steroidogenic cells) is the *direct oxidative pathway*, or *hexose monophosphate shunt* (HMP). The HMP pathway provides pentoses, which are essential components of nucleic acids and nucleotides. This pathway also provides $NADPH_2$, which is important in many reductive biosynthetic processes such as fatty acid and steroid hormone synthesis.

Intracellular glucose is first converted to glucose-6-PO_4 by the enzyme *glucokinase* (Fig. 11.3). Depending on the particular hormonal status of the hepatocyte, the glucose-6-PO_4 may be converted to glucose-1-PO_4 by phosphoglucomutase and then combined with uridine diphosphate to form uridine diphosphoglucose (UDPG). Through the action of the enzyme *glycogen synthetase*, a glucose moiety is transferred to existing glycogen polymers through a glycosidic linkage. Hormonal stimulation of hepatic *phosphorylase* may subsequently cleave the glycogen polymer into monomeric glucose-1-PO_4 units. The glucose-1-PO_4 produced through *glycogenolysis* is converted to glucose-6-PO_4, which can then follow one of two pathways: it may be converted to glucose through the action of glucose-6-phosphatase (an enzyme specific to liver and kidney) and be released from the

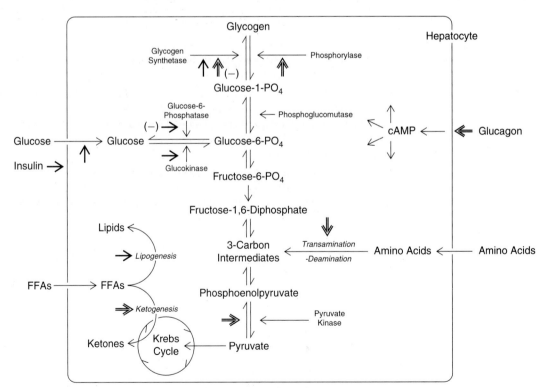

Figure 11.3 General scheme of hormonal regulation of hepatic carbohydrate metabolism. The more prominent actions of insulin (solid arrows) and glucagon (open arrows) are indicated.

cell, or it may be metabolized through a number of enzymatic steps to pyruvate [33]. Pyruvic acid is then converted to acetyl-CoA, which can enter into the *Krebs (citric acid) cycle* or be utilized in fat biosynthesis (lipogenesis).

Glycogen formation and deposition within hepatic cells provides an important storage form of readily utilizable carbohydrate for energy production through the glycolytic pathway and the citric acid cycle. Similar depositions of glycogen are found within skeletal muscle cells and other cells that require immediate sources of this substrate for energy production. Hormones play key roles in the conversion of these metabolites into more readily available and usable energy substrates.

Molecular interconversion between carbohydrates, proteins, and fats provides metabolic intermediates for use within the Embden-Meyerhoff pathway and the citric acid cycle. For example, glycerol derived from the breakdown of fats (lipolysis) can enter the glycolytic pathway. *Deamination* of amino acids or *transamination* between certain amino acids and keto acids may provide intermediates, such as pyruvic acid or α-keto-glutaric acid, that can be used within the glycolytic pathway or citric acid cycle, respectively (Fig. 11.4). Lactate (and pyruvate) released from muscle is transported to the liver, where it serves as a gluconeogenic precursor (Cori cycle). Alanine can flow from muscle to liver where it, too, serves as a gluconeogenic precursor (glucose-alanine cycle). Use of noncarbohydrate substrates, such as amino acids, provides a glucose-sparing action, and the molecules may also be employed directly in glucose formation (*gluconeogenesis*).

Free fatty acids (FFAs) absorbed from the gut may be reformed within mucosal cells into monoglycerides, diglycerides, or triglycerides and complexed with phospholipids and proteins within these cells into small micelles referred to as *chylomicrons*. These particles circulate initially within the lymphatic ducts and are then delivered to the blood vascular system. Through the action of the enzyme *lipoprotein lipase,* localized within the endothelium of the capillaries, the chylomicrons are cleared from the circulation. The released FFAs are then taken up by adipose cells to be re-esterified into triglycerides. Most of the glycerol required for fat synthesis is derived from the glycolytic metabolism of glucose within adipocytes. Within these cells the fats are stored in the form of one or more large fat globules. Through the initial action of *triglyceride lipases* and the subsequent action of diglyceride and monoglyceride lipases, these fats are converted back to FFAs and glycerol and released into the bloodstream.

Within the liver the glycerol liberated by fat breakdown within adipocytes is converted to phosphoglyceraldehyde and used within the glycolytic pathway by catabolism to pyruvic acid or by conversion through glucogenic processes to glucose. The FFAs are broken down by β-oxidation within mitochondria to acetyl-CoA. The acetyl-CoA is then used within the Krebs cycle, another example of a glucose-sparing mechanism. Free fatty acids are also derived de novo from acetyl-CoA through a lipogenic pathway present in many cells. Fatty acid synthesis stops in most cells when the chain is 16-carbon-atoms

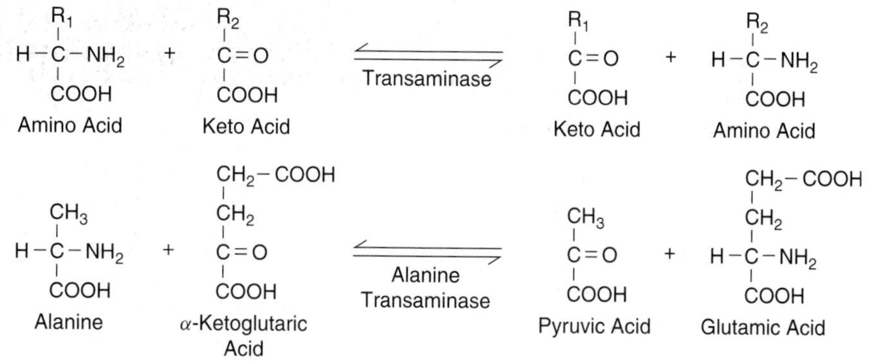

Figure 11.4   General (top) and specific (bottom) scheme of amino acid–keto acid transamination.

long. Within fat cells the FFAs are combined with glycerol to form neutral fats. Fatty acids are also combined with phosphoric acid and other cellular components to form phospholipids, which may comprise important structural elements of cell membranes or other organelles.

Amino acids derived from the breakdown of proteins within the digestive tract are actively transported across the intestinal mucosal cells and delivered to the liver, where they are used after deamination or transamination processes in carbohydrate metabolism (Fig. 11.4). They also pass through the liver to the general circulation to be used by other cells as energy substrates, or they can be employed as building blocks in protein synthesis, particularly in muscle cells. The entrance of amino acids into cells involves an active transport mechanism that is stimulated by insulin and other growth hormones.

INSULIN

Insulin is one of a number of hormones that is required for normal growth and development (see Chap. 12). In addition it is the only hormone that directly lowers blood glucose levels. Most other hormones, if they have an effect on glucose metabolism, tend to elevate blood levels of the sugar. Insulin is a dominant metabolic regulatory factor. Absolute insulin deficiency results in unrestrained glucose production, lipolysis, ketogenesis, proteolysis and, ultimately, death. Massive insulin excess results in hypoglycemia with consequent brain failure and again, ultimately, death. Clearly, insulin is a potent and critically important hormone [11]. An understanding of the chemistry and biological actions of insulin is necessary, therefore, before normal and abnormal physiology of carbohydrate metabolism can be understood.

Synthesis, Chemistry, and Metabolism

Insulin is a polypeptide consisting of an A and a B chain of 21 and 30 amino acids, respectively [45]. The two chains of the dimer are linked through a pair of disulfide bonds; an intrachain disulfide bond connects the sixth and eleventh amino acids within the A chain. There are minor differences in the primary structure of insulin from different vertebrate species. In mammals these differences most often are restricted to the 8, 9, and 10 positions within the intrachain disulfide bond of the A chain and to position 30 of the B chain (Fig. 11.5). Although these differences do not alter considerably the biological potency of the mammalian insulins used in replacement therapy for diabetes mellitus, they are sufficient to make insulin antigenic in some patients. Individuals who become resistant to insulin from one species of animal usually respond to insulin from another source.

Insulin is synthesized from a *proinsulin* molecule where the two chains are united by a connecting peptide, in the human usually consisting of 31 amino acids, not counting the pair of basic residues at the sites of cleavage (Fig. 11.6). Studies on the translation of insulin mRNA have demonstrated that proinsulin is itself derived from a *preproinsulin* precursor. After removal of a C-terminal 23-amino-acid sequence, the proinsulin structure folds onto itself to provide disulfide linkage between the two presumptive individual chains. Enzymatic action then cleaves the connecting peptide to yield the definitive hormonal product (Fig. 11.6). Under conditions of excessive stimulation, proinsulin is also secreted by vesicular exocytosis, along with insulin from the β cells. Because of its slower disappearance rate, proinsulin may constitute up to 50% of the insulinlike material in the blood in the basal state.

Proinsulins and C-peptides have been isolated and sequenced from several mammalian species. The high interspecies variability of mammalian C-peptides is considered to be the result of an evolutionary rate many times that of insulin. Such structural variation might be expected since this portion of the molecule is a by-product of insulin production. Nevertheless, this structural heterogeneity has allowed for the evolution of the insulinlike growth factors (Chap. 12).

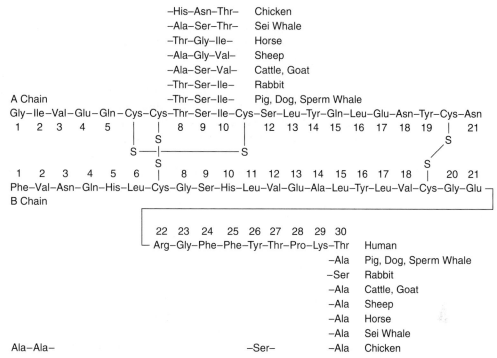

Figure 11.5 Comparative primary structures of the vertebrate insulins.

Insulin is complexed with zinc within the β cells of the pancreas and, in some species, in the form of rhombic crystals within the secretory vesicles. Insulin is normally degraded within the liver and kidneys, having a half-life of about 5 minutes in the human. The major enzyme responsible for insulin degradation is *hepatic glutathione insulin dehydrogenase*, which disrupts the hormone into its individual A and B chains. The transhydrogenase acts in conjunction with *glutathione*, a cysteine-containing tripeptide, which acts as a cofactor for the transhydrogenase and reduces the individual half-cysteine moieties of the interchain disulfide bonds.

Physiological Roles

In response to elevated glucose levels, insulin is promptly released from the pancreatic islets. Insulin interacts with plasmalemmal receptors of a number of different cell types.

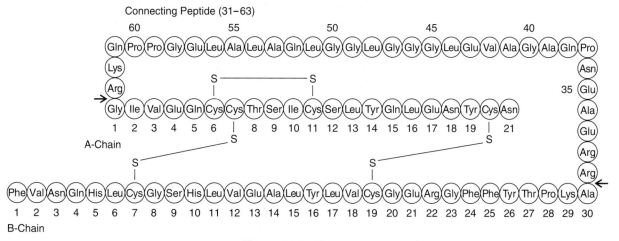

Figure 11.6 Primary structure of porcine proinsulin.

Most important are the actions of insulin on hepatic cells, muscle cells, and adipose tissue cells. In each case the effect of insulin is to enhance the uptake of glucose into the cells where it is metabolized and stored as glycogen or used as an energy substrate in the synthesis of proteins or fats.

Within the liver, insulin activates glycogen synthetase, which produces a direct flow of glucose toward glycogen formation. Glucokinase activity is enhanced, which provides a pool of glucose-6-PO_4 that is then converted to glucose-1-PO_4 and to uridine diphosphoglucose. Conversion of intracellular glucose to glucose-6-PO_4 prevents glucose release from hepatocytes.

In fat cells insulin-stimulated glucose uptake results in enhanced catabolism of the sugar to glycerol [35]. Insulin activation of endothelial cell lipoprotein lipase results in the release of FFAs from chylomicrons. These fatty acids are transported into fat cells where they combine with glycerol to form triglycerides and are added to the lipid droplets within the fat cells. Lipid synthesis is stimulated by insulin via an activation of citrate lipase, acetyl-CoA carboxylase, fatty acid synthase, and glycerol-3-phosphate dehydrogenase [12].

Insulin stimulates the active transport of glucose and amino acids into muscle cells and, by an unknown mechanism, protein synthesis is enhanced. Glycolysis and oxidative phosphorylation of glucose derivatives provide the energy required for such metabolic activity.

Insulin plays an important role in potassium homeostasis. Insulin is stimulatory to K^+ uptake by cells and, at excessively high concentrations, causes extracellular hypokalemia. Low levels of insulin appear to have a permissive effect in the cellular uptake of K^+. Infusion of somatostatin, which reduces fasting insulin levels, is associated with an increase in basal serum K^+ concentration in the human.

Mechanisms of Action

Insulin, like other growth factors (see Chap. 12), mediates its action through a novel plasma membrane receptor [25, 27]. These receptors possess kinase activity but the details of the mechanisms leading to a cellular response are ill-defined.

Insulin Receptor.   The insulin receptor consists of an α subunit that contains the insulin-binding domain and a β subunit that contains a tyrosine kinase domain [18]. The insulin receptor is composed of two α and two β subunits held together covalently by both inter- and intrasubunit disulfide bridges (Fig. 11.7). Both subunits are derived from a common polypeptide precursor, and both are glycosylated in their native forms. The α subunits provide the binding sites for insulin and are wholly extracellular, being anchored by virtue of covalent attachment to the β subunit. The β subunit is a transmembrane protein with globular domains at both the extracellular and cytosolic surfaces. It must be assumed that the intracellular signal(s) elicited by the insulin receptor arise from the activity of the cytosolic domain of the β subunit, after the activation via conformational changes transmitted from the α subunit and the membrane and cytosolic domain of the β subunit.

Insulin binding to the α subunit activates autophosphorylation of the β subunit. Once phosphorylated, the β subunit is an activated tyrosine kinase. The details of other forms of phosphorylation of the insulin receptor and, subsequently, of its substrates are not well understood. The binding of insulin and receptor autophosphorylation appear to be events necessary to trigger insulin action.

When insulin binds to cell-surface receptors on cultured or freshly isolated cells, the hormone receptor complex is internalized. Subsequently, a series of intracellular events ensue that can dissociate the hormone from its receptor. Internalization is the major mechanism by which cell surface insulin receptors are down-regulated. The structures involved in endocytosis appear to be relatively nonspecific and similar for many other peptide hor-

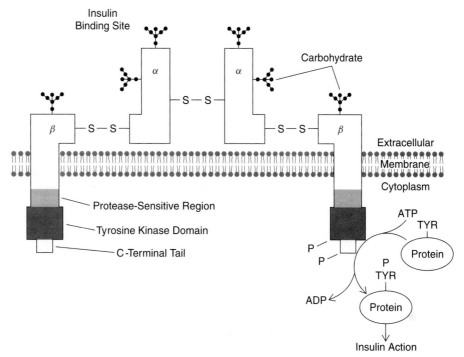

Figure 11.7 Diagrammatic structure of the insulin receptor.

mones. Insulin is initially localized in coated pits on the cell surface, which invaginate, fuse, and then fission to form coated vesicles. These vesicles progressively become larger noncoated structures called endosomes. The acidification of endosomes promotes dissociation of the ligand receptor complex, permitting the ligand and receptor to be processed independently.

The receptor appears to be recycled predominantly from this endosomal compartment. The receptor can also be recycled from other vesicular structures such as lysosomes. Certain types of receptors, such as the LDL receptor (Chap. 15), recycle continuously, whereas internalization and recycling of the insulin receptor predominantly requires ligand binding. Thus down-regulation of the receptor is determined primarily by the rate of receptor endocytosis and the rate of receptor recycling. In the short term, binding of insulin may therefore cause some reversible redistribution of receptor between plasma membrane and subcellular pools, which is manifested as a decrease in the number of cell-surface binding sites. If a substantial fraction of receptors is occupied, this may (in the longer term) lead to accelerated degradation of the internalized receptor pool, resulting in a net loss of receptors from the cell surface.

Second Messengers of Insulin Receptor Activation. Despite extensive studies, the mechanism by which insulin elicits its various intracellular effects remains unknown [42]. Recent data implicate the intrinsic tyrosine kinase activity of the insulin receptor in the initiation of many of the biological responses to insulin. However, other proposed pathways include the generation of a novel second messenger, effects via Ca^{2+}, or possibly even a direct effect of insulin on subcellular organelles. Because the well-recognized mechanisms of signal transduction for other hormones appear not to be central to insulin action, investigators have searched for a novel second-messenger system. A low-molecular-weight substance has been identified that mimics certain actions of insulin on metabolic enzymes. This substance has an inositol glycan structure and is produced by the insulin-sensitive hydrolysis of a glycosyl-phosphatidylinositol in the plasma membrane. This hydrolysis reaction, which is catalyzed by a specific phospholipase C, also results in the production of a structurally distinct diacylglycerol that may

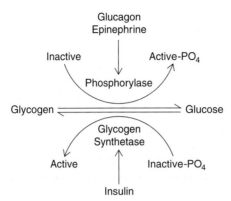

Figure 11.8 General scheme for the control of glycogen synthesis and degradation.

selectively regulate one or more PKCs. The glycosyl-phosphatidylinositol precursor for the inositol glycan enzyme modulator is structurally analogous to the recently described glycosyl-phosphatidylinositol membrane protein anchor. Other proteins anchored in this fashion may be released from cells by a similar insulin-sensitive phospholipase-catalyzed reaction.

A major physiological role of insulin is formation of glycogen from glucose in a number of tissues. Glycogen formation is controlled by the activity of a glycogen synthetase. This enzyme is active in the dephosphorylated state and inactive in the phosphorylated state. Hepatic phosphorylase, the enzyme responsible for activating glycogenolysis, is, on the other hand, activated upon phosphorylation by action of a cAMP-dependent protein kinase (Fig. 11.8). An attractive hypothesis has been that insulin mediates its action by an inhibition of the phosphorylated state of these two enzymes. In both muscle and liver it has been shown that insulin acts to regulate glycogen synthetase by a mechanism not directly related to tissue cAMP concentration. Cyclic AMP-dependent protein kinase (PKA) is known to phosphorylate glycogen synthetase and to decrease its activity. The question was raised as to whether PKA might, therefore, be a target for insulin; this was shown not to be the case. When glycogen-synthetase kinases (GSKs) were discovered it then appeared that insulin might trigger an inhibition of one or more of these enzymes. Instead, it was finally determined that insulin probably stimulated glycogen synthesis by activating a phosphatase that dephosphorylates (and activates) glycogen synthetase [8].

Lipoprotein lipase (LPL) is an enzyme that is synthesized within the parenchymal cells of a tissue and is then transported to the capillary endothelial cells where it has its site of action, for example, to hydrolyze triglycerides from circulating chylomicrons and very low-density lipoproteins (VLDLs). The fatty acids are then transported into the adjacent parenchymal cells. Insulin activates LPL and thus facilitates local transport of FFAs into tissues. Severe uncontrolled diabetes is associated with hypertriglyceridemia and low plasma LPL activity, both of which revert to normal levels upon insulin treatment. Insulin appears to stimulate both the transcription and translation of the enzyme. In addition, insulin induces rapid release of LPL from cells by the activation of a specific phospholipase that hydrolyzes a glycosyl phosphatidylinositol (PI) molecule. The insulin-sensitive glycosyl-PI is structurally similar to the glycolipid membrane anchor of a number of proteins. LPL appears to be anchored to the cell surface by glycosyl-PI, and its rapid release by insulin may be due to activation of a glycosyl-PI-specific phospholipase C.

Glucose Transporter Systems. Glucose homeostasis involves glucose uptake by the liver, muscle, adipose cells, and brain and release of glucose stored in the liver as glycogen or synthesized de novo by hepatic gluconeogenesis into the blood. A key element in the regulation of blood glucose levels is the detection of ambient glucose by α and β cells of pancreatic islets and the consequent secretion of either glucagon, which stimulates glucose release from the liver, or insulin, which induces glucose storage in the liver and stimulates glucose uptake by muscle cells and adipocytes. These mechanisms of glucose uptake, release, and sensing require the presence of membrane proteins known as facilitated-diffusion glucose transporters (GTs), which transport D-glucose and closely related sugars down the chemical concentration gradient. Isoforms of this transporter are expressed in a tissue-specific manner and comprise a family of structurally and functionally related molecules. Their tissue distribution, differences in kinetic properties, and differential regulation by ambient glucose and insulin levels suggest they play specific roles in the control of glucose homeostasis.

All cells express at least one transporter isoform in a constitutive fashion, because a certain level of glucose uptake is an absolute necessity, regardless of influences by various regulatory factors. The level of the constitutive transporter, usually the erythroid glucose-transporter isoform, can be regulated by environmental factors, for example, nutrition. Certain cells express unique transporter isoforms, the quantitatively most important of which is the muscle-adipocyte glucose-transporter isoform that functions in response to insulin to clear most of the blood glucose after a meal. Most commonly, insulin causes a modest (50%) to dramatic (>30-fold) increase in the rate of glucose uptake, depending on the cell type. The most physiologically important aspect of glucose-transport regulation occurs in muscle cells and adipocytes and involves an acute 20- to 40-fold stimulation of transport rates by circulating insulin. This response does not require new protein synthesis and is fully manifest in 10–20 minutes. The major insulin target tissues appear to be uniquely able to produce this transporter isoform, sequester it in a unique organelle, and bring it to the cell surface in which they are inserted by an exocytotic process in response to insulin (Fig. 11.9) [3, 47].

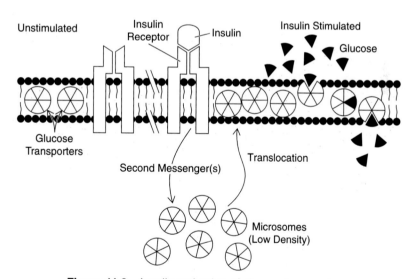

Figure 11.9   Insulin activation of glucose transporters.

The diversity of glucose transporters expressed in mammalian tissues presumably reflects the importance of glucose as a source of metabolic energy, and different glucose transporters have evolved to allow its dietary uptake and tissue-specific utilization. For example, the Na^+-glucose cotransporter is able to actively absorb glucose from the lumen of the small intestine and proximal nephron; the glucose is then passively transferred across the antiluminal surface of the cell. Glucose uptake by other tissues and cells is mediated by transporters whose properties are suited to the specific requirements of the tissues and their cells for glucose and their role in the maintenance of glucose homeostasis.

GLUCAGON

A second important pancreatic hormone that regulates glucose homeostasis was discovered by Kimball and Murlin [28]. Numerous workers had noted that injections of pancreatic extracts into diabetic animals produced a transient hyperglycemia before the hypoglycemic effects of the extracts were observed. Collins and Murlin [10] suggested that besides insulin the extracts might contain a physiologically relevant hyperglycemic factor, which they named glucagon. Glucagon is essential for the complete metabolic syndrome of severe diabetes, previously attributed entirely to the direct consequences of insulin deficiency.

Synthesis, Chemistry, and Metabolism

Mammalian pancreatic glucagon is a single-chain polypeptide of 29 amino acid residues, which bears a striking structural similarity to secretin, gastric inhibitory peptide (GIP), and vasoactive intestinal peptide (VIP) (see Fig. 10.3). Glucagon is derived from a large precursor (preprohormone) that then undergoes a number of posttranslational modifications to yield the definitive hormone. The amino acid sequences of glucagons derived from a number of mammalian species (bovine, ovine, rabbit, rat), including the human, are identical (Fig. 11.10). Glucagons from turkeys and chickens are identical and differ from mammalian glucagons by substitution of the penultimate asparagine (position 28) by serine. Duck glucagon differs from human glucagon by two residues: the asparagine at position 28 is again replaced by serine and the serine at position 16 is replaced by threonine. Such a high degree of structural conservation within the glucagons from these diverse species suggests that the integrity of most of the molecule is necessary for its biological activity.

Physiological Roles

The classical experiments of Foa demonstrated conclusively the role of glucagon in glucose homeostasis [15, 16]. In cross-circulation experiments, the pancreatoduodenal vein of one dog (A) was anastomosed to a femoral vein of a second dog (B) and a return flow was established between a femoral artery of dog B and a femoral vein of dog A. Reduction of plasma blood glucose levels in dog A by insulin resulted in an elevation of blood glucose levels in dog B. Conversely, when hyperglycemia was induced in dog A by administration of glucagon or glucose, a rapid hypoglycemia developed in dog B. These results demonstrated that a reduction or an elevation of blood glucose in dog A was the stimulus to glucagon or insulin secretion, respectively, in dog B. From these experiments, the importance of pancreatic glucagon, along with insulin, in the control of blood glucose levels was elucidated. Subsequent experiments showed that glucagon had a direct effect on glycogenolysis and gluconeogenesis in the isolated perfused liver.

The biological actions of glucagon are essentially the opposite of those of insulin (Fig. 11.3). Glucagon stimulates hepatic glucose release through a glycogenolytic action or through gluconeogenesis. The glycogenolytic action is particularly important in main-

```
                    5                        10                   15
His–Ser–Gln–Gly–Thr–Phe–Thr–Ser–Asp–Tyr–Ser–Lys–Tyr–Leu–Asp

                   20                    25                   29
Ser–Arg–Arg–Ala–Gln–Asp–Phe–Val–Gln–Trp–Leu–Met–Asn–Thr   Mammals
                                                –Ser–       Chicken, Turkey
–Thr–                                           –Ser–       Duck
```

Figure 11.10 Primary structure of mammalian glucagon and related structures of avian glucagons.

taining the short-term levels of blood glucose in well-fed animals that have available stores of liver glycogen. Under conditions of prolonged fasting, exercise, or during neonatal life, the gluconeogenic actions of glucagon are crucial to the maintenance of glucose homeostasis.

Glucagon at physiological levels stimulates the conversion of amino acids to glucose within the liver. Glucagon also promotes the conversion of amino acids and glycerol into glucose by affecting the enzymes in the gluconeogenic and glycolytic pathways in the liver (Fig. 11.3). Glucagon has a lipolytic action on adipose tissue: the FFAs and glycerol liberated from fat cells are used to a minor extent within the hepatocyte in gluconeogenesis. Insulin is such a potent inhibitor of fat cell lipolysis that the actions of glucagon may be manifested only when insulin concentrations are low. The ability of administered glucagon to stimulate lipolysis has nevertheless been demonstrated in the human diabetic.

During fasting the prevention of hypoglycemia is not due solely to decreased insulin secretion; decrements in insulin are probably important, but insulin is not the only relevant glucoregulatory hormone. Glucagon plays a primary counterregulatory role. Adrenal catecholamines compensate and become critical when glucagon is deficient. Adrenomedullary epinephrine is probably the relevant catecholamine [11, 12].

Mechanisms of Action

The major target tissues of glucagon are liver and adipose tissue. Cardiac muscle may also be an action site under certain conditions. The actions of the hormone are at the level of the plasma membrane to stimulate adenylate cyclase production of cAMP; this initial action of the hormone is followed by activation of PKA and subsequent substrate phosphorylation. The actions of glucagon on the hepatocyte are similar to those of epinephrine, but each hormone mediates its effects through separate receptors and different second messengers (see Chap. 14). In the hepatocyte a cascade of protein (enzyme) phosphorylations eventually results in the release of individual glucose-1-PO_4 units from the glycogen polymer (Fig. 11.11). Conversion of inactive (dephosphophosphorylase) phosphorylase to the active enzyme is the final, key step in this cascade phenomenon. At the same time phosphorylation of glycogen synthetase inactivates this enzyme (Fig. 11.8). While catabolic pathways are often activated by direct phosphorylation of rate-controlling enzymes (e.g., hepatic phosphorylase by PKA), in the case of inhibition of biosynthetic pathways by cAMP the mechanism is often more indirect. In the best-studied cases, that is, glycogen biosynthesis, PKA may act by inhibiting protein phosphatases that dephosphorylate sites phosphorylated by other protein kinases [9].

Glucagon also stimulates gluconeogenesis within the hepatocyte; again its action is mediated through the intracellular messenger cAMP. The actions of the cyclic nucleotide block the flow of carbohydrate substrates from glucose-6-PO_4 to pyruvate, specifically by inhibiting enzyme activities between pyruvate and phosphoenolpyruvate and between fructose-6-PO_4 and fructose 1,6-diphosphate. Within the hepatocyte, glucagon also prevents the conversion of FFAs to ketone bodies. The control site of hepatic ketogenesis is at the level of the enzyme carnitine fatty acid transferase. This enzyme promotes the reversible coupling of long-chain fatty acids to carnitine, which is required for the translocation of fatty acids into mitochondria for oxidation. The use of ketones for production of ATP by oxidative phosphorylation within mitochondria provides a glucose-sparing action. Figure 11.3 summarizes the actions of glucagon on a hepatocyte.

Although glucagon is a potent lipolytic hormone, there is great species variation with respect to the sensitivity of adipose tissue to the hormone. Here, as for the hepatocyte, cAMP formation is increased in response to glucagon. In the adipocyte activation of one or more *hormone-sensitive* lipases (triglyceride, diglyceride, and monoglyceride lipases) results in the release of fatty acids and glycerol from fats. These metabolic products of lipolysis circulate to the liver where they subserve substrate roles in gluconeogenic

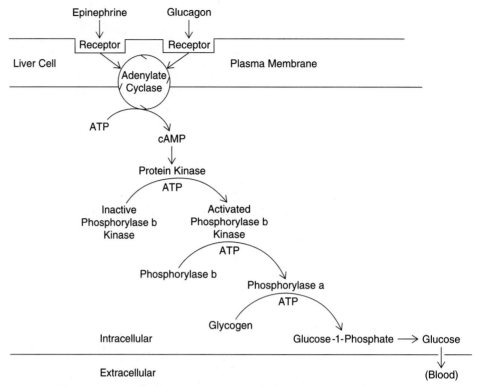

Figure 11.11   Glucagon activation of hepatic adenylate cyclase and the subsequent events in glucose formation.

processes. By the actions of glucagon on adipocytes and hepatocytes, plasma glucose levels are elevated; thus under pathological conditions of pancreatic function the actions of the hormone are diabetogenic.

OTHER PANCREATIC PEPTIDE HORMONES

The α and β cells are the predominant cell types within the pancreas. Nevertheless, using immunocytochemical methods, at least two other peptide hormone-containing cells have been demonstrated to be present within the islets. The control of insulin and glucagon secretion from the islets is much more complicated than described and may be regulated or modulated by these more recently discovered pancreatic peptide hormones.

Somatostatin (SRIF)

Immunoreactive SRIF was shown by immunofluorescence to be localized to a discrete population of cells (D cells) of the endocrine pancreas. The juxtaposition of SRIF-containing D cells to the α and β cells of the islets (Fig. 11.2) is consistent with a local or paracrine role for the hormone. Somatostatin is a tetradecapeptide containing a disulfide bond (see Fig. 6.6); in the pancreas the hormone is derived, as for insulin and glucagon, from a preprohormone.

Somatostatinlike immunoreactivity is elevated in the arterial plasma of dogs that have received a protein meal, suggesting that SRIF may function as a humoral messenger in the control of GI function. Infusions of SRIF, at a rate approximating the postprandial increase in endogenous plasma somatostatinlike activity, markedly lower postprandial triglyceride levels. In addition neutralization of circulating SRIF by antibodies to the peptide is accompanied by higher levels of plasma triglycerides. Somatostatin may, therefore,

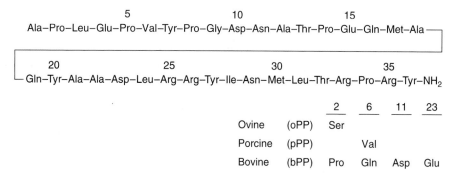

Figure 11.12 Primary structure of human pancreatic polypeptide. Variations within ovine, porcine, and bovine PP sequences are shown.

function as a splanchnic (visceral) humoral hormone that regulates the movement of nutrients from the gut to the internal environment. According to one hypothesis, the function of pancreatic SRIF may be to restrain the rate of nutrient entry into the body by inhibiting various digestive events in response to signals from enteric hormones and rising nutrient concentrations. This would allow the islet hormones, with their movement from the extracellular space into the various tissues, to coordinate the influx of nutrients from the gut.

Pancreatic Polypeptide (PP)

A linear polypeptide has been isolated from the human, pig, cow, sheep, and chicken pancreas (Fig. 11.12) [20, 21]. Avian and beef pancreatic polypeptide (PP) exhibit homology at 16 of 36 amino acid residues, whereas some of the mammalian polypeptides differ by only 2 to 3 residues. Rat PP also contains 36 amino acids; however, there are 8 amino-acid substitutions compared with human PP.

The physiological functions of these pancreatic polypeptides are not clearly delineated, but some of the hormone actions in the chicken have been described [20]. In chickens avian PP decreases liver glycogen, apparently by stimulating hepatic lipogenesis. Avian PP decreases plasma glycerol and FFAs in chickens by inhibiting adipose tissue lipolysis, apparently by reducing fat cell cAMP levels [21]. In humans PP suppresses secretion of SRIF from the gut and pancreas. Similarly, there is a postprandial rise in plasma PP in humans, which can be suppressed by infusions of SRIF. Administration of antisera to SRIF in dogs increases plasma PP levels, suggesting that an inhibitory control of PP secretion by SRIF takes place under physiologic conditions. It was suggested, therefore, that the SRIF-containing D cells and PP-containing F cells control the secretory activity of each other (and probably of insulin and glucagon) within the pancreatic islets by a paracrine mechanism.

Ingestion of a protein meal is a stimulus to PP secretion in humans. Because intravenous infusions of amino acids only modestly elevate plasma PP levels, protein digestion within the GI tract is most likely the stimulus to PP secretion from the pancreatic islets. Acute hypoglycemia is a stimulus to PP secretion, whereas hyperglycemia is associated with a decrease in plasma PP levels. Vagal cholinergic innervation of the pancreas is important in the regulation of PP release. For example, secretion of PP in response to insulin-induced hypoglycemia in humans is abolished by cholinergic (atropine) blockade. Electrical stimulation of the vagus nerve increases portal levels of PP in pigs, a response that is partially inhibited by cholinergic blockage. Protein-rich meals may activate the release of some factor, possibly cholecystokinin, which enhances the release of PP, possibly in concert with vagal activation of pancreatic F cells. Despite the very dramatic effects of meal ingestion on circulating levels of PP, a biological role for PP has not been clearly established. The only clearly documented physiologic effects of PP in humans are inhibition of gallbladder contraction and pancreatic enzyme secretion.

CONTROL OF PANCREATIC ISLET FUNCTION

Although insulin secretion from the pancreatic islets is controlled by endocrine, neural, and metabolic factors, blood glucose is the most important regulator. The temporal hyperglycemia, which develops after an exogenous carbohydrate source, is stimulatory to insulin and inhibitory to glucagon secretion (Fig. 11.13 a).

Catecholamines of neural (ANS) or endocrine (adrenal) origin play a major role in the control of pancreatic islet cell secretion (Chap. 14). Pancreatic A and B cells possess different adrenergic receptors that produce opposite effects on cellular cAMP levels and that are thus primarily responsible for the divergence in the rate of glucagon and insulin release known to occur in several physiological and pathological conditions.

Epinephrine of adrenal origin inhibits insulin secretion under physiological states such as stress. The effects of the catecholamine are mediated through α-adrenergic receptors of the islet B cells. During stress, insulin secretion is depressed so that glucose, rather than stored as glycogen or fat, is more readily available to tissues, such as the liver, muscle, and brain, that are particularly active under such conditions. Glucagon secretion, on the other hand, is stimulated by epinephrine and norepinephrine activation of β receptors of pancreatic A cells; this response provides a mechanism of activating hepatic glucose production and release.

The amino acids arginine and leucine, as well as such keto acids as acetoacetic acid, are also stimulatory to insulin secretion. Insulin is important in the use of these substrates in protein and fat synthesis, respectively. It is interesting to speculate that stimulation of insulin secretion by these metabolic substrates is adaptive in nature and that the insulin released is stimulatory to their use in protein and fat synthesis. Most amino acids stimulate (aminogenic action) the secretion of insulin and glucagon (Fig. 11.13 b). The enormous structural differences within the R-chain of the active amino acids argue against a

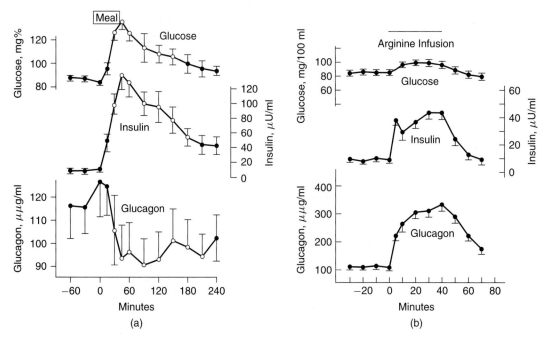

Figure 11.13 (a) The effect of a large carbohydrate meal on the plasma concentration of pancreatic glucagon, insulin, and glucose in 11 normal humans. (b) The effect of an infusion of arginine on the peripheral venous plasma levels of pancreatic glucagon, insulin, and glucose in normal humans. (From Müller et al. [37]. Reprinted, by permission of the *New England Journal of Medicine*, vol. 283, pp. 109–115, 1970.)

structure-activity relationship involving a specific receptor activation. Aminogenic insulin secretion is important, at least from a teleological viewpoint, in that the secreted insulin is available to stimulate incorporation of amino acids into proteins in muscle and other tissues. The concomitant release of glucagon may serve to prevent hypoglycemia as a consequence of the insulin secretion. Aminogenic glucagon secretion is abolished whenever exogenous glucose accompanies the influx of amino acids, such as occurs when carbohydrate is ingested with protein during a meal. In carnivores the release of glucagon as well as insulin in response to a protein meal would be of obvious adaptive value.

Orally administered glucose is a greater stimulus to insulin secretion than intravenously-injected glucose. Glucose is stimulatory to gastric inhibitory peptide (GIP) secretion from the GI tract, which, through circulation to the pancreatic islets, is then stimulatory in conjunction with glucose to insulin secretion (Chap. 10). Glucagon-like peptide 1 (GLP-1) is another member of a class of circulating hormones that subserve humoral communication between the GI tract and the pancreas (the entero-insular axis). The timing of the secretion of GLP-1 is such that circulating levels of the hormone rise coincident with the postprandial increase in the concentration of blood glucose. By binding to specific β-cell receptors and stimulating cAMP production, GLP-1 synergizes with glucose to induce insulin secretion, thereby increasing the concentration of circulating insulin to a level above and beyond that attributable to glucose alone. β cells secrete insulin in response to glucose only when they are "glucose-competent" [22]. Glucose competence is proposed to result from the conditioning influences of circulating insulinotropic hormones (e.g., GLP-1) that render the β-cell glucose-signalling system capable of responding to glucose. Of special significance to the "glucose competence concept" is the existence of a reciprocal relationship between the concentrations of glucagon and GLP-1 in the bloodstream. This is a consequence of the inhibition of glucagon secretion from the α cells of the islets when blood concentrations of glucose and insulin rise. Such a fall in circulating glucagon levels would ultimately lead to diminished β-cell glucose competence if it were not for the compensatory ability of GLP-1 to maintain the glucose-signalling system in a fully functional state. The action of GLP-1, therefore, contrasts with that of glucagon in that GLP-1 confers glucose competence to β cells during the feeding state [22, 49].

The pancreas receives neural innervation from the sympathetic and parasympathetic divisions of the autonomic nervous system [32]. Secretions from the exocrine and endocrine components of the pancreas can be increased by parasympathetic vagal stimulation or by sympathetic stimulation. Neurotransmitters of cholinergic (acetylcholine) and adrenergic (norepinephrine) neurons directly affect pancreatic insulin secretion. Both cholinergic and adrenergic neuronal fibers can be detected in the endocrine and exocrine pancreas. Electron microscopic histochemical studies reveal that both types of neurons innervate the α and β cells of the islets. Transplantation experiments reveal, however, that the pancreatic β cells do not require an intact innervation for functioning. Similarly, unilateral or bilateral vagotomy does not result in observable effects on depression of insulin secretion due to an intravenous glucose load. Nevertheless, cholinergic drugs potentiate glucose-induced insulin release, and the insulin-releasing effect of electrical vagus stimulation increases with the blood-glucose concentration. Probably the vagal nerve modulates the responsiveness of β cells to blood sugar variations in vivo. Furthermore, nervous input to the pancreas may represent a trophic influence of importance for islet cell growth and function over an extended period, and there are data to support such an hypothesis.

Islet α and β cells have been purified from the rat pancreas and examined for their respective sensitivity to somatostatin. Both SRIF-14 and -28 inhibited glucagon and insulin release through direct interactions with the corresponding cell types. A dose-dependent suppression of the secretory activities was paralleled by a reduction in cellular cAMP formation.

Galanin is a 29-amino-acid glucagonlike peptide that is widely distributed within the body and exerts a variety of effects. Immunocytochemistry has revealed that galanin occurs in intrapancreatic nerves in the dog. The nerves were found in the endocrine as well as in the exocrine portion of the pancreas and around blood vessels. The strongest fluorescence was observed in close association with nerves innervating the pancreatic islets. This finding supports an earlier observation of galaninlike immunoreactivity in the rat and pig pancreas, as determined by RIA. Galanin may have a major influence on islet hormone secretion.

The discovery that glucagon stimulates insulin (β-cell) secretion and conversely that insulin suppresses glucagon (α-cell) secretion has led to the hypothesis of an intra-islet, negative-positive, insulin-glucagon feedback. It was originally proposed that, because of their anatomical juxtaposition, the β and α cells might interact with one another via diffusion through intercellular spaces. This concept was bolstered by the observations that somatostatin (D cell) is a potent inhibitor of α-cell and β-cell secretion; thus the extended "paracrine" hypothesis proposed that α, β, and D cells mutually regulate the secretion of each other via the interstitium in order to facilitate metabolic homeostasis. A physiologically functional "directed" microvascular circulation within the islets has been conclusively established with a strict sequence of perfusion of β cells, then α cells, then D cells. Abnormalities in glucagon secretin in diabetes mellitus might be explained by a deficiency in intra-islet microvascular insulin. This intra-islet "sequenced" microcirculation plays a major role in islet regulation and, therefore, metabolic homeostasis [52].

There is evidence that the pancreatic glucose sensor may be solely a component of the β cell. The "liver-type" glucose transporter is present in the insulin-producing β cells of rat pancreatic islets but not in other islet endocrine cells. These results support a possible role for this glucose transporter in glucose sensing by β cells [3, 47]. In response to glucose, information may be conveyed to the α cells directly by way of tight junctions or through the release of insulin, which may then interact with receptors on the α cells. In either case glucose release would be lowered by the action of insulin on its target tissues, such as liver, adipose tissue, and muscle, and additionally through its inhibition of glucagon secretion. In the absence of β cells, as in certain types of diabetes, both these effects of insulin would be lacking. Indeed, the α cell may then be hyperactive; in the juvenile diabetic (who lacks insulin) glucagon levels are elevated even in the presence of hyperglycemia. The observation that glucagon is increased relative to insulin levels in all known forms of endogenous hyperglycemia supports the view that glucagon participates in the marked hepatic overproduction of glucose that is characteristic of the insulin-deficient state [52].

A number of neural or endocrine influences affect glucose homeostasis and glucose intolerance in the diabetic. Somatotropin, in particular, is diabetogenic, but its exact mode of action is undetermined. GH is stimulatory to insulin secretion, but at the same time this hormone reduces the sensitivity of peripheral tissues (e.g., muscle and adipose tissues) to insulin. Acromegalics have increased circulating levels of GH and exhibit abnormal glucose tolerance due to severe insulin resistance. Somatotropin-induced insulin release may be indirect because of the developing hyperglycemia resulting from inhibition of glucose uptake by peripheral tissues. Elevated plasma glucose levels would then be stimulatory to insulin secretion; elevated insulin levels, however, would lead to down regulation of peripheral tissue insulin receptors (insulin resistance) and the vicious cycle would continue.

Glucocorticoid secretion is increased in Cushing's syndrome (see Chap. 15); the effect of these adrenal steroids is generally to increase gluconeogenesis in the liver. In addition glucocorticoids have a catabolic action on muscle and adipose tissues. The liberated amino acids and FFAs provide substrates for increased gluconeogenesis within the liver. Glucocorticoids also enhance the actions of adrenal catecholamines on their target tissues; for example, the lipolytic actions of catecholamines on adipose tissue are enhanced. All these glucocorticoid actions are hyperglycemic in nature and, therefore, are potentially diabetogenic over a prolonged period. Diabetes mellitus is thus a usual sequelae of hypercortisolism (Cushing's syndrome).

Glucose Counterregulation

Glucose is the major metabolic substrate for the brain, and since the brain cannot synthesize or store glucose or increase its capacity to take up glucose from the circulation, the prevention or correction of hypoglycemia is critical to survival. Therefore physiological mechanisms have evolved to effectively prevent or correct the hypoglycemic state [12]. Most important is the decline in insulin secretion in the absence of the β-cell stimulatory actions of glucose. Concomitantly, low levels of glucose are stimulatory to α-cell secretion of glucagon. Under more extreme conditions of hypoglycemia adrenal medullary release of epinephrine is crucial. Epinephrine is both stimulatory to α-cell glucagon secretion and inhibitory to β-cell insulin secretion. Both glucagon and epinephrine are stimulatory to hepatic glycogenolysis and glucose output [37]. In addition, both hormones are stimulatory to adipose cell lipolytic mechanisms that release glycerol and FFAs for hepatic use (glucogenesis). Other hormones such as somatotropin and cortisol also play roles in defense against prolonged hypoglycemia [12].

PANCREATIC ISLET PATHOPHYSIOLOGY

Diabetes mellitus was first described about 1500 B.C. in Egypt [34]. *Mellitus*, the Latin word for honey, characterizes the high sugar content of the urine of diabetics. The word *diabetes*, derived from the Greek for siphon, refers to the copious excretion of water that characterizes the disease. For centuries the disease was known as "the pissing evil" in England, an epithet that appropriately characterizes its most observable symptom [34]. Although diabetes mellitus is generally thought to result from a lack of insulin, it can, however, be considered a heterogeneous group of diseases (Table 11.1).

Insulin-dependent and Noninsulin-dependent Diabetes Insipidus

In patients with *insulin-dependent diabetes mellitus* there is a marked decrease in the number of insulin-containing β cells. The pathogenesis may result from the development of islet cell-surface antibodies [22]. The cues responsible for the production of cytotoxic antibodies are not known. Autoantibodies play a role in the pathogenesis of several other endocrine-based disease states. Juvenile-onset diabetes develops in youth; the symptoms begin rather abruptly, and control of the disease almost always requires insulin replacement therapy. There is evidence that juvenile-onset diabetes may be caused by a virus, but initiation may require more than a single virus infection. The symptoms may only be manifested when sufficient damage has been caused by a number of infections such as mumps and rubella.

There are about 10 million people with diabetes mellitus in the United States. About 80% of these people have noninsulin-dependent diabetes. NIDDM is much more prevalent among Native Americans than among American Caucasians, African-Americans, or Hispanic-Americans [7, 56]. In particular, the Pima Indians of Arizona have the highest reported prevalence of the disease of any population in the world [6, 14, 17]. More than half of these Native Americans over 35 years of age have the disease [6]. The vast majority of diabetics who suffer from *maturity-onset diabetes* generally have above normal levels of insulin, but their tissues do not respond to the hormone. This phenomenon, referred to as *insulin resistance*, may be due to multiple causes [12, 19, 38].

Understanding of the mechanisms of insulin actions allows the division of the mechanisms of insulin resistance into three groups: prereceptor, receptor, and postreceptor insulin resistance. Type A insulin resistance is due to a decrease in the number of insulin receptors, whereas patients with type B insulin resistance have circulating antibodies against some portion of their insulin receptors, and this results in impaired binding

TABLE 11.1   Pathology of the Endocrine Pancreas

Type I (Insulin-Dependent Diabetes Mellitus, IDDM)
   Juvenile-onset diabetes. Viral-induced β-cell destruction.
   Cytotoxic autoantibodies to β cells lead to β-cell destruction [23].

Type II (Noninsulin-Dependent Diabetes Mellitus, NIDDM; Previously Called Adult (Maturity) Onset Diabetes)

   Insulin Resistance [1, 48, 51]
     Pre-Receptor Resistance
       Antibodies against insulin
       Mutant insulin structures
         Defect in primary structure of insulin B chain at one or more positions.
         Familial hyperproinsulinemia [55]
           B-C proinsulin: mutation at the cleavage site between the B chain and the connecting (C) peptide.
           A-C proinsulin: mutation at the cleavage site between the A chain and the connecting (C) peptide.
     Receptor Resistance [48]
       Type A. Decrease in insulin receptor number and/or affinity for the hormone.
         Point mutation in insulin receptor gene prevents processing of the receptor precursor [53].
         Impaired expression of receptor tyrosine kinase activity [46].
         Point mutation blocks insertion of mature receptor into plasma membrane.
       Type B. Receptor blocked by circulatory antibodies to the receptor.
       Leprechaunism
         An autosomal recessively inherited disorder of insulin function that leads to severe intrauterine growth retardation, characteristic dysmorphic features and a disturbed glucose homeostasis. The process underlying this disease is a structural defect in the insulin receptor.
     Post-Receptor Resistance
       Decreased capacity of pancreatic β cells to compensate for the underlying insulin resistance by increased secretion of insulin [51].
         Possible underexpression (down regulation) of β-cell glucose transporters (therefore failure to recognize and respond to hyperglycemia) [50].
         Mutation of the glucokinase gene may prevent uptake and metabolism of glucose necessary for the mechanism of insulin secretion. May be responsible for a young onset Type II diabetes (MODY) [24].

Islet Cell Tumors
   Insulinoma. Excess insulin secretion from β-cell pancreatic tumor (severe hypoglycemia).
   Glucagonoma syndrome. Excess glucagon secretion from α-cell pancreatic tumor.
   Somatostatinoma. Excess somatostatin secretion from D-cell pancreatic tumor.

Hypoglycemic Disorders
   Hypoglucagonemia (isolated glucagon deficiency). Possibly due to autosomal recessive inheritance.
   Hyperinsulinemia (β-cell tumor) [40].
   Antibodies (stimulatory) to the insulin receptor (increased glucose uptake by cells).

---

of insulin to target cells. The majority of insulin resistance is of the postreceptor type due to the extraordinary complexity of the intracellular pathways of insulin action [7]. Noninsulin-dependent diabetes mellitus (NIDDM) is readily distinguishable from insulin-dependent diabetes mellitus (IDDM). NIDDM used to be called adult-onset diabetes mellitus and is also referred to as Type II diabetes mellitus. NIDDM characteristically occurs in middle-aged to elderly adults. Patients with NIDDM, in contrast to patients with IDDM, retain the ability to normally synthesize, store, and release insulin to virtually all insulin secretagogues with the single exception of intravenous glucose. This and other observations strongly support the notion of abnormal glucose recognition by the pancreatic islet as a fundamental defect in NIDDM [33, 41, 54].

    The phosphorylation of glucose in mammalian tissues is mediated by a family of hexose phosphotransferases, which includes glucokinase and hexokinases. Glucokinase is expressed only in the insulin-secreting pancreatic β cells and in hepatocytes. Glucokinase catalyzes the phosphorylation of glucose and plays a key role in the regulation of insulin secretion by pancreatic β cells and glucose metabolism in hepatocytes [24]. Mutations in the gene encoding of this key regulatory enzyme of glycolysis are a common cause of an autosomal dominant form of NIDDM that often has an onset during childhood. The association of mutations in the glucokinase gene with impaired pancreatic β-cell function underscores the importance of glycolysis in the regulation of insulin secretion. The demonstration that mutations in the glucokinase gene can cause diabetes suggests that NIDDM may be, at least in part, a disorder of glucose metabolism, which implies that genes encoding other glycolytic and gluconeogenic enzymes, especially those enzymes that control rate-limiting steps in these pathways, are candidates for contributing to the development of this genetically heterogenous disorder [4].

The circulating levels of insulin rise in individuals who have insulin resistance and in pancreatic islets that function normally. Some patients treated with exogenous insulin develop antibodies to the hormone, and these proteins inhibit access of the active hormone to its receptors. Insulin resistance may also develop in individuals who produce an abnormal hormone that has decreased receptor affinity. In the abnormality of *familial hyperproinsulinemia*, for example, individuals possess elevated circulating levels of a partially cleaved proinsulin. This abnormality is inherited as an autosomal dominant and probably involves a mutation of arginine 32 at the cleavage site connecting the B chain to the C peptide. Another defect resulting in hyperproinsulinemia involves a mutation at the cleavage site connecting the C peptide to the A chain (Fig. 11.6). A biologically defective insulin molecule was produced in another hyperinsulinemic patient, most likely by a single-point mutation (probably a single base change in the DNA), resulting in substitution of leucine for phenylalanine at position 24 or 25 of the insulin B chain. These positions are known to compose part of the active receptor-binding region of insulin that is responsible for its biological activity.

In the absence of insulin most activities described relating to the actions of insulin are reversed. Failure to activate hepatic glycogen synthetase increases the levels of glucose-6-PO_4, and this substrate is now available for dephosphorylation by glucose-6-phosphatase to glucose. The concomitant decreased activity of glucokinase results in the loss of glucose from the hepatocytes and, more important, impedes the flow of glucose into the cells, thus failing to provide substrates for glycolysis and ATP production by way of the Krebs cycle. This sets up a situation within hepatocytes and all other cells where, although there are increased circulating levels of glucose, there is little intracellular glucose for ATP production. Thus cellular famine exists in the midst of plenty. Indeed, polyphagia is a characteristic behavioral trait of these energy-starved individuals. The resulting excess of sugar in the blood leads to the excretion of large amounts of urine (polyuria), which in turn leads to dehydration and intense thirst (polydipsia).

The unavailability of glucose for lipogenesis within fat cells results in increased lipolysis; the released FFAs and glycerol are now available to liver cells as substrates for glucogenesis, which enhances the hyperglycemia, the cardinal symptom of diabetes mellitus [35]. The FFAs released from the fats stored within adipocytes undergo β-oxidation within hepatocytes with resultant production of acetyl-CoA. Although this high-energy compound is available for entry into the Krebs cycle, the increased levels of this substrate may result in condensation of acetyl-CoA moieties into acetoacetyl-CoA. Subsequent condensation of acetoacetyl-CoA with another molecule of acetyl-CoA results in formation of β-hydroxyl-β-methylglutaryl-CoA. In the liver deacylase activity converts acetoacetyl-CoA to acetoacetic acid. This β-keto acid can then be converted to β-hy-droxybutyric acid and to acetone (Fig. 11.14). These ketones, acetoacetate and β-hy-droxybutyrate, are normally used as energy substrates. If, however, the entry of acetyl-CoA into the citric acid cycle is depressed, the rate of ketone formation may exceed the tissue oxidation of these substrates. They then accumulate within the bloodstream, which is followed by an elevation of ketone bodies in the urine (ketonuria). This diabetic ketosis may result in a fatal metabolic acidosis [14, 26]. The urinary ketone bodies are excreted as Na^+ salts and large volumes of water are osmotically removed from the plasma, thus intensifying the dehydration already present due to the hyperglycemic diuresis. The loss of Na^+ disturbs the bicarbonate buffering

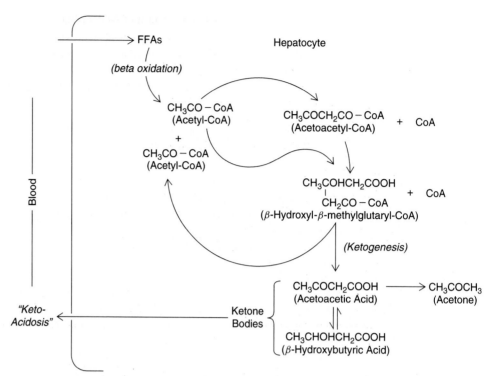

Figure 11.14   Scheme of ketone biosynthesis: the hydroxymethylglutaryl-CoA cycle.

system of the plasma, thus intensifying the blood acidosis. Ketones are also removed through the lungs, producing the characteristic fruity smell of the diabetic in a state of ketosis.

In the absence of insulin, amino acids and glucose cannot enter muscle cells, which results in protein catabolism. The amino acids released through proteolysis from muscle in the diabetic are now available through deamination and transamination for glucose formation within the liver. Use of amino acids in hepatic gluconeogenesis results in a *negative nitrogen balance*. The protein catabolism results in protein depletion and tissue wasting; failure to grow is a symptom of diabetes in children. The protein depletion and accompanying hyperglycemia of the diabetic are also associated with poor resistance to infections.

Obesity and Diabetes

Body fat distribution is recognized as an important predictor of the metabolic complications of obesity [39]. Although obesity results in metabolic abnormalities, upper-body obesity is most strongly associated with hyperlipidemia, hypertension, and NIDDM, whereas lower-body obesity is usually not. It has been discovered that fat cells from women with lower body obesity were of normal size but their numbers were greatly increased. Excessive numbers of adipose cells may be produced by overeating during certain critical periods of childhood. In contrast, upper body obese women were found to have normal numbers of fat cells, but of greatly increased size. This pattern of cell size may be produced by overeating during adulthood. It has been shown that enlargement of fat cells reduces the number of insulin receptors on their surface. The body then produces more insulin to compensate for the lower numbers of receptors; the hyperinsulinemia may then result in down-regulation of insulin receptors in other tissues. This may account for the elevated blood glucose levels (hyperglycemia) that is the cardinal symptom of diabetes mellitus.

Men tend to have only one pattern of fat distribution: they gain more weight around and above the waist. Maturity-onset diabetes is generally more common in obese men than in obese women but less than that of upper body obese women. Since upper body obese women have higher levels of male hormones this suggests that androgens may stimulate the deposition of fat in a pattern similar to that of men. Testosterone has indeed been found to increase the incidence of diabetes, and that may be a contributing factor to NIDDM in these women.

Islet Cell Tumors

Because of the profound effects of pancreatic hormones on nutrient homeostasis, one should expect that malignancies or neoplasms of pancreatic islet cells would have profound effects on carbohydrate, protein, and fat metabolism. Three neoplasms of the islets are insulinoma, glucagonoma, and somatostatinoma. Other tumors (e.g., gastrinomas, VIPomas) of unknown cellular origin within the pancreas may secrete other peptide hormones that cause dire GI tract disturbances.

Benign and malignant insulin-secreting tumors exhibit complete autonomy of insulin release. If mild, the resulting hypoglycemia can be controlled by an increase in food intake; if severe and intractable, it can lead to convulsions and death if the tumor is not surgically removed. The excessive release of glucagon from an α-cell tumor leads to hyperglucagonemia, and the metabolic disturbances that prevail vary with the capability of the individual to secrete insulin. Development of a somatostatinoma results, not unexpectedly, in hypersomatostatinemia. Patients with such tumors may exhibit hypoinsulinemia and hypoglucagonemia. Because somatostatin may perform a number of functions within the GI tract, it is not surprising that digestive tract functioning may also be impaired. Excessive amounts of VIP are released by all VIPomas and most multiple endocrine adenomas. Multiple endocrine neoplasia is characterized by tumors that often occur synchronously in a number of endocrine glands. One type predominantly involves the parathyroid and pituitary glands, and the pancreatic islets.

Insulin Replacement Therapy

In the past, porcine or other mammalian sources of insulin have provided the replacement therapy required by the diabetic. These nonhuman sources of insulin often prove to be immunogenic in some individuals and other sources must be provided. There is hope that DNA recombinant technology will provide a plentiful supply of human insulin (see Chap. 3). Two general approaches have been used. Sequences of DNA encoding for the A and B peptide chains of insulin have been ligated separately into the *Escherichia coli* β-galactosidase gene. The individual polypeptide chains produced by the bacterium are then released by enzymatic cleavage from the translation product and purified and recombined to form the biologically active insulin (see Fig. 3.6). An alternate approach has used human preproinsulin DNA inserted into a plasmid that was then used to transform a strain of *E. coli*. The preproinsulin polypeptide sequence was synthesized and correctly cleaved by the bacterium. The polypeptide could then be successfully converted to an insulinlike component by tryptic digestion. This method has proven feasible for the production of adequate amounts of human insulin for therapeutic purposes.

There is also hope that islet transplantation may prove effective in treating insulin-dependent diabetes. Immunoisolation is a potentially important approach to transplanting islets without the need for immunosuppressive drugs. Systems have been designed in which the transplanted tissue is separated from the host's immune system by an artificial barrier (Fig. 11.15). Immunoisolation systems may provide a solution to the problem of human islet procurement by permitting use of the islets isolated from animal pancreases. These devices are referred to as biohybrid artificial organs because they combine synthetic, selectively permeable membranes that block immune rejection with living transplants [30].

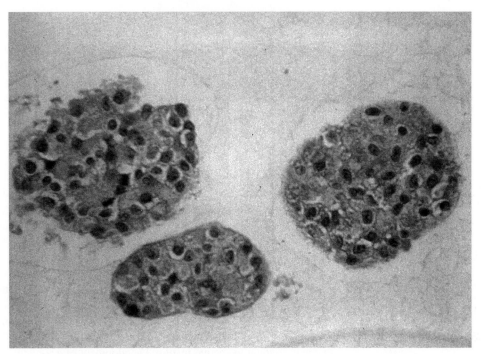

Figure 11.15   Canine islets retrieved from a vascular device after >1 year in a diabetic dog. After device removal, the exogenous insulin requirement of the animal increased >20 units/day (Hematoxylin/eosin, × 400). (From Lanza et al. [30], used with permission from *Diabetes* 41:1503–1510, 1992.)

REFERENCES

[1]   Accili, D., A. Cama, F. Barbetti, H. Kadowaki, T. Kakowaki, and S. I. Taylor. 1992. Insulin resistance due to mutations of the insulin receptor gene: an overview. *J. Endocrinol. Invest.* 14:857–64.

[2]   Banting, F. G., and C. H. Best. 1922. The internal secretion of the pancreas. *J. Lab. Clin. Med.* 7:465–80.

[3]   Bell, G. I., C. F. Burant, J. Takeda, and G. W. Gould. 1993. Structure and function of mammalian facilitative sugar transporters. *J. Biol. Chem.* 268:19161–4.

[4]   Bell, G. I., F. Froguel, S. Nishi, S. J. Pilkis, M. Stoffel, J. Takeda, N. Vionnet, and K. Yasuda. 1993. Mutations of the human glucokinase gene and diabetes mellitus. *TEM* 4:86–90.

[5]   Bliss, M. 1989. J. J. R. Macleod and the discovery of insulin. *Quart. J. Exp. Physiol.* 74:87–96.

[6]   Bogardus, C., and S. Lillioja. 1992. Pima Indians as a model to study the genetics of NIDDM. *J. Cell. Biochem.* 48:337–343.

[7]   Clauser, E., I. Leconte, and C. Auzan. 1992. Molecular basis of insulin resistance. *Horm. Res.* 38:5–12.

[8]   Cohen, P. 1993. Dissection of the protein phosphorylation cascades involved in insulin and growth factor action. Ciba Medical Lecture. *Biochem. Soc. Trans.* 21:555–67.

[9]   Cohen, P., and D. G. Hardie. 1991. The actions of cyclic AMP on biosynthetic processes are mediated indirectly by cyclic AMP-dependent protein kinase. *Biochem. Biophys. Acta* 1094:292–9.

[10] Collins, W. S., and J. R. Murlin. 1929. Hyperglycemia following the portal injection of insulin. *Proc. Soc. Exp. Biol. Med.* 26:485–90.

[11] Cryer, P. E. 1991. Regulation of glucose metabolism in man. *J. Int. Med.* 229:31–9.

[12]   ———. 1993. Glucose counterregulation: prevention and correction of hypoglycemia in humans. *Amer. J. Physiol.* 264:E149–55.

[13]   Dubois, P. M. 1989. Ontogeny of the endocrine pancreas. *Horm. Res.* 32:53–60.

[14]   Fleckman, A. M. 1993. Diabetes ketoacidosis. *Endocrinol. Metabol. Clin. N. Amer.* 22:181–207.

[15]   Foà, P. P. 1973. Glucagon: an incomplete and biased review with selected references. *Amer. Zool.* 13:613–23.

[16]   Foà, P. P., G. Galansino and G. Pozza. 1957. Glucagon, a second pancreatic hormone. *Rec. Prog. Horm. Res.* 13:473–510.

[17]   Gohdes, D., S. Kaufman, and S. Valway. 1993. Diabetes in American Indians. An overview. *Diabetes Care* 16:239–43.

[18]   Goldstein, B. J. 1993. Regulation of insulin receptor signalling by protein-tyrosine dephosphorylation. *Receptor* 3:1–15.

[19]   Hamman, R. F. 1992. Genetic and environmental determinants of non-insulin-dependent diabetes mellitus (NIDDM). *Diabetes Metab. Rev.* 8:287–338.

[20]   Hazelwood, R. 1990. *The endocrine pancreas.* Englewood Cliffs, N.J.: Prentice Hall Publishing Co, Inc.

[21]   Hazelwood, R. L. 1993. The pancreatic polypeptide (PP-fold) family: gastrointestinal, vascular, and feeding behavioral implications. *Proc. Soc. Exp. Biol. Med.* 202:44–63.

[22]   Holz, G. G., and J. F. Habener. 1993. Signal transduction crosstalk in the endocrine system: pancreatic β-cells and the glucose competence concept. *TIBS* 17:388–93.

[23]   Inman, L. R., C. T. Mcallister, L. Chen, S. Hughes, C. B. Newgard, J. R. Kettman, R. H. Under, and J. H. Johnson. 1993. Autoantibodies to the GLUT-2 glucose transporter of β cells in insulin-dependent diabetes mellitus of recent onset. *Proc. Natl. Acad. Sci. USA* 90:1281–4.

[24]   Iynedjian, P. B. 1993. Mammalian glucokinase and its gene. *Biochem. J.* 293:1–13.

[25]   Kahn, C. R., and A. B. Goldfine. 1993. Molecular determinants of insulin action. *J. Diabetes Complications* 7:92–105.

[26]   Kecskes, S. A. 1993. Diabetic ketoacidosis. *Pediatr. Clin. North Amer.* 40:355–63.

[27]   Keller, S. R., L. Lamphere, B. E. Lavan, M. R. Kuhne, and G. E. Leinhard. 1993. Insulin and IGF-I signaling through the insulin receptor substrate 1. *Mol. Reprod. Develop.* 35:346–52.

[28]   Kimball, C. P., and J. R. Murlin. 1923. Aqueous extracts of pancreas. III. Some precipitation reaction of insulin. *J. Biol. Chem.* 58:337–46.

[29]   Korc, M., D. Owerbach, C. Quinto, and W. J. Rutter. 1981. Pancreatic islet-acinar cell interaction: amylase messenger RNA levels are determined by insulin. *Science* 213:351–53.

[30]   Lanza, R. P., S. J. Sullivan, and W. L. Chick. 1992. Islet transplantation with immunoisolation. *Diabetes* 41:1503–10.

[31]   Le Dourain, N. M. 1988. On the origin of pancreatic endocrine cells. *Cell* 53:169–71.

[32]   Magee, D. F. 1989. Does the sympathetic nervous system regulate the exocrine pancreas? *Int. J. Pancreat.* 5:107–16.

[33]   Marie, S., M.-J. Diaz-Guerra, L. Miquerol, A. Kahn, and P. B. Iynedjian. 1993. The pyruvate kinase gene as a model for studies of glucose-dependent regulation of gene expression in the endocrine pancreatic β-cell type. *J. Biol. Chem.* 268:23881–90.

[34]   Maurer, A. C. 1979. The therapy of diabetes. *Amer. Sci.* 67:422–32.

[35]   McGarry, J. D. 1992. What if Minkowski had been ageusic? An alternative angle on diabetes. *Science* 258:766–70.

[36]   Minkowski, O. 1989. Historical development of the theory of pancreatic diabetes. *Diabetes* 38:1–6.

[37]   Müller, W. A., G. R. Faloona, E. Aguilar-Parada, and R. H. Unger. 1970. Abnormal alpha cell function in diabetes. Response to carbohydrate and protein injection. *New Engl. J. Med.* 283:109–15.

[38]   Müller-Wieland, D., R. Streicher, G. Siemeister, and W. Krone. 1993. Molecular biology of insulin resistance. *Exp. Clin. Endocrinol.* 101:17–29.

[39]   O'Dea, K. 1992. Obesity and diabetes in "the land of milk and honey." *Diabetes/Metab. Rev.* 8:373–88.

[40] Phillips, L. S., and D. G. Robertson. 1993. Insulin-like growth factors and non-islet cell tumor hypoglycemia. *Metabolism* 42:1093–101.

[41] Robertson, R. P. 1992. Defective insulin secretion in NIDDM: integral part of a multiplier hypothesis. *J. Cell. Biochem.* 48:227–33.

[42] Romer, G., and J. Larner. 1993. Insulin mediators and the mechanism of insulin action. *Adv. Pharmacol.* 24:21–50.

[43] Sanger, F. 1959. Chemistry of insulin. *Science* 129:1340–44.

[44] Skandalakis, L. J., J. S. Rowe Jr., S. W. Gray, and J. E. Skandalakis. 1993. Surgical embryology and anatomy of the pancreas. *Surg. Anat. Embryol.* 73:661–97.

[45] Stein, R. 1993. Regulation of insulin gene transcription. *TEM* 4:96–101.

[46] Taira, M., M. Taira, N. Hashimoto, F. Shimada, Y. Suzuki, A. Kanatsuka, F. Nakamura, Y. Ebina, M. Tatibana, H. Makino, and S. Yoshida. 1989. Human diabetes associated with a deletion of the tyrosine kinase domain of the insulin receptor. *Science* 245:63–66.

[47] Takata, K., M. Kasahara, Y. Oka, and H. Hirano. 1993. Review: mammalian sugar transporters: their localization and link to cellular functions. *Acta Histochem. Cytochem.* 26:165–78.

[48] Taylor, S. I. 1992. Molecular mechanisms of insulin resistance: lessons from patients with mutations in the insulin-receptor gene. *Diabetes* 41:1473–1490.

[49] Thorens, B., and G. Waeber. 1993. Glucagon-like peptide-1 and the control of insulin secretion in the normal state and in NIDDM. *Diabetes* 42:1219–25.

[50] Unger, R. H. 1991. Diabetic hyperglycemia: link to impaired glucose transport in pancreatic β cells. *Science* 251:1200–5.

[51] Unger, R. H. 1992. GLUT-2 and the pathogenesis of type II diabetes. *Diab. Nutr. Metab.* 5:65–9.

[52] Unger, R. H., P. Raskin, C. B. Srikant, and L. Orci. 1977. Glucagon and the A cells. *Rec. Prog. Horm. Res.* 33:477–517.

[53] Yoshimasa, Y., S. Seino, J. Whittaker, T. Kakehi, A. Kosaki, H. Kuzuya, H. Imura, G. I. Bell, and D. F. Steiner. 1988. Insulin-resistant diabetes due to a point mutation that prevents insulin proreceptor processing. *Science* 240:784–86.

[54] Weir, G. C. 1993. The relationship of diabetes, loss of glucose-induced insulin secretion, and GLUT2. *J. Diabetes Complications* 7:124–9.

[55] Yano, H., N. Kitano, M. Morimoto, K. S. Polonsky, H. Imura, and Y. Seino. 1992. A novel point mutation in the human insulin gene giving rise to hyperproinsulinemia (Proinsulin Kyoto). *J. Clin. Invest.* 89:1902–7.

[56] Young, T. K. 1993. Diabetes mellitus among Native Americans in Canada and the United States: an epidemiological review. *Amer. J. Human Biol.* 5:399–413.

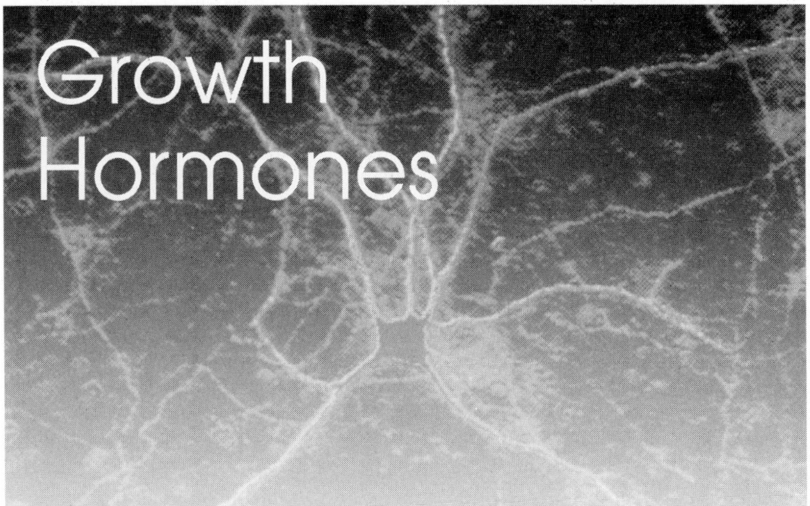

Growth Hormones

12

*A number of hormones are essential to normal body growth through their actions on bone and other organs such as the gonads and the mammary glands. Although pituitary growth hormone (GH, somatotropin or STH) is clearly associated with growth (Chap. 5), most of its actions are mediated indirectly through peptide hormones, the **somatomedins**. Besides the important actions of insulin on carbohydrate and fat metabolism, this hormone also plays an important role in growth regulation. **Prolactin** is necessary for mammary gland growth and development during the latter stage of pregnancy. **Placental lactogen** may prove to be significant in maternal and fetal growth during pregnancy. Other putative growth factors affect the growth, proliferation, and differentiation of specific cell types: nerve growth factor, erythrocyte-stimulating factor (erythropoietin), epidermal growth factor and platelet-derived growth factor, and a number of thymic factors.*

Growth-inhibiting factors, chalones, have been described. When more is known about their origin, synthesis, release, metabolism, and mechanisms of action, some of these factors may be considered to be hormones. Certain steroid hormones, particularly androgens, play crucial roles in normal growth processes. Other hormones, such as the glucocorticoids, and the thyroid hormones, are essential (permissive) for the growth-promoting activities of the peptide growth hormones. The individual roles of growth hormones and the integrated actions of the hormones in growth and development will be discussed.

GROWTH AND CELLULAR PROLIFERATION

All cells in the body are derived from a single cell, the fertilized egg. Although each cell possesses the same genetic information, there are many different kinds of cells. After repeated divisions of the egg to produce cells of a smaller, more uniform size, the cells migrate and continue to divide to produce the embryo. During this process of cell division and subsequent tissue and organ formation, certain genes (proto-oncogenes) are turned on or off, a process that provides the regulatory cues for individual cell differentiation and function. Certain cells are specialized to provide specific functions: some make hemoglobin, some synthesize keratin, some produce antibodies, and others, such as the hepatocyte, participate in a wide spectrum of cellular activities.

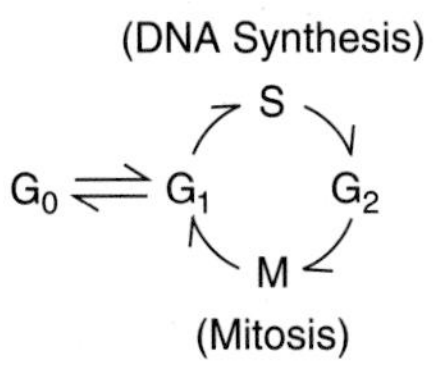

Cells pass through specific stages in their life cycle. The fully mature cell (e.g., skeletal muscle or nerve) is said to be in G_0 (G stands for gap) and is not committed to division (Fig. 12.1). These cells have varying life spans depending on their specific activities. Erythrocytes survive about 120 days in humans; some epithelial cells of the gut live

(DNA Synthesis)

$$G_0 \rightleftharpoons G_1 \quad S \quad G_2$$

$$M$$

(Mitosis)

Figure 12.1 The mammalian cell cycle.

257

only a few days, and certain neurons in the brain may be as old as the individual. G_1 is a growth phase preparatory to S, the synthetic phase where the DNA is duplicated. The G_2 phase is not clearly defined functionally, but it is a short period (3 to 4 hours) where some protein synthesis occurs. During this time preparations are made for entry into the complex events of the next phase, mitosis (M). Following mitosis, the daughter cells may reenter the proliferation cycle or may become resting G_0 cells.

The control point of cell division is believed to be at the transition from G_0 to G_1. Because chemical messengers affect cell division as well as differentiation, it is important to determine whether hormone effects are specific to certain phases of the cell cycle. Hormone receptors may vary in number and/or function throughout the cell cycle and thus affect the responsiveness of the cells to the actions of hormones.

Growth, often defined as simply an increase in size, may occur as a result of three processes: cells may enlarge (become hypertrophic), cells may increase in number (become hyperplastic), and intercellular substances (extracellular matrix) may be produced. These are orderly processes that require exogenous substrates from fuel and from structural components of muscle, bone, adipose tissue, and other organs. Hormones are critical in making these materials available to cells and in stimulating cell division and the secretion of materials (e.g., collagen) for the extracellular framework of the body.

With few exceptions, most hormones stimulate tissue and organ growth, and in their absence target tissues atrophy. For example, in response to MSH integumental melanocytes (in the frog *Xenopus laevis*) increase in number from as few as 10/mm^2 of epidermis to as many as 1000 to 2000 mm^2 (see Fig. 8.11). In the absence of MSH the melanocytes soon atrophy and disappear from the skin. The size of the human adrenal cortex (see Chap. 15) is drastically affected by the levels of ACTH secreted by the pituitary gland.

SOMATOTROPIN AND THE SOMATOMEDINS

The pivotal role of pituitary growth hormone (GH), also known as somatotropin (STH), in the control of growth has been firmly established. Congenital failure to synthesize and secrete GH leads to dwarfism (short stature); hypersecretion of GH, on the other hand, leads to gigantism if overproduction of the hormone is initiated early in life, or to acromegaly if oversecretion occurs in the adult.

Somatotropin causes growth of the epiphyseal regions of the long bones. Growth of bone can be monitored by measuring the incorporation of sulfur (^{35}S) into the epiphyseal cartilage. When bones from young animals are incubated in a medium containing normal serum and the radioactive isotope of sulfur, the sulfur is incorporated into the sulfated polysaccharides of the cartilage. However, when bones are incubated in serum from hypophysectomized animals, no incorporation of ^{35}S takes place. This was initially considered to be due to the lack of GH in the serum. When GH was added to serum from hypophysectomized animals, incorporation of the radioactive sulfur into cartilage still failed to occur. If, however, hypophysectomized animals were injected with GH some hours before blood collection, the serum supported the incorporation of the radioactive sulfur into bone. The conclusion was drawn that GH acts indirectly on bones by way of the production of a *sulfation factor*.

The sulfation factor is now known to consist of several peptides referred to as *somatomedins*. Injected radiolabeled GH rapidly localizes to the liver rather than to the epiphyses of the long bones. Somatomedin is generally used to refer to those growth factors found in the plasma that are under the control of GH, have insulinlike properties, and promote the incorporation of sulfate into cartilage (the "somatomedin hypothesis"). Two substances isolated from the plasma in pure or rather pure form fulfill these criteria: insulinlike growth factors I and II (IGF-I and IGF-II). The peptides bear some structural

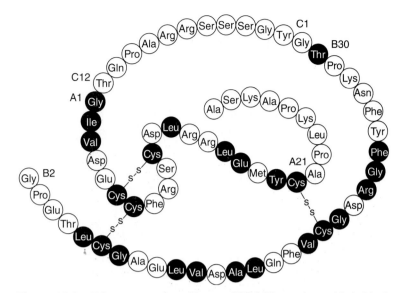

Figure 12.2   Primary structure of human IGF-I. The amino acids in black circles denote those in identical position in the A and B chain of human insulin. (From Humbel and Rinderknecht [22], by permission.)

relationship to proinsulin and, therefore, exhibit some affinity for insulin receptors [29]. Conversely, insulin at high concentration will bind to somatomedin receptors. IGFs are secreted by the liver and by some other tissues in response to GH stimulation. The somatomedins are not, however, stored within the liver; hence, the liver is not a source of extractable growth factors. The growth activity present in the blood cannot be neutralized by antibodies against insulin. The amino acid sequences of these insulinlike growth factors, IGF-I and IGF-II, nevertheless reveal a high degree of similarity to insulin. These polypeptides in the human consist of 70 and 67 amino acid residues, respectively [22, 45], and have a proinsulinlike structure with a shorter connecting peptide of 12 amino acids and an extension of 8 residues at the A-chain terminus (Fig. 12.2). IGF-II is three times more abundant in the adult circulation than IGF-I, yet its origin and function are less well defined.

Insulin is more potent in stimulating metabolic effects in insulin target tissues than are IGF-I and IGF-II. On the other hand, insulin is a less potent stimulator of cell proliferation than these growth factors. From an evolutionary point of view, one precursor hormone of insulin and of IGF-I must have existed that, millions of years ago, was responsible for both the acute regulation of metabolism and the stimulation of the slow processes of growth. Later, a gene duplication must have taken place leading to the diversion of these two functions, leaving the second-to-second metabolic regulation to insulin and regulation of growth to IGF-I. Although the classical actions of IGFs are thought to be endocrine, physiologically important IGF concentrations may be generated at the tissue level. The functions of IGFs are meditated by two main classes of IGF receptors. The IGF-I receptor exhibits ligand-dependent tyrosine kinase activity and autophosphorylation and has considerable structural and functional similarity to the insulin receptor, but higher affinity for IGF-I and IGF-II than for insulin (Fig. 12.3). The IGF-II receptor, in contrast, has a different structure and is homologous with the human mannose-6-phosphate receptor [47]. It has a higher affinity for IGF-II than IGF-I and does not bind insulin. Both IGF-I and IGF-II can bind, although at low potency, to the insulin receptor.

According to the somatomedin hypothesis, GH does not have a direct effect on cartilage but rather stimulates chondrogenesis and subsequent growth indirectly by way of somatomedins. Nevertheless, local injection of GH into the epiphyseal growth plate of the proximal tibia of hypophysectomized rats stimulates unilateral longitudinal bone growth.

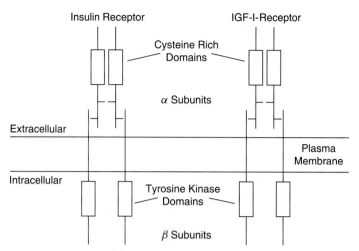

Figure 12.3 The insulin and IGF-I receptors are structurally related heterotetrameric glycoproteins consisting of two α and two β subunits. The α subunits lie entirely extracellularly, contain cysteine-rich regions, and bind the ligands. The transmembrane β subunits are joined to the α subunits by disulfide bonds and contain a tyrosine kinase domain in their cytoplasmic portion. The level of amino acid similarity between these two receptors is particularly high (85%) in the tyrosine kinase domains [29].

The number of IGF-I immunoreactive cells in the proliferative zone is increased. It was concluded that IGF-I is produced in proliferative chondrocytes in the growth plate in response to GH and that the number of IGF-I-containing cells is directly regulated by expansion of differentiated chondrocytes as stimulated locally through autocrine or paracrine mechanisms or both [36, 39].

GH can induce local IGF-I production in the epiphyseal plate at the level of both mRNA and protein. In vitro studies of epiphyseal chondrocytes indicate that GH and IGF-I have different target cells; they bind to different cell populations and give rise to different clonal types in soft agar suspension cultures. Therefore GH, but not IGF-I, stimulates the multiplication of the slowly cycling (label-retaining) cells in the germinal layer of the epiphyseal plate. IGF-I acts only on the proliferation of the resulting chondrocytes. GH, but not IGF-I, stimulates the multiplication of label-retaining cells located in the top layer of the epiphyseal plate. The fact that locally infused IGF-I is able to increase epiphyseal width as well as longitudinal bone growth, together with the finding that IGF-I was unable to increase the number of label-retaining cells in the germinal layer, indicates that the target cells for IGF-I are located in the proliferative cell layer. The cells of the germinal layer may be regarded as the stem cells of the growth plate and the proliferative chondrocytes as "transient amplifying" cells. The growth demonstrated by local or by systemic IGF-I administration could probably be explained by a stimulation of the proliferative cell layer, where extra cell divisions within the transient amplifying cells could result in significant growth. Data support the theory that GH simulates a low differentiated stem cell-like population to start dividing, which gives rise to a clonal expansion, and that IGF-I, on the other hand, enhances the clonal expansion of an already GH-primed cell population [38].

Both T_3 and IGF-I interact with epiphyseal chondrocytes and both substances affect cell proliferation and maturation and therefore longitudinal bone growth. IGF-I is important for proliferation of the cells, while T_3 may initiate the terminal differentiation of epiphyseal chondrocytes [38].

It is likely that the actions of GH on a variety of tissues are mediated by the local production of IGF-I or possibly other somatomedins. In the *dual effector theory* of somatotropin action, GH directly stimulates the differentiated state of certain cell types. For

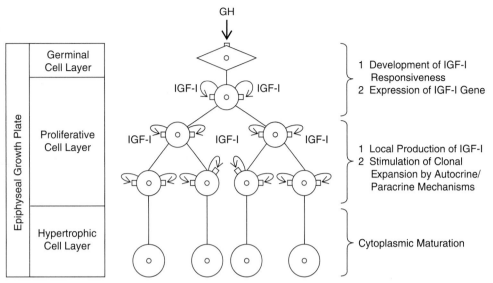

Figure 12.4   Model of the dual-effector hypothesis of GH action. (From Isaksson et al. [23], with permission.)

example, GH, but not IGF-I, directly promotes the differentiation of cultured pread-ipocytes to adipocytes. The newly differentiated adipocytes were shown to be much more sensitive to the mitogenic actions of IGF-I than were the precursor cells. The results of IGF-I action is, therefore, a selective multiplication of young differentiated cells (a so-called clonal expansion). In this dual-effector system, the target cells of IGF-I action are created by the initial direct action of GH [59]. A model for the direct and indirect actions of GH is provided (Fig. 12.4).

Pituitary growth hormone is essential for normal growth in humans and probably most vertebrates. Growth hormone secretion is regulated by stimulating (somatocrinin) and inhibiting (somatostatin) factors from the hypothalamus. Diverse stimuli mediate pituitary GH secretion by their initial actions within the hypothalamus (see Chap. 6). In the adult, excess GH secretion results in acromegaly. There is controversy concern-ing the role of the central nervous system (CNS) in the pathogenesis of acromegaly. The central issue is whether pituitary tumor formation occurs as a consequence of neo-plastic transformation in a somatotroph cell(s) or secondary to excessive stimulation by somatocrinin. Recent molecular biologic studies of two different tumor types support the "pituitary hypothesis." Analysis of these adenomas suggests that these tumors are monoclonal, implying that a mutation preceded the tumor's clonal expansion. In other studies, the sequence of the α subunit of the guanine nucleotide binding (regulatory) protein (G_s) in 35–40% of somatotroph adenomas has been shown to contain a com-mon point mutation at one of two sites that is crucial for its intrinsic GTPase activity [41, 50]. The mutations produce a single amino acid substitution that leads to consti-tutive activation of adenylate cyclase, resulting in enhanced cAMP production (see Figs. 21.13 and 21.14). Cyclic AMP has been implicated as a mitogen, as well as a stimulus, to both the synthesis and release of GH. Although results from several stud-ies argue in favor of a pituitary defect in the etiology of acromegaly, they do not exclude a contribution from the CNS, and it is possible that somatotrophs subjected to stimulation by excessive somatocrinin secretion might be more likely to undergo neo-plastic transformation [19].

IGF-I stimulates hypothalamic somatostatin release and inhibits stimulated pituitary GH release. In addition, intracerebroventricularly injected preparations of IGFs cause a marked decrease in GH secretion. A model for the control of GH secretion and somatomedin production is shown in Fig. 12.5.

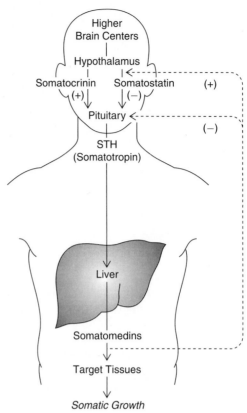

Figure 12.5 Model for the control of somatotropin GH secretion by somatostatin and somatocrinin.

Growth hormone mediates its growth indirectly through hepatic IGF-I production. IGF-I then affects growth through its action on skeletal tissues and many other
connective tissues and organs. Several hormones (e.g., prolactin, placental lactogen,
insulin) may also exert part of their growth-promoting activity through effects on hepatic IGF production. The structures of hPL and PRL are similar to that of GH. IGF
levels remain normal in hypophysectomized pregnant rats even in the absence of PRL
and GH; these levels decline promptly postpartum. Thus other GH-related factors may
be important in IGF production during particular physiological states, such as pregnancy.

Growth hormone has a direct action on a number of target cells in addition to its
action on hepatic IGF production. These GH actions have been described as diabetogenic
in nature. For example, GH stimulates lipolysis [12], which provides substrates for glucose formation, and thus has a sparing effect on direct glucose utilization (see Chap. 11).
The direct and indirect actions of GH are depicted in Fig. 12.6.

Figure 12.7 depicts the relationship between GH and plasma levels of IGFs. Hypopituitary dwarfs, as might be expected, have very minimal plasma levels of IGF-I and IGF-
II. Although levels of IGF-I are greatly increased in acromegalics, levels of IGF-II did not
differ from controls. Like IGF-I, IGF-II production is GH dependent; but this relationship
becomes apparent only when GH levels fall below normal. These results indicate that production of the two IGFs is regulated differently. Some short children with low spontaneous
GH secretion and high percent increase in serum IGF values in response to provocative GH
stimulation benefit from GH or IGF-I treatment by an increased growth rate [18].

Dwarfism in German shepherds may be genetically transmitted by a simple recessive mode of inheritance. Dwarfism in these dogs is caused by GH deficiency resulting in

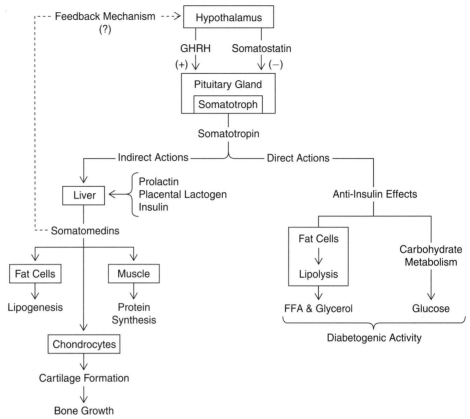

Figure 12.6 Summary scheme of the direct and indirect actions of somatotropin (growth hormone) on growth and metabolism.

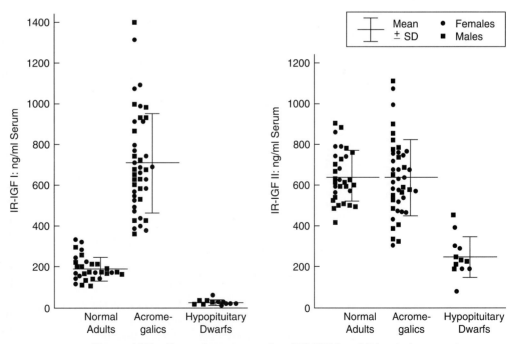

Figure 12.7 Serum immunoreactive (IR) IGF-I and II levels in normal adults, acromegalic patients, and patients with isolated GH deficiency. (Reproduced from Zapf et al. and used by permission from *The Journal of Clinical Investigation*, 1981, vol. 68: 1321–1330. ©The American Society for Clinical Investigation.)

low circulating levels of IGF-I. In the dwarf mouse strain, "little," decreased growth is associated with a partial deficiency of GH production. The pituitaries of these mice are completely insensitive to somatocrinin. GH secretion can, however, be stimulated by DcAMP or agents that increase cAMP levels. These observations suggest a defect in the early stage of somatocrinin-stimulated GH release related either to receptor binding or to a defect in receptor signal transmission.

Short stature in the African Pygmy has been an enigma for centuries. Short stature in the Pygmy might be due to end-organ resistance to IGFs, but it has also been shown that Pygmies have decreased circulating levels of IGF-I (Fig. 12.8). Plasma levels of IGF-II are, in contrast to hypopituitary dwarfs, within the range found in normal adults [5, 33, 34]. Thus normal serum levels of IGF-II are inadequate for promotion of normal growth in the absence of IGF-I, at least in Pygmies. The role of IGF-II in growth remains to be clarified. These findings in the African Pygmy may be consistent with undernutrition.

The amino acid sequences of rabbit and human GH receptors have been deduced from their respective cDNA sequences. There is strong localized sequence identity between the two receptors in both the extracellular and cytoplasmic domains, suggesting that the two receptors originated form a common ancestor. The receptor contains a single membrane-spanning domain and shares sequence with PRL receptors of a variety of species [1].

The growth hormone receptor is activated on binding of GH to stimulate the growth and metabolism of muscle, bone, and cartilage cells. This receptor is a member of a group of receptors that are found on various cell types and are generally involved in cell growth and differentiation. All these receptors are grouped together in the hematopoietic super-family [20]. Like the receptor tyrosine kinases, members of the hematopoietic receptor superfamily have a three-domain organization comprising an extracellular ligand binding domain, a single transmembrane segment, and an intracellular domain of unknown function, which is not homologous within the family. Like the receptor tyrosine kinases, the mechanism through which information from the ligand binding event is transmitted through the membrane to evoke a cellular response is unknown. The nature of intracellular messenger(s), if involved, is also undetermined [13]. A model for GH action is depicted (Fig. 12.9).

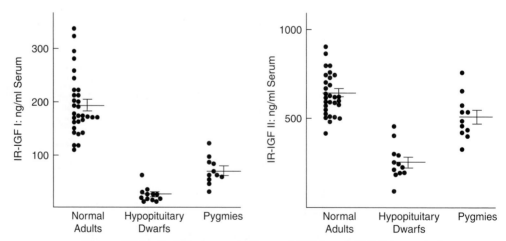

Figure 12.8 Serum concentrations of IGF-I and IGF-II in controls, hypopituitary dwarfs, and Pygmies. IGF-I and IGF-II were measured in the same adult controls. Lines and bars denote means ± S.E.M. Note that only one Pygmy has an IGF-I value within the lower normal range, whereas all but one have IGF-II values within the normal range. All values are corrected for cross-reactivity. (From Merimee, Zapf, and Froesch, reprinted by permission of *New England Journal of Medicine*, vol. 305, pp. 965–968, 1981.)

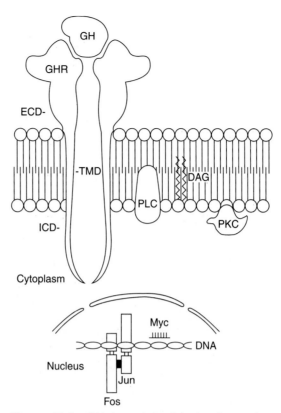

Figure 12.9 GH (somatotropin) signal transduction pathway. GH brings about receptor dimerization by binding first to the extracellular domain (ECD) of one receptor molecule and then to that of another receptor molecule. The signal of GH-binding is probably transmitted via the transmembrane domain (TMD) to bring about conformational changes in the intracellular domain (ICD). Following this, several early biochemical events have been recorded, including phospholipase C (PLC)-mediated DAG production, protein kinase C (PKC)-induced phosphorylation of the GHR, and possibly some cellular proteins. Induction of *Fos, Jun* and *Myc* genes are also observed. (Used by permission from Maharajan and Maharajan, "Growth hormone signal transduction." *Experienta* 49:980–7, 1993, Birkhauser Verlag AG, Basel, Switzerland.)

Laron syndrome is due to an autosomal recessive disorder occurring in consanguineous families, and affected individuals are resistant to the effects of endogenous and exogenous GH. Growth hormone from these individuals is, by chemical and biochemical criteria, similar to GH from normal individuals. Unlike short stature due to isolated GH deficiency, individuals with the Laron syndrome have elevated levels of circulating GH. The affected individuals have markedly reduced circulating levels of IGF-I. Laron syndrome is caused by hepatic unresponsiveness to circulating GH due to a defect in the GH receptor [1, 43, 54]. An inbred population with a high incidence of GH receptor deficiency, which is a type of the Laron syndrome, has been described, with the predominance of the affected individuals being females, "the little women of Loja," (Fig. 12.10), and may be the result of the genetic defect being linked to a trait resulting in early fetal death of most affected males.

The defect in the GH receptor is an extreme example of the Laron syndrome; several different abnormalities of the GH receptor gene have been demonstrated in this condition: a point mutation in one family, a deletion of a large portion of the extracellular domain of the receptor gene in two other cases [1]. The defect also affects the high affinity GH-BP (GH-binding protein); complete absence of GH-binding activity has been demonstrated in the plasma of patients with the Laron syndrome. A high-affinity binding protein has been characterized as a fragment of the GH receptor. The assay of the GH-BP can be used as a tool for diagnosis; Laron syndrome being the only situation in which a complete absence of GH-binding activity is observed [17]. This hypothesis has, however, been re-evaluated because of the recent description of patients displaying the classical features of the Laron syndrome except for the presence of GH-BP activity similar to that of normal subjects. In this variant form of the Laron syndrome, there appears to be a normal GH receptor and signal transmission for GH-BP production but a defect in the post-receptor mechanism for the generation of IGF-I.

The physiological significance of the GH-binding activity and its variations measured in human plasma is an important question. The high-affinity BP corresponds to the

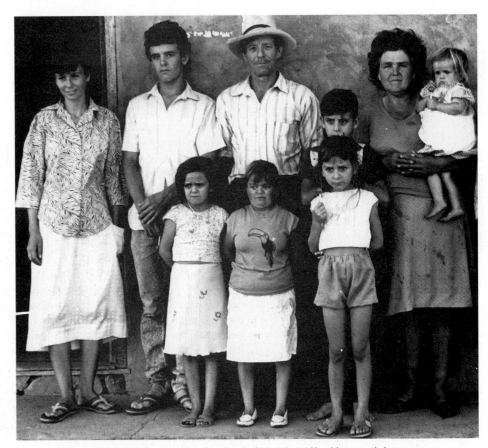

Figure 12.10   The family of patients (#8, #9, #10) with growth hormone receptor deficiency. This photograph shows, from left to right, a sister, 25 years old (height, 158.8 cm); a brother, 18 years old (164.7 cm); Patient 9 (16 years old, 107.1 cm); the father, 52 years old (165 cm); Patient 8 (21 years old, 106.2 cm); a brother, 12 years old (135.9 cm); a sister, 8.5 years old (115.4 cm); and the mother, 46 years old (156.7 cm), holding Patient 10 (6.5 years old, 72 cm). (From A. L. Rosenbloom, J. Guevara Aguirre, R. G. Rosenfeld, and P. J. Fiedler. "The little women of Loja—growth hormone-receptor deficiency in an inbred population of southern Ecuador." Reprinted by permission of *The New England Journal of Medicine*, 323:1367–74, 1990.)

extracellular binding domain of the receptor. The GH-binding activity may reflect the tissue concentration of GH receptors. Results on the regulation of the GH-BP in humans support a parallel regulation of liver membrane receptors and plasma BP. The regulation of the human plasma BP by GH can be compared with the increase in the number of hepatic GH receptors observed in rats infused with rat GH. In rats it has also been shown that GH is necessary to maintain its own receptors in adipocytes. Testosterone, which is able to decrease the level of GH-BP in human plasma, also affects the binding of GH to rat liver membranes. The binding of GH to liver microsomal membranes of castrated male rats is higher than that of age-matched male animals [17].

About 40–50% of circulating GH is complexed to the BP in normal human plasma. The GH-BP complex represents a hormone reservoir and the presence of the BP modifies the amount of hormone that can have access to the receptors. GH-BP generation in the human probably results from the proteolytic cleavage of the liver membrane receptor. On the other hand, in the rat alternate splicing of a single primary DNA transcript may give rise to distinct mRNAs, one encodes the full-length membrane receptor, the other a truncated receptor (the extracellular binding domain) [17].

Binding proteins are important modulators of the ligand-receptor interaction on target cells [6, 7, 44]. IGFs circulate in the serum as high molecular weight complexes. The majority of the IGFs are complexed as a 150-kDa GH-dependent binding protein complex. Lower molecular-weight binding proteins occur in fetal plasma and other extracellular fluids. Only low levels of free IGFs are detected in plasma, raising the question as to whether physiologically active IGF is the free or complexed form. The "free hormone hypothesis" as postulated for steroid and thyroid hormones would allow IGF-binding proteins a merely passive role, that of physically transporting the IGFs and of inactivating the IGFs by their being bound. Studies now indicate a more dynamic role for the IGF-binding proteins, that of interacting with target cells and thus facilitating the delivery of hormones to their receptors. IGF-binding proteins themselves bind to some cell surfaces and thus deliver IGF to adjacent IGF receptors [40]. Figure 12.11 illustrates the anatomical and physiological factors related to growth-hormone disorders.

Ethical Issues. Growth hormone is already accepted as the conventional treatment for short stature in children with GH deficiency [18], but it is now being given to increasing numbers of children who do not fulfill the classic criteria of growth deficiency. GH will augment the growth of many of these children, however, the effect on final adult heights is as yet unknown. Before trials of GH deficiency are extended beyond children with the classic growth deficiency, ethical and other issues should be considered [46]. There are dangers, for example, that GH might be used to alter people to fit a social norm rather than to treat a disease. Also, it has been questioned whether society should spend resources on "something that really isn't a problem" [51].

Safety of Growth Hormone for Animal Use. An independent committee appointed by the National Institutes of Health has examined the available data and concluded that the overall composition and nutritional quality of milk and meat from bGH-treated cows is equal to that from untreated cows. Similarly, the FDA has concluded that the use of bGH presents no increased health risk to consumers. In addition, there is compelling evidence to indicate that GH poses no increased health risk to the target animal. Thus, GH treatment of farm animals is not only an effective technology for increasing productive efficiency, but one that poses no health risk for either the consumer or the target animal [16].

INSULIN

Although insulin plays the dominant role in the control of carbohydrate metabolism in humans and other vertebrates, it also profoundly affects growth processes in animals.

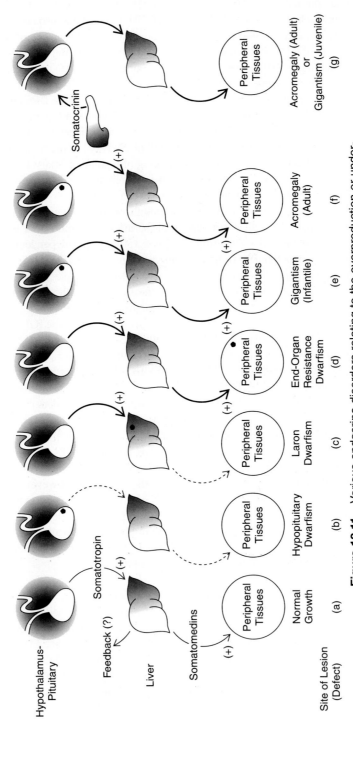

Figure 12.11 Various endocrine disorders relating to the overproduction or under-production of pituitary GH or to inadequate hepatic or peripheral tissue response to GH or somatomedins.

Children with diabetes, for example, fail to grow even though GH levels are normal, whereas infants of diabetic mothers with islet hyperplasia and hyperinsulinism are of increased stature. This might not be too surprising considering the structural similarities between insulin, the IGFs and their receptors. The growth-promoting actions of insulin are amply documented, and protein catabolism is accelerated in the absence of insulin. Insulin is required for the full anabolic effect of GH, an action that may be because insulin, through its action on glucose uptake by muscle, provides the energy substrates necessary for protein synthesis. However, insulin also increases the incorporation of amino acids into muscle by an action that is independent of its effects on glucose metabolism. This may result from the direct action of insulin on the transport of amino acids into cells, as well as activation of ribosomal translational capacity, as protein synthesis per se is not dependent on glucose availability or RNA synthesis. Insulin stimulates the growth of immature hypophysectomized rats, but this action is manifested only when the protein-sparing action of insulin is enhanced by the concomitant feeding of a high carbohydrate diet.

Insulin at a high concentration, as in familial insulin resistance, stimulates general body growth through low-affinity binding to IGF receptors. Although there is insulin-receptor deficiency in this endocrinopathy, the number of IGF receptors appears to be normal. The high circulating levels of insulin thus cause acral (affecting the extremities) overgrowth as well as enlargement of the kidney and adrenal glands; these actions of insulin may result from cross-reactivity with IGF receptors (Fig. 12.3) [42].

PROLACTIN

In humans prolactin (PRL) plays an important role in milk synthesis, a function that of necessity requires development and growth of the mammary glands. Because of the close structural similarity between PRL and GH, it is not surprising that many effects of PRL are growth related; most are usually involved in reproductive processes of the individual (see Chaps. 5 and 19).

Prolactin, along with estrogens and adrenal steroids, is essential for ductile branching during the prepubertal and postpubertal period to form the fully developed system of the mammary glands of the mature female. Large amounts of PRL, even in the absence of adequate amounts of estrogens (as occurs in PRL-secreting tumors in men or postmenopausal women), are usually associated with clinically evident enlargement of the breasts. PRL also stimulates production of somatomedins by the rat liver and could conceivably affect general body growth by an GH-like action.

PRL also has important stimulatory effects on the immune system; it serves as a growth factor for lymphocytes and accelerates T-cell-dependent immune responses. Hyperprolactinemia has been reported in association with autoimmune thyroiditis and systemic lupus erythematosus in humans [55]. PRL is also synthesized and secreted by human blood mononuclear cells and may be an autocrine growth factor for lymphoproliferation [48].

Prolactin also directly affects the growth and function of the ovaries and testes, in some cases by modulating the action of gonadotropins on the gonads. In nonmammalian vertebrates PRL has growth-related actions such as stimulation of tail and gill growth in amphibians. PRL is required for limb regeneration in the salamander and tail regeneration in lizards. Many structural changes in the skin of the salamander related to "water drive" involve the actions of PRL. Hypertrophy of the pigeon crop-sac mucosa, as well as epidermal hyperplasia related to brood patch formation in the dove, are regulated by PRL. Other physiological actions of this hormone are discussed in Chaps. 5 and 19.

The amino acid sequences of human GH and PRL receptors have been deduced from their respective cDNA sequences. There is strong localized sequence identity between the two receptors in both the extracellular and cytoplasmic domains, suggesting that the two receptors originated from a common ancestor. As is true for GH, no means of signal transduction has been identified for PRL. There are no clear effects of PRL on cAMP, cGMP, inositol phospholipids, phosphorylation, calcium ions, or ion channels. Neither the GH nor the PRL receptor appears to be a tyrosinase kinase.

PLACENTAL LACTOGEN

During pregnancy the placenta secretes hormones that augment maternal pituitary and gonadal functions. In addition to chorionic gonadotropin and a number of steroids, the placenta also synthesizes and secretes chorionic somatomammotropin. Although similar to somatotropin in structure, this hormone lacks significant growth-promoting activity but displays considerable lactogenic activity; it is therefore referred to as placental lactogen (PL). In the human, PL is found in the maternal plasma as early as the sixth week of pregnancy and reaches a concentration three orders of magnitude greater than that of GH during the second trimester. Placental lactogen is synthesized within the *syncytiotrophoblastic* epithelial cells of the chorionic villi of the placenta (see Chap. 19).

Placental lactogen increases sulfate uptake into cartilage in hypophysectomized rats, both in vivo and in vitro, and also stimulates growth and induction of milk protein synthesis in mouse mammary explants. Development and maturation of the testes of immature and genetically dwarf mice is also stimulated by PL. All these biological actions are similar to the actions of human PRL. Placental lactogen mimics the action of GH on most of its target tissues but is much less potent than pituitary GH. There is no evidence that PL can increase linear growth in hypopituitary dwarfs. It might be expected, however, that this hormone evolved to play some specific role(s) related to pregnancy and reproductive processes. PL secretion during the second trimester of human pregnancy may supplement the action of choriogonadotropin on the corpus luteum, which is diminishing. The primary role of PL may be to stimulate the development of the mammary glands during pregnancy without actually causing milk secretion. Pituitary PRL then initiates milk secretion soon after parturition. PL may also alter the maternal metabolism so that adequate supplies of glucose, amino acids, and minerals are available to the fetus during the latter part of pregnancy, a time when fetal growth requirements are rapidly increasing. During the second half of pregnancy, PL is one of several factors that counter the effect of insulin in the maternal circulation, thereby facilitating glucose and amino acid availability to the fetus. In this manner, the placental secretion of this hormone indirectly stimulates intrauterine growth. PL may also directly stimulate fetal growth. Ovine PL stimulates glycogenesis in hepatocytes of the fetal rat and sheep and aminoisobutyric acid uptake in diaphragm muscle of the fetal rat. It also stimulates ornithine decarboxylase activity in fetal rat liver and somatomedin secretion in fetal and adult tissue. These observations indicate a role for PL in fetal growth and development (Fig. 12.6).

Human PL and GH are both single-chain polypeptides containing 191 amino acid residues. Both hormones are internally cross-linked through two disulfide bridges and are identical throughout 85% of their primary structures; 162 residues in each polypeptide are identical and occupy similar positions in the hormones. The high degree of structural similarity between hPL and human and ovine GH suggests that the polypeptide arose from a relatively recent duplication of an GH gene (Fig. 12.12), rather than from the more distantly related lactogenic hormones. A placental lactogen immunologically simi-

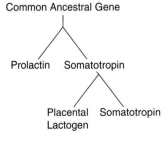

Figure 12.12 Hypothetical scheme for the evolution of somatotropin, prolactin, and placental lactogen.

lar to hPL is present in the plasma of the rhesus monkey, baboon, chinchilla, hamster, goat, cow, sheep, and a number of other mammalian species. In general the level of the placental lactogen begins to rise at or before midpregnancy and usually remains elevated until term.

NEUROTROPIC GROWTH FACTORS

Several peptide growth factors regulate the differentiation and growth of both the central and peripheral nervous systems. The etiological basis of one or more disorders (e.g., Alzheimer's disease) may relate to these neurotropic factors.

Nerve Growth Factor

Growth and differentiation of sensory and motor components of the peripheral nervous system are enhanced by factors released from peripheral target tissues [9]. On the other hand, an intact innervation and release of supporting substances from nerve endings are essential for normal development of the innervated target tissues. There is accumulating evidence that specific chemical messengers are important in these reciprocal actions between nerves and target tissues.

Certain mouse sarcomas induce a pathologic hypertrophy of chick embryonic sensory and sympathetic ganglia. This neuronal hypertrophy depends on a humoral protein factor released by the transplanted tumors. This substance was named nerve growth factor (NGF), and its chemistry and biological roles have been well characterized [30]. NGF is also present in snake venom and in the submandibular (submaxillary) salivary glands of adult male mice. NGF is synthesized within tubular cells of the submandibular gland and its production is androgen dependent. Salivary gland NGF levels in female mice rise during pregnancy and lactation when androgen levels are elevated. Testosterone given to female mice causes tubular cell hypertrophy and the content of salivary gland NGF rises markedly. In contrast, castration of male mice causes tubular atrophy and the salivary gland content of NGF falls dramatically.

The early discovery that mouse submandibular glands synthesize and release into the saliva large quantities of NGF, that the synthesis of the protein molecule is under the control of testosterone and of thyroxine, and that the NGF protein content is about tenfold higher in male than in female mice long remained a puzzling and unexplained finding. The conflicting but negative attempts to reveal the presence of this molecule in the circulating blood, and the lack of any adverse effects on sympathetic and sensory cells by removal of these glands, which deprived these rodents of such a large NGF source, did not support the hypothesis that salivary NGF gains access to their target cells. An alternative biological function for salivary NGF has now been hypothesized. Intraspecific fighting experimentally induced in adult male mice by 6–9 weeks of social isolation results in massive NGF release into the blood stream, an event prevented by previous salivary gland removal. Since injections of NGF induce weight and size increase of the adrenal glands and stimulate the synthesis of tyrosine hydroxylase, the key enzyme in catecholamine synthesis (see Chap. 14), it was suggested that the release of salivary NGF may be instrumental in defense and/or offense mechanisms of vital significance for male mice that engage in intraspecific fighting among individuals of the same sex [30].

Peripheral sympathetic postganglionic neurons of the autonomic nervous system (see Chap. 14) are the primary target cells for NGF and respond to the protein throughout life. Injections of NGF antiserum in newborn mice or chick embryos cause almost complete destruction of the sympathetic nervous system (immunosympathectomy). Exposure in utero to maternal antibodies to NGF, in addition to producing immunosympathectomy, destroys peripheral nervous system sensory neurons in the dorsal root ganglia. These neurons may depend on NGF for survival during prenatal development. Other dorsal root cells may manifest a temporal difference in their dependence on NGF. NGF antiserum administration to adult animals causes deleterious effects on sympathetic neurons that are reversible after antiserum treatment is stopped. Thus it appears that an endogenous NGF is critical for sympathetic nervous system development, and NGF may function in the maintenance of sympathetic neurons throughout life.

Mouse salivary gland NGF is a molecular complex consisting of three types of polypeptide chains, designated α, β, and γ. Each of these subunits consists of a pair of identical molecules. The β subunit is held together by noncovalent bonds. Only the β subunit possesses nerve growth-promoting activity. The biological activity of NGF is dependent upon the dimeric structure of the molecule. NGF is synthesized as a precursor peptide, a proNGF. The individual β chains of NGF are then cleaved by the γ subunit, which is an endopeptidase. The α subunits may also play a role in maintaining the functional integrity of the molecular complex of NGF in the secretory granule.

There is homology between NGF and proinsulin and there are also striking similarities between the biological activities of the two molecules. Both hormones bind initially to cell membranes, which results in an enhancement of a number of ensuing anabolic processes, such as RNA synthesis, polysome formation, and protein and lipid synthesis, characteristic of cellular growth. NGF may be viewed as a hormone whose structural gene may have evolved from an ancestral proinsulin gene and whose mode of action on neurons might, therefore, be somewhat similar to that of insulin on its target tissues. To a limited extent, insulin and proinsulin can compete for the binding of NGF to its receptor, further emphasizing the relationship of NGF to proinsulin.

After an initial interaction with the cell plasma membrane. NGF is internalized and, by retrograde axonal transport, apparently carried to the soma of the cell. Retrograde transport of NGF is specific as other proteins of similar size and charge are transported to a much lesser extent. It is interesting that insulin may be similarly internalized in its target cells to invoke its cellular effects. Binding of NGF is specific to target tissue surface receptors because motor neurons that can internalize and transport tetanus toxin fail to do so with NGF. Similarly, cholinergic parasympathetic nerves, which like motor neurons are refractory to the biological actions of NGF, do not transport NGF.

NGF exerts a pleiotropic effect on nerve cells, which includes the synthesis of specific enzymes, tyrosine hydroxylase and dopamine β-hydroxylase, involved in adrenergic nervous transmission. The stimulation by NGF of nerve fiber outgrowth is reflected in the accumulation of large masses of neurofilaments that are found in developing axons. Neurite outgrowth in response to NGF is an RNA-independent event, which suggests that NGF may stimulate fiber outgrowth by acting in a selective fashion on protein synthesis at a stage after transcription. Ornithine decarboxylase is a key enzyme in the biosynthesis of polyamines and may serve an important regulatory role in cell division and growth. In the brain the intraventricular injection of NGF leads to a marked increase in the activity of this enzyme. Adrenal glucocorticoids appear to be required for NGF to enhance the activity of ornithine decarboxylase.

Clearly, NGF functions in the survival of peripheral sympathetic and spinal sensory neurons during defined periods of their ontogenesis. In addition NGF directs growing sympathetic nerve fibers toward their corresponding target tissues. The role of NGF as a retrograde messenger between peripheral target tissues and innervating sympathetic and neural crest-derived sensory neurons is supported by the observations that the interruption of the retrograde axonal transport has the same effects as the neutralization of endogenous NGF by anti-NGF antibodies, and the close correlation between the density of innervation by fibers of NGF-responsive neurons and the levels of NGF and mRNA in their target organs. In situ hybridization experiments have demonstrated that a great variety of cells in the projection field of NGF-responsive neurons synthesize NGF, among them epithelial cells, smooth muscle cells, fibroblasts, and Schwann cells. The continued availability of NGF to sympathetic neurons is nevertheless essential for neuron survival. A common misconception is that NGF stimulates neuronal cell division. Despite its name, NGF is not mitogenic for neurons. NGF directs neurite outgrowth and guidance to targets; it promotes cell survival in only a few cell populations, which include sympathetic and neural crest-derived sensory neurons [11].

NGF may also have a physiological role in the mammalian central nervous system as a neurotropic factor. There is evidence that the brain contains NGF, NGF messenger RNA, NGF receptors, and NGF-responsive neurons. One function of NGF in the CNS appears to be the regulation of the differentiation of the cholinergic projection neurons found within various nuclei of the basal forebrain. NGF also prevents the retrograde degeneration of cholinergic neurons within the medial septum of the rat brain that normally occurs following axotomy of these neurons. Lesioned animals suffer from deficits in learning and memory. NGF infusion into the brain of these rats counteracts their learning deficiencies, presumably by prevention of neuronal losses. There is hope that the deterioration of the cholinergic neurons in the brains of Alzheimer's patients might be prevented or retarded by treatment with NGF or some drug that mimics NGF activity in the brain [28].

Other Neurotropic Factors

Considering the diversity of neuronal cell types, it is not unexpected that a number of other neurotropic factors have been identified (see Cover photographs and caption).

The NGF Family and Its Receptors.   The gene family of neurotropins includes nerve growth factor (NGF), brain-derived neurotropic factor (BDNF), neurotropin-3 (NT-3), and neurotropin-4 (NT-4). Recently, neurotropin-5 (NT-5), a possible mammalian homologue to NT-4 described in the frog, *Xenopus*, has been cloned in humans and rats. These factors are produced in limited amounts in target tissues and mediate the cell interaction regulating neuron survival during the period of naturally occurring neuronal death in development. The release of these proteins is believed to regulate not only the survival of neurons but also the extent of innervation of the target tissues. As well as being important in neuronal development, neurotrophic factors also have a function in the adult nervous system [15].

These trophic factors are synthesized as precursor polypeptides that are subsequently cleaved to yield the mature neurotrophins. These molecules are homodimers of 115 to 130 amino acid residues that share at least 50% sequence identity, including six conserved cysteine residues. The recent resolution of the crystal structure of NGF has revealed that the two subunits associate through a flat surface formed by three antiparallel β strands, whereas most variable residues are clustered in three β hairpin loops located in the outside regions of the molecule, presumably involved in receptor recognition [2].

The purification of brain-derived neurotrophic factor (BDNF), the elucidation of its primary structure, and the subsequent identification of neurotrophin-3 (NT-3) ended the monopoly of NGF as the only well-characterized, target-derived neurotrophic molecule. NGF, BDNF, and NT-3 are members of a gene family called neurotrophins. They have strictly conserved domains that determine their basic structure. However, they also have distinctly variable domains that determine their different neuronal specificity mediated by different high-affinity receptors and that share a common low-affinity subunit. These similarities and dissimilarities between the members of the neurotrophin gene family are also reflected by their regional distribution, cellular localization and developmental regulation [53].

All neurotropins stimulate survival and differentiation of a range of target neurons by binding to cell-surface receptors. The structure of NGF has recently been determined from crystallographic data. The similarities between the different neurotropins are substantial within the variable regions, giving specificity to each of the family members. A 140-K tyrosine protein kinase encoded by the proto-oncogene *trk* has been found to bind NGF with high affinity and to evoke the cellular neurotropic responses. In addition, a protein encoded by the *trk*-related gene *trk*B has been shown to bind BDNF. Recently, a third member of the *trk* family, *trk*C, has been cloned and demonstrated to function as a high-affinity receptor for NT-3 [15]. Since NGF acts directly through *trk* tyrosine phosphorylation, many other crucial activities, such as neurite outgrowth, cell survival, chemotaxis, neurotransmitter synthesis and regulation, may be influenced by protein phosphorylation [11].

Although NGF and NGF receptors have so far not been described in invertebrates, NGF seems to have effects on neurons from the snail *Lymnaea stagnalis*. Thus evolution of neurotrophic factors and receptor systems mediating neurotrophic interactions in developmental and neuroplasticity processes may well have begun in ancestors common to several major metazoan phyla. No doubt the flexible system of several neurotropins with partially overlapping activities combined with several receptors has been adopted to fulfil various functions during vertebrate evolution. It may thus be anticipated that the neurotropins and their receptors act differently in different groups of vertebrates and also have taken distinct roles in separate organ systems [15].

Target-derived Neurotropic Factor.   Treatment of chick embryos in vivo with crude and partially purified extracts from embryonic hindlimbs (days 8 to 9) during the normal cell death period (days 5 to 10) rescues a significant number of motoneurons from degeneration. The survival activity of partially purified extract is dose-dependent and developmentally regulated. The survival of sensory, sympathetic, parasympathetic, and a population of cholinergic sympathetic preganglionic neurons was unaffected by treatment with hindlimb extract. The massive motoneuron death that occurs after early target (hindlimb) removal is partially ameliorated by daily treatment with the hindlimb extract. These results indicate that a target-derived neurotropic factor is involved in the regulation of motoneuron survival in vivo.

Insulin and IGFs.   Insulin and insulin-like growth factors I and II (IGF-I and IGF-II) are required for optimal growth and proliferation of a number of cell types. These factors also stimulate proliferation of cultured sympathetic neuroblasts, implicating a regulatory role in the mitogenic cycle of neuroblasts during fetal development. As neurons differentiate terminally they cease to divide, but they still express receptors for insulin, IGF-I and IGF-II. In mature brain all three factors can be detected immunochemically, but expression in the brain appears to be restricted to IGF-II and, much less abundantly, to IGF-I. These observations suggest that insulin and IGFs play a role also in the mature nervous system, which seems to include functional maintenance and survival of neurons [41].

Apoptosis

Apoptosis is a mode of cell death in which single cells are deleted from tissues. Apoptosis can be viewed as an equal and opposite force to mitosis and, as such, plays an essential role in the maintenance of renewable tissues. Apoptosis accounts for most or all of the programmed cell death responsible for tissue remodeling in vertebrate development, for the cell loss that accompanies atrophy of adult tissues following diminished endocrine and other stimuli, and for the physiological death of cells in normal tissue turnover. The homeostatic balance of cell number is brought about through the presence or absence of specific hormones or growth factors, such as NGF. The extensive deletion of lymphocytes of the β and T lineages during negative selection in the immune response is effected by apoptosis, as is a proportion of the target cell death of cell-mediated immune killing [58]. Lymphocytolysis evoked by glucocorticoids is a good example of hormone-mediated cell death. This physiologically mediated cell death is to be contrasted with necrotic death resulting from accidental trauma. Drugs that block protein synthesis prevent apoptosis, suggesting that this programmed cell death requires specific proteins ("suicide proteins").

HEMATOPOIETIC GROWTH FACTORS

Hematopoiesis is the process of renewal and replacement of the cells and formed elements of blood. Erythropoiesis is a subset of this larger scheme and includes only these events that lead from the appearance of the committed erythroid progenitor cell through the formation of mature red blood cells. Red and white blood cell differentiation and production are regulated by a number of hormones, as will be discussed below.

Erythropoietin

The circulating red cell mass in adult humans is remarkably constant. It has been estimated that a 70-kg individual has about 2.3×10^{13} red blood cells, and that, under normal conditions, they are synthesized at a rate of about 2.3×10^6 per second. Exposing individuals to high altitudes (low oxygen tension, or hypoxia), however, results in increased *erythropoiesis* (from the Greek, *poietin*, to make), whereas hypertransfusion (hyperoxia) results in reduced erythropoiesis. The presence of an erythropoietic factor was implicated in a parabiotic experiment where subjection of one rat to hypoxia resulted in increased erythropoiesis in its parabiotic partner. Transfusion of plasma from anemic animals into normal animals causes erythropoiesis, thus suggesting the existence of a humoral erythropoietic factor (*erythropoietin*, erythrocyte-stimulating factor, EP). Erythropoietin is elevated by conditions that create tissue hypoxia and decreased by conditions that create tissue hyperoxia. Agents that increase the metabolic rate and oxygen consumption, such as thyroid hormones, or pharmaceutical agents, such as dinitrophenol (an uncoupler of oxidative phosphorylation), produce a state of increased need for oxygen. Under these conditions EP is produced, which leads to increased erythropoiesis. Thus the ratio of oxygen supply to oxygen need appears to determine the level of EP formation and, therefore, the stimulus to erythropoiesis (Fig 12.13).

Bilaterally nephrectomized rats, unlike intact animals, do not respond to phlebotomy (blood withdrawal) or red blood cell destruction by increased EP production. In humans EP levels are low in the serum of anephric patients, but, after successful renal transplantation, EP increases in the blood. Erythropoietic activity is detected in perfusates from isolated kidneys and is also produced by renal cell cultures in vitro. These data establish the kidney as a source of the erythropoietic factor. Erythropoietin levels are diminished after hypophysectomy and, like the somatomedins, is increased in response to growth hormone. EP is also produced in response to androgen stimulation (see Chap. 17). Administration of EP antiserum to normal mice decreases erythropoiesis, providing support for the control of normal erythropoiesis by EP.

EP affects erythroid progenitors in the bone marrow by binding to the EP receptor. Early- and late-stage erythroid progenitor cells differ in their responsiveness to EP. This is due to the fact that they express either a truncated (T) or full-length (F) EPR, EP-T and

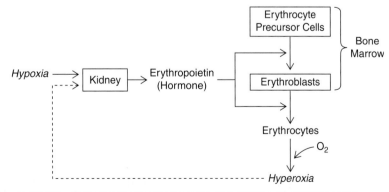

Figure 12.13   Scheme for the biogenesis and actions of erythropoietin.

EP-F, respectively. A majority of the early-stage erythroid progenitors expressing EPR-T may die of apoptosis, but the late-stage erythroid progenitors expressing EPR-F may survive and differentiate into mature erythrocytes in the presence of the same physiological concentration of EP. Thus, a mechanism exists that, under normal conditions, seemingly wastes many early-stage erythroid progenitors but helps to form a large reservoir of late-stage erythroid precursors, which can be mobilized quickly to restore erythrocyte numbers in response to sudden bleeding or hypoxia [35].

An intrarenal O_2 sensor is thought to monitor the availability of O_2 and to translate this parameter into an altered rate of EP production [3]. Changes in oxygen flux may be detected by the tubular epithelial cells and transmitted to the adjacent peritubular endothelial cells, resulting in an induction of the gene for EP. An alternate hypothesis is that the proximal tubule cells release prostaglandin E_2, which then acts as the chemical messenger to activate EP-producing cells. The severity of hypoxia has no influence on the kinetics of the EP response, which would seem to indicate that the trigger mechanism that activates EP production in the kidney operates in an all-or-none fashion. Factors other than EP may have a stimulatory effect on erythropoiesis and may be necessary for the expression of the EP gene under hypoxic conditions. IGF-I, for example, stimulates erythropoiesis directly, as well as indirectly by increasing EP formation [4].

EP mRNA should be localized to those cells that produce EP. Two groups using a radioactive probe for the EP mRNA, in situ hybridization, and autoradiography demonstrated that a peritubular interstitial cell, outside the tubular basement membrane, was the renal cell that synthesized EP mRNA either under baseline conditions or after hypoxia. These cells were found in the cortex or outer medulla. When the number of interstitial cells with EP mRNA was measured in relation to increasing anemia, these cells increased in an exponential manner in parallel with the exponential increase in total EP mRNA and serum EP. Thus increased EP production was related to increased numbers of cells producing the EP mRNA rather than to increased production of the mRNA by the individual EP-producing cells. It was estimated that 20% to 30% of the total interstitial cell population of the inner cortex, but less than 10% of the interstitial cells in the subcapsular cortex, produced EP. Thus EP-producing cells may represent a specialized cell type within the cortical interstitium rather than a generalized cell type, such as a peritubular capillary endothelial cell [27].

Although the kidney is the primary source of EP, EP is also known to originate in other tissues. Evidence has shown that a low basal rate of erythropoiesis is maintained by both anephric patients and those with chronic renal failure. This extrarenal source of EP may be the liver; because the liver is the primary producer of fetal erythropoietin, it may maintain some degree of that function until adulthood. In the presence of intact kidneys the liver would play an insignificant role in EP production, but if the kidneys were nonfunctional or removed, the liver's role would be of greater importance. Recently two striking and controversial observations regarding extra-renal EP synthesis have been made. Evidence has been obtained for secretion of EP by bone marrow macrophages. Indeed, this work would suggest that EP production by these macrophages may be a principle source of the hormone in the bone marrow micro-environment under normal (nonanemic) conditions [52].

Plasma EP is a sialoprotein consisting of 165 amino acids. This glycoprotein contains over 40% carbohydrate, consisting of sialic acid and a number of sugars. The sialic acid residues are necessary for biological activity in vivo as in the asialo form it is cleared too rapidly by the liver. Erythropoietin is found in the plasma and urine of many mammalian species, as well as in birds and fishes.

The effects of EP are not noted until 2 to 3 days after stimulation, due to the time it takes for reticulocytes to mature. The half-life of EP, however, is only about 5 hours. This implies that a continuous supply of erythropoietin is not necessary for developing erythroblasts; all that may be needed is a priming stimulus. The role of EP is to enhance proliferation of erythrocyte precursor cells in bone marrow (or fetal liver) into erythroblasts (cells determined to become erythrocytes) and to stimulate proliferation of newly formed erythroblasts. Stimulation of RNA synthesis is the primary event in the mechanism of EP action. Experiments suggest that EP has its primary effect on the cytoplasmic membrane of marrow cells to produce an active cytoplasmic protein intermediate that interacts with the nucleus to stimulate synthesis of a variety of RNAs. DNA synthesis, cell division, and maturation (hemoglobin synthesis) in the responsive cells follow. The molecular mechanism of EP signal transduction remains largely undefined.

The possible role of the EP in human diseases has been studied in a variety of clinical conditions. Anemia results from any of a number of events that lead to hemorrhage, hemolysis, or decreased red blood cell production by bone marrow. Some patients with rheumatoid arthritis, chronic infection, and other malignancies may become anemic because of lowered EP levels. Neuraminidase (a sialase enzyme) inactivates EP and may play a role in producing anemia. Chronic renal disease with progressive loss of renal mass also results in decreased production of EP.

Polycythemia (above normal red cell number) is due to several etiologic factors; in some cases an inappropriate increase in EP production is the causative factor. A structurally abnormal EPR gene has been identified in a human erythroleukemia cell line. In polycythemia vera, red cell progenitors exhibit exaggerated sensitivity to EP and express only low-affinity EP receptors. Some cases of hereditary polycythemia may be due to a mutant EPR conferring enhanced EP sensitivity. Other pathologic conditions may also be associated with abnormalities of the EPR or its associated molecules. Soluble, immunoreactive EPR is detectable in human serum, but its physiological significance is unknown [57].

Because EP induces marked reticulocytosis and pronounced increases in the circulating red cell mass, EP has potential therapeutic value in the management of certain anemias in which responsive stem cells and erythroid precursors are available but EP plasma levels are low. Commercially produced recombinant human EP is used routinely in the care of patients with renal failure. Patients with renal failure are usually very anemic, and a major factor contributing to their anemia is insufficient production of endogenous EP. Almost all patients respond to the administration of recombinant EP, and frequent transfusions of blood that had been required previously in their care, will no longer be needed. EP therapy is being tested in patients with anemias due to a wide variety of causes other than renal failure, and its role in clinical medicine will almost certainly increase in the future [26].

Thymic Hormones

The thymus gland is a lobular organ that lies in the upper thorax above the heart and in front of the aorta (Fig. 12.14). In humans and other mammals the thymus begins to atrophy shortly after puberty [49]. Removal of the gland in the adult animal usually causes no harmful effects. On this basis the thymus was considered to be an organ without a function. It is now realized that the thymus is an endocrine organ that plays a pivotal role in the development of immunological competence [31].

Thymectomy of mice immediately after birth results in a wasting disease characterized by severe depletion of white blood cells, specifically lymphocytes. Certain lymphocytes synthesize antibodies and, without such molecules, an animal cannot mount an immunological defense. In addition, in the absence of antibody production an immune imbalance may contribute to the etiology of several diseases. Reimplantation of the thymus into young mice prevents the animals from developing the wasting disease; lymphocytes are produced and the animals are capable of developing an immunological response. In experiments, however, a rather puzzling observation was that the lymphocytes in animals receiving a thymus graft were of host origin. It had been thought that the thymus was the source of all the animal's lymphocytes. The results suggested that the thymus was responsible for stimulating proliferation of host lymphocytes. Was the thymus gland the

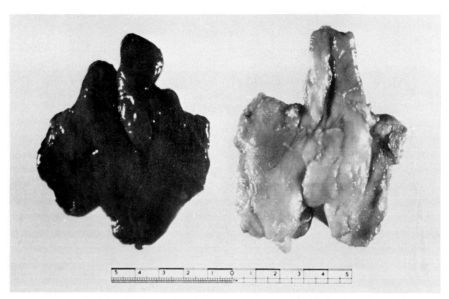

Figure 12.14   Thymus glands from a 9-year-old girl (left) and an 80-year-old man (right). Although size and shape were similar, the gland from the older person was yellow in color and fatty. (From Kendall, Johnson, and Singh [24], "The weight of the human thymus gland at necropsy." *J. Anat.* 131:485–499, 1980.)

source of a lymphocyte-stimulating hormone? The definitive answer came from an experiment where a thymus gland was placed in a small plastic capsule with pores so small that no thymus or other cells could escape or enter. Molecules could, however, pass freely in and out through the pores of the capsule. Young mice receiving only a plastic capsule implant developed the wasting disease. Mice receiving a capsule containing a thymus gland, on the other hand, grew and survived like normal animals and were capable of developing an immunological response. The results clearly indicated that the thymus might produce a hormone whose role was to activate lymphocytes for antibody production. An attempt to isolate such a factor from the thymus would be the next step to determine if it indeed were capable of stimulating lymphocyte antibody production.

It was eventually demonstrated that a partially purified thymus gland preparation, termed *thymosin fraction five*, could correct some of the immunological deficiencies resulting from a lack of thymic function in a number of animal models, as well as humans with primary and secondary immunodeficiency diseases. This thymosin fraction induced lymphocyte differentiation and enhanced immunologic function in genetically athymic mice, adult thymectomized mice, and strains of mice with autoimmune reactions. Several thymosin fractions are active in various immunological assays, but only a few have been chemically characterized.

Generalized Roles.   White blood cells (leukocytes) are produced in the bone marrow. Stem cells in this hemopoietic tissue give rise to the following white blood cell types: granulocytes (neutrophils, eosinophils, basophils), monocytes (which give rise to some macrophages), and lymphocytes. Lymphocytes may reside within the thymus gland or pass on through to compose a body of circulating T (thymus-derived) lymphocytes. Other lymphocytes of bone cell origin (B lymphocytes) establish themselves in other lymphoid tissues where they can become transformed into plasma cells that secrete antibodies.

The T lymphocytes become competent to participate in the immune response either by actual passage through the thymus, where they come into contact with one or more thymic hormones, or, alternatively, they are stimulated to become immunologically com-

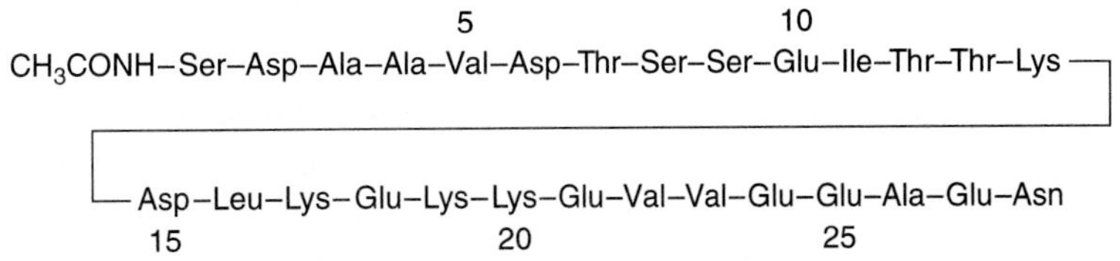

$$\text{5} \qquad\qquad\qquad \text{10}$$
$$\text{CH}_3\text{CONH–Ser–Asp–Ala–Ala–Val–Asp–Thr–Ser–Ser–Glu–Ile–Thr–Thr–Lys} \rightharpoondown$$

$$\text{Asp–Leu–Lys–Glu–Lys–Lys–Glu–Val–Val–Glu–Glu–Ala–Glu–Asn}$$
$$\text{15} \qquad\qquad\qquad \text{20} \qquad\qquad\qquad \text{25}$$

Figure 12.15   Primary structure of bovine thymosin α_1.

petent in response to humoral factors (hormones) released by the thymus. Both processes may be components of the maturation process of T lymphocytes. The fully differentiated T cells play a variety of roles in the immune response: they function as killer cells to combat tumor cell development; they release substances (lymphokines) that affect macrophage function; and they may function as helper cells with B cells in antibody production. The lymphocytes are considered to represent a complex group of cells derived from a common origin that are related by a linear or a branching differentiation. The processes that determine the commitment to any one of the pathways of differentiation may be under hormonal control. Clearly, the thymus may be a key element in the complex program, culminating in the fully developed immune system. Abnormalities of thymic function may, on the other hand, be responsible for some pathologies related to the immune system. Excess activity of certain lymphocytes may lead to hyperimmune conditions whereas impaired function may lead to immunological deficiencies such as agammaglobulinemia (total inability to produce antibodies). Failure of the thymus to develop is manifested in DiGeorge's syndrome, which is characterized by a seriously deficient immune system, usually revealed by an abnormal reaction to vaccination.

The Thymosins.   Thymosin is generally used to designate a biologically active class of substances found within extracts of the thymus gland. Subfractionation and purification of these extracts have yielded specific thymosin polypeptides whose primary structures have been determined.

A thymosin polypeptide (thymosin α_1) was isolated from calf thymus that consists of 28 amino acid residues and is highly active in several bioassay systems (Fig. 12.15). This polypeptide is probably derived from a larger precursor molecule and appears to be identical to a similar polypeptide derived from other species (human, pig, sheep, chinchilla, and mouse). The structure of thymosin β_4 has also been reported (Fig. 12.16). This polypeptide appears to act on stem cells to form prothymocytes, whereas thymosin α_1 may act on prothymocytes to induce their differentiation to more mature T cells [21]. Thymosin β_4 is also found in high concentrations in tissues other than the thymus.

Thymosins are being used in clinical tests with children who have primary immunodeficiency diseases. No undesirable side effects have been noted, and significant clinical improvement has been indicated [21]. Immune modulation using thymosins is being considered in the field of immunotherapy for the treatment of cancer. Thymosins appear to

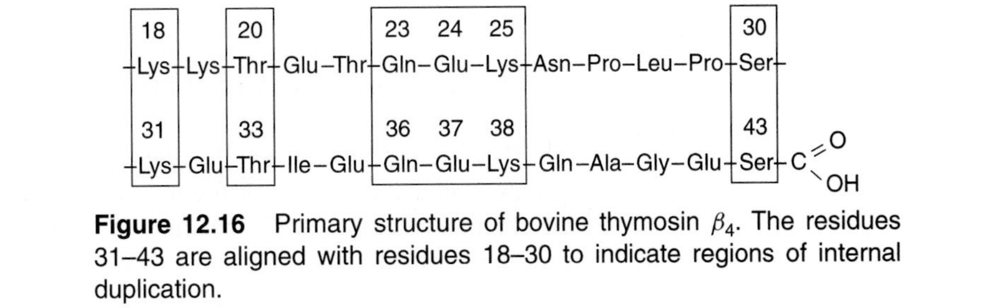

$$\text{CH}_3\text{–C} \overset{\text{O}}{\underset{\text{H}}{{<}}} \quad \overset{\text{1}}{} \qquad\qquad \overset{\text{5}}{} \qquad\qquad\qquad \overset{\text{10}}{} \qquad\qquad\qquad \overset{\text{15}}{}$$
$$\text{N–Ser–Asp–Lys–Pro–Asp–Met–Ala–Glu–Ile–Glu–Lys–Phe–Asp–Lys–Ser–Lys–Leu–}$$

18		20			23	24	25					30	
Lys	Lys	Thr	Glu–Thr	Gln–Glu–Lys	Asn–Pro–Leu–Pro	Ser
31		33			36	37	38					43	
Lys	Glu	Thr	Ile–Glu	Gln–Glu–Lys	Gln–Ala–Gly–Glu	Ser–C $\overset{\text{O}}{\underset{\text{OH}}{{<}}}$

Figure 12.16   Primary structure of bovine thymosin β_4. The residues 31–43 are aligned with residues 18–30 to indicate regions of internal duplication.

trigger maturational progression of several early stages of T-cell development and to augment the capacity of certain mature T cells to respond to antigens. One action of the thymosins may be to act through cGMP to induce the expression of alloantigens (antigen occurring in some, but not all, members of the same species) on the surface of T cells as they develop their functional capacity for immunological competence.

Platelet-derived Growth Factor

Whole blood serum is a requirement for the growth of certain cells (smooth muscle, fibroblasts, 3T3, and glial) in culture. Although there are many factors present in serum that are necessary for viability and growth of cells in culture, serum prepared from cell-free plasma has little or no mitogenic activity. This activity can, however, be restored by adding material released from blood platelets to sera. Thus the mitogen principle in whole blood serum may be derived from platelets. This *platelet-derived growth factor* (PDGF) is released from platelets during platelet aggregation in the process of blood clot formation. At sites of wounding, the platelets adhere to the endothelial lining of the vessel in such a way as to plug the defect. Platelets also release one or more chemical messengers that stimulate contraction of the injured vessels to prevent further loss of blood. At sites of injury, platelets release PDGF in response to thrombin. The role of PDGF at these sites may be to induce proliferation of smooth muscle cells within the arterial wall—the intima—as a component of a wound-healing process. Animals made thrombocytopenic with an antiplatelet serum fail to produce smooth muscle proliferative lesions in response to vessel injury. These lesions also fail to form in animals whose platelet function is inhibited by drugs (e.g., dipyridamole) that prevent platelet adhesion and granule release at sites of endothelial injury. PDGF is localized within α granules of the platelet; interaction of platelets with localized surfaces of damaged blood vessels provides for a site-specific release mechanism of PDGF to act as a local hormone. The wide distribution of smooth muscle cells throughout the body would, indeed, necessitate such a specialized mode of hormone delivery.

Atherosclerosis is recognized as a principal cause of death in the Western Hemisphere. Atherosclerotic lesions are localized to the innermost layers of the artery wall, the tunica intima and tunica media. This disease process, which results from endothelial disruption due to a number of possible causes, involves smooth muscle proliferation, formation of large amounts of a collagen matrix by the proliferated smooth muscle cells, and the deposition of lipids within these cells and the surrounding connective tissue. These atherosclerotic plaques impede blood flow in affected vessels, which may lead to brain stroke, heart attack, or other complications, depending on the particular vascular bed concerned. Although PDGF serves an important role in the healing process of the vascular system, it may play a dominant part in the development of atherosclerosis. It has been demonstrated that PDGF is also a potent vasoconstrictor, and it is possible that this peptide may be responsible, in part, for the increased vasoreactivity that occurs primarily at the site of atherosclerotic lesions.

PDGF consists of a family of molecules wherein each peptide is a heterodimer composed of an A and B chain. The two chains share 60% sequence identity and can dimerize to form PDGF-AA, PDGF-BB, and PDGF-AB. All three dimer forms have been identified in nature and shown to be biologically active. Analysis of the dimer composition of PDGF isolated from human platelets has shown that PDGF-AB is the predominant form obtained, but PDGF-AA and PDGF-BB are also present. There are two PDGF receptor subtypes: one that recognizes all three PDGF varieties and a second that binds only the BB variety. It is believed that the existence of two receptor forms is biologically important and that they have different functions. The existence of genes encoding two PDGF receptors that interact in a distinct manner with three different PDGF isoforms likely confers considerable regulatory flexibility in the functional responses to PDGF.

OTHER PEPTIDE GROWTH FACTORS

Other peptide growth factors have been discovered, and it is likely still others will be found in the future. Although their physiological roles are unclear, these factors are important peptides for the study of the growth requirements of cells maintained in tissue culture. These peptides also provide important insights into evolution of hormone structure and common mechanisms of hormone action. These growth factors may eventually prove to be of immense medical importance.

Epidermal Growth Factor

Administration of partially purified nerve growth factor (NGF) from mouse submaxillary glands to newborn mice results in an early opening of the eyelids and precocious eruption of the teeth. A heat-stable protein, distinct from NGF, was isolated from these extracts that possessed the ability to accelerate tooth eruption and eyelid opening in neonatal mice and rats. The biological activity was subsequently found to be due to a direct stimulation of the proliferation and keratinization of epidermal tissue. Autoradiography using [^{3}H]thymidine revealed that this epidermal growth factor (EGF) enhanced cell proliferation in the basal layer of the skin.

Mouse EGF consists of 53 amino acids and is conformationally restricted by three intrachain disulfide bonds (Fig. 12.17). EGF is found within the salivary gland combined with an EGF-binding protein that is an arginine esterase. This observation is interesting because NGF is also found within the submaxillary glands. NGF is associated with other proteins, and one of the subunits of this complex is also an arginine esterase, which may be similar but not identical to the EGF-binding esterase as the latter does not complex with NGF. EGF and NGF appear to be derived from inactive precursors, and the biosynthesis and activation of both may be similar, perhaps under the control of the same genetic locus. This is further substantiated by the discovery that the synthesis of both peptides is androgen dependent.

Release of the peptide from the salivary glands (in mice) may be under nervous system control because α-adrenergic agonists (see Chap. 14) increase serum levels of EGF, as does electrical stimulation of the superior cervical ganglia. Although mouse EGF is found in duct cells of the submaxillary glands, these glands are not the sole source of the peptide, as removal of the glands does not eliminate immunoreactive EGF-like material from the blood.

In addition to effects on tooth eruption, eyelid opening, and skin proliferation in the neonate and embryo, EGF stimulates growth in a number of cultured normal epithelial

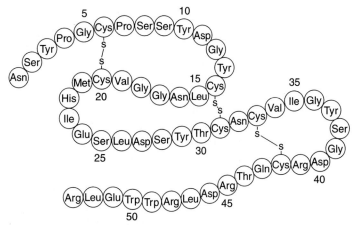

Figure 12.17 Primary structure of mouse epidermal growth factor (EGF).

cells. In epithelia, EGF rapidly stimulates the transport of small molecules into cells, followed by an increase in the rate of RNA synthesis and a conversion of pre-existing ribosomes into polysomes. One consequence of the binding of EGF to membrane receptors is a rapid activation of a cAMP-independent phosphorylating system.

Some known biological effects of EGF in the mammal include the following:

- enhanced proliferation and differentiation (keratinization) of the epidermis
- increased growth and maturation of the fetal pulmonary epithelium
- stimulation of ornithine decarboxylase activity and DNA synthesis in the mucosa of the digestive tract
- acceleration of the healing of wounds of the corneal epithelium, and phosphorylation of membrane and nuclear proteins.

Human milk is mitogenic to a number of cultured cell lines, an activity that is neutralized by antibodies to human EGF. These observations and other experimental results identify EGF as a major growth-promoting agent in breast milk [25]. Because EGF is not entirely destroyed in the digestive tract, it might act directly on tissues of the digestive tract.

Most interesting is the discovery that EGF promotes plant-shoot growth and possibly growth of roots. It has been hypothesized, therefore, that EGF or EGF-like substances may control plant community productivity [14]; that is, the presence of a growth factor, such as EGF, in the saliva of an herbivorous animal might provide the stimulus for plant regrowth after grazing.

Many animals lick their wounds. Is it possible that the EGF present in the saliva of some animals may be a stimulus to the wound-healing process? Several lines of evidence suggest that salivary EGF plays a role in wound healing of the skin and gastric mucosa. It has been shown that wound healing of the skin is enhanced by licking, that is, transfer of saliva to the wound. In addition, topical application of EGF to the skin promotes wound healing. Healing of gastric ulcer is retarded in rats by sialoadenectomy (removal of the submandibular glands) and can be restored by intragastric administration of EGF but not EGF-free saliva. EGF produced in the submandibular glands also promotes wound healing of the tongue. It is suggested that EGF-rich excreta such as saliva, duodenal juice, and tears may play important roles in the promotion of wound healing [37].

A surprising finding is that peptic ulcer in humans undergoes remission during pregnancy, and urine contains a potent inhibitor of gastric acid secretion. This substance, *urogastrone*, consists of a single polypeptide chain of 53 residues with three disulfide bonds. It was then discovered that mouse EGF is of the same length and differs from urogastrone in only 16 of the 53 residues (see Fig. 10.11). Urogastrone is a gastrointestinal peptide that is inhibitory to gastric acid (HCl) secretion directly at the level of the gastric mucosa. Urogastrone, like EGF, induces premature opening of eyes in young mice. Both peptides stimulate DNA synthesis within human fibroblasts, and at submaximal concentrations their effects are additive. Binding data also reveal that they share the same receptor site on fibroblasts. Immunocytochemical studies indicate that cells of the human submandibular gland contain urogastronelike activity. In the GI tract urogastrone appears to be localized to cells of Brunner's glands. Urogastrone in the human and EGF in the mouse are known to be elevated during pregnancy. Because androgen levels are also elevated during pregnancy, it is possible that elevated levels of these peptides in the blood reflect the changing hormonal status of the female. Present evidence suggests, therefore, that urogastrone is the human hormonal equivalent of mouse EGF.

Activation of the EGF receptor initiates a cascade of cellular events. On binding ligand, the intrinsic tyrosine kinase activity is triggered, and this is immediately followed by a rise in cytosolic Ca^{2+} concentration and receptor internalization, which results in receptor degradation. Specific gene transcription is stimulated within minutes. Hours later, DNA synthesis and cell division occur. It has been shown that the tyrosine kinase activity of the receptor is necessary for all subsequent receptor actions, including internalization [56].

Angiogenic Factors

Angiogenesis is the formation of blood vessels in situ and involves the orderly migration, proliferation, and differentiation of vascular cells. For tumors to grow they must become vascularized to provide the nutrients and oxygen necessary for cellular proliferation. It was shown experimentally that tumor cells isolated within a Millipore filter could induce the growth of new capillary vessels despite separation of the cells from the vascular bed of the host. This provided evidence for the release of a diffusible tumor-derived *angiogenic factor*, although an alternative explanation might be that the tumor enhanced the degradation of an inhibitor of tumor growth. The *angiogenins* fall into two groups: those that act directly on vascular endothelial cells to stimulate locomotion or motility, and those that act indirectly through mobilizing host cells (cellular elements of the blood) to release endothelial growth factors. The angiogenic peptides are not restricted to tumors but are also present in normal tissues. Their release must therefore be tightly regulated. Besides fibroblast growth factor, these polypeptides include *angiogenin* and *transforming growth factors* (TGFs).

In addition to the angiogenesis induced by tumors, it now appears that a number of non-neoplastic diseases may be considered angiogenic diseases because they are characterized by the pathologic growth of capillary blood vessels. It will be important to now determine whether angiogenic factors administered in vivo, either locally or systemically, can be used to accelerate the healing of wounds and fractures, or to increase neovascularization of the ischemic or infarcted heart.

Fibroblast Growth Factors.   The fibroblast growth factor (FGF) family consists of polypeptide growth factors characterized by amino acid sequence homology, heparin-binding avidity, the ability to promote angiogenesis, and mitogenic activity towards cells of epithelial, mesenchymal, and neural origin. Members of the FGF family appear to have roles in development, tissue repair, maintenance of neurons, and the pathogenesis of disease. Aberrant expression of FGFs may cause cell transformation by an autocrine mechanism. Moreover, FGFs may enhance tumor growth and invasiveness by stimulating blood vessel growth into the tumor or by inducing production of proteases such as plasminogen activator.

The FGF family includes acidic and basic FGFs, the keratinocyte growth factor, and several other peptides. The actions of acidic and basic FGF are mediated through binding to high-affinity cell surface receptors. It is not known whether each FGF interacts with a different receptor or whether the different forms of FGF share the same receptor. Of all the growth factors that have been identified to date, none have such a wide range of effects on so many cell types.

bFGF is a single-chain peptide composed of 146 amino acids that can also exist in a NH_2-terminally truncated form missing the first 15 amino acids. The truncated form of bFGF is as potent as the native form, thus indicating that this NH_2 terminus region of bFGF is not involved either in biological activity or in binding to FGF cell surface receptors. Acidic FGF is a 140-amino-acid peptide that can also exist in a NH_2-terminally truncated form missing the first six amino acids. bFGF has been well conserved through evolution. In the case of bovine and human bFGF, only two of the 146 amino acids are different, giving an overall amino acid sequence homology of 98.7%. Avian bFGF has the same amino acid composition and cross-reacts on an equimolar basis with bovine bFGF in RIA. This suggests that homologous epitopes are well conserved across species. aFGF seems to be less well conserved, and the bovine form differs from the human by 11 of the 140 residues. The high degree of homology between aFGF and bFGF suggests that they are derived from a single ancestral gene. The recent cloning of the genes and analysis of the complementary DNA (cDNA) sequences of both bFGF and aFGF suggest that through processes of gene duplication and evolutionary divergence, they have become separate gene products.

bFGF has been purified from many mesoderm- and neuroectoderm-derived tissues that have been shown to be FGF sensitive either in vitro or in vivo. These include the brain, pituitary, retina, corpus luteum, adrenal gland, kidney, placenta, prostate, thymus, bone, immune system (macrophages-monocytes), and various tumors such as melanoma, chondrosarcoma, and hepatoma. Depending on the organ from which it is purified, either the complete (146aa) or truncated (des 1–15aa) forms of bFGF may be present. In the pituitary, brain, and retina, the complete form predominates, while in the kidney and corpus luteum, only the truncated form can be detected. In the adrenal gland and placenta, both forms coexist. It is not known whether these various forms coexist in the tissues, or whether they are artifactually created by specific proteases during FGF extraction and subsequent isolation. So far, aFGF has been found only in the brain and retina. The complete (140aa) and truncated form (des 1–6aa) seem to be present in stoichiometric amounts. Most of the organs from which bFGF has been purified share in common a strong angiogenic potential as well as being heavily vascularized. This suggests that cells of the vascular system might be responsible for bFGF production.

Probably one of the most important questions to be resolved is the in vivo role of FGF. The high degree of structural conservation of bFGF through species as diverse as mammals, birds, and amphibians, as well as its presence in all vertebrates studied to date, including fish, indicates that in vivo FGF could have a primordial role. It has been shown that bFGF can act as a morphogen at one of the earliest embryonic stages, including the transformation of cells designed to be ectodermal into mesenchymal cells. This is consistent with the in vitro properties of bFGF, which have been shown to act as mitogen as well as morphogen for all mesenchymal cells studied to date. It is also in agreement with the ability of bFGF to support the regeneration process in lower vertebrates.

Transforming Growth Factors. Two structurally distinct TGFs, TGF-α and TGF-β, have been purified and their primary sequences determined [10]. TGF-α is composed of 50 amino acids and bears sequence homology to EGF and binds to the EGF receptor. TGF-α exhibits some homology with the amino acid sequences of human and mouse EGFs. If TGF-α plays some role in normal development, one might wonder why there is an apparent duplicity of growth factors such as the TGF-α and EGF. Maybe TGF-α plays a local role under normal conditions requiring autocrine or paractine stimulation of growth, as in embryogenesis and tissue regeneration. EGF, on the other hand, which is secreted by glands may fulfill an endocrine type of role. Topical application of TGF-α in an antibiotic cream to partial thickness second-degree burns increased the rate of epidermal regeneration. This finding suggests that topical application of selected growth factors may be useful in accelerating the healing of wounds.

TGF-β is a homodimer consisting of 112 amino acids per chain. TGF-β occurs in two related forms (TGF-β_1 and TGF-β_2). TGF-β has been shown to show some structural homology to inhibin (see Chap. 16) and to Müllerian regression factor (see Chap. 18). It is of interest that both inhibin and MRF, like TGF-β, exhibit strong growth-inhibitory activities. Depending upon the experimental condition, TGF-β can stimulate or inhibit growth of certain nonendothelial cells depending upon whether the cells are anchored or not and whether EGF is present or absent.

It has been suggested that TGF-β acts as a bifunctional regulator of cell growth in vitro. In fact, "transforming growth factor" may be a misnomer, since TGF-β more often than not has an inhibitory effect on the proliferation of most cell types, with the exception of fibroblasts. It is possible that the loss of responsiveness of cells to TGF-β may contribute to the uncontrolled division of cancer cells. Human breast cancer cells produce several growth-promoting factors, including TGF-β. Breast cancer patients who have estrogen-dependent tumors may be treated with drugs that block the hormone's effects (see Chap. 19). Antiestrogens, for example, increase TGF-β production, an effect that may contribute to their ablity to inhibit growth. Estrogens themselves decrease TGF-β production. TGF-β might be considered to be a chalone, as discussed later. Although TGF-β inhibits the proliferative actions of some hormones on cells, it does not inhibit protein synthesis induced by these hormones; thus the action of TGF-β is to stabilize the differentiated state induced by other hormones and to allow cellular hypertrophy and phenotypic expression.

Normal skeletal growth results from a balance between the processes of bone matrix synthesis and resorption. These activities are regulated by both systemic and local factors. Bone turnover is dynamic, and skeletal growth must be maintained throughout life. Although many growth promoters are associated with bone matrix, it is enriched particularly with TGF-β activity. Experimental evidence indicates that TGF-β regulates replication and differentiation of mesenchymal precursor cells, chondrocytes, osteoblasts, and osteoclasts. TGF-β activity in skeletal tissue may be controlled at multiple levels by other local and systemic agents. Consequently, the intricate mechanisms by which TGF-β regulates bone formation are likely to be fundamental to understanding the processes of skeletal growth during development, maintenance of bone mass in adult life, and healing subsequent to bone fracture [10].

Cytoplasmic determinants influence the development of embryonic cells. A critical early stage in the development is formation of the three germ layers, known as the endoderm, the ectoderm, and the mesoderm, from which the specific tissues of the organism later differentiate. The TGF-β family of peptides has now been linked to early embryonic development of the frog egg, specifically to mesoderm formation. TGF-β is made at the appropriate site, the cells of the vegetal pole of the egg, and at the right time in development for mesoderm induction. Transforming growth factor β_2 (TGF-β_2, but not TGF-β_1, was active in α-actin induction, while addition of fibroblast growth factor had a small synergistic effect. Medium conditioned by *Xenopus* XTC cells (XTC-CM), known to have powerful mesoderm-inducing activity, was shown to contain TGF-β-like activity as measured by a radioreceptor-binding assay, colony formation in NRK cells, and growth inhibition in CCL64 cells. The activity of XTC-CM in mesoderm induction and growth inhibition of CCL64 cells was inhibited partially by antibodies to TGF-β_2 but not by antibodies to TGF-β_1. Thus a TGF-β_2-like molecule may be involved in mesoderm induction. Both TGF-β and bFGF are produced by the amphibian egg and induce mesoderm formation.

Cytokines

A cytokine may be defined as a soluble protein, synthesized by immune or nonimmune cells, that mediates intercellular communication. Cytokines transmit information to target cells through receptor-ligand interactions and thereby regulate immunologic and physiologic events. This class of mediators is represented by growth and differentiation, cytolytic, chemotactic, and immunoenhancing factors. Many of these factors appear to have multifunctional immunologic and physiologic activities. Interleukins may be the best known but least understood group; the eight known interleukins have diverse biologic activities. The term interleukin originally described a leukocyte-derived protein with activity for other leukocytes. It is now understood that both immune and nonimmune cells synthesize interleukins and other cytokines that are important in inflammation. Indeed, many cytokines have physiologic and immunologic activities far beyond those originally discovered.

Chalones

Many hormones stimulate synthetic processes within cells of their target tissues. An increase in cell function and cell size (hypertrophy) is often followed by cell proliferation (hyperplasia). As noted, growth factors are potent mitogens. Mitotic activity of the many tissues of the body is variable. Brain cells, for example, seldom divide, whereas epithelial cells, especially those of the epidermis or the intestinal lining, divide at a much higher rate to replace those cells lost from the surface. When epidermal cells are destroyed by tissue damage, the rate of cell production in the basal layer increases to restore the lost cells. A balance of cellular mitotic activity could probably not be maintained unless controlled by some type of feedback mechanism. The critical moment in the life of an epidermal cell may be when it emerges from mitosis: it must prepare for division again or for keratin synthesis and death.

When the epidermis is damaged the mitotic rate of nearby cells is enhanced. It was thought that mitosis was in response to a "wound hormone." The opposite view is now favored: the epidermis normally contains a mitotic inhibitor whose loss from the damaged area permits the increase in mitotic activity of the adjacent cells. It has been proposed that these substances be referred to as *chalones* (from the Greek, *chalan*, to slacken, slow down), which suggests that they act as mitotic inhibitors. A number of classic experiments have provided strong support for the chalone hypothesis.

GROWTH FACTORS, RECEPTORS, AND CANCER

Neoplastic transformation in some cases may relate to cellular growth factors and their receptors. It has become evident that cells stimulated by growth factors and cells transformed by viruses are quite similar, suggesting common stimulation pathways of cellular proliferation in viral-transformed and growth-factor-stimulated cells. Oncogenes are genes whose coding sequence contains the information necessary to initiate and maintain neoplastic proliferation. Oncogenes were first discovered in transforming viruses, but it is now appreciated that these genes were actually acquired from normal host genes (proto-oncogenes) of infected cells by genetic transduction. Proto-oncogenes can be expressed in many different tissues and provide a potential for malignant transformation. These proto-oncogenes are probably the same genes that were once activated through inductive processes during embryonic development. The inadvertent activation of these genes in the differentiated state by mutational mechanisms may lead to their irreversible activation, and through ensuing cellular proliferation may lead to cancer growth and metastases. Proto-oncogenes can release growth-factorlike peptides that are released extracellularly and then stimulate proliferation of cells through autocrine and paracrine mechanisms.

Proto-oncogene activation within virally infected cells is another way for cancerous cellular proliferation to become manifested. A relationship between growth-factor receptors and transforming proteins of oncogenes has also been noted. There is a marked homology between certain growth-factor receptors (e.g., for EGF) and proteins coded for by certain viruses. Viral-induced transformation might relate to the overproduction and expression of growth-hormone receptor proteins by infected cells, thus leading to their uncontrolled proliferation.

The role of protein kinase C (PKC) in signal transduction was reviewed in Chap. 4. Activation of PKC is a stimulus to cellular proliferation. Phorbol esters—like diacylglycerol, which is the natural second messenger of PKC activation—also activate the enzyme. Phorbol esters share a structural similarity to diacylglycerol, and this probably explains their mitogenic actions. These observations point out how exogenous ligands (carcinogens) can be responsible for cellular activation, possibly leading to tumor growth and spread.

Rapidly growing transformed cells, which frequently secrete growth-promoting polypeptides, also produce high amounts of proteolytic activity. Since high proteolytic activity is usually associated with malignant or proliferating cells, a possible explanation is that malignant cells produce autocrine growth factors or other factors that regulate their proteolytic activity. A few growth factors have previously been found that affect the proteolytic balance of cultured cells. Recent work has indicated that, in fact, several growth factors have an ability to modulate the expression of proteolytic enzymes. However, disturbances in proteolytic balance and overexpression of proteolytic enzymes by malignant cells may result from inappropriate regulation of these activities and can be related to excessive production of certain growth factors or inadequate production of other ones.

REFERENCES

[1]   Amselem, S., P. Duzuesnoy, M. L. Sobrier, and M. Goossens. 1991. Molecular defects in the growth hormone receptor. *Acta Paediatr. Scand.* 377:81–6.

[2]   Barbacid, M. 1993. Nerve growth factor: a tale of two receptors. *Oncogene* 8:2033–42.

[3]   Bauer, C. 1991. Physiologic determinants of erythropoietin production. *Sem. Hematol.* 28:9–13.

[4]   Bauer, C., and A. Kurtz. 1989. Oxygen sensing in the kidney and its relationship to erythropoietin production. *Annu. Rev. Physiol.* 51:845–56.

[5]   Baumann, G., M. A. Shaw, and T. J. Merimee. 1989. Low levels of high-affinity growth hormone-binding protein in African pygmies. *New Engl. J. Med.* 320:1705–9.

[6]   Baxter, R. C. 1991. Insulin-like growth factor (IGF) binding proteins: the role of serum IGF-BPs in regulating IGF availability. *Acta Paediatr. Scand.* 372:107–14.

[7]   ———. 1993. Circulating binding proteins for the insulinlike growth factors. *TEM* 4:91–6.

[8]   Bowen, I. D. 1993. Apoptosis or programmed cell death? *Cell Biol. Intern.* 17:365–80.

[9]   Bradshaw, R. A., T. L. Blundell, R. Lapatto, N. Q. McDonald, and J. Murray-Rust. 1993. Nerve growth factor revisited. *Trends Biochem. Sci.* 18:48–52.

[10] Centrella, M., M. C. Horowitz, J. M. Wozney, and T. L. McCarthy. 1994 Transforming growth factor-B gene family members and bone. *Endocr. Rev.* 15:27–39.

[11] Chao, M. V. 1992. Neurotrophin receptors: a window into neural differentiation. *Neuron* 9:583–93.

[12] Deitz, J., and J. Schwartz. 1991. Growth hormone alters lipolysis and hormone-sensitive lipase activities in 3T3–F442A adipocytes. *Metabolism* 40:800–6.

[13] De Vos, A. M., M. Ultsch, and A. A. Kossiakoff. 1992. Human growth hormone and extracellular domain of its receptor: crystal structure of the complex. *Science* 255:306–12.

[14] Dyer, M. I. 1980. Mammalian epidermal growth factor promotes plant growth. *Proc. Natl. Acad. Sci. USA* 77:4836–7.

[15] Ebendal, T. 1992. Function and evolution in the NGF family and its receptors. *J. Neurosci. Res.* 32:461–70.

[16] Etherton, T. D. 1991. The efficacy and safety of growth hormone for animal agriculture. *J. Clin. Endocrinol. Metab.* 72:957A–957C.

[17] Fontoura, M., J. F. Hocquette, J. P. Clot, A. Tar, R. Brauner, R. Rappaport, and M. C. Postel-Vinay. 1991. Regulation of the growth hormone binding proteins in human plasma. *Acta Endocrinol.* (Copenhagen) 124:10–3

[18] Froesch, E. R., H.-P. Guler, C. Schmid, K. Binz, and J. Zapf. 1990. Therapeutic potential of insulinlike growth factor I. *TEM* 1:254– 60.

[19] Frohman, L. A. 1991. Clinical review 22. Therapeutic options in acromegaly. *J. Clin. Endocrinol. Metab.* 372:1175–81.

[20] Fuh, G., B. C. Cunningham, R. Fukunaga, S. Nagata, D. V. Goeddel, and J. A. Wells. 1992. Rational design of potent antagonists to the human growth hormone receptor. *Science* 256:1677–80.

[21] Goldstein, A. L., T. L. K. Low, G. B. Thurman, M. M. Zatz, N. Hall, J. Chen, S. K. Hu, P. B. Nayler, and J. E. McClure. 1981. Current status of thymosin and other hormones of the thymus gland. *Rec. Prog. Horm. Res.* 37:369–415.

[22] Humbel, R. E., and E. Rinderknecht. 1979. From NSILA to IGF (1963–1977). In *Somatomedins and growth,* eds. G. Giordano, J. J. Van Wyk, and F. Minuto, pp. 61–65. London: Academic Press, Inc.

[23] Isaksson, O. G. P., A. Lindahl, A. Nilsson, and J. Isgaard. 1988. Action of growth hormone: current views. *Acta Paediatr. Scand. (Suppl).* 343:12–18.

[24] Kendall, M. D., H. R. M. Johnson, and J. Singh. 1980. The weight of the human thymus at necropsy. *J. Anat.* 131:485–99.

[25] Koldovsky, O., and W. Thornburg. 1987. Hormones in milk. *J. Pediat. Gastroenterol. Nutr.* 6:172–96.

[26] Koury, J. M., and M. C. Bondurant. 1992. The molecular mechanism of erythropoietin action. *Eur. J. Biochem.* 210:649–63.

[27] Krantz, S. B. 1991. Erythropoietin. *Blood* 77:419–34.

[28] Kromer, L. F. 1987. Nerve growth factor treatment after brain injury prevents neuronal death. *Science* 235:214–6.

[29] LeRoith, D., M. Adamo, H. Kato, and C. T. Roberts, Jr. 1992. Divergence of insulin and insulin-like growth factor-I signalling pathways. *Pediatr. Adolescent Endocrinol.* 24:346–58.

[30] Levi-Montalcini, R. 1987. The nerve growth factor: thirty-five years later. *Biosci. Rpts.* 7: 681–99.

[31] Levy, R. H. 1964. The thymus hormone. *Sci. Amer.* 211(1):66–77.

[32] Maharajan, P., and N. Maharajan. 1993. Growth hormone signal transduction. *Experientia* 49:980–7.

[33] Merimee, T. J., J. Zapf, and E. R. Froesch. 1981. Dwarfism in the pygmy. *New Engl. J. Med.* 305:965–8.

[34] Merimee, T. J., J. Zapf, B. Hewlett, and L. L. Cavalli-Sforza. 1987. Insulinlike growth factors in pygmies: the role of puberty in determining final stature. *New Engl. J. Med.* 316:906–11.

[35] Nakamura, Y., N. Komatsu, and H. Nakauchi. 1992. A truncated erythropoietin receptor that fails to prevent programmed cell death of erythroid cells. *Science* 257:1138–41.

[36] Nilsson, A., J. Isgaard, A. Lindahl, A. Dahlstrom, A. Skottner, and O. G. P. Isaksson. 1986. Regulation by growth hormone of number of chondrocytes containing IGF-I in rat growth plate. *Science* 233:511–4.

[37] Noguchi, S., Y. Ohba, and T. Oka. 1991. Effect of salivary epidermal growth factor on wound healing of the tongue in mice. *Amer. J. Physiol.* 260:E620–5.

[38] Ohlsson, C., A. Nilsson, O. Isaksson, J. Benthan, and A. Lindahl. 1992. Effects of tri-iodothyronine and insulin-like growth factor-I (IGF-I) on alkaline phosphatase activity, [^{3}H]thymidine incorporation and IGF-I receptor mRNA in cultured rat epiphyseal chondrocytes. *J. Endocrinol.* 135:115–23.

[39] Ohlsson, C., A. Nilsson, O. Isaksson, and A. Lindahl. 1992. Growth hormone induces multiplication of the slowly cycling germinal cells of the rat tibial growth plate. *Proc. Natl. Acad. Sci. USA* 89:9826–30.

[40] Ooi, G. T. 1990. At the cutting edge. Insulin-like growth factor-binding proteins (IGFBPs): more than just 1,2,3. *Mol. Cell. Endocrinol.* 71:C39–43.

[41] Pahlman, S., G. Meyerson, E. Lindgren, M. Schalling, and I. Johansson. 1991. Insulin-like growth factor I shifts from promoting cell division to potentiating maturation during neuronal differentiation. *Proc. Natl. Acad. Sci. USA* 88:9994–8.

[42] Pessin, J. E., and A. L. Frattali. 1993. Molecular dynamics of insulin/IGF-I receptor transmembrane signalling. *Mol. Reprod. Develop.* 35:339–45.

[43] Phillips, J. A., III. 1992. Molecular biology of growth hormone receptor dysfunction. *Acta Paediatr.* 383:127–31.

[44] Postel-Vinay, M. C., M. Fontoura, K. Freed, and S. Villares. 1993. The human growth hormone binding protein. *Pediatr. Adolescent Endocrinol.* 24:106–13.

[45] Rinderknecht, E., and R. E. Humbel. 1978. Primary structure of insulin-like growth factor II. *FEBS Lett.* 89:28–86.

[46] Ron, E., G. Gridley, Z. Hrubec, W. Page, S. Arora, and J. F. Fraumeni, Jr. 1991. Acromegaly and gastrointestinal cancer. *Cancer* 68:1673–7.

[47] Roth, R. A. 1988. Structure of the receptor for insulin-like growth factor II: the puzzle amplified. *Science* 239:1269–71.

[48] Sabharwal, P., R. Glaser, W. Lafuse, et al. 1992. Prolactin synthesized and secreted by human peripheral blood mononuclear cells: an autocrine growth factor for lymphoproliferation. *Proc. Natl. Acad. Sci. USA* 89:7713–6.

[49] Schuurman, H.-J., L. Nagelkerken, R. A. De Weger, and J. Rozing. 1991. Age-associated involution: significance of a physiologic process. *Thymus* 18:1–6.

[50] Spada, A., M. Arosio, D. Bochicchio, N. Bazzoni, L. Vallar, M. Bassetti, and G. Faglia. 1990. Clinical, biochemical and morphological correlates in patients bearing growth hormone-secreting pituitary tumors without or with somatic mutation in the alpha-chain (αs) of the stimulatory regulatory protein of adenylyl cyclase (Gs). *J. Clin. Endocrinol. Metab.* 1421–6.

[51] Stone, R. 1992. NIH to size up growth hormone trials. *Science* 257:739.

[52] Sytkowski, A. J. 1991. Control of erythropoietin production. *Blood Rev.* 15–8.

[53] Thoenen, H. 1991. The changing scene of neurotrophic factors. *TINS* 14:165–70.

[54] Vaccarello, M. A., F. B. Diamond Jr., J. Guevara-Aguirre, A. L. Rosenbloom, P. J. Fielder, S. Gargosky, P. Cohen, K. Wilson, and R. G. Rosenfeld. 1993. Hormonal and metabolic effects and pharmacokinetics of recombinant insulin-like growth factor-I in growth hormone receptor deficiency/Laron syndrome. *J. Clin. Endocrinol. Metab.* 77:273–80.

[55] Walker, S. E., S. H. Allen, and R. W. McMurray. 1993. Prolactin and autoimmune disease. *TEM* 4:147–51.

[56] Wells, A., J. B. Welsh, C. S. Lazar, H. S. Wiley, G. N. Gill, and M. G. Rosenfeld. 1990. Ligand-induced transformation by a noninternalizing epidermal growth factor receptor. *Science* 247:962–4.

[57] Winkelmann, J. C. 1992. The human erythropoietin receptor. *Intern. J. Cell Cloning* 10:254–61.

[58] Wyllie, A. H. 1993. Apoptosis. *Br. J. Cancer* 67:205–8.

[59] Zezulak, K. M., and H. Green. 1986. The generation of insulin-like growth factor-I-sensitive cells by growth hormone action. *Science* 233:551–3.

13

Thyroid Hormones

Anatomists of the fifteenth and sixteenth centuries described the thyroid gland in detail, and an enlargement of the thyroid as the anatomical basis for goiter was subsequently noted [24]. The etiological basis for goiter, however, was discerned centuries later after a number of important discoveries in chemistry. Courtois, a French pharmacist, discovered iodine in 1811 and Davy, an English chemist, discovered its elemental nature in 1813. Gay-Lussac named the element iodine in 1814. Iodine was discovered to be abundant in seaweed and other marine products; if eaten, these marine substances had a beneficial effect on goiter. Burnt sponge was recommended as a treatment for goiter in the mid-thirteenth century. It was subsequently surmised and proven correct that iodine might aid in the cure of goiter. Evidence for a connection between iodine deficiency and endemic goiter was obtained from studies of several European locales; the suggestion was put forward in 1849 that the disease was due to a deficiency of iodine in drinking water [21, 24].

*In 1895 Magnus-Levey demonstrated that the feeding of dried animal thyroids to normal men increased their metabolic rate. This suggested that the thyroid gland might contain a substance that affected the cellular activity of other organs. It was hypothesized that thyroid tissue might contain iodine, which was known to be beneficial to hypothyroid individuals. In 1895 Kocher of Bern demonstrated the high amount of iodine in a thyroid concentrate. He named this substance iodothyrin. Iodothyrin was active in hypothyroid patients, whereas an iodine-free fraction of the thyroid was not. In 1918 Kendall isolated the active component of the thyroid that he named thyroxin (**thyroxine**), and proposed its structural formula. Harrington in England revised the constitution of thyroxine and synthesized the definitive structure of L-thyroxine (Fig. 13.1). Thyroxine was later isolated from the thyroid gland in pure form.*

*It was soon discovered that the physiological activity of thyroid material could not be accounted for entirely by its thyroxine content. Kendall suggested that the "active" hormone might contain less iodine than thyroxine. Gross and Pitt-Rivers were then able to isolate a triiodinated thyronine from animal thyroid glands. In 1952 **triiodothyronine** (Fig. 13.1) was synthesized and found to be more active than thyroxine. It was then suggested that triiodothyronine was the peripheral physiological hormone and thyroxine its precursor [35].*

THE THYROID GLAND

The thyroid gland is derived from endoderm of the cephalic portion of the embryo's alimentary canal [16, 27]. A saclike diverticulum first appears in the midline of the ventral surface of the pharynx. This glandular organ becomes bilobed but remains connected to

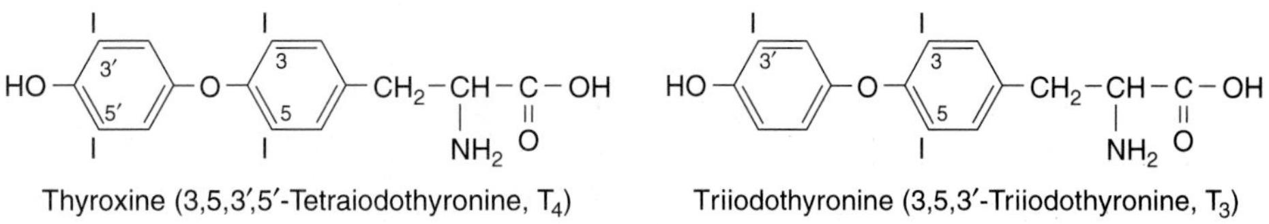

Thyroxine (3,5,3′,5′-Tetraiodothyronine, T_4)   Triiodothyronine (3,5,3′-Triiodothyronine, T_3)

Figure 13.1 Structures of thyroxine (T_4) and triiodothyronine (T_3).

the pharynx by a thyroglossal duct. The thyroglossal duct becomes a solid stalk that usually atrophies. The two lateral lobes of the human thyroid become solid masses of tissue and remain connected to each other by a narrow isthmus of tissue. The thyroid tissue in mammals lies over the trachea at a position just below the cricoid cartilage (see Fig. 9.1). A pyramidal lobe near the isthmus of the thyroid may persist as a remnant of the thyroglossal stalk (Fig. 13.2). The thyroid gland of humans weighs about 15 to 20 g. In nonmammalian species the thyroid gland consists of a pair of glands separated from each other at varying distances lateral to the esophagus.

The functional components of the thyroid gland are the individual thyroid follicles, which consist of a cuboidal epithelium arranged as a single layer surrounding a lumen that contains a colloid material (Fig. 13.3). In humans an individual thyroid follicle may reach a diameter of almost 1 cm. The follicular cells of the normal thyroid gland are not identical among themselves; they are highly individual metabolic units, a trait that is transferred from the mother cell to its progeny. Daughter follicles produced from mother follicles during goitrogenesis arise from a few predestined follicular cells endowed with an inherited propensity to replicate at higher than average rates. Whenever a thyroid gland is forced to grow, that is, to generate new follicles, the daughter follicles may differ from their ancestors in as many different ways as the cells that comprise the mother follicle differ among themselves [45].

In the mammal, so-called clear (C) cells are present within the follicular wall and the extracellular space between the follicles. These cells are the source of calcitonin, an important hormone involved in Ca^{2+} homeostasis in some animals (see Chap. 9) [32].

The follicular cells synthesize a protein, *thyroglobulin*, which is released into the colloid space by vesicular exocytosis. Thyroglobulin is important as substrate for tyrosine iodination and the subsequent synthesis of thyroid hormones. In response to endocrine stimulation follicular cells engulf the colloid by phagocytosis. The colloid within the endocytotic vesicles is enzymatically degraded to yield thyroid hormones that are released from the follicular cells into the extracellular space where they enter the abundant capillaries.

The thyroid of some mammalian species, including humans, is richly supplied with sympathetic postganglionic neurons that not only serve a vasomotor function, but appear to innervate the individual follicular cells. In mice unilateral sympathetic stimulation induces secretion of thyroid hormones from those areas of the thyroid supplied by the stimulated nerve. Sympathetic innervation of the thyroid may provide a means for effecting

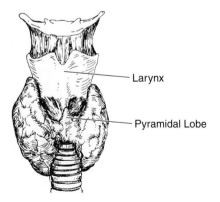

— Larynx

— Pyramidal Lobe

Figure 13.2 The human thyroid gland.

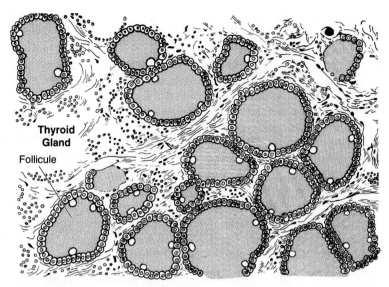

Figure 13.3 Diagrammatic histological representation of the human thyroid gland.

prompt, short-term alterations in the rate of thyroid hormone secretion [30]. Amine-containing mast cells are present between the thyroid follicles of mammals; they respond to TSH by releasing histamine and serotonin (5-hydroxytryptamine, 5-HT), as well as other substances. The released biogenic amines may act directly on the follicle cells to initiate thyroid hormone secretion or to increase blood flow through the thyroid gland.

SYNTHESIS AND CHEMISTRY

Thyroid hormones are unique in that they are complexed through covalent bonds to iodine. The availability of iodine to the terrestrial vertebrate is limited and, therefore, some interesting cellular mechanisms have been adopted for the ultimate utilization and conservation of the element. The thyroid follicular cells are able to trap iodide at the base of the cell and transport it against an electrical gradient across the cell. Accumulation of iodide by the thyroid is known to be an energy-requiring mechanism. Its Na^+ dependence was soon recognized and a Na^+-I^- cotransport system was demonstrated. Iodide uptake into the thyroid cell (thyrocyte) is an example of a secondary active transport mechanism, sometimes improperly referred to as the "iodide pump." The Na^+-I^- cotransport is inserted into the basolateral membrane of the thyrocyte. Its activity is dependent on the Na^+ gradient across the membrane and therefore on Na^+/K^+-ATPase [18].

Iodide is then converted by a *peroxidase* at the luminal surface of the cell, to an oxidized species of iodine that is incorporated into tyrosyl groups of thyroglobulin (TG) as monoiodotyrosine (MIT) and diiodotyrosine (DIT) residues. Within the TG, iodinated tyrosines undergo an *oxidative coupling* that results mainly in the formation of T_4 and smaller amounts of T_3. This oxidative coupling may be catalyzed by the same peroxidase responsible for conversion of iodide to iodine. Iodination of TG tyrosyl residues and subsequent oxidative coupling to form *iodothyronines* may be facilitated by intraluminal ciliary action and the subsequent movement of TG to reactive sites of the apical surface of the follicular cells [42].

Through the processes of micropinocytosis and macropinocytosis, the colloid is engulfed by follicular cell pseudopods and transported into the cells as *colloid droplets*. These colloid-containing vesicles that then fuse with lysosomes are referred to as *secondary lysosomes*. Much of the TG within these vesicles is degraded by lysosomal proteolytic enzymes. The thyroid hormones are then released (presumably by diffusion) into the cytoplasm and enter the extracellular space by diffusion, apparently through the basal or lateral follicular membranes [48]. Exocytosis of vesicular products, including T_3 and T_4, is not excluded as TG is also secreted into the circulation. The iodinated tyrosines that are released into the cytosol through lysosomal proteolysis are then deiodinated by a *deiodinase* and recycled for use within the cell. The scheme of the events involved in thyroid hormone synthesis and secretion is depicted (Fig. 13.4).

Thyrotropin Stimulation of Thyroid Hormone Synthesis

Follicular thyroid hormone synthesis is regulated through the action of thyrotropin (TSH) (see Chap. 5). Continued stimulation of the thyroid by TSH results in a great increase in the quantity and activity of the synthetic machinery (rough endoplasmic reticulum and Golgi) of the follicular cells [49]. The cells become columnar in shape and the luminal content of the colloid is greatly decreased. In the absence of TSH, synthesis of thyroid hormones is minimal or nonexistent. Subsequently, there is a loss of most protein-synthesizing elements of the cell; the individual follicular cells become flattened and the lumen remains enlarged and full of colloid.

In response to TSH there is an immediate activation of follicular cell thyroid-hormone-synthesizing activity (Fig. 13.4). TSH interacts with follicular-cell membrane receptors with resulting activation of adenylate cyclase and cAMP production [26]. The thyrotropin receptor has been cloned and its primary structure determined. The TSHR and the receptor for luteinizing hormone/choriogonadotropin constitute a subfamily of G

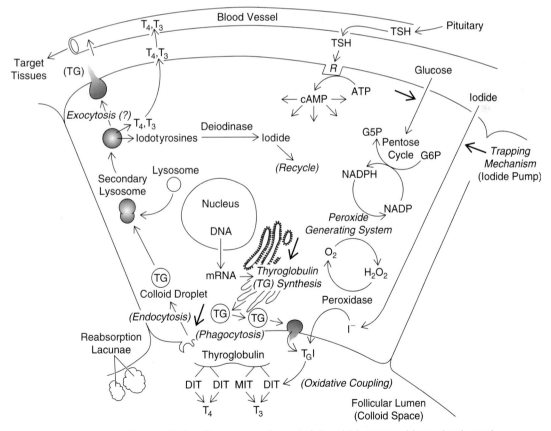

Figure 13.4 Summary scheme of thyroid hormone biosynthesis and secretion. The actual oxidative coupling of iodinated tyrosine residues probably takes place at the apical surface of the follicular cell, rather than in the lumen [48].

protein-coupled receptors with distinct sequence characteristics (see Fig. 19.2). All the subsequent follicular activities may be mediated through cAMP phosphorylation of substrate proteins, as theophylline and cAMP analogs added to thyroid tissue mimic most actions of TSH. TSH stimulates the in vitro incorporation of radiolabeled iodide into thyroglobulin, which suggests that the iodide pump and peroxidase activities are stimulated by the hormone. In response to TSH oxygen consumption is increased in incubated thyroid tissue and glucose is taken up from the medium and metabolized via the *pentose monophosphate shunt*. In this pathway NADPH is generated from NADP; this reduced adenine nucleotide is required for the reduction of molecular oxygen to hydrogen peroxide. The H_2O_2 is then used in the oxidation of iodide to an active form. The reaction is catalyzed by a thyroidal peroxidase that may be present within the Golgi-derived vesicles containing newly synthesized TG. Conversion of iodide to active iodide and organification of iodide into tyrosine residues of TG may occur as TG is secreted into the follicular lumen.

Immediately upon stimulation of the thyroid by TSH, there is enhanced pinocytotic activity at the apical follicular membrane. Thus colloid is actively engulfed and carried into the cell by this endocytotic process. The active removal of colloid from the lumen can be visualized as so-called *reabsorption lacunae* (Figs. 13.3 and 13.4).

Thyroglobulin is made of two identical subunits, each containing a 330 kDa polypeptide. The primary structure of the subunit has been determined [10]. Although tyrosyl residues are essential for iodine incorporation, the actual amount of tyrosine within TG is low (about 2%). The main intrathyroidal storage form of thyroid hormones is TG, and the individual iodinated thyronines are liberated from TG as T_4 and T_3 within the colloid droplets by the action of proteolytic enzymes. Iodination of TG initially requires the conversion of inorganic iodide to some molecular species of "active iodide." This active iodide then reacts with tyrosine moieties of the TG. Incorporation of a single iodide into the phenolic ring of tyrosine yields a 3-monoiodotyrosine (MIT). A second iodide may be incorporated into the 5 position to yield a 3,5-diiodotyrosine (DIT). Iodination specifically involves initial iodination of the 3 position, which is usually followed by iodination of the 5 position as 5-monoiodotyrosine is never formed.

Coupling of iodinated tyrosyl residues within TG is undoubtedly assisted by the three-dimensional structure of TG, but the exact mechanism remains undetermined. For example, the extent to which intramolecular or intermolecular coupling by tyrosyl moieties predominates is unknown. Coupling is enzymatically controlled and apparently involves the cleavage of a phenolic ring from tyrosine, and its incorporation through an ether (—O—) linkage, to another iodinated tyrosine. Coupling usually involves the joining of two DIT moieties to form 3,5,3',5'-tetraiodothyronine, T_4, while the addition of MIT to a DIT residue yields 3,5,3'-triiodothyronine, T_3. All iodinated tyrosines do not become coupled, and much extractable organic iodide remains in the form of MIT or DIT.

One suggested coupling scheme involves free radical formation. In this model free DIT radicals are generated within the TG matrix through the action of thyroperoxidase. In this particular pathway a serine residue would remain in the position formerly occupied by the phenolic residue cleaved from the tyrosine (Fig. 13.5). The formation of T_3 may occur by a similar scheme, except the coupling would be between MIT (contributing a phenolic group) and DIT [19].

Antithyroid Drugs

Certain drugs inhibit thyroid function by antagonizing formation of thyroid hormones. These drugs are generally classified into those compounds that inhibit iodide transport (iodide trapping) into the thyroid gland and those that inhibit iodine incorporation into tyrosine. Univalent inhibitors of iodide transport include thiocyanate and other monovalent anions (perchlorate, chlorate, periodate, etc.). Even iodide in large doses is transiently inhibitory to thyroid function (Wolff-Chaikoff effect), but the mechanism of this

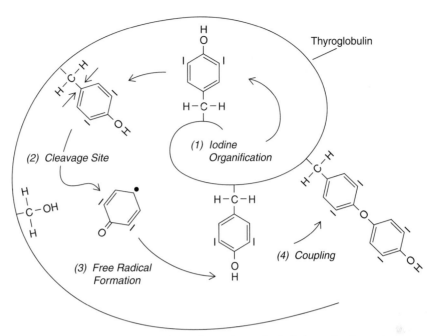

Figure 13.5 Hypothetical coupling scheme for iodothyronine formation.

inhibition remains unexplained. Iodide pump inhibitors probably antagonize iodide transport through *competitive inhibition*. Other antithyroid compounds include the thionamides, the sulfonamides (e.g., para-aminobenzoic acid), and the sulfonylureas (carbutamide, tolbutamide). Maintenance of an effective concentration of these antithyroid drugs for a sufficient time will usually cause thyroid hypertrophy and goiter. These agents are therefore often referred to as *goitrogens*. A number of these drugs are of clinical importance in the treatment of excess thyroid hormone production (thyrotoxicosis) (Fig. 13.6).

Dietary goitrogens may be responsible for *endemic goiter* in certain parts of the world. Certain *cyanogenic glucosides* (found in cassava, sorghum, sweet potatoes, maize, apricots, cherries, almonds) are hydrolyzed by glucosidases in the gut and release free cyanide that is converted to thiocyanate. Thioglucosides found in certain plants (e.g., genus *Brassica*: cabbage, Brussels sprouts, cauliflower, turnips, and rutabagas) are metabolized within the body to thiocyanates and isothiocyanates (Fig. 13.7). These plant products are usually not consumed in large enough quantities to produce goiter, although they may augment endemic goiter in areas deficient in iodine. Involvement of dietary goitrogens in the pathogenesis of human goiter has been discovered in a population of natives in Zaire, Africa [14]. Cassava forms an important part of the natives' diet, and it has been shown that ingestion of cassava from this area depresses radioiodide uptake by the normal human thyroid. The nature of the putative goitrogen remains unclear. Congenital goiter in lambs of ewes fed various mustard greens has also been reported.

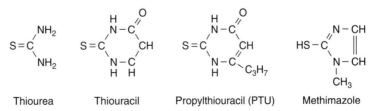

Thiourea   Thiouracil   Propylthiouracil (PTU)   Methimazole

Figure 13.6 Structures of some thionamide type antithyroid drugs.

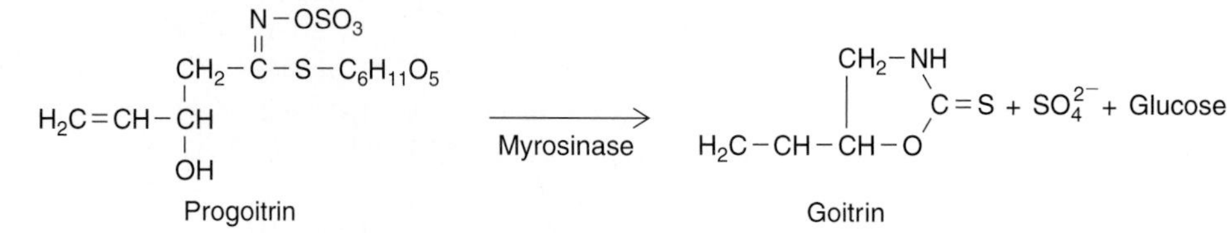

$$
\begin{array}{c}
N-OSO_3 \\
\parallel \\
CH_2-C-S-C_6H_{11}O_5 \\
H_2C=CH-CH \\
\mid \\
OH
\end{array}
\qquad
\xrightarrow[\text{Myrosinase}]{}
\qquad
\begin{array}{c}
CH_2-NH \\
\mid \\
H_2C-CH-CH-O \\
\end{array}
C=S + SO_4^{2-} + \text{Glucose}
$$

Progoitrin   Goitrin

Figure 13.7 Synthesis and structure of goitrin.

THYROID HORMONES OR THYROID HORMONE?

Normally, thyroxine (T_4) is produced in greater quantity than triiodothyronine (T_3). In human serum the concentration of T_4 is about 50 times greater than the T_3 level. Because T_4 is converted to T_3 in athyreotic human subjects, extrathyroidal monodeiodination of T_4 appears, therefore, to be the major source of T_3 in the body. If T_3 is the physiologically relevant hormone, is T_4 therefore the prohormone of T_3? Is it possible that both T_4 and T_3 are hormones, each with its own specific target tissues? There is strong evidence that T_3 is the major physiologically active thyroid hormone regulating cellular activity in many species, but T_4 is thought to exert a negative feedback action on the hypothalamus. In newborn infants serum T_3 levels are very low in cord blood, whereas T_4 concentrations are high, suggesting that T_4 may serve a direct functional role during certain developmental stages of animals. In this text the term *thyroid hormones* will refer to the putative activities of both T_3 and T_4, but it must be understood that T_3 is the most effective thyroid hormone under normal serum levels of iodothyronines, at least in mammals [46].

OTHER IODOTHYRONINES IN BIOLOGICAL FLUIDS

Although T_4 and T_3 are the major thyroid hormones in the human circulation, other iodothyronines are also present [46] (Fig. 13.8). The relative concentrations of these iodinated thyronines vary in healthy and diseased states, but the significance of these dif-

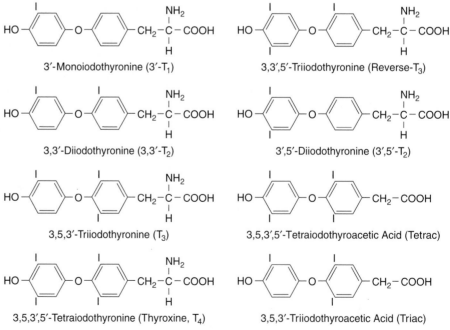

Figure 13.8 Structural formulas of iodothyronines found in human plasma.

ferences is presently unknown. T_3, T_4, triac (3,5,3'-triiodothyroacetic acid), and tetrac (3,5,3',5'-tetraiodothyroacetic acid) have calorigenic activity; the relative potency of these compounds is approximately 300 : 100 : 21 : 11, respectively. Although reverse triiodothyronine (3,3',5'-triiodothyronine, rT_3) has little thermogenic activity, it is more potent than T_3 in a number of systems [11]. Nevertheless, it is argued that the concentrations of these iodothyronines required to cause physiological responses in vitro exceed by several orders of magnitude those concentrations present in vivo. Thus the physiological significance, if any, of the actions of these iodothyronines is questionable.

The T_3 and rT_3 present in body fluids are derived from monodeiodination of T_4 within peripheral tissues. Subsequent metabolism of these iodothyronines provides the major sources of the T_2's and $3'$-T_1. Ultimately, these iodinated thyronines are made soluble through sulfation or glucuronide formation within the liver and are excreted in the urine or with bile salts. Recent evidence suggests that high concentrations of T_0 (completely deiodinated thyronine) are present in the plasma and urine and may represent a major end product of thyronine deiodination in humans.

CONTROL OF THYROID HORMONE SECRETION

Thyroid hormone secretion is regulated by TSH from the pituitary gland that, in turn, is controlled by TRH of hypothalamic origin (see Chap. 6). Thyroid hormones feed back at the pituitary and hypothalamic levels to inhibit TSH secretion (Fig. 13.9). TSH secretion is inhibited by stress in a number of species, including humans [42]. The action of TRH follows its specific high-affinity binding to the thyrotroph plasma membrane receptor. Hydrolysis of phosphatidylinositol followed by altered intracellular Ca^{2+} is the proximate event in the secretion of TSH, while cAMP appears not to be involved [12].

In many mammals activation of the pituitary-thyroid axis occurs during exposure to a lowered ambient temperature. Acute cold exposure of the rat, for example, leads to a rapid release of TSH, probably involving a neuroendocrine reflex mechanism. TSH release in response to a cold stimulus occurs in infants but is minimal or absent in adult humans. Present evidence suggests that an acute neuroendocrine reflex exists for TSH release in some mammals and in human infants and is mediated initially by peripheral sensory receptors, then relayed to the hypothalamus where stimulation of TRH release occurs. This is substantiated by the observation that prior administration of T_4 inhibits pituitary TSH release in response to a cold stimulus. In addition, peripheral plasma levels of TRH increase in hypophysectomized cold-exposed rats. Finally, TRH synthesis is increased in vitro in hypothalamic tissue taken from cold-exposed rats.

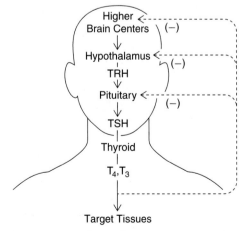

Figure 13.9 Central nervous system pituitary-thyroid axis.

In addition to the well-established negative feedback action of T_4 on pituitary thyrotropin (TSH) production, T_4 controls thyrotropin-releasing hormone (TRH) synthesis by regulating gene expression of the TRH prohormone in the "thyrotrophic area" of the hypothalamus. The negative feedback effect of T_4 on the synthesis of the TRH-prohormone is specific for TRH-producing neurons located in the medial division of the paraventricular nucleus (PVN), whereas TRH neurons elsewhere in the hypothalamus or in extrahypothalamic locations are not affected by changes of thyroid status. For example, TRH in the hypothalamus, but not olfactory lobe, is regulated by thyroid hormone. In the hypothalamus, hypothyroidism enhances not only proTRH synthesis but also release of TRH and another proTRH-derived peptide [6].

CIRCULATION AND METABOLISM

The thyroid hormones are water-insoluble molecules that require specific binding proteins in the plasma and the cell cytosol to gain access to nuclear receptors. This protein-bound iodine (PBI) consists of two major thyroxine-binding proteins present in human plasma: *thyroxine-binding prealbumin* (TBPA) and *thyroxine-binding globulin* (TBG). Prealbumin has a molecular weight of 55,000 and is composed of four identical subunits, each consisting of 127 amino acid residues arranged in a tetrahedral symmetry and possessing a pair of T_4-binding sites. These binding sites are located deep inside a cylindrical channel that runs completely through the molecule and are almost completely removed from the surrounding medium. TBG consists of a single polypeptide chain; although it is similar in molecular weight to TBPA, much less is known about its chemical constitution. About 70% to 75% of T_4 is bound to TBG, 15% to 20% to TBPA, and 5% to 10% may be bound to albumin. These binding proteins are synthesized within the liver.

During pregnancy in humans there is a doubling of TBG concentration, which may result from estrogen stimulation of binding protein synthesis within the liver. Increased TBG production is followed by increased thyroid T_4 synthesis and secretion, but the plasma concentrations of unbound iodothyronines remain unchanged. In normal individuals less than 0.5% of the total serum T_4 and about 0.3% of the serum T_3 are present in the free or unbound state. Any factor that alters the serum-binding proteins, particularly thyroxine-binding globulin (TGB), may affect the total T_4 concentration in the absence of thyroid dysfunction. Pregnancy and estrogen-containing medications increase TBG concentrations; testosterone, corticosteroids, severe illness, cirrhosis, and nephrotic disorders can lower TBG concentrations [23]. Teleost fishes lack high-affinity T_4-binding plasma proteins. If one function of the binding proteins is to provide a large extrathyroidal pool of iodide, these proteins may not be required in a marine environment where iodide is always abundant.

PHYSIOLOGICAL ROLES

The first scientific experiment to determine the role of the thyroid gland was reported in 1858 and involved the removal of the gland from dogs. The animals died soon after. Transplantation of thyroid tissue from a thyroidectomized animal into the body cavity resulted in survival of the animals for a long duration, thus demonstrating that death was due to an absence of the thyroid rather than to the operation itself. Many experiments led to the erroneous belief that the thyroid gland is essential to life. Only later was it realized that death from thyroidectomy was due to removal of the parathyroid glands present within the thyroid tissue. The essential role of the thyroid glands in the control of numerous physiological processes is now well documented.

Thyroid hormones influence most bodily functions [19]. They directly affect a number of physiological processes and, although without observable actions, they are often required (permissive) for the actions of other hormones on these processes. For example, they are obligatory, along with somatotropin, for early growth and development. Thyroid hormone deficiencies in humans produce major abnormalities in growth, development, reproduction, behavior, and metabolism. Thyroid hormones are unique in that they exert effects within almost every tissue of the body throughout the life of an individual.

Growth and Development

The absence of thyroid hormones results in severe growth retardation, which is associated with arrest of bone elongation as well as retarded bone maturation. Somatotropin secretion is diminished in the absence of thyroid hormones and renewed when thyroid hormones are administered. Thus one cause of growth retardation is the absence of circulating levels of GH. Nevertheless, administration of GH to hypothyroid individuals is without effect if thyroid hormones are not also given. Thus the role of thyroid hormones in normal growth is twofold; they are required both for the production of GH and for its systemic actions.

Levels of hyaluronic acid are high in proliferating tissue and decrease as division ceases and the cells become more differentiated. The enzyme *hyaluronidase* (an endoglycosidase), which splits hyaluronic acid into smaller oligosaccharides, is apparently induced at a time when tissues mature and may, therefore, serve as a signal for differentiation. Thyroid hormones stimulate tadpole tissue differentiation, which is paralleled by a decrease in hyaluronic acid levels and an increase in hyaluronidase concentrations. In myxedematous tissue from subjects with hypothyroidism there is an increase in hyaluronic acid. These observations suggest that thyroid hormones stimulate differentiation through stimulation of hyaluronidase production.

Thyroid hormones in concert with prolactin play an important role in the regulation of mouse mammary gland development. Decreased serum levels of thyroid hormones result in retarded growth of the ductal system and little or no alveolar development. Thyroid hormones may also be required for the synthesis of normal levels of PRL by the pituitary gland. Thyroid hormones are required for the normal development of the brain; without them there is decreased protein synthesis, decreased myelinogenesis, and retarded axonal ramifications. These developmental processes, unlike general body growth, are irreversibly compromised and lead to mental deficiency, as is evident in cretins. Nerve growth factor (NGF) induces dendritogenesis and regeneration of sympathetic neurons (see Chap. 12). It may be significant, therefore, that thyroid hormone administration increases the concentration of NGF in the brain. These observations suggest that thyroid hormones may control CNS development through stimulation of NGF biosynthesis. Thyroid hormones also accelerate axonal regeneration in the cerebrum of lesioned adult rats, and the hormones appear to be selectively concentrated within adrenergic nerve terminals.

Thermogenesis

The evolution from poikilothermy to homeothermy required the acquisition of some mechanism for heat production. Active sodium transport uses a high proportion (possibly as much as 20% to 40%) of the total cellular energy supply. In the process of ATP hydrolysis by the Na$^+$ pump, heat is liberated, which contributes greatly to the maintenance of an elevated body temperature in homeotherms (sodium pump theory of thermogenesis). The activity of the sodium pump requires a source of ATP, which is produced mainly within the mitochondria. Thyroid hormones stimulate mitochondrial oxygen consumption and production of ATP. The T$_3$-induced increase in Na$^+$/K$^+$-ATPase activity results from an increase in the number of enzyme sites rather than a change in the affinity of the enzyme for substrates or in the catalytic properties of the enzyme. Na$^+$/K$^+$-ATPase expression is controlled at multiple levels, including transcriptional, translational, and post-translational levels; T$_3$ regulation of this important enzyme is highly tissue specific and may be mediated by one or more of these regulatory mechanisms operating simultaneously [22, 43]. Inhibition of Na^+/K^+-ATPase activity by ouabain and other sodium pump antagonists markedly reduces the action of thyroid hormones on heat production and oxygen consumption.

Diet and Thyroid Hormone Function

The increase of caloric intake (mixed diet or carbohydrates) in individuals results in an increased diet-induced thermogenesis [12]. The production of T_3 is increased during short-term overfeeding; the increased serum levels of T_3 apparently derive from altered (increased) peripheral conversion of T_4 to T_3 and a decreased conversion of T_3 to rT_3. Individuals fed isocaloric diets low in carbohydrates or containing no carbohydrates develop changes in T_3 and rT_3 opposite to those resulting from feeding excess carbohydrates. Here may be an adaptation in which the resting metabolic rate is increased in the presence of excess poor-quality food (carbohydrates) to provide enough of a scarce nutrient, such as protein or even minerals, and not be burdened with a weight gain.

Plasma levels of T_3 decrease during prolonged fasting, which is correlated with a decrease (down regulation) in hepatic nuclear T_3 receptors. A decrease in serum T_3 concentration per se does not diminish hepatic nuclear T_3 receptor content as brain T_3 receptor number is not concomitantly changed. A particular cell type may be able to modify its nuclear T_3 receptor content in response to its own metabolic status, which "infers the possibility of individual target cell acceptance or rejection of the hormonal directive" [39]. This may represent a homeostatic protective mechanism to prolong survival of the organism under conditions of food deprivation.

Thyroid Hormones and Aging. Food restriction alters the aging process. In rats long-term reduction in food consumption increases longevity, decreases the frequency of occurrence and severity of age-related diseases, and retards much of the physiological decline seen with aging. The mechanism by which food restriction exerts its anti-aging action is not known, but it has been suggested that its effects on aging are mediated by altering endocrine and/or neural regulatory systems. The thyroid hormone system represents one potential coupler of food restriction with aging. Since this endocrine system is sensitive to changes in food consumption, several studies have suggested that the thyroid is involved in the aging process per se [44].

Permissive Actions

Thyroid hormones are required for the actions of other hormones on target tissues. This permissive action of thyroid hormones is also a characteristic of gonadal and adrenal steroids on some of their target tissues. Because thyroid and steroid hormones mediate most of their actions at the level of the genome to induce protein synthesis, it is likely that these proteins function as substrates in the action pathway of other hormones (see Fig. 4.12).

Thyroid hormones induce GH production in cultured rat pituitary tumor (GH_1) cells. Glucocorticoids also stimulate GH synthesis, but only in the presence of thyroid hormones. There is a dramatic synergistic activation of GH production when both hormones are present together in the medium, suggesting that the ability of glucocorticoids to stimulate GH synthesis is controlled by thyroid hormones. This is another example of the permissive action of thyroid hormones.

The enzyme ornithine decarboxylase (ODC) is essential for polyamine biosynthesis and is intimately related to the regulation of nucleic acid and protein biosynthesis. Somatotropin stimulates ODC activity in brain tissue, but only in the presence of thyroid hormones. Thyroid hormones do not, however, stimulate brain ODC activity. This demonstrates dramatically the permissive action of a hormone. In the liver, in contrast, GH and thyroid hormones stimulate ODC activity independently. These results demonstrate the

TABLE 13.1   Some Physiological Roles and Actions of Thyroid Hormones in Mammals

---

Feedback inhibition of pituitary TSH secretion
Permissive to the action of many other hormones:
   Enhances lipolytic response of adipose tissue to hormones
   Required for the growth-promoting activity of GH
Increases activity of the sympathoadrenal system
Regulates basal metabolic rate:
   Increases mitochondrial oxidative phosphorylation
Required for hepatic conversion of carotenes to vitamin A
Required for bone growth and maturation
Required for nervous system differentiation in early development
Required for pituitary prolactin and growth hormone synthesis
Increases the rate of intestinal glucose absorption
Increases human red blood cell Ca^{2+}-ATPase activity
Induces enzyme synthesis:
   Na^+/K^+-ATPase (or a protein component or activator of the sodium pump)
   Carbamoyl phosphate synthetase (a phosphotransferase)
   α-Lactalbumin (lactose synthetase system proteins)
   Hepatic pyruvate carboxylase (converts pyruvate to oxaloacetate)
   Chromatin protein kinase
   Mitochondrial α-glycerophosphate dehydrogenase
   Malic dehydrogenase (converts malic acid to oxaloacetate)
   Hyaluronidase (dissolves intercellular ground substance)
Induction of cellular proteins (other than enzymes):
   Prolactin, growth hormone, lung surfactants, brain nerve growth factor (NGF)

---

tissue specificity to these hormones within an individual animal. Some of the more prominent actions of thyroid hormones are summarized in Table 13.1.

MECHANISMS OF ACTION

The action of T_3 is analogous to the model for steroid hormone action (see Chaps. 4, 9, 15 and 18) [5, 25, 50].

There are two known thyroid hormone receptor (TR) genes: thyroid hormone receptor β (TRβ) on chromosome 3 and thyroid hormone receptor α (TRα) on chromosome 17. Both genes encode isoform products by alternative mRNA splicing. The TRβ gene produces TRβ1 and TRβ2 proteins, and the TRα gene produces TRα1 and an α2 isoform. The TRβ1, TRβ2, and TRα1 proteins appear to be physiologic thyroid hormone receptors that avidly bind T_3 and regulate subsequent thyroid hormone-responsive gene transcription. The α2 isoform does not bind T_3 and is thus not a receptor, but is believed to inhibit the transcriptional effects of TRβ1, TRβ2, and TRα1. TRβ1 and TRα1 receptors are present in many tissues, but TRβ2 appears to be restricted to the pituitary gland and some areas of the central nervous system. The TRs are intranuclear proteins (ligand-activated transcription factors) that have distinct domains for binding to T_3 and DNA and for forming homodimers with nearby TRs or heterodimers with other nuclear receptors (retinoic acid receptors, retinoid X receptors), or thyroid hormone receptor auxiliary proteins (TRAPs). Under normal circumstances, circulating T_4 and T_3 traverse the cell membrane by an energy-dependent process. T_4 is then converted to T_3, which enters the nucleus where it binds to the TR. The T_3-TR complexes bind as monomers, homodimers, or heterodimers to specific thyroid-response elements present in thyroid hormone-regulated genes. This initiates the activity of RNA polymerase, which controls transcription of the structural gene regions into mRNA. Subsequently, mRNA is translated into protein products that ultimately mediate thyroid hormone tissue effects (Fig. 13.10).

The actions of T_3 may not be restricted to a genomic locus; rather, they may induce effects on the plasma membrane and mitochondria [13]. Thyroid hormones stimulate

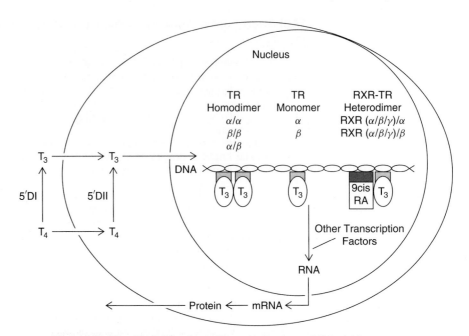

Figure 13.10 Model for the action mechanism of thyroid hormone on target tissues. The active form of thyroid hormone, triiodothyronine (T_3), is produced by deiodination of thyroxine (T_4) by the enzymes $T_4$5'-deiodinase (5'-D) types I and II. Type I $T_4$5-deiodinase is found predominantly in the liver and kidneys; its action is responsible for the production of two-thirds of the total T_3 in the body. Type II $T_4$5'-deiodinase is responsible for most of the T_3 found in the pituitary, the brain, and brown fat. T_3 enters the cell or is produced locally and then transported into the nucleus. Transcriptionally active forms of thyroid hormone receptors (TR) include monomers, homodimers, and heterodimers with nuclear protein partners, such as the retinoid X receptor (RXR). The T_3-receptor complex interacts with specific sequences in DNA regulatory regions and modifies gene expression. T_3 causes both increases and decreases in gene expression and may also influence the stability of messenger RNA (mRNA). 9-*cis* RA denotes 9-*cis*-retinoic acid, the ligand for RXR. (From Brent [5], with permission. Reprinted by permission of *The New England Journal of Medicine.* "The molecular basis for thyroid hormone action." 331:847–853. ©1994 Massachusetts Medical Society.)

human red cell Ca^{2+}-ATPase activity, which clearly documents the extranuclear actions of these hormones. Thyroid hormones stimulate the rapid uptake of amino acids into cells, an action not blocked by actinomycin D or puromycin. These results again suggest a direct action of thyroid hormones at the level of the plasma membrane. In addition 2-deoxyglucose (a nonmetabolizable glucose substrate) uptake into cells is rapidly stimulated by T_3 at physiological concentrations. These effects are also not blocked by inhibitors of transcriptional and translational processes. Thyroid hormones also stimulate plasmalemmal Na^+/K^+-ATPase (the sodium pump). This enhanced activity may be an indirect action of the hormones and result from an increased number of pump units rather than any direct increase in the activity of the ATPase. It is believed that newly synthesized ATPase derives from actions of the thyroid hormones at the level of the genome.

For many years there was argument whether thyroid hormones mediated their effects through direct actions on mitochondria. The following data provide convincing evidence that, indeed, mitochondria are another site of thyroid hormone action. In the hypothyroid state mitochondria are altered both morphologically and functionally, and the uptake of ADP by mitochondria is increased after administration of T_3 or T_4 to thyroidectomized rats. A specific receptor for T_3 and T_4 is a component of the inner mitochondrial membrane, which is known to be the site of oxidative phosphorylation. These receptors are present in mitochondria from thyroid hormone-responsive tissues, but not in spleen and testes, tissues known to be refractory to thyroid hormones. Most interesting is the observation that mitochondria from neonatal rat brain, but not from brain tissues of older animals, possess thyroid hormone receptors. These data are compatible with the known temporal responsiveness of this tissue to thyroid hormones. Finally, mitochondrial oxygen consumption is increased in vitro by thyroid hormones. This effect is not inhibited by cycloheximide, an inhibitor of protein synthesis, suggesting an acute action of the hormones on the mitochondria. The marked changes in mitochondrial nucleic acid synthesis in vivo that are associated with altered thyroid states suggest that thyroid hormone action in mitochondria may involve both acute and long-term actions, the latter involving mRNA and protein synthesis.

In summary thyroid hormones act on a number of cellular receptor sites. The actions of most hormones that mediate their effects at the plasmalemma involve changes in the intracellular levels of one or more cyclic nucleotides or other second messengers, whose activities appear restricted to substrate phosphorylation. There appears to be no single intracellular effector mechanism for thyroid hormone action; rather, several pathways contribute to an integrated cellular response of these hormones. The nuclear actions of thyroid hormones may be related to slower anabolic effects such as those involved in growth and differentiation. The actions of thyroid hormones on the plasmalemma (sodium pump hypothesis) and mitochondria (mitochondrial receptor hypothesis) are rapidly initiated events that control increased heart rate, oxygen consumption, and ATP production.

PATHOPHYSIOLOGY

Because thyroid hormones affect many physiological processes and are necessary for the optimal activity of numerous hormones, it is not surprising that abnormalities of thyroid function lead to gross alterations in the normal physiology of an individual [32, 40]. Thyroid hormone underproduction or overproduction, referred to as hypothyroidism or hyperthyroidism, respectively, can occur at birth (congenital) or later in life. A defect at the level of the pituitary or hypothalamus would result in decreased or increased production and secretion of TSH with resulting secondary or tertiary hypothyroidism or hyperthyroidism, respectively. Abnormalities of thyroid function may be familial (genetic) in nature and involve failure in growth or normal function of the thyroid gland. Other genetic defects may result in biosynthetic defects related to thyroid hormonogenesis, which may involve a defect in iodine trapping or organification, defective thyroglobulin synthesis and secretion, and other abnormalities [29].

In certain cases, idiopathic central hypothyroidism may result from the secretion of a biologically inactive thyrotropin. It has been determined experimentally that the TSH secreted in these cases indeed lacks biological activity, as evidenced by impaired binding to thyroid cell receptors. TRH treatments can correct this defect. The evidence suggests that TRH regulates not only the secretion of TSH but also its specific molecular and conformational features required for hormone action [2]. In the *low T_3 syndrome,* hypothyroidism results from a failure in the peripheral conversion of T_4 to T_3, which is the physiologically relevant thyroid hormone [8].

TSH is a member of a group of closely related glycoprotein hormones, all of which are heterodimeric molecules consisting of common α and specific β subunits. Several cases have been found that show congenital, isolated TSH deficiencies associated with cretinism, displaying severe mental and growth retardation with the failure to go through puberty. One family with two patient siblings has been analyzed intensively. These patients showed no TSH in the blood even in the hypothyroid state, but showed normal levels of other glycoprotein hormones, such as luteinizing hormone (LH) and follicle-stimulating hormone

(FSH), which share the same α subunit with TSH. Upon administration of TRH, a dramatic increase of the α subunit was observed in the bloodstream, but not of the heterodimeric TSH or the free β subunit, suggesting that the patients do not produce active β subunits. The absence of the β subunit could either be due to a failure to produce the polypeptide or to the production of an inactive subunit. It was shown that the patients' β subunit genes carry a mutation in the 29th amino acid codon, and that the mutant gene may produce a conformationally abnormal β subunit that cannot associate with the α subunit [20].

Overstimulation of the thyroid may result from an autoimmune response involving antibodies to the TSH receptor [9]. *Long-acting thyroid stimulator* (LATS) is the name given to the antibody believed responsible for TSH receptor stimulation. This type of hyperthyroidism has been referred to as Graves' disease [7, 38], but a large number of affected patients have no measurable plasma levels of LATS. Present evidence is that LATS is probably not the etiologic factor in Graves' disease. Graves' thyrotoxicosis is uniquely associated with an exophthalmos (protruding of the eyes). In rare instances hyperthyroidism may result from the ectopic production of TSH or even from a trophoblastic (placental) tumor secreting either excessive amounts of choriogonadotropin (structurally somewhat related to TSH) or a TSH-like molecule. Primary hyperthyroidism may derive from development of a thyroidal adenoma or carcinoma and involve gross overproduction of thyroid hormones.

Cretins are individuals who suffer from a deficiency or total absence of thyroid hormones. *Athyreotic cretinism* may result from an in utero (congenital) thyroiditis or from a failure in thyroid development. Thyroid dysgenesis is responsible for decreased thyroid function in most infants with hypothyroidism and is most prevalent in females. Although sporadic, it may be familial in origin and may also occur in association with maternal autoimmune thyroiditis. Congenital goiter may also be associated with thyroid dyshormonogenesis due to hereditary defects in hormone synthesis or metabolism. The major symptoms of cretinism are failure of skeletal growth and maturation and a marked retardation in development of intellect. Hypothyroidism in the adult is referred to as *myxedema* (from the Greek, *myxa*, mucus and *oidema*, swelling) because of the characteristic mucinous protein deposit in the subcutaneous tissues.

A genetic failure in development of thyroid hormone receptors results in a familial peripheral (end organ, target tissue) resistance with resulting hypothyroidism [37]. Generalized resistance to thyroid hormone (GRTH), in which most or all of the tissues of the body are variably resistant to thyroid hormone, has been described in more than 200 cases. Selective pituitary resistance to thyroid hormone (PRTH), in which predominantly the pituitary gland is resistant, has been reported in at least 32 cases, and selective peripheral resistance to thyroid hormone (PerRTH), in which only peripheral tissues are resistant, has been described in one individual [28, 47].

The clinical manifestations of tissue resistance to the action of thyroid hormones differ dramatically depending on the tissues involved. Individuals with the general resistance syndrome are clinically euthyroid; they may have goiter and plasma levels of thyroid hormones may even be elevated. The variable biochemical defects responsible for end organ thyroid hormone resistance may be caused by the following: (1) decreased binding affinity; (2) decreased binding capacity (decrease in receptor number); and (3) an abnormal postreceptor mechanism. For example, a genetic defect in development of thyroid hormone receptors results in a familial peripheral resistance with resulting clinical hypothyroidism that is not, however, characterized by goiter. On the other hand, individuals with a pituitary (thyrotroph) resistance to thyroid hormone feedback are hyperthyroid and, as might be expected, plasma TSH and thyroid hormone levels are elevated. This example of TSH-dependent hyperthyroidism represents one of the *syndromes of inappropriate TSH secretion.*

Failure of the thyroid to produce T_4 and T_3 may lead to the development of a goiter (Fig. 13.11) as, in the absence of any negative feedback to the hypothalamus and pituitary gland, there is excessive secretion of TSH. In the absence of thyroid hormone production TSH stimulation continues to lead to hypertrophy of the thyroid follicular cells. Thyroid glands from such hypothyroid individuals are hyperplastic and exhibit grossly columnar

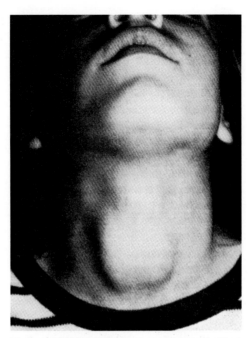

Figure 13.11 Diffuse thyromegaly (goiter) in a 12-year-old girl with euthyroid autoimmune thyroiditis. (From Foley [17], with permission. *Endocrinology and Metabolism Clinics of North America* 22:593–606, 1993.)

follicular cells with a decreased amount of colloid (due to enhanced engulfment and degradation). Goiters may also develop under conditions of thyroiditis due to autoantibodies against thyroid TSH receptors. In the past a lack of iodine in the diet resulted in hypothyroidism; with the general availability of iodized salt this problem has been eradicated throughout much of the world. Clinically, endemic (simple) goiter is treated with iodized salt, but prolonged hypothyroidism may lead to irreversible stunting and cretinism.

About one billion people worldwide are potentially at risk from iodine-deficiency disorders. Endemic goiter is the most common manifestation, and its prevalence rises directly with the degree of iodine lack, reaching 100% in communities with severe iodine deficiency. The greatest morbidity of severe iodide deficiency arises not by its primary consequences on thyroid gland enlargement, but by its secondary effects on thyroid hormone homeostasis acting on fetal and neonatal brain development. This is expressed clinically in its extreme as endemic cretinism, a disorder of profound mental and physical disability [3, 4, 31].

The integrity of the TG structure as a protein is essential for adequate synthesis of thyroid hormone. Also a large supply of iodine and of thyroid hormone is stored in the TG molecule and is therefore available for secretion on demand. Mutations in TG gene or hyposialylated TG, due to defective sialytransferase activity, cause a structurally defective protein and severely impairs the function of TG. Defective TG synthesis and secretion can cause goiter and hypothyroidism [29].

Thyroxine has been used as replacement therapy in hypothyroidism. For the treatment of thyrotoxicosis, such antithyroid drugs as propylthiourea, methimazole, or carbimazole are used most commonly (Fig. 13.6). These thionamide-type drugs inhibit the coupling of iodotyrosyl residues in thyroglobulin to form T_4 and T_3. Propylthiourea (PTU) is the preferred drug as, in addition to the effects in the thyroid common to all these drugs, it blocks the peripheral conversion of T_4 to T_3 in the liver. Radioactive (cytoxic) iodine, administered one time only, is a preferred treatment of hyperthyroidism in patients who have difficulty adhering to the medical regimen of taking antithyroid drugs three times a day for a year or more.

TABLE 13.2   Major Physiological Manifestations of Hyperthyroidism and Hypothyroidism

Hyperthyroidism	Hypothyroidism
Elevated T_4-T_3 levels	Decreased (or absent) T_4-T_3 levels
Elevated basal metabolic rate (BMR) (hypermetabolism)	Low basal metabolic rate (BMR) (hypometabolism)
Increased perspiration	Decreased perspiration
Rapid pulse (increased cardiac output, hypertension)	Slow pulse (decreased cardiac output, hypotension)
Increased body temperature (sensation of warmness)	Lowered body temperature (sensation of coldness)
Heat intolerance	Cold intolerance
Warm, moist palms	Coarse, dry skin, subdermal thickening
Nervousness, anxiety, excitability, restlessness, insomnia	Lethargy, decreased mentation, depression, paranoia, sleepiness, tiredness
Weight loss	Weight gain
Muscle wasting	Loss of hair, dry and brittle texture
Increased appetite	Edema of face and eyelids
Menstrual irregularities	Menstrual irregularities
Exophthalmos (in some individuals)	Carotenemia (increased plasma levels of carotenes)
Goiter (primary or secondary origin)	Goiter (may or may not be present)

The general symptoms of hypothyroxinemia and thyrotoxicosis are summarized in Table 13.2. Many general manifestations of underproduction or overproduction of thyroid hormones relate to decreased or increased activity of the sympathoadrenal system (see Chap. 14). A summary of the general etiology of hypothyroidism and hyperthyroidism is provided in Table 13.3 and Fig. 13.12.

TABLE 13.3   Pathophysiology of the Human Thyroid Gland

HYPOTHYROIDISM (Hypothyroxinemia)
    Primary hypothyroidism
        Familial or congenital thyroid dysgenesis
        Failure of thyroid hormonogenesis (usually of genetic origin)
    Secondary hypothyroidism
        Hypothalamic hypothyroidism (tertiary hypothyroidism)
    Cretinism (childhood hypothyroidism)
        Goitrous cretinism (endemic; lack of dietary iodide)
        Athyreotic cretinism (congenital absence of thyroid; thyroid dysgenesis)
    Myxedema (adult hypothyroidism)
        Simple goiter (endemic; lack of dietary iodide)
        Primary myxedema
            Idiopathic (atrophic thyroiditis of unknown origin)
            Iatrogenic (surgical removal or chemical inactivation)
            Spontaneous (autoimmune destruction: Hashimotos thyroiditis)
    Familial peripheral (end-organ) resistance to thyroid hormones (e.g., lack of or defective T_3, T_4 receptors)
    Familial thyroid hormone-binding globulin (TBG) deficiency syndrome
    Low T_3 syndrome (failure of peripheral conversion of T_4 to T_3)
    Thyroid gland resistance to TSH

HYPERTHYROIDISM (Thyrotoxicosis)
    Primary hyperthyroidism
        Neoplasia (adenoma, carcinoma neoplasia producing excessive TSH)
    Secondary hyperthyroidism
        Hypothalamic hyperthyroidism (tertiary hyperthyroidism)
        TSH-dependent hyperthyroidism (pituitary thyrotroph unresponsiveness to T_3 feedback inhibition)
        Ectopic TSH secretion (rare)
        Long-acting thyroid stimulator (LATS) (autoimmune agonistic antibodies of thyroid TSH receptors) (Graves disease) [9, 38]

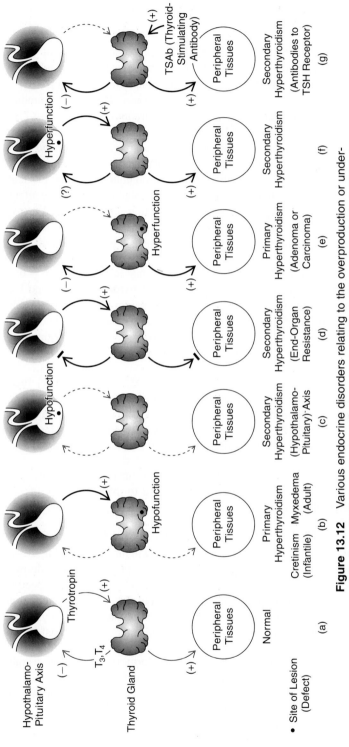

Figure 13.12 Various endocrine disorders relating to the overproduction or underproduction of TSH or to inadequate thyroid- or peripheral-tissue responses to TSH or thyroid hormones.

Tests for Thyroid Function

A variety of tests are used to determine the functional status of the thyroid gland. These tests are generally designed to identify the particular site of malfunction in the hypothalamic-hypophysial-thyroid axis.

Plasma T_4, T_3 Levels.   Plasma concentrations of T_4 and T_3 are measured by radioimmunoassay. As noted, most serum content of thyroid hormones is bound to one or more serum proteins. It is the minute quantities of free T_4 and T_3 that best reflect the tissue metabolic activities of these hormones. The most commonly used tests of thyroid metabolic function measure the concentrations of total serum TBG-bound T_4 and T_3, and some measure the quantities of the free T_4 and T_3 moieties. An important consideration is the total amount of serum proteins available to bind T_4 and T_3 and the extent to which these protein-binding sites are saturated by thyroid hormones.

Any factor that alters the serum-binding proteins, particularly thyroxine-binding proteins, especially thyroxine-binding globulin (TGB), may affect the total T_4 concentration in the absence of thyroid dysfunction. Pregnancy and estrogen-containing medications increase TBG concentrations; testosterone, corticosteroids, severe illness, cirrhosis, and the nephrotic syndrome can also lower TBG concentrations [23].

Serum Thyrotropin.   In the normal individual there is usually an inverse correlation between the serum concentrations of thyroid hormones and TSH. Serum levels of TSH are elevated in patients with primary hypothyroidism and are usually undetectable in thyrotoxicosis of primary or autoimmune origin. A discrepancy in the reverse correlation between serum thyroid hormone levels and TSH concentrations might be suggestive of pituitary or hypothalamic dysfunction (secondary and tertiary hypothyroidism or hyperthyroidism).

Tests of Pituitary TSH Reserve.   In this test an increase in serum TSH in response to administration of synthetic TRH is measured. Thyroid hormones, also released in response to the TSH, are measured as an increase in plasma levels of T_4 and T_3. The TRH test clearly distinguishes between a hypothalamic or pituitary defect in TSH secretion as functional thyrotrophs will usually respond by releasing TSH [36].

TSH Stimulation Test.   This test measures the ability of the thyroid to respond to exogenous TSH. It was originally used to differentiate primary hypothyroidism due to thyroid gland failure from other defects in the pituitary thyroid axis.

Tests of Thyroid Gland Activity and Hormone Synthesis.   Radioisotopes of iodine, ^{131}I and ^{125}I, are used to assess a number of facets in the pathway of thyroid gland hormonogenesis. Increased or decreased uptake of these radioisotopes is associated with excessive or diminished production of thyroid hormones, respectively. The isotope is given intravenously or orally, and the amount of radioactive iodine accumulated by the thyroid at various times following administration is measured by epithyroid radioisotope decay detection. Other tests are designed to determine the intrathyroidal organification of iodine.

Tissue Sensitivity to Thyroid Hormones.   Numerous other tests are used in clinical medicine to determine other aspects of thyroid function. For example, to determine tissue responses to thyroid hormones an increase in basal metabolic rate is often measured.

COMPARATIVE ENDOCRINOLOGY

Some classical experiments in endocrinology were performed early this century on amphibian larvae, most often the anuran (frog, toad) tadpole. These experiments established a role for the thyroid in the control of metamorphosis in the amphibian [1, 41]. The following experimental observations were made:

1. Preparations (desiccated tissue) of the thyroid gland fed to frog tadpoles induced metamorphosis.

2. Removal of the thyroid glands prevented metamorphosis of tadpoles.

3. Implantation of thyroid glands into tadpoles caused accelerated development.

4. Hypophysectomy of tadpoles resulted in thyroid gland atrophy and prevented metamorphosis.

5. Injections of pars distalis extracts induced metamorphosis of hypophysectomized tadpoles.

6. Implantation of the pars distalis, but not the neurointermediate lobe, accelerated development in normal and hypophysectomized larvae, but not in thyroidless tadpoles.

The conclusion that emerged was that "metamorphosis is due to the combined action of both the anterior lobe of the hypophysis and the thyroid gland" [1]. Evidence has now shown that a thyroid-stimulating hormone (TSH) is specifically produced by thyrotrophs of the pars distalis and that thyrotropin of any source will stimulate metamorphosis of larval amphibians. Both thyroxine and triiodothyronine induce metamorphosis of amphibian larvae, and they are the likely thyroid hormones controlling metamorphosis in these animals.

Metamorphosis involves radical changes in body structure and function to allow successful transition of the amphibian from an aquatic to a terrestrial habitat (Fig. 13.13). The following metamorphic changes occur in amphibians:

1. Loss of the tail as a locomotory organ and acquisition of the characteristic tetrapod appendages.

2. Change in the integument from a smooth, moist skin (for respiration and increased locomotion) to a thicker, keratinized skin that is more resistant to water loss.

3. Loss of the major respiratory structure, the gills, and acquisition of lungs.

4. Radical changes in structural components of the GI tract: loss of the horny, rasping beaklike mouth and development of a new mouth with distensible tongue; shortening of the long intestine (needed for an essentially vegetarian diet) to a much shorter one for a generally carnivorous diet.

5. Development of corneal reflex, eyelids, and ocular muscles to control eye movements (eye movements in larvae are essentially nonexistent).

6. Biochemical changes in numerous organs:

    (a) From predominantly amylase to protease production within the GI tract.

    (b) From larval hemoglobins to adult hemoglobins. Larval hemoglobins bind more avidly to O_2 than do adult hemoglobins because O_2 is usually more limiting in the aquatic environment than in the terrestrial habitat.

    (c) From larval visual pigments to those of the adult, a change from predominantly rhodopsin to mostly porphyropsin.

    (d) From ammonia excretion (ammonotelism) to urea excretion (ureotelism).

Amphibian larvae are voracious omnivores and spend most of their time eating and converting the ingested metabolic substrates into body structures, essentially proteins. After reaching a particular body size, or in response to environmental cues, larvae undergo irreversible metamorphic changes that ultimately lead to their adult forms. Clearly, thyroid hormones control metamorphic change, but what are the particular endocrine events involved? Are circulating levels of thyroid hormones increased? If so, what physiological events are responsible for such changes? What causes the destruction

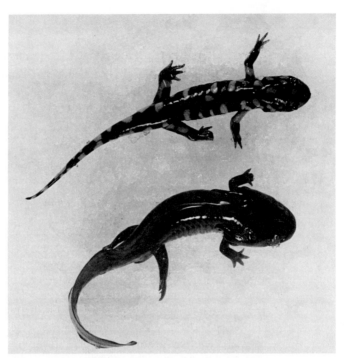

Figure 13.13 Metamorphic change of the salamander, *Ambystoma tigrinum*, as induced by thyroxine (T_4) added to the aquarium water.

of one tissue (e.g., the tail) and the development of another (e.g., tongue)? The activity of the thyroid gland (amount of rough ER, follicular height) is clearly increased at metamorphic climax. A popular hypothesis is that the low circulating levels of thyroid hormones in the premetamorphic tadpole cause a slow maturation of hypothalamic neurosecretory centers, in time resulting in greater thyroid hormone secretion. The increase in these hormones, in turn, provides a positive feedback to the hypothalamus, which causes an accelerated maturation of the hypothalamus and its neurosecretory neurons. The resulting activation of TRH secretion and subsequent stimulation of pituitary TSH secretion would provide the final stimulus to thyroid gland maturation and maximal T_4-T_3 secretion [15]. Injection of a minute amount of T_4 directly into the hypothalamus is capable of activating the hypothalamo-hypophysial-thyroid axis in larval salamanders [33].

A body of evidence suggests that prolactin is a larval growth hormone with antimetamorphic actions in amphibians. Normal metamorphic processes may depend on an interplay between PRL and thyroid hormones. For example, thyroxine-induced metamorphosis in the frog is accelerated by injections of antiserum to PRL. Hypophysectomized larval amphibians administered PRL continue to grow with time, even beyond their normal size range; although they never metamorphose, they may be made to do so by injections of high concentrations of thyroid hormones. Both in vivo and in vitro experiments have provided data that PRL antagonizes the action of thyroid hormones on metamorphic processes. For example, thyroxine added to tadpole tails incubated in vitro causes their resorption, a process that normally takes place in the intact animal during metamorphosis. In contrast, PRL added to the incubation medium inhibits the actions of thyroid hormones on tail resorption. It was proposed that the actions of the PRL are also exerted at the level of the thyroid to inhibit thyroid hormone synthesis and secretion (a goitrogenic action). In the *hypothalamic maturation model of metamorphosis* the action of thyroid hormones at the level of the hypothalamus would also involve the establishment of an inhibitory influence on the release of pituitary PRL secretion. This might be effected by the developmental acquisition of functional PRL-inhibiting factor neurons, resulting in establishment of a tonic inhibitory control over pituitary PRL secretion, as in mammals [15].

Acceleration of the metamorphic process may involve more than an increase in circulating levels of thyroid hormones. There appears to be an increased sensitivity of target tissues, such as the tail, during the progress of metamorphosis. Experimental evidence suggests that the number of binding sites for T_3 in nuclei from tail tissue increases during spontaneous metamorphosis; nuclear receptors for T_3 increase after exposure of intact cells to thyroid hormones. It has been proposed, therefore, that the elevated levels of endogenous thyroid hormones at the onset of metamorphic climax in the tadpole regulate the number of their own nuclear receptors, thus increasing tissue sensitivity to the hormones.

Further evidence for thyroid hormone-prolactin interactions during amphibian metamorphosis is available and provides interesting insights into the developmental roles of these two hormones. Certain urodeles, such as the red-spotted newt (*Notophthalmus viridescens*), undergo a second metamorphosis. After an initial metamorphosis from an aquatic larva to a terrestrial tetrapod, the young salamander migrates back to water (so-called "water drive"). Young newts can be induced to undergo precocious water drive by injections of PRL. Thyroid hormones, on the other hand, antagonize the actions of PRL. All actions of PRL and thyroid hormones are not exerted in opposition to each other; their actions are indeed often synergistic. For example, binding of PRL to the kidney of the bullfrog tadpole increases during metamorphic climax and in response to treatment with thyroxine. It was suggested that, during metamorphosis, the role of PRL as a growth-promoting agent is lost, along with its ion regulation of the gill. The osmoregulatory function of PRL may nevertheless persist beyond the larval period and be directed through the actions of the thyroid hormones from the gills (which are lost) to the kidneys.

Role of the Thyroid in Other Vertebrates

Evidence is lacking for a clearly defined role of the thyroid gland in cyclostomes and elasmobranchs. In teleost fishes the thyroid gland is required for normal gonadal maturation. Thyroxine increases the sensitivity of the teleost olfactory epithelium to detection of salinity [34]. Thyroid hormones also increase O_2 consumption in fishes and amphibians, but the increase in metabolic activity is easily obscured by other factors. In reptiles a calorigenic action of thyroid hormones has been documented under certain environmental conditions. Thyroid hormones in birds appear to assume roles similar to those in mammals. In amphibians, reptiles, and birds, thyroid hormones have prominent effects on the growth and differentiation of the integument and are required for moulting of feathers and shedding of skin. Thyroxine is involved in the normal moulting of the pelage in mammals; in addition it stimulates the rate of hair growth in rodents and increases the rate of wool growth in sheep.

It has been hypothesized that in the evolution of endothermy, thermoregulatory responses to cold, thyroxine, and the sodium pump are related functionally and phylogenetically. In this evolutionary scheme thyroxine was selected as the hormonal regulator because its major role in fishes is ion regulation. Thyroxine increases spontaneous motor activity in all classes of vertebrates; thus thyroxine enhances behavioral thermoregulation through heat generation from muscular activity. Any increase in oxygen demand results in a concomitant stimulation of the Na^+ pump, and it is speculated that the evolution of nonshivering (metabolic) thermogenesis involved a bypassing of behavioral thermogenesis to a direct stimulation of the Na^+ pump by thyroid hormones to produce heat.

Because of the diverse physiological roles of thyroid hormones in mammals, it can be confidently conjectured that the thyroid gland probably subserves many other functions in nonmammalian vertebrates that have not hitherto been documented.

REFERENCES

[1]   Allen, B. M. 1927. Influence of the hypophysis upon the thyroid gland in amphibian larvae. *Univ. Calif. Publ. Zool.* 31:53–78.

[2]   Beck-Peccoz, P., F. Forloni, D. Cortelazzi, L. Persani, M. J. Papandreou, C. Asteria, and G. Faglia. 1992. Pituitary resistance to thyroid hormones. *Horm. Res.* 38:66–72.

[3]   Boyages, S. C. 1993. Clinical review 49. Iodine deficiency disorders. *J. Clin. Endocrinol. Metab.* 77:587–91.

[4]   Boyages, S. C., and J.-P. Halpern. 1993. Endemic cretinism: toward a unifying hypothesis. *Thyroid* 3:59–69.

[5]   Brent, G. A. 1991. The molecular basis for thyroid hormone action. *New Engl. J. Med.* 331:847–53.

[6]   Bruhn, T. O., J. H. Taplin, and I. M. D. Jackson. 1991. Hypothyroidism reduces content and increases in vitro release of pro-thyrotropin-releasing hormone peptides from the median eminence. *Neuroendocrinology* 53:511–5.

[7]   Burman, K. D., and J. R. Baker, Jr. 1985. Immune mechanisms in Graves' disease. *Endocr. Rev.* 6:183–232.

[8]   Burrow, G. N. 1993. Thyroid function and hyperfunction during gestation. *Endocr. Rev.* 14:194–202.

[9]   Buse, J. B., and G. S. Eisenbarth. 1985. Autoimmune endocrine disease. *Vit. Horm.* 42:253–314.

[10] Christophe, D., and G. Vassart. 1990. The thyroglobulin gene. Evolutionary and regulatory issues. *TEM* 2:351–6.

[11] Cody, V. 1988. Thyroid hormone structure-activity relationships: molecular structure of 3,5,3′-triiodothyropropionic acid. *Endocr. Res.* 14:165–76.

[12] Danforth, E., and A. G. Burger. 1989. The impact of nutrition on thyroid hormone physiology and action. *Annu. Rev. Nutr.* 9:201–27.

[13] Degroot, L. J. 1989. Thyroid hormone nuclear receptors and their role in the metabolic action of the hormone. *Biochimie* 71:269–77.

[14] Ermans, A. M., F. Delenge, M. Van Der Velden, and J. Kinthaert. 1972. Possible role of cyanide and thiocyanate in the etiology of endemic cretinism. In *Human development and the thyroid gland*, eds. J. G. Stanbury and R. L. Kroc. New York: Plenum Publishing Corporation.

[15] Etkin, W. 1978. The thyroid: a gland in search of a function. *Perspectives Biol. Med.* 22:19–30.

[16] Fisher, D. A., and D. H. Polk. 1989. Development of the thyroid. *Bailliere's Clin. Endocrinol. Metab.* 3:627–57.

[17] Foley, T. P. Jr. 1993. Goiter in adolescents. *Endocrinol. Metab. Clin. N. Amer.* 22:593–606.

[18] Golstein, P., M. Abramow, J. E. Dumont, and R. Beauwens. 1992. The iodide channel of the thyroid: a plasma membrane vesicle study. *Amer. J. Physiol.* 263:C590–7.

[19] Green, W. L., ed. 1987. *The thyroid.* New York: Elsevier Science Inc.

[20] Hayashizaki, Y., Y. Hiraoka, K. Tatsumi, T. Hashimoto, J.-I. Furuyama, K. Miyai, K. Nishijo, M. Matsuura, H. Kohno, A. Labbe, and K. Matsubara. 1990. Deoxyribonucleic acid analyses of five families with familial inherited thyroid stimulating hormone deficiency. *J. Clin. Endocrinol. Metab.* 71:792–96.

[21] Hoskins, R. G. 1946. *The tides of life.* New York: W. W. Norton & Co., Inc.

[22] Ismail-Beigi, F. 1993. Thyroid hormone regulation of Na,K-ATPase expression. *TEM* 4:152–5.

[23] Kaye, T. B. 1993. Thyroid function tests. Application of newer methods. *Postgrad. Med.* 94:81–90.

[24] Lason, A. H. 1946. *The thyroid gland in medical history.* New York: Frogen Press.

[25] Lazar, M. A. 1993. Thyroid hormone receptors: multiple forms, multiple possibilities. *Endocr. Rev.* 14:184–93.

[26] Magner, J. A. 1990. Thyroid-stimulating hormone: biosynthesis, cell biology, and bioactivity. *Endocr. Rev.* 11:354–85.

[27] Mansberger, A. R., and J. P. Wei. 1993. Surgical embryology and anatomy of the thyroid and parathyroid glands. *Surg. Clin. N. Amer.* 73:727–46.

[28] McDermott, M. T. and E. C. Ridgway. 1993. Thyroid hormone resistance syndromes. *Amer. J. Med.* 94:424–32.

[29] Medeiros-Neto, G., H. M. Targovnik, and G. Vassart. 1993. Defective thyroglobulin synthesis and secretion causing goiter and hypothyroidism. *Endocr. Rev.* 14:165–81.

[30] Melander, A., L. E. Ericson, F. Súndler, and S. H. Ingbar. 1974. Sympathetic innervation of the mouse thyroid and its significance in thyroid hormone secretion. *Endocrinology* 94:959–66.

[31] Moreno-Reyes, R., M. Boelaert, S. El Badawi, M. Eltom, and J. B. Vanderpas. 1993. Endemic juvenile hypothyroidism in a severe endemic goiter area of Sudan. *Clin. Endocrinol.* 38:19–24.

[32] Nelkin, B. D., A. C. De Bustros, M. Mabry, and S. B. Baylin. 1989. The molecular biology of medullary thyroid carcinoma. A model for cancer development and progression. *JAMA* 261:3130–35.

[33] Norris, D. O., and W. A. Gern. 1976. Thyroxine-induced activation of hypothalamo-hypophysial axis in neotenic salamander larvae. *Science* 194:525–27.

[34] Oshima, K., and A. Gorbman. 1966. Olfactory responses in the forebrain of goldfish and their modification by thyroxine treatment. *Gen. Comp. Endocrinol.* 7:398–409.

[35] Pitt-Rivers, R. 1978. The thyroid hormones: historical aspects. In *Hormonal proteins and peptides*, vol. 6, ed. C.H. Li, pp. 391–422. New York: Academic Press, Inc.

[36] Rapaport, R., I. Sills, U. Patel, E. Oppenheimer, K. Skuza, M. Horlick, S. Goldstein, J. Dimartino, and P. Saenger. 1993. Thyrotropin-releasing hormone stimulation tests in infants. *J. Clin. Endocrinol. Metab.* 77:889–94.

[37] Refetoff, S. 1982. Syndromes of thyroid hormone resistance. *Amer. J. Physiol.* 243:E88–E98.

[38] Safran, M., and L. E. Braverman. 1985. Thyrotoxicosis and Graves' disease. *Hosp. Pract.* 20(3A):33–49.

[39] Schussler, G. C., and J. Orlando. 1978. Fasting decreases triiodothyronine receptor capacity. *Science* 199:686–87.

[40] Sessions, R. B. and B. J. Davidson. 1993. Thyroid cancer. *Med. Clin. N. Amer.* 77:517–38.

[41] Shi, Y.-B. 1994. Molecular biology of amphibian metamorphosis. A new approach to an old problem. *TEM* 5:14–20.

[42] Silva, J. E. 1988. Pituitary-thyroid relationships in hypothyroidism. *Baillière's Clin. Endocrinol. Metab.* 2:541–65.

[43] ———. 1993. Hormonal control of thermogenesis and energy dissipation. *TEM* 4:25–32.

[44] Spaulding, S. W. 1987. Age and the thyroid. *Endocrinol. Metab. Clinics* 16:1013–25.

[45] Studer, H., H. J. Peter, and H. Gerber. 1989. Natural heterogeneity of thyroid cells: the basis for understanding thyroid function and nodular goiter growth. *Endocr. Rev.* 10:125–35.

[46] Sypniewski, E. 1993. Comparative pharmacology of the thyroid hormones. *Ann. Thorac. Surg.* 56:S2–8.

[47] Takeda, K., R. E. Weiss, and S. Refetoff. 1992. Rapid localization of mutations in the thyroid hormone receptor-β gene by denaturing gradient gel electrophoresis in 18 families with thyroid hormone resistance. *J. Clin. Endocrinol. Metab.* 74:712–19.

[48] Van Herle, A. J., G. Vassart, and J. E. Dumont. 1979. Control of thyroglobulin synthesis and secretion. *New Engl. J. Med.* 301:239–49, 307–14.

[49] Vassart, G. and J. E. Dumont. 1992. The thyrotropin receptor and the regulation of thyrocyte function and growth. *Endocr. Rev.* 13:596–611.

[50] Yen, P. M., and W. W. Chin. 1994. New advances in understanding the molecular mechanisms of thyroid hormone action. *TEM* 5:65–72.

14

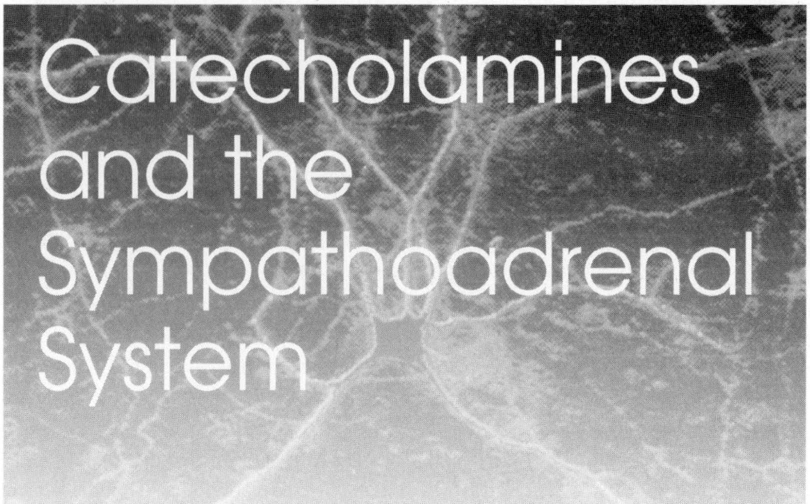

Catecholamines and the Sympathoadrenal System

The physiologically relevant catecholamines are **epinephrine** *(E),* **norepinephrine** *(NE), and* **dopamine** *(DA). The chemical structure of E was the first determined; the structure of NE (also referred to as noradrenaline) was elucidated much later. Although E (also referred to as adrenaline) has generally been considered a classic example of a hormone (a humoral messenger) and NE a truly representative neurotransmitter, it is now realized that both catecholamines function reciprocally as humoral effectors or as neurotransmitters. Dopamine's major physiological roles are relegated to the CNS and certain autonomic nervous system ganglia. A chronological history of research related to the catecholamines provides a fascinating example of the growth and development of endocrine physiology [20].*

HISTORICAL PERSPECTIVE

1895   Oliver and Schafer discovered that extracts of the suprarenal (adrenal) glands (specifically the chromaffin component) of a number of mammalian species produced a pressor response when injected into animals [40].

1899   The pressor principle of the adrenal gland was isolated and named epinephrine by Abel.

1901   The true structural identity of epinephrine was determined by Aldrich (Fig. 14.1).

1898–1901   Lewandowsky and Langley noted that injections of adrenal extracts produced effects similar to stimulation of sympathetic neurons.

1904   Elliot postulated that sympathetic nerve impulses release an epinephrinelike substance onto adjacent effector cells. This was the first suggestion of a neurohumor and the concept of neurotransmission.

1904–1905   Stolz (1904) and subsequently Dakin (1905) synthesized epinephrine.

1905   Administration of epinephrine was found to exhibit both excitatory (vasopressor) and inhibitory (vasodepressor) effects on the cardiovas-

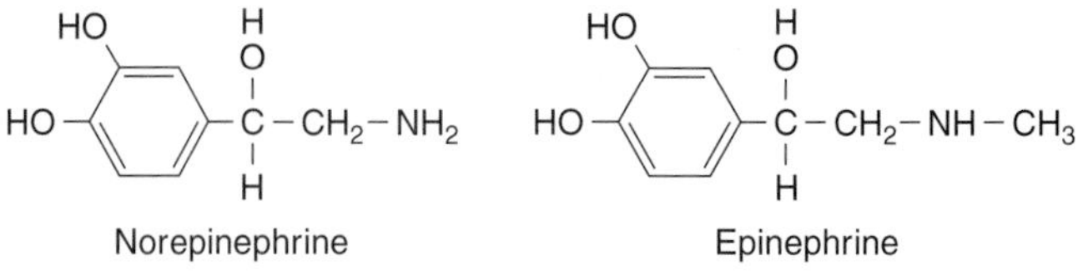

Figure 14.1 Structures of norepinephrine and epinephrine.

cular system. Langley therefore proposed that autonomic effector cells may possess excitatory and inhibitory receptive substances and that the particular response elicited depended on which substance was present.

1906   Dale discovered that a drug, an ergot alkaloid, specifically antagonized the pressor activities of sympathetic nervous stimulation or epinephrine administration [10, 15, 16]. Indeed, the drug actually reversed the actions of such stimuli, producing instead a vasodepressor response. These observations again revealed that epinephrine could elicit two opposing actions, even in the same tissue.

1910   Barger and Dale studied the action of a large number of synthetic amines related to epinephrine in structure and termed the actions of these drugs as sympathomimetic.

1921   Loewi provided evidence that, indeed, an excitatory substance similar to epinephrine is released from the vagus nerve upon electrical stimulation. In this same year Cannon and Uradil noted that although stimulation of certain sympathetic neurons released an epinephrinelike substance that increased blood pressure and heart rate, other smooth-muscle responses differed qualitatively from the effects produced by epinephrine. Cannon and Bacq referred to the substance released as sympathin. Barger and Dale had noted earlier (1910) that the effects of sympathetic nerve stimulation were more similar to those of a primary amine than epinephrine or other secondary amines.

1931   Bacq advanced the thesis that sympathin might be norepinephrine (noradrenaline).

1933   Cannon and Rosenblueth formulated the concept that two sympathins might exist, a sympathin E (excitatory) and a sympathin I (inhibitory) [11].

1935   Although Bacq realized that sympathin was not identical to epinephrine, he objected to the view that both a sympathin E and I existed. Rather, a catecholamine could have opposite effects on the same cell.

1946   Von Euler established that the neurotransmitter released from the postganglionic neurons of the sympathetic system was norepinephrine (Fig. 14.1). Although the chemical nature of sympathin was elucidated, this putative neurotransmitter, norepinephrine, could elicit either smooth muscle contraction or relaxation depending on the particular muscle preparation studied. The hypothesis of two sympathins was still in vogue.

1948   Ahlquist studied a large number of sympathomimetic amines and determined that for each tissue a certain potency ranking could be established for the biological actions of these agents. He formulated the concept of dual adrenoceptors where different receptors controlled smooth muscle contraction and relaxation. These receptive substances were referred to as α- and β-adrenoceptors, respectively. Although the *adrenoceptor hypothesis* was not accepted immediately, the discovery of drugs that specifically inhibit either α- or β-adrenoceptors firmly established the validity of the concept.

1962   Sutherland and his colleagues discovered cAMP and proposed that this cyclic nucleotide be considered an intracellular second messenger of hormone action. It was subsequently revealed that β-adrenoceptor stimulation always leads to cAMP production, whereas in some tissues α-adrenoceptor stimulation lowers cellular cAMP levels.

In retrospect the confusion relating to the roles and actions of the catecholamines is understandable. Both E and NE are similar in structure and are released from the adrenal or from neurons in response to a variety of stimuli. Also, both catecholamines can produce similar or opposing physiological responses within the same tissue; their actions at a particular concentration may even be different. The formulation of the adrenoceptor hypothesis by Ahlquist [1] substantiated the early suggestion of Langley that cells might possess different "receptive substances" (in this context, adrenoceptors) and that the particular response of a cell depended on which substance (receptor) was activated. A more thorough historical discussion of catecholamines and adrenoceptors is available [20].

THE SYMPATHOADRENAL SYSTEM

Epinephrine and norepinephrine are hormones of the adrenal chromaffin tissue and sympathetic neurons, respectively. Because these two catecholamines have similar structures and biological actions, it is customary to discuss their endocrine roles together, as components of the *sympathoadrenal system*. It is first necessary to review the general anatomical components of the autonomic nervous system (ANS), because both sympathetic neurons and chromaffin tissue are integral structural and functional components of the ANS.

The Autonomic Nervous System

The *peripheral nervous system* consists of those nerves that arise from the brainstem and spinal cord—the cranial and spinal nerves, respectively. Cranial and spinal nerves that innervate skeletal (voluntary) muscle make up the somatic component (*somatic nervous system*) of the peripheral nervous system. The cell bodies of the somatic neurons lie within the spinal column, and the long axons of these nerves directly innervate skeletal muscle. The other nerves of the peripheral nervous system make up the ANS. These nerves supply the skin and all visceral organs (heart, blood vessels, GI tract, pancreas, adrenals, kidneys, etc.). These nerves are mainly *vasomotor* and *secretomotor* in function; that is, the neurons innervate smooth muscles of blood vessels, and they innervate exocrine (salivary, pancreas) and endocrine (adrenals, pancreas) glands. Other smooth muscles of the GI tract, gallbladder, urinary bladder, spleen capsule, hair follicles, as well as the cardiac muscle of the heart, are also innervated by neurons of the ANS.

The ANS can be subdivided into nerves that comprise the *parasympathetic nervous system* and the *sympathetic nervous system*. The nerves of both systems are composed of *preganglionic* and *postganglionic* neurons. The cell bodies of the preganglionic fibers of both divisions, which reside within the spinal cord, synapse with a second neuron within various ganglia. The postganglionic neurons then directly innervate the various *autonomic effector organs*. Neurotransmission between preganglionic and postganglionic neurons is effected by *acetylcholine* release from the presynaptic neurons. The neurotransmitter of the postganglionic neurons of the parasympathetic system is also acetylcholine, but the neurotransmitter released by the postganglionic neuron of the sympathetic system is norepinephrine.

Parasympathetic nerves arise in the cranial-sacral segments of the spinal column, whereas sympathetic neurons arise in the thoraco-lumbar region of the spinal cord. The very long parasympathetic preganglionic fibers usually synapse with postganglionic neurons within ganglia located in the autonomic effector organs that they regulate. The sympathetic preganglionic fibers, on the other hand, usually synapse with postganglionic neurons within ganglia located some distance from the target tissues they innervate. The general anatomy of the autonomic system and its effector organs is shown (Fig. 14.2).

The parasympathetic system is concerned mainly with the so-called vegetative (resting) states of the body. Most of its actions are related to those processes concerned with

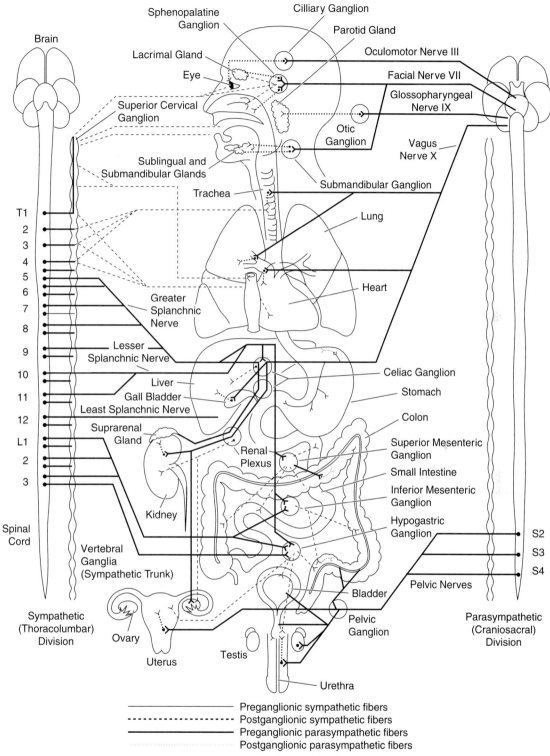

Figure 14.2 The autonomic nervous system. (From William F. Evans, *Anatomy and Physiology* 2nd ed., p. 187. © 1976. Reproduced by permission of Prentice Hall, Inc., Englewood Cliffs, N.J.)

the movement and digestion of food within the GI tract, the transit of metabolic substrates into the body proper, and the conservation (storage) of these substrates within organs such as the liver, adipose tissue, and muscle. The sympathetic nervous system, in contrast, is concerned with those processes related to the more active states of the body and plays a particularly important role under conditions of stress. The sympathetic system generally prepares the body for "fight or flight" [10]. Here for example, the muscular and secretory activities of the GI tract are depressed, whereas the force and rate of the heartbeat are increased, and consequently blood flow is increased, particularly to those areas, such as muscle, that are most active. Blood flow to the brain and coronary arteries is enhanced, whereas circulation to the skin, digestive tract, and kidneys is diminished.

Although the individual actions of acetylcholine and NE are often viewed as opposite, they are actually complementary to each other. For example, NE contracts the heart and forces blood out into the circulatory system. Acetylcholine, on the other hand, relaxes the heart so that it can again fill up with blood. The movement of food through the GI tract results from peristalsis, a process that involves the alternate contraction and relaxation of individual segments of the gut in temporal unison. Contractions of the gut are regulated by acetylcholine, whereas NE relaxes smooth muscles of the gut. Although their actions are opposite in direction, both neurotransmitters participate in the rhythmic (peristaltic) movement of food through the gut.

Adrenal Chromaffin Tissue

The adrenal gland of many vertebrates is composed of two distinct cellular types of different embryological origin that secrete structurally very different hormones [12, 46]. Chromaffin cells (pheochromoblasts) are derived from the neural crest, whereas the steroidogenic component of the adrenal is of mesodermal origin (see Chap. 15). In most mammals the chromaffin tissue is surrounded by an outer adrenal cortex composed of steroid-producing cells. Therefore, the chromaffin tissue is often referred to as the *adrenal medulla*. In most nonmammalian species, however, the chromaffin tissue is not associated with any surrounding mass of cortical tissue; hence the term adrenal medulla is without anatomical justification unless used in reference to a restricted number of mammalian species. The term chromaffin (from the Greek, *chroma* or color, and the Latin, *affinis* or affinity) tissue derives from the observation that the pheochromocytes become brown when placed in contact with oxidizing agents such as chromate.

The human adrenal medulla consists of two cell types: adrenaline (A)-storing cells and noradrenaline (N)-storing cells. Chromaffin cells contain granules composed of catecholamines, adenine nucleotides (mainly ATP), proteins, and lipids. The protein of these granules is referred to as *chromogranin*. Histochemical studies demonstrate that the cells are not biochemically identical: the A cells apparently contain more glycoproteins. The ratio of these two cell types differs between species; the chromaffin tissue of the human and the guinea pig, for example, consists mainly of A cells. Less information is available relative to nonmammalian species, but the same two cell types have been recognized in species of elasmobranchs, amphibians, birds, and reptiles.

Extra-adrenal chromaffin tissue occurs as encapsulated and nonencapsulated masses scattered throughout the abdominal prevertebral sympathetic plexuses of the human fetus. The encapsulated masses predominate and are richly vascularized from adjacent blood vessels. These numerous chromaffin masses are of varying size and are referred to as para-aortic bodies or *paraganglia*. The larger para-aortic bodies lie on the aorta near the origin of the inferior mesenteric artery and are known as the *organs of Zuckerkandl*. These groups of isolated chromaffin cells probably represent neural crest cells that "fail" to migrate into the adrenal during embryonic development. The extra-adrenal chromaffin tissue involutes after birth, but tumors may appear later from this tissue. The para-aortic chromaffin tissue may also proliferate and achieve a functional role if the adrenals are surgically removed or destroyed by disease.

Large amounts of extra-adrenal chromaffin tissue are present in the fetus. Although this tissue only contains NE, it is not known if it is secreted into the fetal circulation. The tissue, however, does have an endocrine appearance. Because the sympathetic nervous system is still incompletely developed at the time of birth, the vascular tone of the fetus may be under humoral control by NE produced by the para-aortic bodies; during postnatal life this function may be replaced by NE of sympathetic origin [13].

Comparative anatomical studies reveal that the distribution of chromaffin tissue and adrenal steroidogenic tissue differs considerably among the vertebrates. In elasmobranchs and teleost fishes the two tissues are well separated, whereas in mammals and birds they are always intermingled. The association of the two tissues in amphibians and reptiles is variable. The functional significance of what appears to have been an evolution of the two tissues to come together as a single anatomical entity—the adrenal gland—is nebulous. There is clearly a biochemical correlation between the degree of anatomical association of the two tissues and the relative amounts of NE and E produced by the chromaffin tissue.

In the dogfish shark, where the chromaffin tissue is entirely separated from steroidogenic tissue, NE is the only catecholamine produced. In the frog, where chromaffin tissue is intermingled with steroidogenic tissue, NE accounts for about 55% to 70% of the catecholamines. In primates and other mammals, where the two tissues are closely intermingled, very little NE is produced and E may be the exclusive product of the chromaffin tissue. From these observations it has been concluded that the proximity of the adrenal steroidogenic tissue determines the degree to which NE is methylated to E in the chromaffin tissue.

Nature and Nurture in ANS Development

Elegant experimental techniques have provided fascinating observations related to the embryology of the ANS and continue to provide new insights into factors that may influence the autonomic neurons and chromaffin cells during development [2, 4, 6, 29]. There are preferential pathways located at precise levels of the embryo that direct neural crest cells to their definitive anatomical destinations. Nevertheless, differentiation of the autonomic neuroblasts is controlled by the environment in which the crest cells become localized at the end of their migration. Neural crest cells destined to populate the ANS express an overt noradrenergic phenotype only upon reaching the primordium of the sympathetic chain. The initial metabolic commitment, however, appears to be mutable (plastic), and further differentiation may be influenced by the environment within which the cells reside. For example, those cells that populate sympathetic ganglia remain noradrenergic, whereas those that invade the adrenal gland begin to synthesize E [4].

The expression of the adrenergic phenotype of chromaffin tissue precursor cells in the embryonic adrenal gland has been studied in some detail. In the 13.5-day-old mouse the medullary precursors lying in the sympathetic ganglia primordia—those migrating toward the adrenal as well as those within the adrenal—express noradrenergic characteristics (tyrosine hydroxylase and dopamine-β-hydroxylase activities). Phenylethanolamine-N-methyltransferase (PNMT), the enzyme required for conversion of NE to E, is not present but is detectable 3.5 days later at 17 days gestation. This initial expression of PNMT is not dependent on normal glucocorticoid levels and cannot be induced prematurely by glucocorticoids; it is also independent of the pituitary adrenal axis [6]. The normal ontogenetic increase in the activity of this enzyme after the initial expression has occurred does require the presence of an intact pituitary-adrenal axis [20]. The synthesis of PNMT within the CNS indicates that development within the adrenal environment is not an absolute requirement for PNMT biosynthesis. Extra-adrenal chromaffin tissue is also capable of expressing PNMT activity in response to glucocorticoid stimulation.

Sympathetic neurons and adrenal chromaffin tissue derive from a common neuroectodermal origin; the morphology and enzymatic profiles of the two cell types, however, differ considerably. Neural crest cell differentiation into sympathetic neurons is controlled by nerve growth factor (NGF). Prenatal and postnatal injections of NGF into rats can divert partially differentiated chromaffin cells into nerve cells that are morphologically and ultrastructurally indistinguishable from sympathetic neurons. NGF can channel chromaffin cell precursors toward nerve cell differentiation, an action that apparently must override the effects of glucocorticoids that normally induce enzymes required for E synthesis. Sympathetic neurons disconnected from their autonomic effector organs die unless supplied with exogenous NGF. Apparently the effector organs normally provide a continuous supply of NGF to the sympathetic neurons, which is a requirement for their structural and functional integrity. In the absence of NGF administration the transformed sympathetic cells undergo destruction (apoptosis); injections of antisera to NGF into the rat fetus produce massive destruction of chromaffin cell precursors. Isolated adrenal medullary cells treated with NGF occasionally develop neurites, sometimes even in the absence of exogenous NGF. Addition of a glucocorticoid to the incubation can inhibit neurite development. These results imply that normal growth and development of adrenal chromaffin tissue may depend on the temporal interactions of NGF and glucocorticoids (see Chap. 12).

SYNTHESIS, CHEMISTRY, AND METABOLISM OF CATECHOLAMINES

The pathways of catecholamine biosynthesis within the CNS, sympathetic postganglionic neurons, and adrenal chromaffin tissue appear to be identical. The number of steps in each pathway, however, depends on the definitive product—DA, NE, or E—to be secreted [20] (Fig. 14.3).

Synthesis.   The conversion of tyrosine to E involves four steps: (1) hydroxylation at the three position of the phenolic ring; (2) side-chain decarboxylation; (3) side-chain hydroxylation; and (4) N-methylation. Hydroxylation of phenylalanine, although essential for tyrosine production, may not make an important contribution to tyrosine availability within sympathetic neurons and chromaffin cells. Tyrosine is transported into the cell where it is converted to dihydroxyphenylalanine (DOPA) by the enzyme *tyrosine hydrox-*

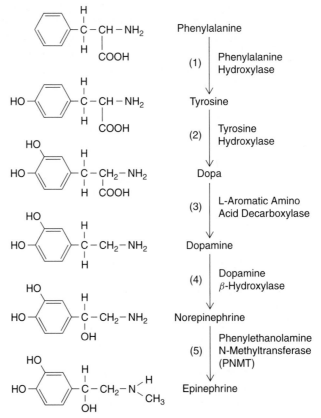

Figure 14.3   Pathway of catecholamine biosynthesis.

ylase. This is the rate-limiting enzyme in catecholamine biosynthesis. The activity of this enzyme is regulated by feedback (end-product) inhibition by cytoplasmic catecholamines. Chronic stimulation of catecholamine synthesis and secretion leads to elevation of cellular tyrosine hydroxylase levels. In the subsequent step DOPA is decarboxylated to DA by DOPA *decarboxylase*, a nonspecific decarboxylase (L-aromatic amino acid decarboxylase) found in many tissues. Dopamine is then hydroxylated by *dopamine β-hydroxylase* (DBH) by addition of an —OH group to the side-chain carbon (β-carbon adjacent to the phenolic ring). Dopamine is an important neurotransmitter within the CNS [3]. In dopaminergic neurons, DA is the final step in catecholamine biosynthesis. In noradrenergic cells or neurons DA is then converted to NE within the chromaffin granule. The NE produced is converted to E by PNMT outside the granule; this enzyme is found only in cells that synthesize E (adrenal chromaffin tissue of many vertebrates, and within specific neuronal tracts in the brain). It should be noted that NE is a primary amine, whereas E is a N-methylated secondary amine; these differences provide an important structural basis for the differing potency of these two catecholamines on adrenoceptors.

In species where the chromaffin tissue is separated from the adrenal steroidogenic tissue, NE is usually the main synthetic product. In those species (e.g., human, rat) where the chromaffin cells are contiguous with steroidogenic tissue, however, E is the predominant catecholamine synthesized. Levels of PNMT decline in hypophysectomized rats, and normal levels are restored by administration of ACTH or glucocorticoids. These results suggest a role for pituitary corticotropin in adrenal medullary catecholamine biosynthesis.

Storage and Release. Catecholamines are stored within granules wherein they are complexed with ATP and a specific protein, *chromogranin*, and DBH [48]. The secretory vesicles are released through a stimulus-secretion coupling requiring calcium (Ca^{2+}). All the contents of the storage granules are released during vesicular exocytosis [37].

Metabolism. Catecholamines are catabolized by two enzymes, catecholamine-O-methyltransferase (COMT) and monoamine oxidase (MAO). Norepinephrine and E are metabolized extracellularly by COMT to normetanephrine and metanephrine, respectively (Fig. 14.4). COMT is localized within the cytosol of sympathetic effector cells and is also found in close proximity to adrenoceptors of autonomic effectors. Increased activity of COMT in response to catecholamines provides a homeostatic mechanism for the rapid

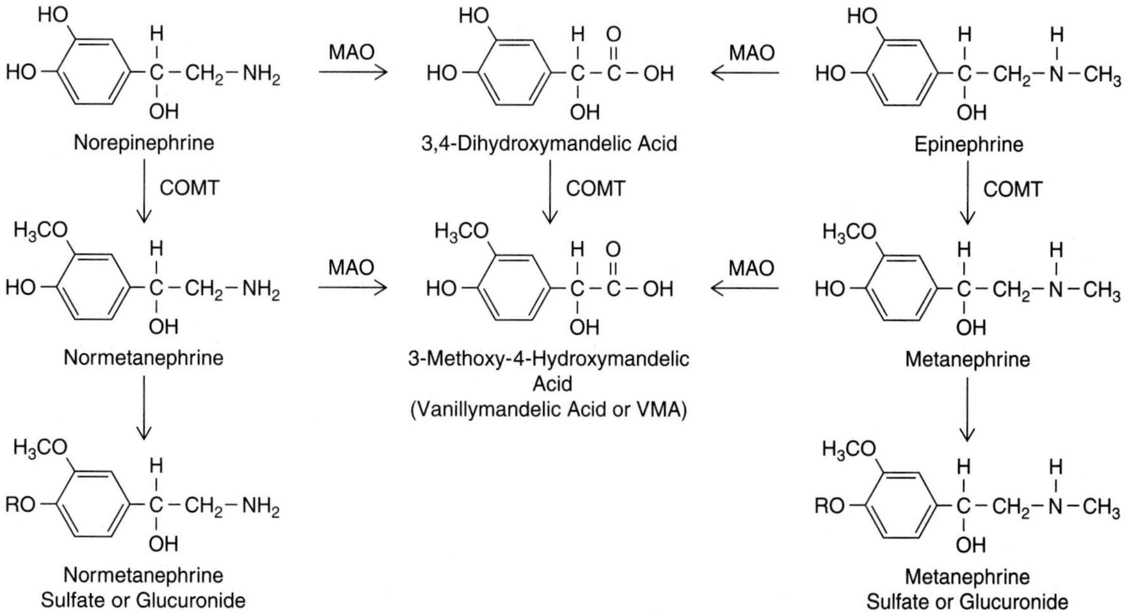

Figure 14.4 Pathways of catecholamine metabolism.

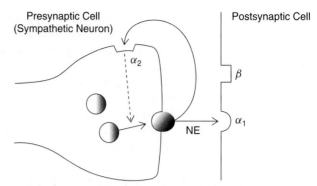

Figure 14.5 Sympathetic negative feedback mechanisms for inhibition of sympathetic neuron secretion.

removal of catecholamines from the circulation and the synaptic cleft. MAO is found in the surface of the outer membrane of mitochondria where it limits the accumulation of catecholamines within the cytoplasm. Because of the sequential action of these two enzymes, the main metabolite of catecholamines excreted in the urine is 3-methoxy-4-hydroxy-mandelic acid (also known as vanillylmandelic acid, VMA) (Fig. 14.4). Most NE released from sympathetic neurons is taken back up into the neuron where it is either transported into the secretory vesicles or destroyed by MAO. The NE accumulated within the synaptic cleft feeds back to α-adrenergic receptors within the presynaptic membrane, and this stimulates uptake and inhibits further synthesis of NE (Fig. 14.5).

SYMPATHOADRENAL SYSTEM RECEPTORS

The terms *adrenergic* and *cholinergic* were introduced by Dale to designate those nerves that release the sympathetic transmitter (unknown at that time) and acetylcholine, respectively. These terms are now used to designate the receptors through which these neurotransmitters of the postganglionic neurons of the sympathetic (norepinephrine) and parasympathetic (acetylcholine) nervous system mediate their effects. These receptors are localized to the postsynaptic membranes of the innervated effector cells (e.g., smooth muscle, salivary gland cells).

Cholinergic Receptors

Cholinergic receptors respond to acetylcholine and several related analogs of acetylcholine [7, 21]. Two plant substances, *nicotine* and *muscarine*, also stimulate cholinergic receptors and are appropriately referred to as *cholinomimetic* agents. The effects of these two cholinergic agonists are tissue specific. Nicotine, for example, stimulates skeletal muscle and autonomic postganglionic neurons. Muscarine, on the other hand, stimulates autonomic effector cells such as smooth muscle. These observations suggest that these nicotinic and muscarinic cholinoceptive receptor sites are not identical. This is further substantiated by the observation that the drug curare (and also tubocurare) specifically blocks *nicotinic* receptors, whereas the drug atropine is inhibitory to acetylcholine stimulation of *muscarinic* cholinergic receptors. For example, the muscles lining the gut of a teleost fish, the tench, are composed of both striated and smooth muscle. Electrical stimulation of the vagus nerve innervating these muscles results in contraction of both types of muscle, producing a recorded response that contains both a quick and a slow component of contraction. After curarization, however, only the slow component can be elicited. After blockade by atropine, on the other hand, only the fast component of contraction is evident. The slow and fast components of muscle contraction are both abolished, however, after administration of both curare and atropine [20]. Autoantibodies against skeletal cholinergic receptors block their normal response to acetylcholine, resulting in a pathological condition known as myasthenia gravis.

Until recently, all muscarinic receptors were thought to be alike. However, at least three different pharmacologically identifiable types and at least five different molecular forms have now been delineated. These glycosylated proteins have single chains of 460 to 590 amino acids and span the plasma membrane seven times, creating four extracellular domains, seven helical hydrophobic transmembrane domains, and four intracellular domains. In structure and evolution, muscarinic receptors are quite distinct from nicotinic receptors and belong to the growing family of seven-helix receptors (see Fig. 4.2). This family includes the adrenoceptors, at least three subtypes of serotonin receptors, substance K receptors, rhodopsin, and opsin. The seven-helix receptors bind the ligand and transduce their intracellular signals through one or more species of guanosine triphosphate-binding proteins (G proteins) [44, 45].

Adrenergic Receptors (Adrenoceptors)

After studying the actions of a number of sympathetic amines on smooth muscle contraction and relaxation, Ahlquist concluded that two types of adrenergic receptors (ARs) might exist: α- and β-ARs or, as they are also designated, α- and β-adrenoceptors [1]. These putative receptors differed in their relative responsiveness (sensitivity) to certain sympathetic amines. The response of α-ARs provided the following potency ranking: epinephrine (E) > norepinephrine (NE) > isoproterenol (ISO). The potency ranking for β-ARs was (ISO) > (E) > (NE). The α-ARs subserve smooth muscle contraction, the β-ARs relaxation. A number of drugs were then discovered that could stimulate specifically the putative ARs or antagonize the response of these receptors to catecholamines. It was noted, for example, that phenylephrine was a very specific agonist of α-ARs, whereas isoproterenol was a very specific β-AR agonist. Used at high (unphysiological) concentrations sympathoamines can usually stimulate either AR, as these agents are structurally related.

After α-AR blockade certain smooth muscle preparations relaxed rather than contracted as they normally did in response to E [38]. This "epinephrine reversal" was reminiscent of that noted by Dale [15] using an ergot alkaloid preparation. The subsequent discovery of a compound that specifically blocked β-AR-stimulated smooth muscle relaxation provided an explanation for the phenomenon of E reversal [5]. E stimulates both α- and β-ARs simultaneously, but the actions of the hormone on α-ARs dominate (Fig. 14.6). However, in the presence of α-AR blockage the response of the "silent" β-AR is revealed. Simultaneous incubation of smooth muscle in the presence of both α- and β-AR antagonists (blocking agents) totally inhibits smooth muscle responses to the agonists. The *dual receptor hypothesis* provided a rational explanation for the contrasting effects of catecholamines on autonomic effectors. It was no longer necessary to think of a sympathin E and a sympathin I to account for the excitatory and inhibitory activities of a

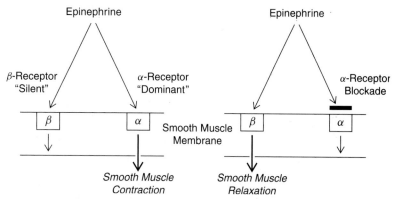

Figure 14.6 Experimental demonstration of epinephrine (catecholamine) reversal.

catecholamine; rather, a single sympathetic neurotransmitter exists whose actions are determined by the nature of the particular ARs stimulated.

The adrenoceptor family consists of nine distinct receptors that mediate the varied effects of only two physiological agonists, E and NE. At least four subtypes of these catecholamine receptors, the α_1-, α_2-, β_1-, and β_2-adrenoceptors (α_1-, α_2, β_1-, and β_2-ARs), have been identified on the basis of their pharmacological properties and physiological effects. Chemical agents that selectively block or stimulate these receptors are used extensively in clinical medicine. The genes encoding the α_1-, α_2-, β_1-, and β_2-AR have been isolated. They belong to a family of homologous genes that encode integral membrane receptors that have seven membrane-spanning domains (see Figs. 4.2 and 14.9) and that are coupled to regulatory G proteins.

Dopamine (Dopaminergic) Receptors.   Dopaminergic receptors are mainly restricted to the brain wherein they subserve a multitude of functions (see Chap. 21). As for other adrenoceptors, DA receptors can be further subdivided into two or more subclasses based on their relative affinities for DA and their relative antagonism by pharmaceutical agents (e.g., DA_1 and DA_2 receptors) [3, 9, 39]. It is now well accepted that in the periphery, specific DA receptors are present in many tissues, including those of the cardiovascular and autonomic nervous system. They seem to be involved in vasodilation of certain vascular beds' inhibition of neurotransmitter release during electrical nerve stimulation, diuresis and natriuresis, renin release and aldosterone release. Peripheral DA receptors have been subdivided into the subtypes DA_1 receptors and DA_2 receptors [9]. Dopaminergic receptors regulate pituitary PRL (see Chap. 19) and α-melanotropin (see Chap. 8) secretion, whereby DA of hypothalamic origin is inhibitory to the secretion of these two hormones.

α-Adrenoceptors.   Arterial vasoconstriction in a wide array of vascular beds is mediated by a mixed population of postjunctional vascular α_1- and α_2-adrenoceptors [43]. The physiologic function and/or distribution of these receptors is beginning o be understood. Using a variety of α_1-selective, α_2-selective, and nonselective α-adrenoceptor antagonists, it was observed that pressor responses to exogenously administered catecholamines were selectively antagonized by α_2-adrenoceptor blockers. Conversely, the pressor response evoked by sympathetic nerve stimulation was selectively antagonized by α_1-adrenoceptor blockers. It was postulated that postsynaptic vascular α-adrenoceptors located at the neuroeffector junction (i.e., junctional receptors) were of the α_1-subtype, while those located away from the neuroeffector junction (i.e., extrajunctional receptors) were of the α_2-subtype. Presynaptic α_2-ARs occur at all noradregeneric synapses where they subserve an autoinhibition (negative feedback) in which released NE inhibits its own further release (Fig. 14.6). The structures of phenylephrine and clonidine, α_1- and α_2-AR agonists, respectively, are shown, as is the structure of a mixed α-AR antagonist, phentolamine (Fig. 14.7).

It is increasingly clear that α-adrenoceptors are not pharmacologically homogeneous. Evidence from radioligand binding studies, functional studies of smooth muscle contractile responses, and studies of receptor-mediated second-messenger accumulation

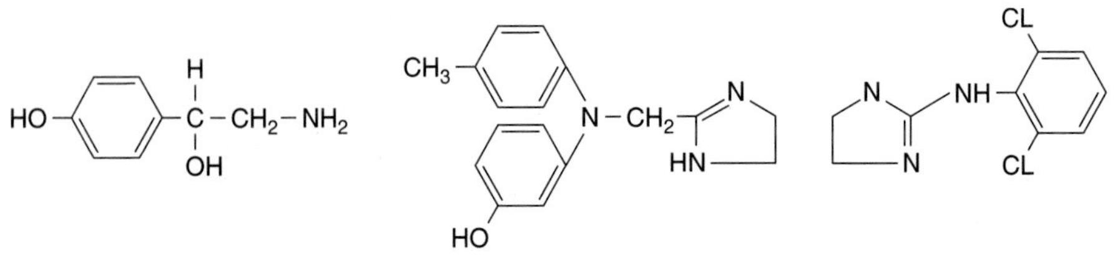

Phenylephrine
(α_1-Agonist)

Phentolamine
(Mixed α-Adrenoceptor Antagonist)

Clonidine
(α_2-Agonist)

Figure 14.7   Examples of α-AR agonist and antagonist structures.

shows substantial differences in the affinities and efficacies of agonists, and the affinities of antagonists for α_1-ARs in different tissues. Based on these differences, the existence of at least two discrete subtypes of α_1-ARs (α_{1A}, α_{1B}) and two subtypes of α_2-ARs (α_{2A}, α_{2B}) seems clear. [33, 43, 44, 45]

   β-Adrenoceptors. There is evidence that β-ARs represent at least two pharmacologically different subgroups. The lipolytic response of adipose tissue and the contraction of cardiac muscle typify β_1-ARs, where the potency ranking for certain agonists is ISO » E ≅ NE. Bronchodilation and vasodepression, on the other hand, are regulated by β_2-ARs, where the agonist potency profile is ISO > E » NE. The major difference between β_1- and β_2-ARs is their sensitivity to norepinephrine. The β_1-receptors respond readily to circulating E or to neurally released NE. On the other hand, the natural agonist of the β_2-ARs is probably E. From these observations it has been suggested that the β_2-receptor is a hormonal AR, whereas the β_1-AR is a neuronal AR.

   β-AR blocking agents do not block responses associated with α-ARs, and they do not inhibit the actions of other hormones or drugs. For example, E and glucagon both stimulate hepatic glycogenolysis, but only the actions of E are antagonized by the blocker (see Fig. 11.11). On the adipocyte, β-AR antagonists block the lipolytic action of E but not ACTH. The structures of β-AR agonists and antagonists bear resemblance to isoproterenol (Fig. 14.8).

   Since the classification of β-adrenergic receptors into β_1 and β_2 subtypes, additional β-ARs have been implicated in the control of various metabolic processes by catecholamines. A human gene has been isolated that encodes a third β-AR, the "β_3-AR." Exposure of eukaryotic cells transfected with this gene to E or NE promotes the accumulation of cAMP; only two of eleven classical β-AR blockers efficiently inhibited this effect, whereas two others behaved as β_3-AR agonists. The potency order of β-AR agonists for the β_3-AR correlates with their rank order for stimulating various metabolic processes in tissues where atypical adrenergic sites are thought to exist.

   The Silent β-AR.   The adrenoceptor hypothesis of Ahlquist adequately explains the vasopressor and vasodepressor responses of smooth muscle to catecholamines. The presence of dominant α-ARs also explains the vasodepressor response to E or NE after α-AR blockade. Nevertheless, catecholamine reversal is a pharmacological phenomenon. The physiological significance of the β-AR in the presence of the dominant α-AR is

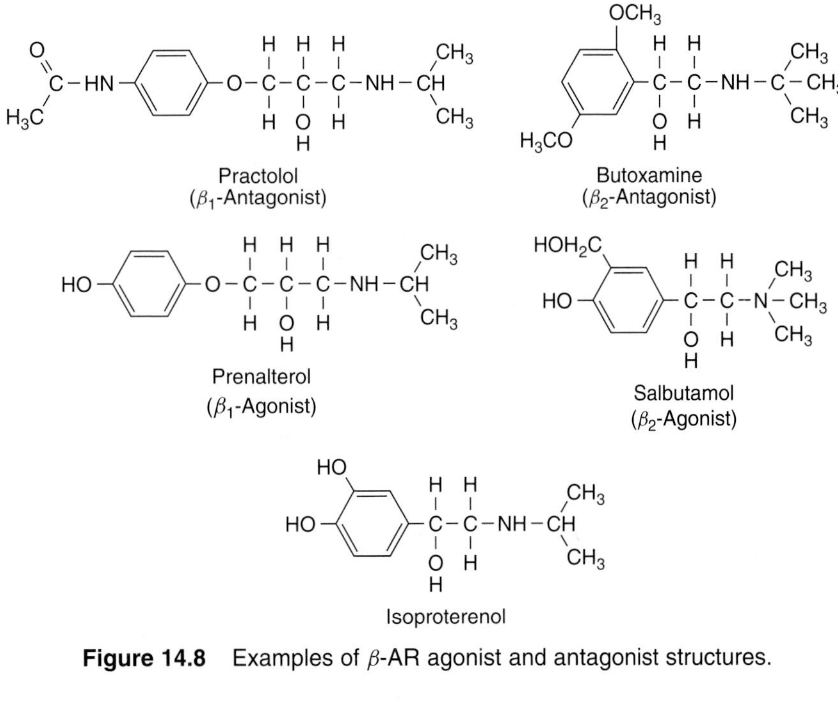

Figure 14.8   Examples of β-AR agonist and antagonist structures.

unclear. Although there are examples of smooth muscles that lack α-ARs and only possess β-ARs, there apparently are no examples of smooth muscles that possess α-ARs in the absence of β-ARs. It is reasonable to hypothesize, therefore, that the β-AR provides a mechanism for *autoinhibition*. For example, although there is an initial smooth muscle contraction in response to dominant α-ARs, there follows a reversal of the vasopressor response due to a slowly developing β-AR response. Autoinhibition can be prevented by β-AR blockade. The silent β-AR may provide a mechanism for protection against continuous vascular vasoconstriction that would lead to oxygen deprivation and gangrene in the peripheral extremities. Indeed, certain drugs, ergot alkaloids, which establish an irreversible vasoconstriction, have been known to cause gangrene of the legs.

ADRENOCEPTOR STRUCTURE

Understanding ligand binding and the coupling of ARs to specific biochemical pathways depends on determining the structures of the family members of these related receptors. Recently the molecular cloning of the gene and complementary DNA (cDNA) for the hamster and human β_2-AR and the cDNA for the human β_1-AR, all of which stimulate adenylate cyclase, was reported [25]. An avian β-AR, which also stimulates adenylate cyclase, and two subtypes of muscarinic cholinergic receptors, which are coupled to stimulation of polyphosphoinositide turnover and the inhibition of adenylate cyclase, have also been cloned. The deduced structures of these receptors reveal that they are homologous to each other and to the visual light pigment, rhodopsin [30, 31].

Analysis of the amino acid sequence of the β-AR has revealed that the protein contains seven regions of hydrophobic amino acids (20–30 residues in length) that may form

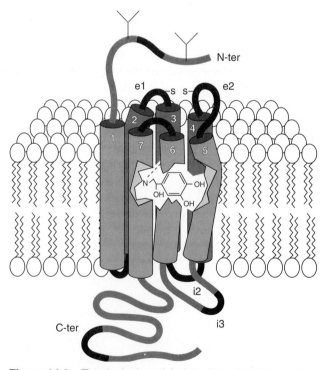

Figure 14.9 Topological model of the ligand-binding pocket of the β_2-adrenergic receptor, which is inserted in the membrane. The ligand-binding region formed by the seven transmembrane domains is buried in the lipidic bilayer. (From Strosberg [45], with permission, from *Molecular Neurobiology* 4:211–50, 1990. ©1992 by Humana Press, Inc.)

membrane-spanning helices (Fig. 14.9). These hydrophobic domains are connected by short hydrophilic segments, which apparently form extramembranous loops. The tertiary structure predicted for the receptor is similar to that proposed for the visual pigment rhodopsin, which acts through G-proteins to stimulate cGMP phosphodiesterase. Further analysis has shown that the receptor shares significant amino acid similarity with rhodopsin. This primary sequence conservation is highest in the putative transmembrane regions that in opsin comprise the binding site for the ligand retinal (Chap. 21). In contrast, there is little or no similarity in sequence within the hydrophilic loop regions. It has been hypothesized that the ligand-binding site lies in the transmembrane domain of the receptor [24] (Fig. 14.9).

The function of specific structural domains of these receptors was determined after construction and expression of a series of chimeric α_2-, β_2-AR genes. Studies with chimeric ARs and muscarinic cholinergic receptors implicate the putative 3i-loop as the major, but not the sole, determinant of selective coupling to their respective G proteins [35]. Chimeric receptors are proving useful for elucidating the structural basis of receptor function [24].

ADRENOCEPTOR SIGNAL TRANSDUCTION

NE or E of neural or humoral origin, respectively, interact with ARs of the plasma membrane of target cells. Depending on the nature of the AR, ligand binding is followed by signal transduction and second-messenger production as described below [22].

A number of neurotransmitter and hormone receptors elicit their responses via biochemical pathways that involve transduction elements known as guanine nucleotide regulatory (G) proteins (Chap. 4). Among these are several types of receptors for E; these adrenergic receptor subtypes are of particular interest because they are coupled to each of the major second-messenger pathways that are known to be linked through G proteins. Thus the β_1- and β_2-ARs stimulate adenylate cyclase; the α_1-AR stimulates breakdown of polyphosphoinositides, and the α_2-AR inhibits adenylate cyclase (Fig. 14.10).

α-Adrenoceptors. It is now well established that activation of α_1-adrenergic receptors by NE or other agonists increases hydrolysis of PIP$_2$, probably through an intermediary G protein. The resulting release of Ins(1,4,5)P$_3$ and diacylglycerol into the intracellular milieu mobilizes Ca^{2+} stored in intracellular pools, such as the endoplasmic and sarcoplasmic reticulum, and activates protein kinase C (see Fig. 4.9). These primary events appear to be responsible for many of the effects of α_1-adrenergic receptor activation in many tissues.

α_1-Adrenergic receptor responses in some tissues may be mediated through a signal transduction mechanism unrelated to breakdown of PIP$_2$. Increases in Ca^{2+} influx,

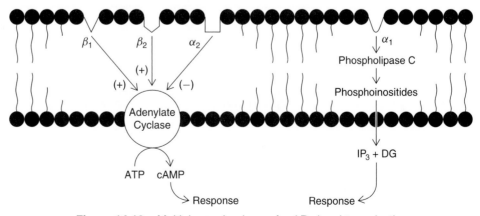

Figure 14.10 Multiple mechanisms of α-AR signal transduction.

arachidonic acid release, and cyclic GMP accumulation [36] have all been reported in response to α_1-AR activation, and some of these effects have been clearly differentiated from activation of inositol phospholipid breakdown. The possibility that different α_1-AR subtypes use different signal transduction mechanisms is increasingly attractive [9]. A hypothesis consistent with most available data is that the α_{1A}-AR primarily promotes influx of extracellular Ca^{2+} through dihydropyridine-sensitive channels, while the α_{1B}-AR initiates signals through the well-characterized inositol phospholipid pathway. Overall, the existence of pharmacologically distinct subtypes of α_1-ARs linked to different signal transduction mechanisms raises interesting questions concerning the basic mechanisms by which receptor activation controls the intracellular, free Ca^{2+} concentration (Fig. 14.10). Further characterization of these subtypes may also lead to the development of more selective and useful therapeutic agents for treating a variety of physiological disorders.

β-Adrenoceptors.   In Sutherland's initial studies it was established that cAMP is the intracellular second messenger in the hepatic glycogenolytic response to β-AR stimulation by E. All subsequent studies have established that cellular response to β-AR stimulation are, without exception, linked to adenylate cyclase activation and cAMP formation. Although both glucagon and E stimulate hepatic glycogenolysis, they do so through separate receptors that are, nevertheless, linked through a common adenylate cyclase (see Fig. 11.11). Similarly E and ACTH stimulate fat cell lipolysis and do so through separate receptors again linked to a common adenylate cyclase (Fig. 14.11). The transduction mechanisms linking these separate receptors to cyclase requires Ca^{2+}, whereas activation of the enzyme through β-AR stimulation is without such a divalent metal ion requirement. This lack of Ca^{2+} requirement for β-AR signal transduction appears to be a common feature of this receptor in many, but possibly not all, tissues.

Adrenoceptor Autoinhibition.   The myometrium of the uterus provides a good model for understanding the role of the cyclic nucleotides in autoinhibition of uterine muscle contractility in response to E. In vitro, the isolated uterus always contracts in response to E, a response that can be blocked by α-AR antagonists. However, the contractile response to subsequent doses of E is usually completely inhibited. This autoinhibition can be prevented by the β-AR antagonist, propranolol; each subsequent addition of

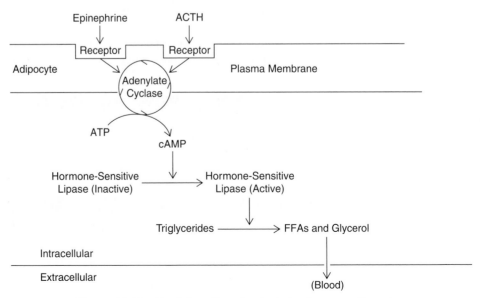

Figure 14.11   Lipolytic action of catecholamines on adipocytes.

E to the uterus will produce a contraction as long as a β-antagonist is present. E stimulates adenylate cyclase activity of uterine muscle, an action antagonized by β-AR antagonists. (Bu)$_2$ cAMP added to the incubation medium mimics the inhibitory action of E. Thus the initial contractile response to the myometrium to E is mediated through α-ARs, but simultaneous stimulation of silent β-ARs elevates the intracellular levels of cAMP, which are then inhibitory to myometrial contractility (autoinhibition).

Adrenoceptor Desensitization. Stimulation of plasma membrane β-ARs with catecholamines results in profound increases in the intracellular levels of cAMP. Detectable increases in the concentration of this second messenger occur within a few seconds of exposure to agonists. Following removal of agonist stimulation of the β-AR, the intrinsic GTPase activity of Gα_s hydrolyzes the bound nucleotide, GTP, to GDP (see Chap. 4). An interesting feature of the cAMP response is that even when the agonist is continuously present, intracellular cAMP levels generally plateau or even return to near basal levels within a few minutes. This waning of the stimulated response in the face of continuous agonist exposure has been termed desensitization. Desensitization has been demonstrated in many other hormone- and neurotransmitter-receptor systems, including those that activate different G proteins and effector systems. In addition, many pharmacological agents targeted at hormone receptors show diminished effectiveness (tachyphylaxis) with time. Desensitization of signal transduction may occur through a variety of processes, including receptor internalization or receptor uncoupling mediated by receptor phosphorylation [17, 35].

Agonist-induced β-AR desensitization appears to be due to a rapid attenuation of the stimulated rate of cAMP generation. Plasma membrane preparations derived from desensitized cells exhibit markedly diminished adenylate cyclase activities upon restimulation by the desensitizing agonists. The molecular mechanisms underlying rapid β-AR desensitization do not appear to require internalization of the receptors, but rather an alteration in the functioning of β-AR themselves that uncouples the receptors from Gα_s. This uncoupling phenomenon involves phosphorylation of the β-AR by at least two kinases, PKA and the β-AR kinase (β-ARK), which are activated under different desensitizing conditions (Fig. 14.12). Receptor phosphorylation by the two kinases leads to desensitization of the receptor response via distinct biochemical mechanisms, and additional cytosolic factors appear to be involved in the case of β-ARK [32, 41].

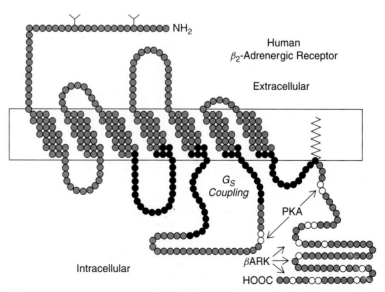

Figure 14.12 Mechanism of β-AR desensitization. (From Hausdorff et al. 1990. "Turning off the signal: desensitization of β-adrenergic receptor function." *FASEB J.* 4:2881–9.)

HORMONAL MODULATION OF ADRENOCEPTORS

The tissue density of ARs varies and depends on the presence or absence of stimulation; ARs increase (up-regulation) in the absence of stimulation and decrease (down-regulation) under continuous stimulation. The density of β_1- and β_2-ARs can be independently regulated, providing strong evidence that the receptors are separate. An increase in the sensitivity of adrenergic effector organs to catecholamines has been noted after denervation. The denervated heart of the dog and the denervated rat pineal, for example, respond to catecholamines by an enhanced production of cAMP over that of intact control tissues. This *denervation supersensitivity* is due to an increase in tissue β-ARs. On the other hand, the density of these receptors decreases in tissues subjected to continued elevated levels of the β-AR agonist, isoproterenol.

Gonadal Steroid Hormones. AR responses to catecholamines are affected by gonadal steroids. Steroid hormones affect sympathetic function by modulating AR responses to catecholamines. Estrogen and progesterone may modulate sympathoadrenal activity by altering catecholamine metabolism and, in addition, produce qualitative changes in the contractile response of smooth muscle to stimulation by catecholamines. The response of the human oviduct and uteri from several species changes from contraction to relaxation, depending on the concentrations of gonadal steroids present. Contraction is mediated through α-ARs in the estrogen-dominated uterus, whereas β-AR-induced relaxation predominates during pregnancy or when incubated in vitro in the presence of progesterone.

Adrenal Steroid Hormones. Glucocorticoids play a permissive role in regulating cAMP-mediated effects of hormones on the liver and other organs. In adrenalectomized rats the stimulation of liver gluconeogenesis and glycogenolysis in response to catecholamines is greatly reduced. The lipolytic response of adipose tissue to epinephrine in vitro is blunted in tissues removed from adrenalectomized animals. Glucocorticoid treatment restores the lipolytic response of fat tissue removed from adrenalectomized animals. Catecholamine-induced pressor effects on the cardiovascular system are dependent on permissive actions of glucocorticoids. One mechanism of glucocorticoid enhancement of cardiovascular responses to catecholamines may involve inactivation of COMT. Glucocorticoids therefore play vital roles in the regulation of tissue responses to catecholamines during stress.

Thyroid Hormones. Thyroid hormones profoundly affect the activity of the sympathoadrenal system. Sympathoadrenal activity is enhanced under conditions of hyperthyroidism and depressed under conditions of low levels of thyroid hormones, as in myxedema. Therefore, the major symptoms of patients with a thyroid dysfunction relate to functional alterations of those organs regulated by the sympathetic nervous system (see Table 13.2).

SYMPATHOADRENAL FUNCTIONS

The role of the sympathoadrenal system is to maintain the constancy of the internal environment of the body [10, 11]. Any decrease in blood pressure, blood glucose level, or oxygen availability leads to an acute enhancement of sympathoadrenal activity with resulting elevation in plasma catecholamines. In addition the sympathoadrenal system is activated in anticipation of events that may affect adversely an individual. Stress is a term generally used to designate the state resulting from events (stressors) of external or internal origin, real or imagined, that tend to affect the homeostatic state. Although an acceptable definition of stress may not be available, in the present context stress refers to any condition tending to elevate plasma catecholamine levels in response to exogenous or endogenous stimuli. For example, the early experiments of Cannon [10, 11] revealed that the barking of a dog was a stimulus to E secretion from the adrenal gland of a cat. In humans, plasma levels of NE and E are immediately elevated upon standing, during exercise, during and after surgery, and whenever plasma glucose levels fall below normal [14].

Norepinephrine is released by sympathetic neurons to provide localized autonomic effector control, whereas E is released from the adrenal as a humoral messenger that may also provide an additional stimulus to autonomic effectors. Since catecholamines communicate with their effector cells through ARs, the distribution and nature of these receptors will determine the response generated. These tissues must therefore possess the "correct" type of AR to provide the response that will be most appropriate (adaptive) under conditions of stress. By inference, therefore, it should be possible to predict the nature of both the response and the type of AR that characterize a particular tissue. The following guidelines should assist in the formulation of such predictions. First, autonomic effector cells may possess α- and β-ARs or only β-ARs in addition to cholinergic receptors. Second, smooth muscle contraction, with few exceptions (intestinal smooth muscle), is regulated through α-ARs, whereas relaxation, with one exception (cardiac muscle), is controlled through β-AR stimulation. Third, where α-ARs are present they dominate (mask) β-ARs. Fourth, β-ARs are generally stimulatory to cellular secretion, whereas α-ARs (with few exceptions) are inhibitory to cellular secretion. Fifth, where β-ARs of smooth muscle control relaxation, cholinergic receptors will regulate contraction. Sixth, when α-ARs regulate smooth muscle contraction, acetylcholine will normally regulate relaxation.

Intermediary Metabolism

Carbohydrate Metabolism. One would expect that under conditions of stress blood glucose levels would need to be elevated to provide this metabolic substrate for energy production within critical tissues (brain, heart, skeletal muscle). Glycogen is available as a storage form of glucose within the liver. E is stimulatory to hepatic glycogenolysis and glucose release through its action on β-ARs. Skeletal muscle may provide an even greater total source of glycogen and, in response to β-AR stimulation, glycogen is converted through the glycolytic pathway to lactic acid. This lactic acid is cycled to the liver and through E-stimulated gluconeogenesis converted to glucose.

Most interesting is the demonstration that catecholamines are inhibitory (through α-ARs) to insulin secretion. On the other hand, catecholamines are stimulatory to glucagon secretion through an action on β-ARs of pancreatic A cells (see Fig. 21.9). Therefore, under conditions of stress, elevated circulating levels of E would be stimulatory to numerous physiological processes that would elevate blood glucose levels. The inhibition of insulin secretion, for example, would prevent removal of glucose from the general circulation.

If the blood glucose concentration is reduced by fasting or administration of insulin, an immediate release of E follows [8]. The denervated adrenal is, however, insensitive to a hypoglycemic stimulus. Adrenal catecholamine secretion in response to hypoglycemia can be blocked by local anesthetic application to the hypothalamus and adjacent brain areas. In addition intracerebroventricular injection of a nonmetabolizable analog, 5-thioglucose, increases sympathoadrenal-mediated hyperglycemia. These observations suggest that some glucoreceptors that regulate sympathoadrenal discharge reside within the brain. The cellular receptors that mediate the hyperglycemic response to glucoprivation are apparently localized caudal to the forebrain [23]

Fat Metabolism. Adipose tissue cells possess β-ARs and, in response to catecholamines of either sympathetic or adrenal origin, lipolysis is stimulated. Epinephrine-induced cAMP production activates a hormone-sensitive lipase, triglyceride lipase, which metabolizes fats into FFAs and glycerol (Fig. 14.11). The FFAs released into the blood are then used directly by certain tissues (brain, cardiac muscle) as sources of energy (a glucose-sparing action), or they may be used within the liver in the formation of glucose.

The demonstration that not all lean individuals gain weight when overfed, coupled with a number of studies pointing to a metabolic defect in the obese, has led to the notion that there are two necessary conditions for the development of obesity: (1) an ample supply of food, and (2) a genetic predisposition for a high efficiency in the conversion of food to body fat. It is toward the latter condition that current pharmaceutical work on obesity is directed; that is to say, there is an active search for drugs that will raise metabolic rate (i.e., thermogenic drugs). The use of thermogenic drugs in the treatment of obesity is now directed toward a search for stimulants of the sympathetic nervous system (SNS). This approach follows several lines of evidence that suggest an important role for the SNS in the control of diet-induced thermogenesis, and that an impairment in its functional state could lead to obesity. A reduced release of norepinephrine (NE), rather than insensitivity to the neurotransmitter, has been implicated in the thermogenic defect of the obese. Drugs that mimic the activity of the SNS and increase metabolic rate therefore offer considerable therapeutic potential and provide a rational approach for the treatment of obesity [18].

Protein Metabolism.   Epinephrine acting through β-ARs and cAMP decreases the release of amino acids from skeletal muscle. A reduced rate of muscle proteolysis appears to be the mechanism which causes adrenergic inhibition of amino acid release. This adrenergic modulation of protein degradation may be of physiological importance to the short-term fight or flight response associated with increased adrenal E secretion. Under these conditions, lactate, glycerol, and glucose levels would be increased and additional gluconeogenic substrates might not be needed.

Thermogenesis

The sympathetic nervous system plays a critical role in the regulation of mammalian thermogenic responses to cold exposure and dietary intake [27]. Both fasting and feeding induce changes in sympathoadrenal activity. In rats, fasting suppresses and overfeeding stimulates the sympathetic nervous system. It was hypothesized that during fasting suppression of sympathetic activity would conserve calories by decreasing metabolism and heat production, whereas during feeding the increased sympathetic activity would expend the excess calories. Increased sympathetic activity might account for some of the increased incidence of cardiac arrhythmias, angina, and hypertension in populations known for overeating.

Shivering Thermogenesis.   Thermogenesis associated with muscular activity is a by-product, rather than a goal, of the activity. The heat produced by shivering, however, has heat production as the major objective. Piloerection (goose pimples) is controlled by the SNS.

Nonshivering (Chemical) Thermogenesis.   Catecholamine-stimulated thermogenesis is mediated by β-ARs [26]. In the rat, brown adipose tissue (BAT) is the major site of metabolic heat production in response to both cold (nonshivering thermogenesis) and diet-induced thermogenesis. Measurements of NE turnover rate in interscapular BAT of the rat demonstrate increased sympathetic activity in response to both cold exposure and overfeeding. Injections of NE trigger a coordinated proliferation of brown adipocytes and endothelial cells in vitro that is similar to those observed after cold exposure. It has also been suggested that cold exposure stimulates BAT growth by increasing the release of NE from sympathetic nerves and that the neurohormone activates mitoses in BAT precursor cells via β-AR pathways [19]. In adult humans, a physiologically significant role for BAT has not been established, but cannot be excluded.

Cardiovascular System

Epinephrine increases both the force and rate of the heartbeat through stimulation of cardiac muscle β-ARs [20]. There are no other examples known where β-ARs induce muscle contraction. From an adaptive standpoint, it is obvious that enhanced pumping of blood through the heart would be desirable. The particular distribution of vascular smooth muscle ARs provides a mechanism for the shunting of blood to various body compartments during stress. For example, blood is shunted from the skin, mucosa, connective tissue, and kidneys; as expected, vascular smooth muscles of these organs possess α-ARs. In contrast, smooth muscle of coronary arteries, as well as skeletal muscle, possess β-ARs. If dominant α-ARs were present, blood flow to these vital organs would be diminished when these organs were maximally active. The decreased blood flow to the kidneys reduces glucose clearance from the circulation, and this reduced clearance may be primarily responsible for the prolonged hyperglycemia induced by catecholamines.

The spleen capsule is contracted through catecholamine stimulation of α-ARs, which increases the circulating levels of erythrocytes. These erythrocytes provide the blood with an increased capacity for oxygen uptake from the lungs. Epinephrine enhances blood platelet adhesiveness and reduces clotting time by its actions on platelet α-ARs.

In those smooth muscles where α-ARs subserve contraction, the parasympathetic nervous system, through the release of its neurotransmitter, acetylcholine, controls relaxation. This holds true for cardiac muscle as well. Since β-ARs also regulate relaxation of smooth muscle [36], acetylcholine regulates the contractile component of the muscle.

Respiratory System

Bronchial smooth muscle is relaxed in response to catecholamines and only β-ARs are present. Relaxation of these muscles dilate the bronchial passageways so that increased amounts of air containing oxygen are made available to the blood under conditions of increased exertion.

Sympathoadrenal Activity and Stress

Both postganglionic sympathetic neurons and adrenal chromaffin cells are directly innervated by cholinergic neurons. Under stress, adrenal chromaffin cell enzymes are regulated by both neuronal and endocrine pathways. Tyrosine hydroxylase and DBH are regulated mainly by neuronal transynaptic stimulation, whereas PNMT is primarily under endocrine control. For example, denervation of an adrenal gland by cutting the splanchnic nerve prevents elevations in tyrosine hydroxylase and DBH in response to stress, whereas PNMT is still enhanced. PNMT and DBH activities in the adrenal decrease following hypophysectomy and can be restored by administration of ACTH or glucocorticoids. Levels of tyrosine hydroxylase, on the other hand, are increased by ACTH, but not by glucocorticoids. Thus in addition to neuronal influences tyrosine hydroxylase activity appears to be directly affected by ACTH.

Discrepancies between perceptions of internal or external circumstances and innate or acquired expectations lead to patterned stress responses involving several homeostatic systems, of which the sympathoadrenomedullary system (SAMS) is one. Severe, generalized threats such as hypoglycemia, hypoxia, hemorrhage, circulatory collapse, and fight/flight situations elicit generalized SAMS activation, including cardiac stimulation; splanchnic, cutaneous, and renal vasoconstriction; and usually preserved skeletal-muscle blood flow. Patterned sympathetic neural responses, resulting in redistribution of blood volume or changes in glandular activity, occur during orthostasis, exercise, altered environmental temperature, the postprandial state, and performance of attention-requiring tasks. In all these situations, SAMS activity is coordinated with that of the parasympathetic nervous system, the pituitary-adrenocortical system, and probably several neuropeptide systems.

NOREPINEPHRINE: HUMORAL HORMONE AND NEUROTRANSMITTER IN HUMANS

Epinephrine, in humans at least, is generally considered the only humoral catecholamine normally serving an endocrine function. Nevertheless, NE does escape into the circulation during sympathetic activity. Is this extrasynaptic NE destined only for metabolic degradation, or might it also subserve some role as a hormone? NE was infused into normal men and a variety of physiological parameters were monitored concomitantly. Only NE levels in excess of 1800 pg/ml caused hemodynamic and metabolic effects. Thus, under usual conditions, NE's biological actions may only relate to its sympathetic neurotransmitter function. Because NE levels can exceed 1800 pg/ml during stress, for example, it is conceivable that NE might subserve some role in stress along with epinephrine of adrenal origin [14]. Also, posturally stimulated NE concentrations occur in normal, and even adrenalectomized individuals, suggesting that the adrenals are not the only source of plasma NE.

SYMPATHOADRENAL PATHOPHYSIOLOGY

β-Adrenoceptor antagonists ("β-blockers") play an important role in the pharmacological therapy of such cardiovascular disorders as hypertension, ischemic heart disease, and arrhythmias. Rapid relief of symptoms is often achieved using β-AR antagonists and with few side effects. The demonstration that ARs can be classed into subgroups based on their selective response to pharmaceutical agonists and antagonists raises hopes that other drugs might be developed that would be selective for these AR subtypes; such selectivity might also decrease the severity of any side effects. β_1 and β_2-ARs are components of many tissues and therefore may limit their effectiveness until further specificities of the receptors are discovered.

Adrenal Chromaffin Tumors.   Neuroblastoma is a highly malignant neoplasm of early life that arises from primitive sympathetic cells and neuroblasts. Tumors may arise within the sympathoadrenal system. Adrenal chromaffin tumors (pheochromocytomas), although generally benign, are nevertheless life-threatening. Although pheochromocytomas are found wherever sympathetic nervous tissue is located, it most often arises from the adrenal medulla or along the sympathetic chain. Pheochromocytomas that contain only E are comprised entirely of A cells, whereas those containing only NE consist entirely of N cells. Both cells are present in mixed pheochromocytomas containing both NE and E. The excessive secretion of catecholamines, characteristic of pheochromocytoma and neuroblastoma, results in severe hypertension, as well as increased basal metabolic rate, increased oxygen consumption, weight loss, psychosis, tremulousness, and increased respiratory rate. Competitive inhibitors of tyrosine hydroxylase, such as α-methyltyrosine, are often effective in the treatment of pheochromocytoma [49].

Adrenoceptor Hypothesis of Asthma.   It has been suggested that the symptoms and pathophysiology of asthma may be explained in terms of reduced pulmonary β-AR function [34]. The status of β-AR function in asthmatics has been extensively investigated for many years, but it remains controversial. Studies both in vitro and in vivo have shown that asthmatics do not necessarily have diminished bronchial β-AR function. Furthermore, it is well established that blockade of β-ARs of nonasthmatics does not induce asthma or bronchial hyperresponsiveness. These findings indicate that β-AR dysfunction is not a fundamental cause of asthma. Since β_2-agonists are widely used and are an effective treatment for asthma, it is also clear that significant β-AR function is maintained in most asthmatics. Nevertheless, a definite decrease in β-AR function has been detected in bronchial smooth muscle removed from severe asthmatics. Evidence suggests that the reduction in β-AR function involves both receptor uncoupling and a decrease in receptor number. The marked worsening of asthma produced by β-blockers illustrates the role of effective β-AR function in maintaining adequate airway caliber in asthmatics. Thus significant β-AR hypofunction, secondary to asthma, may contribute to the further deterioration of this disease by rendering the subject more vulnerable to spasmogens and less responsive to β-agonist therapy.

Adrenoceptors, Fat Cells, and Heart Disease.   ARs play important roles in fat cell metabolism, lipogenesis, and lipolysis. α-AR stimulation results in fat storage, whereas β-AR activation results in catabolic metabolism within the cells. The relative distribution of ARs may determine gender differences in fat distribution in humans. It has been stated that gender differences in distribution of α-ARs may partly explain the tendency of the male to look like an apple rather than like a pear, as does the female. Female shape may have to do with differences in fat cell number and size in the hips, thighs, and buttocks, whereas the male potbelly may be due to a greater number of α-ARs in abdominal adipose tissue [42].

Recent epidemiological studies have confirmed an earlier observation of a relationship between anatomical distribution of fat and the risk of diabetes, hypertension, stroke, ischemic heart disease, and early death. Among individuals with the same degree of relative adiposity, those whose adipose tissue is located predominantly in the upper body (android distribution) have higher rates of diabetes, hypertension, stroke, ischemic heart disease, and early death than those whose fat is located primarily in the hips, buttocks, and thighs (gynecoid distribution). The biological reasons for these epidemiologic associations are not known.

COMPARATIVE ENDOCRINOLOGY

The comparative physiology and pharmacology of ARs in vertebrates has not been studied systematically. Because NE, E, and possibly DA are the only catecholamines produced by the sympathoadrenal system, it might be expected that the ARs of all vertebrates are similar, although the particular response elicited might show some species specificity. (The turkey erythrocyte, for example, has been used for detailed studies on the β-AR.) Melanosome aggregation and dispersion within dermal melanophores of elasmobranchs, teleosts, amphibians, and reptiles are stimulated by catecholamines interacting through α- and β-ARs, respectively. These responses can be blocked by the classical α- and β-AR antagonists (see Chap. 8).

Evidence to date supports the hypothesis that adrenergic and cholinergic receptors existed for hundreds of millions of years and that the same receptor molecules have been put to a variety of uses in different species and tissues. The extent of structural homology among these proteins became apparent with the cloning and sequence analysis of genes encoding adrenergic and muscarinic cholinergic receptors from a variety of species. Gene cloning and sequencing have provided data that have proven that a high degree of structural homology exists between a number of neurotransmitter receptors and the opsins. It has been proposed that an evolutionary relationship exists between adrenergic and muscarinic cholinergic receptors and that they evolved from one common ancestor via gene duplication events [47].

REFERENCES

[1] Ahlquist, R. P. 1948. A study of the adrenotropin receptors. *Amer. J. Physiol.* 153:586–600.

[2] Anderson, D. J. 1992. Cell fate determination in the peripheral nervous system: the sympathoadrenal progenitor. *J. Neurobiol.* 24:185–98.

[3] Andersen, P. H., J. A. Gingrich, M. D. Bates, A. Dearry, P. Falardeau, S. E. Senolles, and M. G. Caron. 1990. Dopamine receptor subtypes: beyond the D_1/D_2 classification. *TIPS* 11:231–6.

[4] Black, I. B. 1982. Stages in development of autonomic neurons. *Science* 214:1198–1204.

[5] Black, J. 1989. Drugs from emasculated hormones: the principle of syntopic antagonism. *In vitro Cell. Develop. Biol.* 25:311–20.

[6] Bohn, M. C., M. Goldstein, and I. B. Black. 1981. Role of glucocorticoids in expression of the adrenergic phenotype in rat embryonic adrenal gland. *Develop. Biol.* 82:1–10.

[7] Brann, M. R., V. J. Klimkowski, and J. Ellis. 1993. Structure/function relationships of muscarinic acetylcholine receptors. *Life Sci.* 52:405–12.

[8] Bray, G. A. 1993. The nutrient balance hypothesis: peptides, sympathetic activity, and food intake. *Ann. N.Y. Acad. Sci.* 676:223–41.

[9] Brodde, O. E. 1990. Subclassification of peripheral dopamine receptors. *J. Auton. Pharmacol.* 10:S5–10.

[10] Cannon, W. B. 1932. *The wisdom of the body.* New York: W. W. Norton & Co., Inc.

[11] Cannon, W. B., and A. Rosenblueth, 1937. *Autonomic neuroeffector systems.* New York: Macmillan, Inc.

[12] Carmichael, S. W., and S. L. Stoddard. 1993. The adrenal medulla, 1989–1991. Boca Raton: CRC Press, Inc.

[13] Coupland, R. E. 1953. On the morphology and adrenaline-noradrenaline content of chromaffin tissue. *J. Endocrinol.* 9:194–203.

[14] Cryer, P. E. 1980. Physiology and pathophysiology of the sympathoadrenal neuroendocrine system. *New Engl. J. Med.* 303:436–44.

[15] Dale, H. H. 1906. On some physiological actions of ergot. *J. Physiol.* 3:163–206.

[16] ———. 1934. Chemical transmission of the effects of nerve impulses. *Br. Med. J.* 1:835–41.

[17] Dawson, T. M., J. L. Arriza, D. E. Jaworsky, F. F. Borisy, H. Attramadal, R. J. Lefkowitz, and G. V. Ronnett. 1993. β-Adrenergic receptor kinase-2 and β-arresting-2 as mediators of odorant-induced desensitization. *Science* 259:825–8.

[18] Dulloo, A. G., and D. S. Miller. 1989. Ephedrine, caffeine and aspirin: "over the counter" drugs that interact to stimulate thermogenesis in the obese. *Nutrition* 5:7–9.

[19] Geloen, A., A. J. Collet, G. Guay, and L. J. Bukowiecki. 1988. β-Adrenergic stimulation of brown adipocyte proliferation. *Amer. J. Physiol.* 254:C175–82.

[20] Gilman, A. G., L. S. Goodman, and A. Gilman. 1980. *Goodman and Gilman's The pharmacological basis of therapeutics.* 6th ed. New York: Macmillan, Inc.

[21] Goyal, R. K. 1989. Muscarinic receptor subtypes: physiology and clinical implications. *New Engl. J. Med.* 321:1022–9.

[22] Hadcock, J. R., and C. C. Malbon. 1993. Agonist regulation of gene expression of adrenergic receptors and G proteins. *J. Neurochem.* 60:1–9.

[23] Himsworth, R. L. 1970. Hypothalamic control of adrenaline secretion in response to insufficient glucose. *J. Physiol.* 206:411–7.

[24] Kobilka, B. K., T. S. Kobilka, K. Daniel, J. W. Regan, M. G. Caron, and R. J. Lefkowitz. 1988. Chimeric α_2-, β_2-adrenergic receptors: delineation of domains involved in effector coupling and ligand binding specificity. *Science* 240:1310–6.

[25] Kobilka, B. K., H. Matsui, T. S. Kobilka, T. L. Yang-Feng, U. Francke, M. G. Caron, R. J. Lefkowitz, and J. W. Regan. 1987. Cloning, sequencing, and expression of the gene coding for the human platelet α_2-adrenergic receptor. *Science* 238:650–6.

[26] Lafontan, M., and M. Berlan. 1993. Fat cell adrenergic receptors and the control of white and brown fat cell function. *J. Lipid Res.* 34:1057–90.

[27] Landsberg, L., M. E. Saville, and J. B. Young. 1984. Sympathoadrenal system and regulation of thermogenesis. *Amer. J. Physiol.* 247:E181–9.

[28] Leclere, J., and G. Weryha. 1989. Stress and auto-immune endocrine diseases. *Horm. Res.* 31:90–93.

[29] Le Douarin, N. M. 1986. Cell line segregation during peripheral nervous system ontogeny. *Science* 231:1515–22.

[30] Levitzki, A. 1988. From epinephrine to cyclic AMP. *Science* 241:800–806.

[31] Liggett, S. B., and J. R. Raymond. 1993. Pharmacology and molecular biology of adrenergic receptors. *Baillières Clin. Endocrinol. Metab.* 7:279–306.

[32] Lohse, M. J., J. L. Benovic, J. Codina, M. G. Caron, and R. J. Lefkowitz. 1990. β-Arrestin: a protein that regulates β-adrenergic receptor function. *Science* 248:1547–50.

[33] Lomasney, J. W., S. Cotecchia, R. J. Lefkowitz, and M. G. Caron. 1991. Molecular biology of α-adrenergic receptors: implications for receptor classification and for structure-function relationships. *Biochim. Biophys. Acta* 1095:127–39.

[34] Lulich, K. M., R. G. Goldie, and J. W. Paterson. 1988. Beta-adrenoceptor function in asthmatic bronchial smooth muscle. *Gen. Pharmacol.* 19:307–11.

[35] Luttrell, L. M., J. Ostrowski, S. Cotecchia, H. Kendall, and R. J. Lefkowitz. 1993. Antagonism of catecholamine receptor signaling by expression of cytoplasmic domains of the receptors. *Science* 259:1453–6.

[36] Nakatsu, K., and J. Diamond. 1988. Role of cGMP in relaxation of vascular and other smooth muscle. *Can. J. Physiol. Pharmacol.* 67:251–62.

[37] Neher, E., and R. S. Zucker. 1993. Multiple calcium-dependent processes related to secretion in bovine chromaffin cells. *Neuron* 10:21–30.

[38] Nickerson, M., and L. S. Goodman. 1947. Pharmacological properties of a new adrenergic blocking agent: *N,N*-dibenzyl-β-chloroethylamine (Dibenamine). *J. Pharmacol. Exper. Ther.* 89:167–85.

[39] O'Dowd, B. F. 1993. Structures of dopamine receptors. I. *Neurochem.* 60:804–16.

[40] Oliver, G., and E. A. Schafer. 1895. The physiological effects of extracts from the suprarenal capsules. *J. Physiol. Lond.* 18:230–76.

[41] Pitcher, J. A., J. Inglese, J. B. Higgins, J. L. Arriza, P. J. Casey, C. Kim, J. L. Benovic, M. M. Kwatra, M. G. Caron, and R. J. Lefkowitz. 1992. Role of $\beta\gamma$ subunits of G proteins in targeting the β-adrenergic receptor kinase to membrane-bound receptors. *Science* 257:1264–7.

[42] Presta, E., R. L. Leibel, and J. Hirsch. 1990. Regional changes in adrenergic receptor status during hypocaloric intake do not predict changes in adipocyte size or body shape. *Metabolism* 39:307–15.

[43] Ruffolo, R. R., Jr., A. J. Nichols, J. M. Stadel, and J. P. Hieble. 1993. Pharmacologic and therapeutic applications of α_2-adrenoceptor subtypes. *Annu. Rev. Pharm. & Toxicol.* 32:243–79.

[44] Strosberg, A. D. 1991. Biotechnology of the β-adrenergic receptors. *Mol. Neurobiol.* 4:211–50.

[45] ———. 1993. Structure, function, and regulation of adrenergic receptors. *Protein Sci.* 2:1198–209.

[46] Tischler, A. S., and R. A. Delellis. 1988. The rat adrenal medulla. I. The normal adrenal. *J. Amer. Coll. Toxicol.* 7:1–21.

[47] Venter, J. C., U. Di Porzio, D. A. Robinson, S. M. Shreeve, J. Lai, A. R. Kerlavage, S. P. Fracek, Jr., K.-U. Lentes, and C. M. Fraser. 1988. Evolution of neurotransmitter receptor systems. *Prog. Neurobiol.* 30:105–69.

[48] Winkler, H., and R. Fischer-Colbre. 1992. The chromagranins A and B: the first 25 years and future perspectives. *Neuroscience* 49:497–528.

[49] Young, W. F. Jr. 1993. Pheochromocytoma: 1926–1993. *TEM* 4:122–7.

15

Adrenal Steroid Hormones

The adrenal gland of most vertebrates is composed of two tissues of different origin that produce two classes of hormones unrelated in structure. Nevertheless, the hormones of both the adrenal steroidogenic tissue and the adrenal chromaffin tissue play important roles in response to stress. The discoveries that led to present knowledge of the adrenal steroidogenic tissue hormones and their role in endocrine physiology are presented in the following chronological summary. A number of treatises on adrenal structure and function are available [32, 33, 57].

HISTORICAL PERSPECTIVE

1815	Meckel described the gross comparative anatomy of the adrenals.
1846	Ecker provided a detailed description of the histology of the adrenal medulla and cortex.
1854	Kölliker recognized the cortex and medulla as functionally different structures in humans.
1855	Addison described a disease (Addison's disease) that involved a degeneration of the adrenals.
1856	Brown-Séquard studied the effects of adrenalectomy in animals and concluded that the glands are indispensable for life.
1866	Arnold described the cellular zonation of the cortex.
1927	Baumann showed that longevity in animals after adrenalectomy was prolonged by injections of sodium salts. Other investigators noted that there was excessive excretion of sodium and chloride by the kidneys in the absence of normal adrenal function.
1927–1930	Smith established that although the adrenals of the rat atrophied after hypophysectomy, they could be restored to normal size by administration of pituitary extracts.
1928–1931	Baumann and colleagues were among the first to employ adrenal cortical extracts as replacement therapy in adrenalectomized animals and in patients with Addison's disease. In 1931 Swingle and Pfiffer, and in 1930 Hartman and Brownell, described the beneficial actions of adrenal extracts on survival of adrenalectomized animals.
1936	Kendall and coworkers obtained crystalline extracts of the adrenal cortex and demonstrated the effectiveness of compound E (cortisone) in ameliorating the symptoms of adrenalectomy in rats.

1936   Selye described the *general adaptation syndrome,* which provided a major impetus to stress research and the subsequent recognition of the essential role of the adrenal in the stress response.

1940   Long and associates established the importance of the adrenal cortex relative to carbohydrate metabolism.

1945   By 1945, 6 active and more than 20 inactive steroids were extracted from the adrenal cortex. The four compounds with greatest biological activity were 11-dehydrocorticosterone, corticosterone, cortisone, and hydrocortisone (cortisol).

1950   Hench and associates described the effectiveness of cortisone in relieving the symptoms of rheumatoid arthritis. It was noted, however, that patients treated with ACTH excreted cortisol rather than cortisone. Cortisol was found to be the principal glucogenic steroid secreted by patients with Cushing's disease.

1951   It was established that cortisol is the major steroid released from the human adrenal gland following stimulation by ACTH.

1952   Tait and Simpson and colleagues demonstrated the presence of an adrenal steroid that is extremely active in retaining sodium.

1954   The structure of the salt-retaining hormone aldosterone was determined by Simpson and Tait and colleagues.

1955   Conn described primary hyperaldosteronism (Conn's disease) [10].

1955   Li and coworkers isolated the pituitary factor ACTH (corticotropin), which regulates adrenal cortisol secretion. As early as 1940 Swann proposed that there were separate controls for adrenal glucocorticoid and mineralocorticoid secretion.

1960   Laragh described the renin-angiotensin system that controls adrenal aldosterone secretion.

These studies established that **cortisol**, *a glucocorticoid, and* **aldosterone**, *a mineralocorticoid, play important roles in carbohydrate and Na+ balance, respectively, in humans and many other vertebrates. Abnormal secretion of either of these hormones has profound pathophysiological consequences in humans.*

THE ADRENAL GLANDS

The adrenal gland is composed of steroidogenic as well as chromaffin tissue. In many mammals the steroidogenic tissue forms a cortical mass surrounding an inner medullary component of chromaffin tissue. In humans and many other mammals these tissue components may appropriately be referred to as the adrenal cortex and adrenal medulla. In many vertebrates, including some mammals, these two tissues are intermingled; in some poikilotherms the two endocrine components are totally separate masses of tissues, therefore, the comparative endocrinologist prefers the functional designations adrenal steroidal and adrenal chromaffin tissue [5, 27].

Anatomy and Embryology

Steroidogenic and chromaffin tissues originate from separate primordia. Chromaffin cells are derived from the neural crest (see Chap. 14), while the steroidogenic tissue arises from the coelomic mesoderm (corticogonadal anlagen) in the genital ridge of the embryo. During migration to definitive anatomical sites, some steroidogenic tissue becomes located in

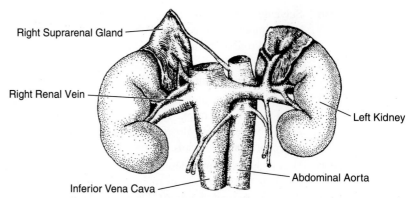

Figure 15.1 Gross anatomy of the human adrenal glands.

extra-adrenal sites. These aberrant adrenal *rests* may hypertrophy and become more active after adrenalectomy. In humans adrenal rests are usually distributed in the celiac plexus and the adjacent fatty tissue, or along the path of the spermatic cord.

In the primate the adrenals are located adjacent to the upper surface of each kidney (Fig. 15.1). Each human adrenal gland weighs approximately 3.5 to 4.5 g and is well vascularized by arterial branches from the aorta. Smaller arterial branches spread over the adrenal capsule, pierce it, and pass as sinusoids between adjacent rows of cortical cells to a subcapsular plexus at the corticomedullary junction. A few venules flow through the medullary chromaffin tissue to a central vein that connects directly or indirectly (via the renal vein) to the inferior vena cava.

The Adrenal Functional Unit. In humans and many other mammals the chromaffin tissue is surrounded by steroidogenic tissue and the vascular relationships are such that the secretory products of the cortex perfuse the medulla through a portal network. In addition sphincterlike muscles in the central adrenal vein may alter the rate of flow of adrenal cortical effluent. Adrenal chromaffin epinephrine synthesis is dependent on steroid hormonal support (Chap. 14). There is evidence that chromaffin tissue has the capacity to carry out many enzymatic reactions characteristic of the cortex and is therefore capable of converting incomplete steroid intermediates passing through the medulla into active glucocorticoids. The close anatomical coupling and the functional interrelationship between the cortex and medulla suggest that these two tissues, although of diverse origin, may constitute an integrated functional unit, at least in higher vertebrates. This relationship may be of particular adaptive importance under conditions of stress when both epinephrine and glucocorticoids are in particular demand.

Histology

In most mammals the adrenal cortical tissue can be divided into three morphologically and functionally different layers: a thin outer *zona glomerulosa;* a thicker middle *zona fasciculata*; and an innermost, moderately thick *zona reticularis* (Fig. 15.2). Steroidogenic cells are filled with lipid droplets (liposomes) containing cholesterol, the substrate for steroid biosynthesis. These droplets are stainable with lipid-soluble dyes such as Sudan red or Sudan black. In the typical alcohol dehydration preparation the cells appear full of vacuoles due to extraction of the lipids from their contained vesicles; these cells are often referred to as spongiocytes. Ultrastructurally, the steroidogenic cells (like those of the gonads) contain abundant mitochondria and an especially conspicuous smooth endoplasmic reticulum. Although the cortical tissue may be grossly divided into three separate regions, the histological picture reveals that the three cell types are parts of the same cords of cells that extend from the capsule to the medulla. These cell cords are surrounded by a capillary network, thus providing steroids ready access into the blood.

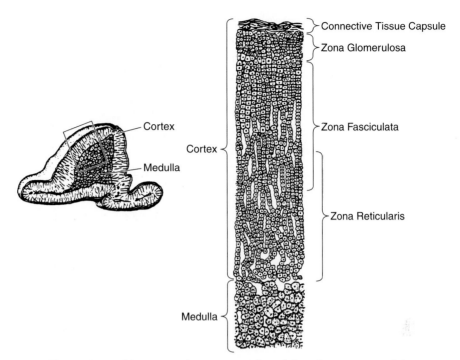

Figure 15.2 Diagrammatic representation of the microanatomy of the human adrenal cortex.

The Fetal Adrenal Cortex and the X Zone

In the fetus a specialized region of the human adrenal cortex has been described between the maturing (permanent) cortex and the medulla. This primate *fetal adrenal cortex* may exceed the size of the kidney; the fetal cortex regresses during the last month of gestation and is then only one-tenth or less the size of an individual kidney. A transient adrenal cortex is also present in the monkey, armadillo, sloth, members of the cat family, elephant seal, and pig [29, 45].

In the mouse the cortex possesses a juxtamedullary zone where morphological expression varies according to sex and age. This zone, generally referred to as the *X zone*, degenerates in the male at maturity and in the female early during the first pregnancy. Castration of the male mouse before puberty allows the X zone to survive, apparently in response to increased secretion of pituitary LH. Injections of LH into the postpubertal castrated mouse re-establish the X zone. The X zone does not disappear in the unmated female. Androgens of gonadal origin appear to be responsible for degeneration of the X zone in some strains of mice, but possibly not in other strains. The adrenal X zone degenerates in Tfm mutant mice whose cells are insensitive to androgens, suggesting that in this strain the X zone atrophy is not directly dependent on androgens [50]. The product(s) that the X zone might secrete is unknown as is the significance of this specialized area.

SYNTHESIS AND CHEMISTRY

Cholesterol, a sterol consisting of 27 carbon atoms, is the precursor for both gonadal and adrenal steroid hormone biosynthesis [43]. The first step in the biosynthetic pathway of steroidogenesis involves cleavage of the terminal six carbons of the side chain of cholesterol, resulting in the formation of pregnenolone. Key enzymes, collectively known as the *desmolase system (cytochrome p450scc)*, are requisite for side-chain cleavage. From pregnenolone a number of pathways [37] lead to the formation of metabolic intermediates that give rise ultimately to the definitive steroid hormones characteristic of the species

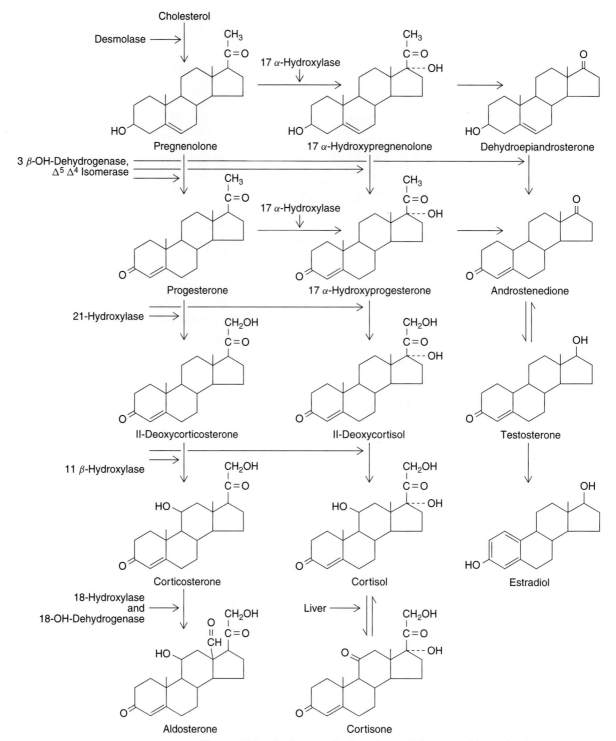

Figure 15.3 Pathways of adrenal steroid hormone biosynthesis.

(Fig. 15.3). The steroid hormones of the adrenal glands may be categorized into three groups according to their principal effects: glucocorticoids, mineralocorticoids, and androgens. Cortisol and aldosterone are the major glucocorticoid and mineralocorticoid hormones, respectively, of humans. Note that all the steroids of the adrenal contain the *cyclopentanoperhydrophenanthrene* nucleus (Fig. 15.4).

The double bond between positions 4 and 5 and the presence of the keto group at position 3 of the A ring are essential for the biological activities of adrenal steroids. Intro-

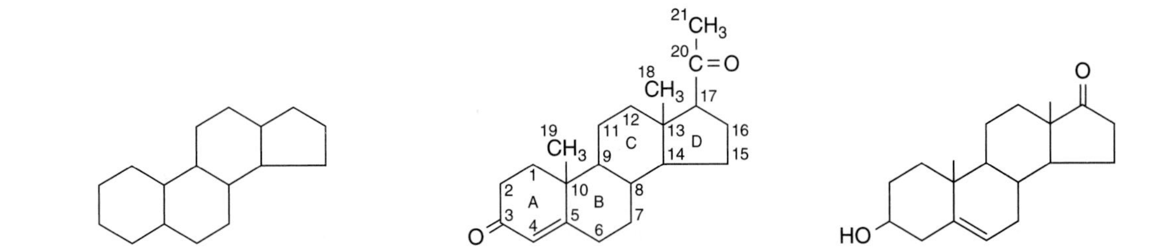

Figure 15.4 Steroid hormone structure and nomenclature.

duction of a 1,2 double bond in cortisone (prednisone, Δ^1-cortisone) or cortisol (prednisolone, Δ^1-cortisol) enhances the ratio of glucocorticoid to mineralocorticoid activity by increasing the former. Incorporation of fluoride into the 9α position enhances both the glucocorticoid and mineralocorticoid activity of cortisol (9α-fluoro-cortisol). Dexamethasone (9α-fluoro-16α-methylprednisolone) is a very potent glucocorticoid with minimal salt-retaining activity.

Conversion of cholesterol to pregnenolone occurs within the mitochondria. Pregnenolone is then released from the mitochondria and, in the smooth endoplasmic reticulum, the double bond is shifted from the 5 to the 4 position and the hydroxyl group at position C-3 is oxidized to a keto group by an enzyme, Δ^5,3-β-hydroxysteroid dehydrogenase-isomerase. All the remaining steps in corticosteroidogenesis consist of additional hydroxylations, at either positions 11, 17, or 21, by various NADPH-dependent hydroxylases. The pathway leading to aldosterone synthesis involves an initial hydroxylation at position 18 followed by dehydrogenase activity, resulting in formation of an aldehyde group at that position.

Several different systems of nomenclature are used to refer to individual steroid structures (Tables 15.1 and 15.2). The Greek capital letter Δ (delta) is often used to indicate a double bond, and it is important to note that a Δ^4 bond is common to nearly all the adrenal steroids. The orientation of hydroxyl groups at either the 11 or 17 position of the

TABLE 15.1 Terms Used in Steroid Nomenclature

Term	Description
Hydroxy-	Indicates an —OH (hydroxyl) group
-ol	Indicates an —OH (hydroxyl) group
Oxy-	Indicates an =O (keto) group
Keto-	Indicates an =O group
-one	Indicates an =O (keto) group
-al	Indicates an aldehyde (—CHO) group
Δ	Signifies location of a double bond in the steroid nucleus (e.g., Δ^4 = double bond between C-4 and C-5 positions)
-ene[a]	Indicates one double bond in the steroid nucleus
-diene	Indicates two double bonds in the steroid nucleus
-triene	Indicates three double bonds in the steroid nucleus
α- and β-	Designates if a substituted group lies below (α) or above (β) the plane of the molecule
Estrane[b]$_{(C18)}$	Indicates basic steroid skeleton with a methyl group attached at C-13 in addition to the 17 carbon atoms of the ring structure
Androstane[b]$_{(C19)}$	Indicates steroid structure with methyl groups at both the C-13 and C-10 positions
Pregnane[b]$_{(21)}$	Indicates basic steroid skeleton with methyl groups at C-13 and C-10 and a two-carbon atom side chain attached at the C-17 position

[a]The suffix -ene is currently used more often than Δ.
[b]Hypothetical parent compound.

TABLE 15.2 Systematic Names of Vertebrate Steroids

Class name	Trivial name	Systematic name
Glucocorticoids	Cortisol (hydrocortisone)	11 β,17 α,21-Trihydroxy-pregn-4-ene-3,20-dione
	Corticosterone	11 β,21-Dihydroxy-pregn-4-ene-3,20-dione
Mineralocorticoids	Aldosterone	11 β,21-Dihydroxy-pregn-4-ene-3,20-dione-18-al
	11-Deoxycorticosterone	21-Hydroxy-pregn-4-ene-3,20-dione
Androgenic steroids	Dehydroepiandrosterone	3 β-Hydroxy-androst-5-ene-17-one
	Testosterone	17 β-Hydroxy-androst-4-ene-3-one
Estrogenic steroids	Estradiol	1,3,5(10)-Estratriene-3,17 β-diol
Progestens	Pregnenolone	3 β-Hydroxy-pregn-5-ene-20-one
	Progesterone	Pregn-4-ene-3,20-dione

steroid nucleus is indicated by a β sign and a solid line (—OH), or an α sign and a dashed line (---OH). The latter designation indicates that the group projects below the plane of the steroid nucleus, while the former indicates that it is above. Cortisol, for example, has a Δ^4-3-keto configuration in the A ring and β- and α-hydroxyl groups at positions 11 and 17, respectively, of the molecule. Aldosterone is unique in having an aldehyde group at the 18 position of the molecule. The systemic names of some steroids are provided in Table 15.2.

The bulk of adrenal cholesterol is derived by uptake from plasma cholesterol rather than by intracellular synthesis as previously believed [4]. Low-density lipoproteins (LDLs) are the major cholesterol transport complexes in human plasma. Cholesterol esters, with triglycerides, are packaged into lipoprotein particles where they form a hydrophobic core surrounded by a monolayer of polar phospholipids and small amounts of proteins called *apolipoproteins.* The apolipoproteins bind to LDL receptors of adrenal target cells, which may stimulate endocytosis and the transport of the lipoproteins into the cells, an event enhanced by ACTH. Subsequent to receptor binding, the lipoproteins are internalized by receptor-mediated endocytosis and catabolized in lysosomes [22]. The number of LDL binding sites is highest in membranes of the adrenal cortex and ovarian corpus luteum, two tissues that synthesize steroids and therefore have a high requirement for cholesterol.

In 1973, studies with cultured human fibroblasts, by Brown, Goldstein, and colleagues [4] showed that receptor-mediated endocytosis of low-density lipoprotein (LDL) is the regulatory event in cellular cholesterol homeostasis. The complete sequence of metabolic events associated with the binding, uptake, and degradation of these cholesterol-rich lipoprotein particles by mammalian cells has been termed the "LDL receptor pathway" [4]. This important process supplies cells with cholesterol, thereby mediating the removal of cholesterol-rich lipoproteins from the circulation. Also, it protects cells from over-accumulation of cholesterol, because the cholesterol derived from lysosomal hydrolysis of LDL cholesterol esters exerts a series of feedback control mechanisms designed to maintain a constant level of cholesterol within the cell. Thus, high extracellular concentrations of LDL reduce cellular synthesis of cholesterol by suppression of the activities of 3 hydroxy-, 3-methyl-glutaryl-CoA synthase and reductase (rate limiting enzymes in cholesterol synthesis); stimulate its re-esterification; and decrease the number of LDL receptors, preventing further cellular entry of cholesterol [47].

A model for cholesterol homeostasis in the adrenal gland is presented in Fig. 15.5. In the basal state the amount of cholesterol delivered to the cell by LDLs is balanced by cholesterol conversion to steroid hormones that are then secreted. The metabolically active pool of free cholesterol is derived from LDL internalization, limited endogenous synthesis (through acetyl-CoA), and hydrolysis of cholesterol esters. In response to ACTH there is an enhancement of intracellular cholesterol synthesis as well as hydrolysis of cholesterol esters. Esterified cholesterol reserves are limited, and endogenous cholesterol synthesis apparently soon returns to basal levels; consequently, extracellular lipoproteins must provide the cholesterol for continued steroid hormone biosynthesis. This is apparently accomplished by an increase in the number of LDL receptors (Fig. 15.5).

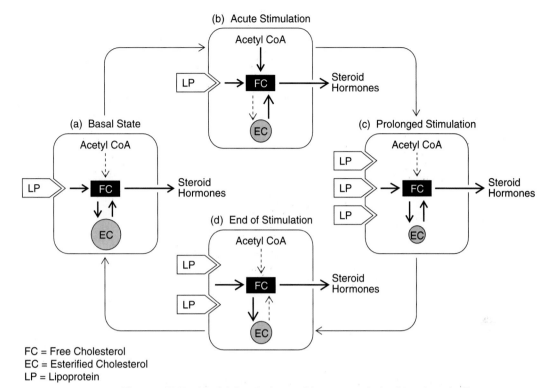

FC = Free Cholesterol
EC = Esterified Cholesterol
LP = Lipoprotein

Figure 15.5   Model for cholesterol homeostasis in the adrenal. (From Brown, Kovanen, and Goldstein [4], with permission.)

Functional Zonation of the Adrenal Cortex

In most mammals mineralocorticoids are produced in the zona glomerulosa, glucocorticoids in the zona fasciculata, and androgens in the zona reticularis. Functional separation of the zones was suggested when Greep and Deane [21] noted that the zona fasciculata may atrophy or become grossly hyperactive without any conspicuous alteration in the zona glomerulosa. These investigators also noted that, on a gross morphological basis, the gland could be separated into two zones, and they were the first to comment on the dual nature of the adrenal cortex control. The mammalian zona glomerulosa lacks a 17 α-hydroxylase and therefore synthesizes corticosterone, a glucocorticoid that does not contain a 17 α-hydroxyl group. Sequential actions by the enzymes 18-hydroxylase and 18-hydroxysteroid dehydrogenase convert corticosterone to aldosterone. The latter enzyme is found only in the glomerulosa. In humans and cattle 17-hydroxysteroids are produced by the zona fasciculata and zona reticularis [57].

CONTROL OF SYNTHESIS AND SECRETION

The biological roles of adrenal glucocorticoids and mineralocorticoids differ considerably. It is not unexpected, therefore, that the control of synthesis and secretion of these two classes of steroid hormones is also different. Adrenal glucocorticoid synthesis and secretion are controlled by pituitary adrenocorticotropin (ACTH), whereas aldosterone secretion is controlled primarily by the *renin-angiotensin system* [51].

Glucocorticoids

Glucocorticoid production by cells of the zona fasciculata is regulated by pituitary ACTH. The release of ACTH is in turn regulated by a hypothalamic corticotropin-releasing

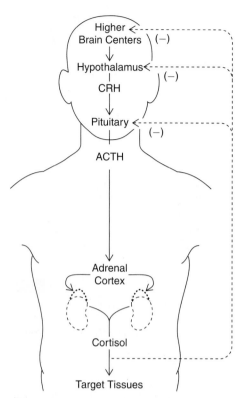

Figure 15.6 Brain-pituitary-adrenal axis.

hormone (CRH) as discussed in Chaps. 5 and 6. Unilateral adrenalectomy is followed by contralateral adrenal hypertrophy and hyperplasia. After bilateral adrenalectomy or in primary adrenal insufficiency (Addison's disease), there is a striking increase in plasma ACTH levels. These elevated levels of ACTH can be returned to normal by administration of glucocorticoids, demonstrating a negative feedback regulation of ACTH secretion by the steroids. Glucocorticoid negative feedback is mediated at the level of the pituitary, hypothalamus, and even higher brain centers (Fig. 15.6).

ACTH interacts with the plasmalemma of zona fasciculata cells to increase intracellular cAMP levels; activation of one or more protein kinases follows. During ACTH stimulation increased cAMP production precedes the steroidogenic event. Calcium is required for ACTH activation of adenylate cyclase, but not for binding of the peptide to adrenal cells. The effects of ACTH on adrenal fasciculata cell steroidogenesis are mimicked by methylxanthines and cAMP analogs, revealing that cAMP is the second messenger regulating ACTH action.

Incubation of primary cultures of human fetal adrenal cells with ACTH or cAMP results in an accumulation of IGF-II mRNA. The time-course and dose-response curves of IGF-II mRNA and P450scc mRNA accumulation rose in parallel. ACTH and other hormones exerted this action on IGF-II production in a strictly tissue-specific fashion: hCG did not affect adrenal cells, and ACTH, PRL, and GH did not affect the IGF-II or p450scc mRNAs in granulosa cells (see Chap. 18). The stimulation of IGF-II mRNA was not secondary to trophic hormone stimulation of steroidogenesis, as exogenously added steroid hormones did not affect IGF-II mRNA. These results suggest that the hypertrophy and hyperplasia of the adrenal seen in response to ACTH may be due to a direct stimulation of IGF-II, which then acts locally as an autocrine/paracrine growth factor (Fig. 15.7). When IGF-I or IGF-II is added to the culture medium, the responses of P450c17 and P450c21 mRNAs to ACTH were not altered compared to controls. By contrast, exogenously added IGF-I or -II significantly reduced the ACTH-stimulated accumulation of IGF-II mRNA in the same cells. This experiment supports the hypothesis that trophic hor-

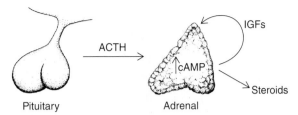

Figure 15.7   Model for the role of IGFs in the control of adrenal steroidogenesis.

mones stimulate adrenal growth via stimulation of IGF-II, which is autoregulated by short-loop feedback [51].

In humans there is a diurnal rhythm of ACTH and 17-hydroxycorticoid excretion (e.g., cortisol). The regularity of this rhythm appears to be a function of the sleep–wake habits of the individual. In those individuals who sleep regularly at the same hours each day, a sharp increase in ACTH-cortisol secretion occurs during the third to fifth hour of sleep and becomes maximal about an hour after awakening. Minimal levels of these hormones are reached a few hours before and after resumption of sleep. In humans this rhythm of activity is first established at about 3 months of postnatal life. The circadian rhythm has a cycle length of about 24 hours and cannot be synchronized with environmental lighting regimes. In a free-running environment with an absence of clues to the true local time, the rhythm persists but is slightly and consistently longer or shorter than 24 hours.

Aldosterone

Aldosterone secretion from the zona glomerulosa is mainly controlled by *angiotensin II* (AII, Ang II), an octapeptide that is derived from a decapeptide, angiotensin I, through the action of a *converting enzyme*. Angiotensin I (AI) is derived from a precursor protein, appropriately designated as *angiotensinogen* (or renin substrate), which originates in the liver. The conversion of angiotensinogen to AI results from the enzymatic action of an enzyme, *renin*, which is released from specialized granular cells, *juxtaglomerular (JG) cells*, in the afferent arteriole of the vascular pole of the renal glomerulus. The action of AII on adrenal glomerulosa cells is terminated by *angiotensinases,* which split the octapeptide into smaller inactive fragments (Fig. 15.8). Extrarenal sources of renin, *isorenins*, have been described (brain, uterus, adrenal glands), but their significance is undefined [46]. Angiotensin I converting enzyme has been localized to a variety of vascular beds. The presence of this enzyme in these vessels may be indicative of a functional role of angiotensins in the local control of blood flow. These extrarenal sites of angiotensin production make up so-called tissue angiotensinogenase systems [17, 23].

Renin is secreted in response to hypovolemia or to an increase in the osmolarity of the blood [24]. According to the *baroreceptor hypothesis*, the afferent arteriole

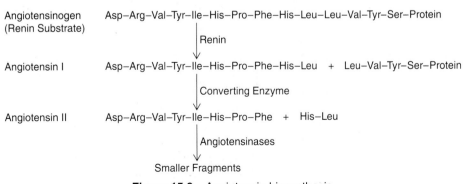

Figure 15.8   Angiotensin biosynthesis.

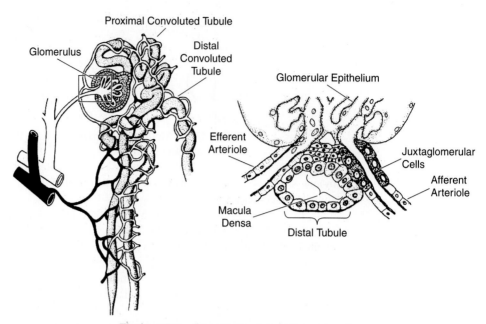

Figure 15.9   Renal juxtaglomerular apparatus.

responds to a change in mean renal perfusion pressure. These changes result in either a stretching or a decreased transmural (vessel-wall) pressure in the afferent arteriole, which results in an observable altered JG cell granularity (the granules being the cellular source of renin). In this theory the JG cells are modified smooth muscle cells and function as baroreceptors.

Another theory suggests that specialized cells of the distal tubular epithelium play a pivotal role in the control of renin release. These cells are in close apposition to the JG cells; they may function as chemoreceptors and monitor the urinary Na+ load within the distal tubule. According to the *macula densa theory*, this information is in some manner relayed to the JG cells where appropriate modifications of renin release take place. The renal functional unit of renin secretion, which consists of the macula densa cells and the JG cells, is referred to as the *juxtaglomerular apparatus* (Fig. 15.9).

Renin secretion is also regulated by the ANS. Renin release is increased in response to sympathetic nerve stimulation, and catecholamines stimulate renin release from kidney slices incubated in vitro. Norepinephrine released from sympathetic neurons acts on β-adrenoceptors of the JG cells, and the resulting increase in cAMP is the stimulus to vesicular exocytosis of the renin secretory granules.

Vascular smooth muscle contraction and the release of aldosterone from the adrenal gland were the first recognized biological actions of AII. Within the kidney AII is a vasoconstrictor. Both afferent and efferent arteriolar resistances are modulated by AII, and these actions influence glomerular filtration rate.

Removal of the N-terminal aspartic acid residue from AII gives rise to a heptapeptide referred to as angiotensin III. Although originally considered only a degradative product of AII metabolism, this peptide produces levels of aldosterone secretion in the rat similar to that of AII, but possesses very little pressor activity. It has been suggested, therefore, that AIII may serve as a specific hormone for aldosterone secretion. On the glomerulosa cell AIII is as potent as AII.

Recent investigations have focused on the possible role of an intra-adrenal renin-angiotensin system as an important regulator of aldosterone biosynthesis. As in many other tissues, renin, angiotensinogen, and AII have all been demonstrated in the adrenal gland, especially in the zona glomerulosa. Dietary modifications of both K+ loading and Na+ restriction increase adrenal renin content. Therefore the activity of the adrenal renin system may play a role in determining the stimulatory effects of these diets. It has been

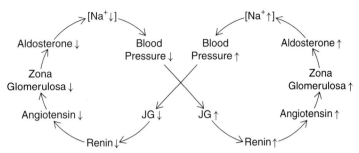

Figure 15.10 Renin-angiotensin system and Na$^+$ homeostasis. Arrows indicate increases ($\uparrow$) or decreases ($\downarrow$) in the factors indicated. (From Goss [20], with permission.)

shown that Na$^+$ restriction increases zona glomerulosa AII content but reduces the content of AI. This suggests that Na$^+$ restriction not only increases angiotensin generation, but also selectivity increases the conversion of AI to AII.

Aldosterone mediates its action at the level of the distal convoluted tubules and possibly, to a lesser degree, the cortical collecting tubules of the kidney [28]. Sodium resorption increases the osmolarity of the blood, which is monitored by the JG cells, and they respond by decreased renin secretion (Fig. 15.10). Increasing the plasma Na$^+$ concentration may be a direct inhibitory stimulus to further aldosterone secretion. In the absence of aldosterone, the ratio of K$^+$ to Na$^+$ increases; high K$^+$ is a direct stimulus to aldosterone secretion. Besides its action on the cells of the zona glomerulosa, AII stimulates vasoconstriction. This adaptive vasopressor response results in elevation of the blood pressure. Afferent sensory neurons respond to the vasoconstriction and, by a reflex mechanism, inhibit sympathetic stimulation of renin secretion.

Renal Kallikrein-Kinin System

Kinins are peptide hormones released from plasma protein precursors by plasma and tissue enzymes termed *kallikreins* [40]. The protein precursors are referred to as *kininogens*, and they serve as substrates for the enzymatic actions of the kallikreins, which may themselves become activated after they are enzymatically released from proenzymes referred to as *prekallikreins*. The kinins are subsequently inactivated by enzymes referred to as *kininases* (Fig. 15.11). Glandular kallikreins are a group of kinin-forming enzymes found in many glands such as the kidney. Glandular kallikreins from diverse tissues differ in primary structure. Activation of these enzymes (isozymes) and their subsequent activation of kininogens may provide a mechanism for the local production of kinins. Within the kidney kallikrein activation leads to the production of a decapeptide, *lysylbradykinin* (Lys-Arg-Pro-Pro-Gly-Phe-Ser-Pro-Phe-Arg), which is then converted (apparently by an angiotensinase) to the nonapeptide *bradykinin* by the removal of the terminal lysine.

In the kidney, renin is derived from an inactive zymogen precursor, a prorenin [30, 39]. There is evidence that renal kallikrein is responsible for the enzymatic activation of

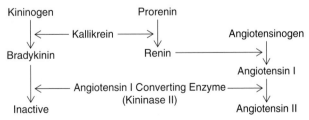

Figure 15.11 Kallikrein role in renin activation and bradykinin production. (From Inagami and Murakami [30], with permission.)

renin from prorenin, in addition to its role in the activation of a kininogen to bradykinin [48]. Most interesting is the discovery that the AI-converting enzyme is apparently identical to kininase II. Thus this enzyme is responsible for the conversion of AI to its active form, AII, as well as the conversion of bradykinin to inactive fragments (Fig. 15.11).

It is interesting that renal kallikrein participates in the activation of two peptides that have vasoactive actions. Angiotensin II can be considered a systemic vasoconstrictor whose direct actions on the arterial tree elevate blood pressure. Within the kidney, on the other hand, bradykinin may function as a localized vascular smooth muscle relaxant. It has been suggested that the concurrent release of two enzymes that produce peptides with diametrically opposing actions would seem counterproductive. However, it would be important that maintenance of blood pressure via constriction does not occur at the expense of renal blood flow. The role of bradykinin would be confined to the renal vascular bed so that kidney perfusion is protected. Thus this dual system would function to maintain a normal renal blood flow and at the same time increase systemic pressure [48].

Within the kidney kallikrein is localized to the basal membrane of the epithelial cells of the distal tubules. There is evidence that aldosterone increases kallikrein excretion in humans and other animals and also enhances renin activity. A stimulus may be required to release prorenin so that it can be acted on by kallikrein. There is strong evidence that bradykinin mediates its renal vasodepressor action through activation of one or more E-series prostaglandins. Bradykinin also increases the concentration of PG-like substances in the renal venous blood. PGs released from renal tissues may therefore participate in the regulation of renin release. Prostacyclin I_2 (PGI$_2$) appears to be the arachidonic acid product that is responsible for renin release. It is possible that the roles of PGE$_2$ and PGI$_2$ vary in different compartments of the kidney. A summary scheme of the possible relationships of aldosterone and the renal kallikrein-bradykinin system to renin production is shown (Fig. 15.12).

Atrial Natriuretic Factor (ANF)

A number of early experimental observations suggested that variations in glomerular filtration rate and aldosterone secretion were insufficient to fully account for renal responses to volume expansion. It was therefore postulated that a humoral substance regulated volume overload by inhibiting reabsorption by the renal tubules, thereby promoting diuresis and natriuresis. There is now evidence that a hormone released by the atria of the heart may mediate some of the physiological responses to volume expansion [6, 56].

This *atrial natriuretic factor* (ANF), also known as atriopeptin, was localized (as its name implies) to the atria [8, 9]. Atrial cardiocytes contain granular inclusions that are the source of ANF. Injections of atrial, but not ventricular, extracts induce a rapid diuresis and

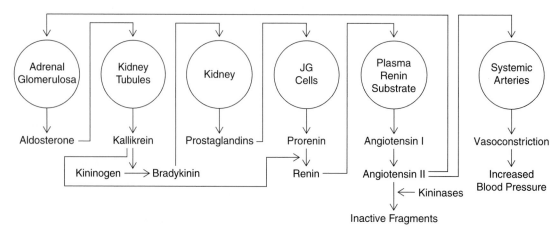

Figure 15.12 Summary scheme of the role of aldosterone in renal renin production.

Amino Acid Sequence of Human ANF Prohormone

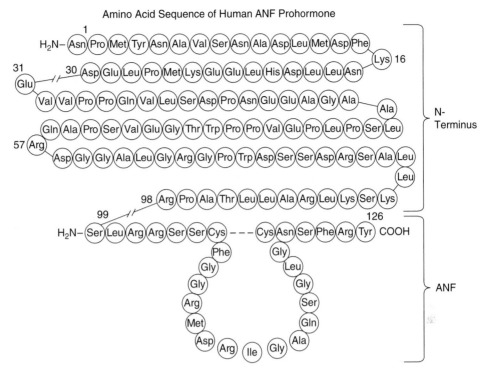

Figure 15.13   Primary structure of atrial natriuretic factor (ANF). (From Vesely [56], with permission.)

natriuresis in experimental animals. Immunohistochemical studies using antibodies to the peptide have localized the hormone to the granules of atrial myocytes. The ventricles as well as the atria of nonmammalian vertebrates contain secretory granules, suggesting that a restriction of the hormone to the atria is a more recent evolutionary acquisition.

ANF is a peptide composed of 28 amino acids and is derived from a 126-amino-acid precursor (pro-ANF) (Fig. 15.13). Most interesting is the observation that proANF gives rise to three structurally unrelated fragments that all exhibit ANF activity to varying degrees [56]. ANF affects diuresis and natriuresis by several physiological actions:

1. it inhibits aldosterone production by the adrenal glomerulosa cells;
2. it inhibits the release of renin (which indirectly stimulates aldosterone secretion);
3. it inhibits vasopressin secretion from the pituitary, as well as the action of vasopressin at the level of the kidney; and
4. it causes relaxation of blood vessels (possibly by antagonizing the vasoconstrictor actions of AII).

All these ANF actions effectively reduce the retention of Na^+ and water, and therefore decrease volume expansion (Fig. 15.14).

In addition ANF may have a central role in suppression of fluid and salt intake (drinking and salt appetite, respectively) and of vasopressin secretion, actions that again would result in processes leading to reduction in body salt and fluid levels and peripheral blood pressure. Conversely, ANF levels (in dogs) are reduced during hypotension due to hemorrhage, thus protecting the hypovolemic organism from further volume loss. Thus ANF contributes to the re-establishment of intravascular volume homeostasis in states of acute volume overload or depletion (Fig. 15.15). It has been shown that ANF has biological effects in humans at physiological plasma homeostatic concentrations.

Although some experimental evidence is consistent with the concept that ANF is an important physiological regulator of renal Na^+ excretion, this hypothesis remains unproven

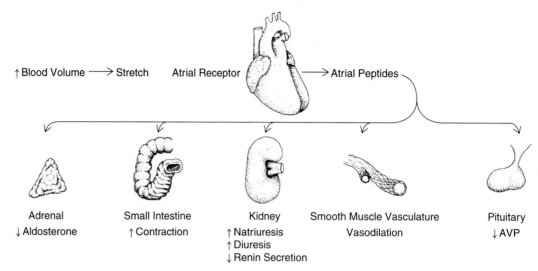

Figure 15.14   Biological roles of ANF. (Revised from Vesely [56].)

[1]. Evidence also suggests that ANF does not contribute to the process that elicits a postprandial natriuresis, a process that presumably is of primary importance in the physiological regulation of Na^+ balance. A number of common physiological, experimental, and pathophysiological conditions reveal that circulating ANF does not correlate with renal Na^+ excretion. This lack of correlation may suggest that systemic ANF is not an important regulator of Na^+ excretion in these situations [19]. Evidence that the kidneys produce their own natriuretic peptide may partly explain why investigations of the effects of endogenous ANF on renal Na^+ excretion often have yielded inconsistent results. This inconsistency has led to a gradual evolution of opinion concerning the functional role of ANF. Based on current data, it is postulated that ANF is primarily a regulator of the cardiovascular system and that renal natriuretic peptide (urodilatin?) participates locally in the intrarenal regulation of Na^+ and chloride transport [19].

ANP was the first described member of a family of polypeptide hormones that regulates salt and water balance and blood pressure. Subsequent to the isolation and characterization of ANP, two related hormones have been described: BNP, isolated from both brain and heart; and CNP, purified from porcine brain. Like ANP, both of these hormones can elicit vasorelaxant, natriuretic, and diuretic responses in bioassay systems. These natriuretic peptides share a common structural motif consisting of a 17-amino acid loop formed by an intramolecular disulfide linkage. Only 5 of the 17 amino acids in the ring

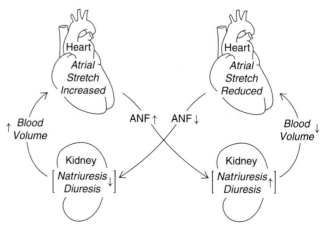

Figure 15.15   The role of atrial natriuretic factor (ANF) in blood volume homeostasis.

differ among the three peptides isolated from the pig, whereas the NH$_2$- and COOH-terminals vary in both amino acid composition and length. Among different species, the structures of both ANP and CNP are highly conserved, whereas the amino acid sequence of BNP varies as much as 50% [34]. The physiological significance of these ANF-related peptides remains to be determined.

CIRCULATION AND METABOLISM

Steroid hormones are only sparingly soluble in water, and most are transported to their target tissues by plasma proteins. Within the plasma, cortisol is reversibly bound to two proteins, *transcortin* or *corticosteroid-binding globulin* (CBG) and, to a lesser extent, an α-2 globulin. About 6% of cortisol is unbound, and it is this pool that apparently represents the hormone available for uptake by target tissues ("free hormone hypothesis"). The bound cortisol provides a larger buffer pool of the corticosteroid that can be made immediately available as the free cortisol [25].

More than 50% of circulating aldosterone is unbound. The biological half-life of cortisol in the human is about 80 minutes, whereas the half-life of aldosterone is about 30 minutes. The short half-life of aldosterone may be because most aldosterone circulates in an unbound form and is therefore readily available for metabolism and excretion. Metabolism of adrenal steroids occurs primarily in the liver, where side-chain and A-ring reductions take place. Structurally altered steroids are then conjugated to glucuronic acid or sulfates to form water-soluble derivatives [26]. One pathway of cortisol metabolism is shown in Fig. 15.16.

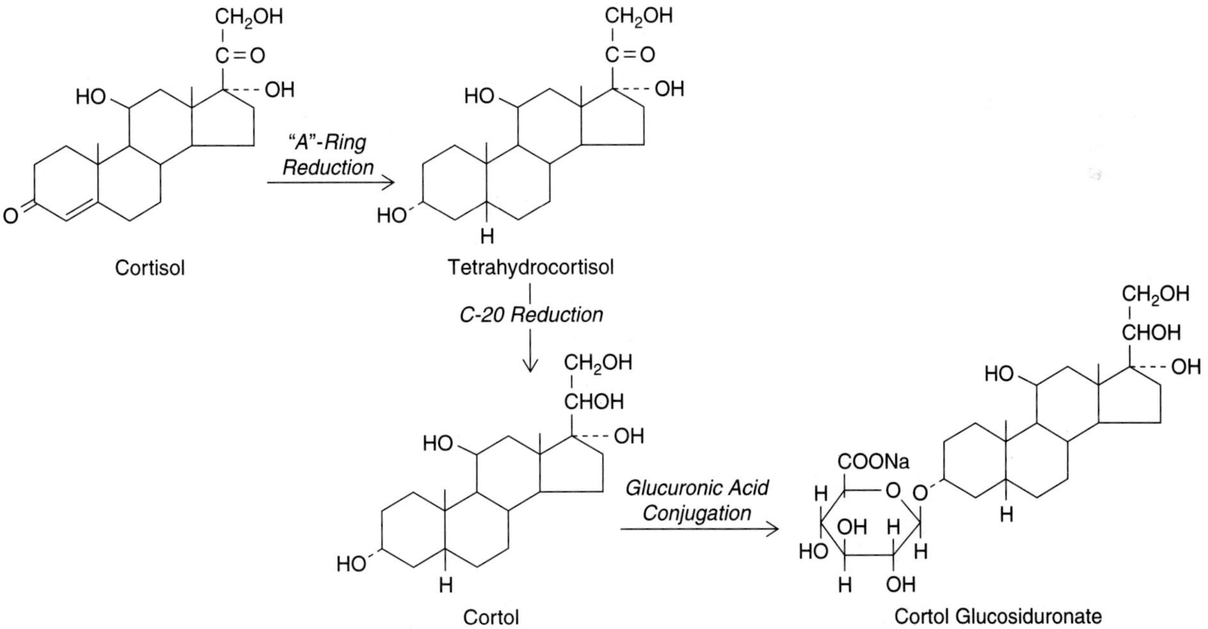

Figure 15.16 One pathway of cortisol metabolism and glucuronide formation.

PHYSIOLOGICAL ROLES

In humans the biological roles of cortisol and aldosterone, the major glucocorticoid and mineralocorticoid, respectively, are quite different. In pathophysiological states of cortisol hypersecretion (Cushing's disease) or aldosterone hypersecretion (Conn's disease),

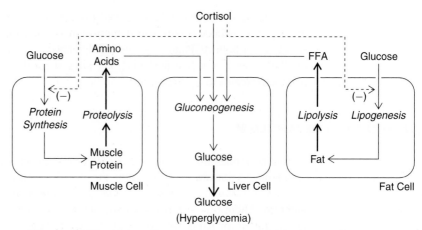

Figure 15.17   Major effects of excess cortisol in intermediary metabolism.

each hormone may, however, exhibit both glucocorticoid and mineralocorticoid activity because they share structural similarities.

Glucocorticoids

Intermediary Metabolism.   Glucocorticoids affect carbohydrate, lipid, and protein metabolism. They increase synthesis of a number of key enzymes in the gluconeogenic pathway within hepatocytes. Although the actions of glucocorticoids on the liver are anabolic, the actions on skeletal muscle and adipose tissue are catabolic. Catabolic actions may result because glucose uptake by these tissues is inhibited by glucocorticoids. In the absence of a metabolic substrate for ATP production, proteolysis of muscle proteins and lipolysis of fat occur. The FFAs and amino acids that are released from these tissues become available as substrates for gluconeogenesis within the liver (Fig. 15.17). The glucose produced is either stored as glycogen or released into the blood. Excessive secretion of glucocorticoids is antagonistic to the actions of insulin and predisposes the individual to diabetes mellitus as the actions of glucocorticoids elevate blood glucose levels. Glucocorticoids also reduce the affinity of certain cells for insulin, which further aggravates the diabetic hyperglycemia.

Permissive Actions.   Most, if not all, effects of glucocorticoids may be considered permissive to the actions of other hormones. In particular, glucocorticoids are required for functioning of the sympathoadrenal system. Under conditions of stress, and in the absence of glucocorticoids, there is vascular collapse, which usually leads to death. Glucocorticoids are necessary for catecholamine synthesis within sympathetic nerve terminals and for the process of catecholamine reuptake from the synaptic cleft; they may also decrease the rate of catecholamine degradation by COMT. Evidence for these statements includes a diminished sympathoadrenal activity in the absence of glucocorticoids. Fat mobilization in response to catecholamines is impaired after hypophysectomy but is corrected by treatment with ACTH or glucocorticoids. Glucocorticoids themselves have little, if any, fat-mobilizing activity, but they apparently maintain levels of lipolytic enzymes that are activated through the actions of catecholamines. Hypothermia usually follows adrenalectomy, and adrenalectomized animals soon die under conditions of cold stress. Glucocorticoids maintain body temperature in homeotherms through their permissive actions on liver gluconeogenesis and adipose tissue metabolism.

Role in Reproduction.   In sheep and other domestic animals the pituitary-adrenal axis is clearly involved in the process of parturition. Plasma levels of corticosterone increase in fetal sheep several days before birth, and infusions of ACTH or dexamethasone induce premature parturition. The fetal adrenal is relatively unresponsive to ACTH until 7 to 9 days before term, but no adequate explanation is available as to why adrenal sensitivity to ACTH changes just prior to parturition (see Chap. 19). Cortisol and prolactin are the principal hormones required for lactogenesis in the mouse mammary gland. In mammary tissue the actions of cortisol are expressed through a specific glucocorticoid receptor. There is about an 85% decrease in the level of casein mRNA after adrenalectomy. A single injection of cortisol can then cause an increase in casein mRNA to a level above that of the adrenalectomized animal.

Nervous System Effects.   Neonatal administration of corticosterone can reduce both the basal level and amplitude of the diurnal rhythm of plasma corticosterone in the adult rat, depending on the age at which exposure to the steroid occurs. This suggests that, as for gonadal steroids, adrenal steroids of fetal or maternal origin may play an important role in early "imprinting" of the CNS (Chap. 16). It is also possible that the presence of maternal steroids in excessive concentrations adversely affect the normal development of the fetal nervous system and thus contribute to birth defects.

Certain hormones influence the survival of neurons in the developing brain and are necessary for maintenance of the structural integrity of the mature brain. The hippocampus, a brain region involved in learning, memory, and a number of neurological disease states, is a target of adrenal steroids and is thought to play a role in the endocrine functions of the adrenal-hypothalamic-pituitary axis. Adrenalectomy of adult male rats results in a nearly complete loss of hippocampal granule cells by 3 to 4 months after surgery. Granule cell loss is selective; that is, there is no apparent loss of hippocampal pyramidal cells or of several types of hippocampal interneurons. The hippocampal CA1 pyramidal cells of adrenalectomized animals exhibit normal electrophysiological responses to afferent stimulation, whereas responses evoked in the dentate gyrus are severely attenuated. Corticosterone replacement prevents both the adrenalectomy-induced granule cell loss and the attenuated physiological response. Thus the adrenal glands play a role in maintaining the structural and functional integrity of the normal adult brain [52].

Steroids can rapidly alter neuronal function and behavior through poorly characterized, direct actions on neuronal membranes. In the classic model of steroid hormone action, steroids bind to intracellular receptors, which act as ligand-dependent transcription factors that regulate gene expression. Steroids may also alter brain functions through nongenomic mechanisms. For example, in rats, short-term exposure to progesterone is associated with rapid changes in behavior, and this effect occurs in the absence of new protein synthesis. Gonadal and adrenal steroid hormones can alter neuronal firing activity within milliseconds to minutes of administration; these responses can occur in brain regions lacking classic steroid receptors or if steroid access to intracellular receptors is blocked. These events appear to be mediated by direct steroid action on neuronal membranes, but there is little information concerning steroid binding to membrane-bound recognition sites in the brain [41].

Anti-inflammatory and Immunosuppressive Actions of Glucocorticoids.   At higher than physiological concentrations, as in Cushing's disease, glucocorticoids inhibit inflammatory and allergic reactions. These actions may result from stabilization of lysosomal membranes that prevents the secretion of enzymes that normally occurs during inflammation. Glucocorticoids inhibit the infiltration of leukocytes into the affected tissue and also exert an immunosuppressive action through their lympholytic actions.

In addition to the catabolic actions of glucocorticoids on muscle tissue and the protein matrix of bone, glucocorticoids cause atrophy of the lymphatic system (lymph nodes, thymus gland, spleen), which results in decreased levels of circulating lymphocytes. Ultimately, this lymphocytopenia results in failure of the body to provide antibodies during an infection. Although glucocorticoids may be useful in combating the undesirable effects of local infections, excessive use of these agents may render the individual susceptible to severe systematic bacterial infection as many protective mechanisms are suppressed, but the underlying cause of the disease remains.

IL-1, a member of a family of polypeptides produced by activated monocytes and other cells, has an important role, not only in stimulating the immune cells, but also in eliciting a variety of physiological reactions observed during infection, inflammation, and injury. Stimulation of ACTH release may be one of these important nonimmune responses that can be induced by the monokine. Stimulation of ACTH release induced by IL-1β may contribute to a homeostatic regulation of the immune function. Increased hypothalamo-pituitary-adrenal activity results in an increased secretion of glucocorticoids that suppress immune responses, and thereby unfavorable overstimulation of the immune reaction, during infection or other conditions. Increased secretion of glucocorticoids could represent a way for the body's natural defense mechanism to control or remedy undesirable symptoms and conditions, such as arthritis, induced by increased production of IL-1β as observed in various infections, such as Lyme disease. These findings suggest that IL-1 may play an important role as a carrier of messages from the immune system to the neuroendocrine system. Numerous other data indicate that there is bidirectional communication between the immune system and the neuroendocrine system.

Glucocorticoids and the General Adaptation Syndrome.   In 1936 Selye published the paper "A Syndrome Produced by Diverse Nocuous Agents." This syndrome was later referred to as the general adaptation syndrome or GAS. In response to stress a body responds in a stereotypic manner, which, if the stress is prolonged, may proceed through a number of stages: (1) an initial *alarm reaction;* (2) *resistance;* and eventually (3) *exhaustion* [49]. These stages may be characterized more precisely if one understands the underlying physiological processes involved in the adaptation syndrome.

In response to stress the sympathoadrenal system is activated (Chap. 14). Through the actions of epinephrine released from the adrenal chromaffin tissue and norepinephrine released from sympathetic nerve endings, the general body metabolic and motor activity is increased (alarm reaction). The basal metabolic rate is elevated and blood flow is increased, particularly to those organs that are more physiologically active. A major effect of circulating catecholamines is the utilization of liver glycogen stores for the production of glucose. This depot source of readily available carbohydrate, though limited, may be sufficient for an immediate stress (alarm) response.

The release of adrenal glucocorticoids is also activated in response to stress. Through the permissive actions of these hormones there is an enhancement of sympathoadrenal activity. In fact, in the absence of adrenal steroids, sympathoadrenal actions are generally depressed, which may lead to the individual's demise. Glucocorticoids enhance the lipolytic actions of catecholamines on adipose tissue. The FFAs released from fat cells provide metabolic substrates necessary for survival in the absence of hepatic glycogen stores. Hepatic glycogen depots are also restored through gluconeogenesis resulting from FAA utilization. The actions of glucocorticoids are slower than the initial rapid actions of catecholamines on metabolic processes, but they provide the secondary response (resistance) necessary for continued sympathoadrenal activity and hepatic gluconeogenesis.

Under prolonged conditions of stress the individual enters the third stage of the adaptation syndrome, exhaustion. In effect, the prolonged hypercortisolism eventually leads to muscle wasting, hyperglycemia (diabetes mellitus), atrophy of the immune system, vascular derangements, gastrointestinal ulceration, and other symptoms of excessive sympathoadrenal activity.

Adrenal Hormones and Self-Regulation of Mammalian Populations.   Within natural populations of animals adrenal hormones may play an important role in the control of population density. Some mammalian populations establish social hierarchies where there is a dominant animal, a second-ranking animal, and so on, to the lowest-ranking animal that is subordinate to all others [7]. Adrenocortical morphology and function (corticosterone output) are negatively related to social rank or dominance in these populations. In subordinate animals adrenal hypertrophy is followed by thymic involution, diminished resistance to disease, and many symptoms related to excessive glucocorticoid and sympathoadrenal activity. Increases in population density also enhance the number of encounters between members of a group that can lead to further subordination of the less dominant individuals. Increased mortality follows, as well as diminished reproductive capacity. Therefore, the ultimate effect of increased population density is, through the actions of adrenal hormones, to inhibit recruitment of new individuals into the population and thus to maintain the population at a level below that which might exhaust environmental resources [7].

It is clear that adrenal steroid hormones are essential for survival under stress. Continued stress eventually leads to gross pathophysiological alterations of bodily processes due to prolonged excessive actions of adrenal hormones. A little stress may be of adaptive necessity; too much, however, may be disastrous.

Aldosterone

Aldosterone's major role is to regulate Na^+ homeostasis and, indirectly, volume homeostasis by influencing water reabsorption from the nephron. Like parathormone, which also regulates blood electrolyte (Ca^{2+}) composition, aldosterone is essential for life.

Sodium/Potassium Homeostasis. Aldosterone accelerates the reabsorption of Na^+ by the kidney distal and cortical collecting tubules, salivary and sweat glands, and GI mucosa. Through its major action on renal tubular Na^+ retention aldosterone also profoundly affects the plasma concentration of K^+ and hydrogen ions. In the nephron the uptake of Na^+ in response to aldosterone is usually balanced by a concomitant loss of K^+ (Fig. 15.18). Under conditions of plasma K^+ deficiency (hypokalemia) there is an increase in distal tubular H^+ secretion, whereas during states of K^+ excess distal tubular secretion of K^+ is enhanced. One of the important elements in acclimatization to heat is the ability of an animal to reduce the amount of Na^+ in sweat. Injections of a mineralocorticoid into an individual not exposed to heat produce a drop in the Na^+ content of sweat within 2 to 3 days. These observations suggest that the Na^+ concentration of sweat is regulated in the human by aldosterone. High affinity sites for aldosterone have been identified in the rat

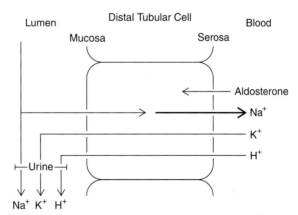

Figure 15.18 Physiological effects of aldosterone on renal distal tubular NA$^+$ resorption and K$^+$ and H$^+$ excretion. In response to aldosterone, sodium is actively transported across the tubular serosal membrane into the peritubular space. Potassium and hydrogen ions are passively shunted across the mucosal membrane in exchange for sodium.

brain. These receptors may represent extrarenal sites of aldosterone action, and one of these may affect salt intake (see Chap. 20).

Adrenal Androgens

The production of androgens by the adrenal is minimal compared to the production of these hormones by the gonads. In the female, adrenal androgens may contribute to pubertal changes (adrenarche), and postmenopausally these androgens may serve as substrates for extragonadal estrogen production. Abnormal adrenal steroid production, due to a defect in the normal steroidogenic pathway or to a tumorous condition, has profound morphogenetic consequences, particularly in the pregnant female. There is evidence that adrenal steroids may help support growth of mammary and prostatic carcinomas. Regression of steroid-dependent tumors, although accelerated after gonadectomy, is further enhanced by adrenalectomy.

MECHANISMS OF ACTION

Adrenal steroid hormones, like other steroid hormones, mediate their actions through a genomic mechanism.

Glucocorticoids

Glucocorticoids regulate the activity of a variety of tissues. Most actions involve de novo synthesis of cellular proteins, most often enzymes. In addition glucocorticoids, as well as other steroid hormones, enhance guanylate cyclase activity at physiological concentrations in a variety of tissues. Glucocorticoids also inhibit prostaglandin synthesis possibly by an inhibition of phospholipase A_2 activity. One mechanism of glucocorticoid action may be to modulate the number of cell membrane receptors for hormones.

Enzyme Induction. Glucocorticoids increase the activity of a number of enzymes. This action could come about either by controlling the number of mRNA templates for enzyme synthesis or by changing the translational efficiency of a fixed level of mRNA. There is evidence that glucocorticoids stimulate the de novo synthesis of mRNA; thus glucocorticoids stimulate both transcriptional and translational processes related to protein synthesis. Many of these enzymes, such as hepatic tyrosine amino transferase, play important roles in the anabolic actions of steroid hormones. A majority of the actions of cortisol are, however, catabolic in nature.

Glucocorticoid Receptors. Glucocorticoids exert their effects on target tissues though intracellular receptors that are hormone-dependent transcription factors. In cells the unliganded receptors are present as heteromeric structures consisting of a pair of steroid-binding proteins attached to a heat-shock protein. On hormone binding they are rapidly activated to a DNA-binding form by a process known as "activation" or "transformation" that involves dissociation of the subunits (see Chap. 4). The activated hormone-receptor complexes translocate to the nucleus, where they are thought to associate as dimers with hormone response elements in the DNA through which they activate or repress regulated genes [42].

Glucocorticoid Resistance. The essential nature of the glucocorticoid receptor in mediating the physiologic effects of glucocorticoid hormones is underscored by the clinical abnormalities that result from receptor deficiency or receptor defects. A rare familial syndrome has been described in which primary cortisol resistance is caused by a glucocorticoid receptor present at normal concentration, but with decreased affinity for cortisol. The syndrome is characterized by hypercortisolism without the features of Cushing's syndrome. In the affected patients, compensatory production of adrenocorticotropic hormone may cause hyperpigmentation, hypertension, hypokalemia, and precocious puberty.

Aldosterone

Both the kidney and the (toad) urinary bladder have been used extensively for studies on the mechanism of aldosterone action. Aldosterone increases the rate of Na^+ transport across epithelial cells of these organs. This movement of Na^+ is generally viewed as a two-step process: (1) there is entry of Na^+ from the fluid bathing the mucosal surface of the cell; and (2) there is subsequent extrusion of Na^+ through the serosal membrane into the interstitial space (Fig. 15.18). Numerous experiments have been directed toward determining which step in the transport process is stimulated by aldosterone.

Aldosterone mediates its action through the induction of the synthesis of proteins within target tissues. Three different mechanisms have been postulated by which these hormone-inducible proteins augment transepithelial Na^+ transport (Fig. 15.19). The sodium pump theory postulates that these proteins directly stimulate the activity of a sodium pump that is localized in the serosal side of the cell. The metabolic theory suggests that the aldosterone-inducible proteins increase the supply of ATP to the pump. In the permease theory these proteins enhance the permeability of the luminal mucosal membrane to Na^+. Experimental evidence strongly supports the view that both the passive apical entry of Na^+ and the active extrusion of Na^+ across the basal-lateral serosal membranes depend on the induction of enzymes that modulate energy metabolism. Aldosterone also stimulates fatty acid synthesis and the turnover of membrane phospholipid fatty acids in the toad bladder. Aldosterone alteration of the lipid composition of membranes may be an important component of its action mechanism.

Vasopressin (AVP) also increases the rate of Na^+ transport and the permeability to water of the urinary bladder of the toad, two responses mediated through cAMP (see Chap. 7). Although aldosterone stimulates Na^+ transport in these tissues, it does so without affecting permeability to water. Aldosterone stimulation of Na^+ transport does not involve cAMP production, but it enhances cAMP-induced Na^+ transport and water permeability. The action of the steroid may involve the inhibition of the degradation of

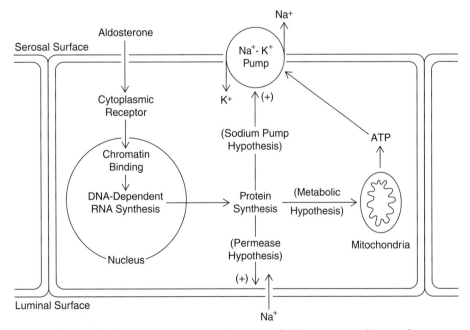

Figure 15.19 Hypothetical mechanisms of aldosterone action on the kidney.

cAMP, as suggested by the following observations. In response to AVP or theophylline, cAMP levels are higher in aldosterone-treated tissues, and the activity of cyclic nucleotide phosphodiesterase, the enzyme that catalyzes the degradation of cAMP, is depressed.

Mineralocorticoid Receptors. Mineralocorticoid receptors, from tissue extracts and when recombinant-derived, have equal affinity for the physiological mineralocorticoid aldosterone and for the glucocorticoids, cortisol and corticosterone, which circulate at much higher concentrations than aldosterone [44]. Such receptors are found in mineralocorticoid target tissues (kidney, parotid, and colon) and in nontarget tissues, such as hippocampus and heart. Given this equal receptor affinity and the much higher circulating levels of cortisol or corticosterone than aldosterone, additional mechanisms must operate to allow selective mineralocorticoid action in mineralocorticoid target tissues. In mineralocorticoid target tissues the receptors are selective for aldosterone in vivo because of the presence of the enzyme 11 β-hydroxysteroid dehydrogenase, which converts cortisol and corticosterone, but not aldosterone, to their 11-keto analogs. These analogs cannot bind to mineralocorticoid receptors [13, 14, 15].

Angiotensin II

The recent availability of pure AII antagonists has established that there are at least two types of angiotensin receptors, now referred to as AT_1 and AT_2 subtypes [53, 58]. The cardiovascular effects of AII are mediated by the AT_1, receptor subtype and include the following actions: aldosterone secretion from the adrenal, pressor and tachycardiac (increased heart beat) responses, increased water intake (polydipsia), and contraction of certain vascular smooth muscles. The role(s) of the AT_2 receptor subtype remains to be defined. The rat AII receptor, AT_1, has been cloned. As for many other peptide hormones, seven hydrophobic domains are postulated to transverse the cell membrane [2, 3]. Numerous second messengers have been implicated in the actions of AII as depicted in Fig. 15.20.

PATHOPHYSIOLOGY

The clinical manifestations of abnormal levels of adrenal glucocorticoids or mineralocorticoids in humans are predictable from an understanding of the biological actions of these corticosteroids (Table 5.3). A total loss of adrenal function may derive from a congenital developmental defect or adrenal destruction during a particular disease state (e.g., tuberculosis). The adrenal abnormality may be of primary origin and involve a failure of glucocorticoid or mineralocorticoid biosynthesis due to a genetic defect related to an absence or faulty structure of a particular enzyme. Overproduction of a particular corticoid may be due to an adrenocortical adenoma or carcinoma, resulting in excess cortisol (Cushing's syndrome) or, as in primary aldosteronism, in excess aldosterone secretion (Conn's disease). Hyposecretion or hypersecretion of adrenal steroids may be of secondary origin and involve a defect in mechanisms involved in the control of cortisol or aldosterone secretion (Fig. 15.21).

Disorders of Cortisol Secretion

Addison's Disease. In a manuscript published in 1855, "On the Constitutional and Local Effects of Disease of the Supra-Renal Capsules," Addison provided the classical description of the disease that bears his name. The disease may be of primary origin and involve total destruction of the glands ("primary adrenocortical failure"). Most often the etiology is due to bilateral tubercular destruction of the glands. Atrophy due to

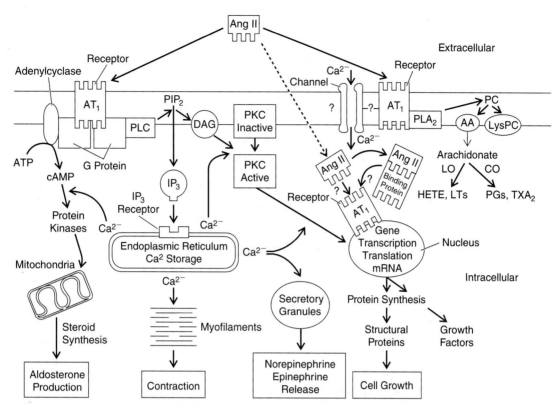

Figure 15.20   All receptor-cellular response coupling. PLC, phospholipase C; DAG, diacylglycerol; IP$_3$, inositol triphosphate; G protein, guanosine triphosphate-binding protein; PKC, protein kinase C; AA, arachidonic acid; PC, phosphatidylcholine; LysPC, lysophosphatidylcholine; LO, lipoxygenase; CO, cyclooxygenase; HETE, hydroxyeicostatetraenoic acid; TXA$_2$, thromboxane A$_2$; PGs, prostaglandins (e.g., prostaglandin E$_2$); channel; calcium channel; PIP$_2$, phosphatidylinositol diphosphate; LTs, leukotrienes. (From Timmermans et al. 1993. "Angiotensin II receptors and angiotensin II receptor antagonists." *Pharmacological Res.* 45:205–51, used by permission.)

tuberculosis involves the medulla as well as the cortex, whereas in idiopathic (unknown cause) atrophy usually only the cortex is affected. The most frequent symptoms of Addison's disease include weakness, increased melanin pigmentation of the skin, weight loss, hypotension, salt craving, and hypoglycemia. These symptoms result from a combination of both glucocorticoid and mineralocorticoid deficiencies. The increased integumental pigmentation, a cardinal symptom of the disease, is because in the absence of cortisol feedback to the hypothalamus, excessive amounts of ACTH are secreted. Because nearly the complete structure of α-MSH is contained within the ACTH molecule (see Fig. 8.1), it is probable that ACTH acts on integumental melanocytes to increase melanin production of the skin. In Addison's disease of secondary or tertiary origin the defect may reside at the level of the pituitary or hypothalamus, respectively. A failure of the hypothalamus to secrete CRH or the absence of functional pituitary corticotrophs could explain the etiology of some forms of adrenal insufficiency (Fig. 15.21).

Cushing's Syndrome.   This disease, first described by Cushing in 1932, refers to any clinical entity due to excessive and prolonged secretion and action of glucocorticoids, although the cause of the disease may relate to any one of a number of origins. Primary hypercortisolism may be due to an adrenal cortical tumor (adenoma or carcinoma). Cushing's disease of secondary origin may derive from a pituitary tumor secreting an excess of

TABLE 15.3 Endocrine Pathophysiology of the Adrenal Cortex

Adrenocortical Hypofunction
  Addisons disease
    Primary adrenocortical insufficiency
    Secondary adrenocortical insufficiency
      Pituitary origin (no ACTH secretion)
      Hypothalamic origin (no CRH secretion?)
  Hypoaldosteronism
    Primary (adrenocortical insufficiency)
    Secondary
      Hyporeninemic hypoaldosteronism
Adrenocortical Hyperfunction
  Syndromes of excess cortisol secretion (Cushings disease)
    Cushings syndrome (primary origin)
      Adrenal adenoma or adenocarcinoma
    Cushings syndrome (secondary origin)
      Bilateral adrenal hyperplasia
        Pituitary origin (microadenoma-secreting ACTH, Nelsons Syndrome)
        Hypothalamic origin
        Ectopic ACTH syndrome
  Syndromes of excess aldosterone secretion
    Primary hyperaldosteronism, Conns syndrome (adrenal adenoma, aldosteronoma)
    Secondary hyperaldosteronism
      Bartters syndrome (hyperreninism)
      Malignant hypertension (due to decreased renal perfusion pressure)
      Renin-secreting tumor
      Glucocorticoid-suppressible aldosteronism (GSA)
  Syndromes of excess adrenal androgen secretion (virilizing adrenal tumors)
    Male (precocious pseudopuberty in the preadolescent boy)
    Female (masculinization)
  Syndromes of excess estrogen production (feminizing adrenal tumor)
    Male (gynecomastia)
    Female (precocious puberty in the preadolescent girl)
Adrenal Enzyme Deficiency Syndromes
  Congenital (lipoid) adrenal hyperplasia (fatal)
  Congenital virilizing adrenal hyperplasia
    3 β-Dehydrogenase deficiency
    11 β-Hydroxylase deficiency (hypertensive form)
    21 β-Hydroxylase deficiency (salt-losing form)
  Congenital 17 α-hydroxylase deficiency
  Corticosterone methyl oxidase (type II) deficiency (hypoaldosteronism)
  Syndrome of apparent mineralocorticoid excess

ACTH, or to ectopic ACTH production, or to pituitary corticotroph hyperplasia. The simultaneous measurement of plasma ACTH and cortisol is useful in differentiating between adrenal hyperplasia (due to excess pituitary ACTH stimulation) and adrenal tumors as the cause of Cushing's syndrome. In patients with adrenal tumors plasma cortisol levels are high but the concentration of ACTH is low or undetectable. In contrast, both cortisol and ACTH plasma levels are elevated in bilateral adrenal hyperplasia, and both can be lowered by exogenous dexamethasone (a synthetic glucocorticoid) administration. A summary scheme of the etiological basis for Cushing's disease is shown (Fig. 15.21).

Some symptoms of cortisol excess are central (trunkal) obesity, hypertension, glucose intolerance, hirsutism, osteoporosis, polyuria, and polydipsia. The hyperglycemia resulting from excess glucocorticoids leads to a so-called "steroid diabetes," where prolonged elevated levels of glucose may, in time, lead to pancreatic β-cell exhaustion (diabetes mellitus). The change in fat distribution is due to the lipolytic action of ACTH and glucocorticoids on the normal fat depots. The redistribution of fat may not be due to the direct actions of glucocorticoids but rather to the insulin that is secreted in response to increased hepatic glucose formation. Although the actions of insulin on the normal fat

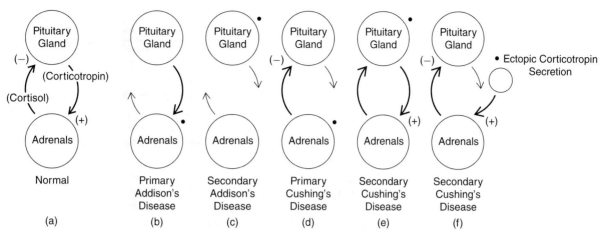

Figure 15.21   Summary scheme of the etiology of hypocortisolism and hypercortisolism.

depots are apparently antagonized by cortisol, insulin appears able to exert a lipogenic effect in other areas of the body, such as the face, upper back, and supraclavicular fat pads. The catabolic actions of glucocorticoids on skeletal muscle cause thinning of the extremities. Loss of the protein matrix of bones causes severe osteoporosis, which may severely affect the spinal column. The excess androgens produced are the cause of hirsutism in the female. Again, the hyperpigmentation that may be present in Cushing's disease of secondary origin may be due to the presence of increased circulating levels of ACTH. Polyuria and polydipsia are due to the loss of large volumes of water as a result of solvent drag during the process of excessive glucose excretion by the kidneys.

Disorders of Aldosterone Secretion

Conn's Syndrome.   In 1955 Conn published a classical report, "Primary Aldosteronism: A New Clinical Syndrome" [10]. The cause of aldosterone hypersecretion is almost always an adrenal adenoma, but in some instances it may be due to adrenal carcinoma, hyperplasia, or other unknown causes. The oversecretion of aldosterone increases renal distal tubular secretion of K^+ (K^+ diuresis) and H^+ in exchange for reabsorbed Na^+. This leads to the cardinal findings of plasma *hypernatremia* and *hypokalemia;* because hydrogen ions are also lost, this leads to serum *alkalosis* and nephropathy. The hypernatremia is usually associated with water retention, leading to severe hypertension. Therefore, plasma renin levels are low in primary aldosteronism.

Renin-secreting Tumors.   The rare but fatal occurrence of a renin-secreting tumor is associated with hypertension, due to excessive renin secretion (primary reninism). Renin-secreting tumors show that, in humans, hypertension can be produced and maintained by hypersecretion of renin, as shown by the complete reversal of hypertension after removal of the tumor. The hypertension can be totally reversed, even if the duration of hypertension lasted more than 10 years [12].

Malignant Hypertension.   This disease state develops whenever renal damage decreases the flow of blood to the afferent arteriole of the glomerulus. The localized decrease in blood pressure is the stimulus to renin secretion that becomes excessive due to the constancy of the restricted blood flow to the glomerulus. The resulting overproduction of AII, due to increased renin secretion, causes a chronic hypertension.

Hyporeninemic Hypoaldosteronism.   As the clinical name implies, this disease state is associated with reduced plasma renin levels. It is not known, however, whether the etiology involves a defect in stimulatory cues to renin secretion or resides at the level of the JG cell itself. Clinical evidence suggests that in some cases the defect involves destructive lesions of the JG cells, most often associated with diabetes mellitus.

Bartter's Syndrome.   Hyperaldosteronism due to hyperreninism has been associated with hyperplasia of the JG cells in some individuals. This disease is usually associated with increased urinary excretion of E-series prostaglandins. The increased production of these PGs may contribute to several functional abnormalities usually associated with this syndrome. Prostacyclins are directly stimulatory to JG cell renin secretion and may be implicated in JG cell hyperplasia.

Glucocorticoid-Suppressible Aldosteronism (GSA).   This is a rare form of hyperaldosteronism inherited as an autosomal dominant trait. The unique feature of this disorder is that the hypersecretion of aldosterone and the elevation of blood pressure are corrected by chronic glucocorticoid therapy. Aldosterone secretion in these patients is regulated by ACTH. During adrenal cell migration, it is likely that during the transition from one type of cells to another, intermediate cell type(s) are formed. These hybrid cells will have some of the characteristics of glomerulosa and fasciculata cells, and they have been called "transitional cells." In the normal adrenal cortex, a small population of such transition cells co-exist between the well-developed glomerulosa and fasciculata cells. Thus, these cells are able to synthesize cortisol and aldosterone, as well as the hybrid steroids (18-hydroxycortisol and 18-oxocortisol), having both 17- and 18-hydroxylation by the action on cortisol of the same enzyme(s) responsible for the final steps of aldosterone synthesis [16, 35, 36].

Disorders Due to Adrenal Enzyme Defects

Genetic defects can lead to inherited inborn errors of metabolism that lead to specific enzymatic deficiencies in the biosynthesis of adrenal steroids. The severity of such a defect depends on whether the block occurs early or late in the steroidogenic biosynthetic pathway.

Congenital Adrenal Lipoidal Hyperplasia.   This rare and fatal condition results from a defect in the conversion of cholesterol to pregnenolone. In the absence of cortisol production and negative feedback to the hypothalamus or pituitary, there is enhanced secretion of ACTH. Corticotropin stimulates adrenal cortical cells; although cholesterol is taken up, it is not used as substrate for steroid hormone production. This leads to a condition referred to as adrenal lipoidal hyperplasia. This defect in enzyme activity in the initial stage of steroid biosynthesis would also involve a concomitant failure in synthesis of gonadal steroids.

Congenital Virilizing Adrenal Hyperplasia.   A defect in 3 β-hydroxysteroid dehydrogenase, 11 β-hydroxylase, or 21 β-hydroxylase leads to virilizing syndromes of differing severity, depending on whether the defect is partial or complete. In the absence of 3 β-hydroxysteroid dehydrogenase activity there is impaired formation of both cortisol and aldosterone, thus this defect in steroidogenesis is usually fatal. Because ACTH secretion is elevated and the desmolase system is intact, as is 17 α-hydroxylase activity, the major product formed is dehydroepiandrosterone. Although a weak androgen with minimal masculinizing activity, excessive levels of this androgen are indeed masculinizing. Excessive androgen production causes virilization of affected newborns. About two-thirds of the cases have an associated mineralocorticoid defect leading to impaired renal tubular resorption of sodium ("salt losing") that can result in shock and death.

In the absence of 11 β-hydroxylase activity, diminished cortisol secretion leads to excessive ACTH secretion, resulting in adrenal cortical hyperplasia. The subsequent excessive production of cortisol precursors leads to an increased availability of substrates for androgen production (mainly androstenedione), causing excessive virilization in both male and female. There is enhanced deoxycorticosterone production (at the expense of cortisol synthesis), and the excessive secretion of this mineralocorticoid leads to hypertension. Glucocorticoid replacement therapy will correct the abnormal steroid synthesis and secretion by suppressing the excessive pituitary ACTH production.

A defect in 21 β-hydroxylase may be partial or complete. In the female the excessive secretion of androgens may lead to complete masculinization of the external genitalia (see Chap. 16). In the salt-losing form of the syndrome there is an almost total lack of 21 β-hydroxylase activity essential for mineralocorticoid production. Both mineralocorticoid and glucocorticoid replacement therapies are essential for survival.

Corticosterone Methyl Oxidase (Type II) Deficiency. Hypoaldosteronism, due to an inborn error in the terminal step of aldosterone biosynthesis, has been discovered within related members of a family. These individuals exhibit hyperreninemia and elevated plasma and urinary levels of specific 18-hydroxysteroids. The genetic basis for this disease involves a defect in the function of corticosterone methyl oxidase (type II), the enzyme (see Chap. 16) involved in the oxidation of the hydroxyl group at the C-18 position to the aldehyde [18, 38, 55].

17-Hydroxylase Deficiency. Deficient activity of 17-hydroxylase results in deficient biosynthesis of cortisol and androgens. The enzymic defect is also in ovarian tissue and, as testosterone is the precursor to estradiol synthesis, estrogen deficiency is also present, resulting in primary amenorrhea and defeminization (breast and genital atrophy), depending on whether the defect is congenital or occurs later in life. With diminished 17-hydroxylase activity adrenal metabolism is shunted toward increased production of aldosterone, as well as the production of the precursor mineralocorticoids, 11-deoxycorticosterone, and corticosterone. Absence of glucocorticoid feedback to the brain results in an aggravated production of precursors to mineralocorticoid synthesis (Fig. 15.22). The resulting hypertension can be alleviated by the administration of dexamethasone, which feeds back to the hypothalamus, resulting in decreased ACTH secretion.

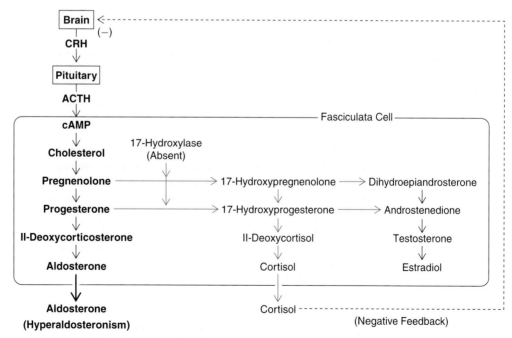

Figure 15.22 Genetic defect in 17-α-hydroxylase activity leading to hyperaldosteronism.

Syndrome of Apparent Mineralocorticoid Excess.   This disorder has thus far been reported only in children and young adults. Its clinical presentation is like that of primary aldosteronism with hypertension, hypokalemic alkalosis, and suppressed plasma renin activity. The response of these clinical manifestations to spironolactone suggest the presence of a circulating mineralocorticoid; however, levels of aldosterone and all known mineralocorticoids are either very low or absent. It is likely that the functioning mineralocorticoid in this disorder is cortisol, circulating in normal amounts, but exerting a mineralocorticoid effect because of incomplete metabolism at target tissues. Normally, cortisol has little mineralocorticoid activity in vivo or in mineralocorticoid receptor preparations. It has been shown that the pure mineralocorticoid receptor, as well as preparations from nonmineralocorticoid target tissues, possesses equal affinity for both mineralocorticoids and glucocorticoids. The abnormality in steroid metabolism in the syndrome appears to be due to a decreased intracellular conversion of cortisol to cortisone. Normally, a reversible 11 β-hydroxy oxidoreduction leads to an equilibrium mixture of approximately equal amounts of cortisol and cortisone. Cortisone itself is biologically inactive [54].

Lipoprotein Receptors and Atherosclerosis

The term atherosclerosis encompasses a range of degenerative phenomena that affect the arterial wall. Lipid, though present in variable amounts, plays a key role in the development of atherosclerotic plaques. Numerous clinical studies have shown a close association between lipoprotein abnormalities and coronary heart disease (CHD) susceptibility. The primary carrier of cholesterol in the blood is LDL. Epidemiological studies have clearly implicated elevated serum LDL levels in the premature development of CHD. LDL is formed by the action of lipoprotein lipase on its precursor, intermediate-density lipoprotein. Both LDL and intermediate-density lipoprotein are recognized by a specific receptor called the LDL receptor.

There is now compelling evidence linking a defect in the activity of the LDL receptor to the etiology of atherosclerosis [31, 47]. The link between the two comes from an "experiment of nature" called familial hypercholesterolemia (FH). In this genetic disorder there is a relative or absolute deficiency of LDL receptor function leading to accumulation of cholesterol in the plasma and resulting in the occlusive vascular disease. Most afflicted individuals are heterozygous for the disease and possess only about half the normal complement of hepatic LDL receptors. The liver possesses most of the body's LDL receptors. In true receptor-negative homozygous FH, no receptors are present. The LDL receptor is expressed in virtually all cells, but the hepatic expression of LDL receptor is primarily responsible for modulating cholesterol homeostasis in vivo. Transplantation of a liver that expresses normal levels of LDL receptors into patients with homozygous deficiency leads to near normalization of serum cholesterol level, illustrating the importance of hepatic LDL receptor expression. Traditional pharmacologic therapy for hypercholesterolemia in LDL receptor-expressing patients is, in fact, based on up-regulation of residual hepatic LDL receptor function. Drugs such as 3-hydroxy-3-methylglutaryl coenzyme A reductase inhibitors and bile acid binders result in diminished intracellular hepatic-free cholesterol, which leads to derepression of the LDL receptor gene, increased LDL catabolism, and decreased serum cholesterol level [22].

Apolipoprotein E, a protein constituent of several plasma lipoproteins, serves as a high-affinity ligand for the LDL receptor. A major function of apo-E is the transport of lipids (especially cholesterol) among various cells of the body from sites of synthesis or absorption to sites of utilization (peripheral tissues) or excretion (liver). Equally important is its role in the local redistribution of lipid within a tissue during normal cholesterol homeostasis, especially during injury and repair. The elaborate system for storing, releasing, and reusing cholesterol depends on a coordinated regulation of apo-E synthesis and LDL receptor expression. Genetic variability of apo-E, resulting from different alleles coding for proteins with single amino acid substitutions, has been most informative in defining, at a cellular and molecular level, the role of this protein in normal and abnormal lipoprotein metabolism. The genetic disorder type III hyperlipoproteinemia, which is associated with premature atherosclerotic disease, is secondary to the presence of a variant apo-E that does not bind normally to the LDL receptors [31].

Adrenal Steroid Hormone Pharmacology

A number of drugs have been produced that are useful in the treatment of overproduction or underproduction of adrenal steroids or their actions. One approach to secondary hyperaldosteronism is to prevent the production of AII from its precursors by inhibition of AI converting enzyme activity (ACE inhibitors). Potent and specific renin inhibitors would constitute an interesting alternative to ACE inhibitors for two reasons: (1) the first step in the renin-angiotensin system, the hydrolysis of angiotensinogen by renin, is rate limiting; and (2) renin has a unique specificity for angiotensinogen, as there is no other known substrate for this enzyme. Inhibitors with an exceptionally high specificity and affinity for renin have been developed in recent years; however, most of the structures are peptidic in nature and have relatively large molecular weights, which might explain their low oral availability and their rapid metabolism [11]. Other enzyme inhibitors have been developed to prevent specific enzyme-related hydroxylations in the aldosterone biosynthetic pathway. Renin secretion may normally be regulated by a renal prostaglandin; indomethacin, an inhibitor of PG synthesis, has been used successfully in some cases to lower renin secretion and aldosterone production in Bartter's syndrome.

Spironolactone, an aldosterone antagonist, is a competitive inhibitor of aldosterone binding to receptors, primarily those of the distal renal tubule. Spironolactone is used clinically to suppress the action of excess aldosterone on renal Na$^+$ retention. Metyrapone, an inhibitor of cortisol production, is used to test the capacity of the pituitary to respond to decreased circulating levels of plasma cortisol. Metyrapone is particularly useful in the differential diagnosis of Cushing's syndrome, as it will usually enhance ACTH secretion if the disease is of pituitary origin but not if the excess cortisol is due to ectopic production of ACTH.

REFERENCES

[1] Awazu, M., and I. Ichikawa. 1993. Biological significance of atrial natriuretic peptide in the kidney. *Nephron.* 63:1–14.

[2] Berstein, K. E., and R. W. Alexander. 1992. Counterpoint: molecular analysis of the angiotensin II receptor. *Endocr. Rev.* 13:381–6.

[3] Botarri, S. P., M. De Gasparo, and N. R. Levens. 1993. Angiotensin II receptor subtypes: characterization, signalling mechanisms, and possible physiological implications. *Front. Neuroendocrinol.* 14:123–71.

[4] Brown, M. S., P. T. Kovanen, and J. L. Goldstein. 1979. Receptor-mediated uptake of lipoprotein-cholesterol and its utilization for steroid synthesis in the adrenal cortex. *Rec. Prog. Horm. Res.* 35:215–57.

[5] Callard, I. P., and G. V. Callard. 1978. The adrenal gland in reptilia. In *General, comparative and clinical endocrinology of the adrenal cortex,* vol. 2, eds. I. Chester Jones and I. W. Henderson, pp. 419–94. New York: Academic Press, Inc.

[6] Cantin, M., and J. Genest. 1986. The heart as an endocrine gland. *Sci. Amer.* 254:76–81.

[7] Christian, J. J. 1971. Population density and reproductive efficiency. *Biol. Reprod.* 4:248–94.

[8] Christensen, G. 1993a. Cardiovascular and renal effects of atrial natriuretic factor. *Scand. J. Clin. Lab. Invest.* 53:203–9.

[9] ———. 1993b. Release of atrial natriuretic factor. *Scand. J. Clin. Lab. Invest.* 53:91–100.

[10]   Conn, J. W. 1955. Primary aldosteronism: a new clinical entity. *J. Lab. Clin. Med.* 45:3–17.

[11]   Corvol, P., D. Chauveau, X. Jeunemaitre, and J. Menard. 1990. Human renin inhibitor peptides. *Hypertension* 16:1–11.

[12]   Corvol, P., F. Pinet, F. X. Galen, P. F. Plouin, G. Chatellier, J. Y. Pagny, M. T. Corvol, and J. Menard. 1988. Seven lessons from seven renin secreting tumors. *Kidney Int.* 34:S38–44.

[13]   Funder, J. W. 1993a. Aldosterone action. *Annu. Rev. Physiol.* 55:115–30.

[14]   ———. 1993b. Mineralocorticoids, glucocorticoids, receptors and response elements. *Science* 259:1132–3.

[15]   Funder, J. W., P. T. Pearce, R. Smith, and A. I. Smith. 1988. Mineralocorticoid action: target tissue specificity is enzyme, not receptor, mediated. *Science* 242:583–5.

[16]   Ganguly, A. 1991. Glucocorticoid-suppressible hyperaldosteronism: a paradigm of arrested adrenal zonation? *Clin. Sci.* 80:1–7.

[17]   Ganong, W. F. 1993. Blood, pituitary, and brain renin-angiotensin systems and regulation of secretion of anterior pituitary gland. *Front. Neuroendocrinol.* 14:233–49.

[18]   Globerman, H., A. Rosler, R. Theodor, M. I. New, and P. C. White. 1988. An inherited defect in aldosterone biosynthesis caused by a mutation in or near the gene for steroid 11-hydroxylase. *New Engl. J. Med.* 319:1193–7.

[19]   Goetz, K. L. 1991. Renal natriuretic peptide (urodilatin?) and atriopeptin: evolving concepts. *Amer. J. Physiol.* 261:F921–32.

[20]   Goss, R. J. 1978. *The physiology of growth.* New York: Academic Press, Inc.

[21]   Greep, R. O., and H. W. Deane. 1947. Cytochemical evidence for the cessation of hormone production in the zona glomerulosa of the rat's adrenal cortex after prolonged treatment with desoxycorticosterone acetate. *Endocrinology* 40:417–25.

[22]   Grossman, M., and J. M. Wilson. 1992. Frontiers in gene therapy: LDL receptor replacement for hypercholesterolemia. *J. Lab. Clin. Med.* 119:457–460.

[23]   Guillery, E. N., and J. E. Robillard. 1993. The renin-angiotensin system and blood pressure regulation during infancy and childhood. *Pediat. Clin. North Amer.* 40:61–78.

[24]   Hackenthal, E., M. Paul, D. Ganten, and R. Taugner. 1990. Morphology, physiology, and molecular biology of renin secretion. *Physiol. Rev.* 70:1067–116.

[25]   Hammond, G. L. 1990. Molecular properties of corticosteroid binding globulin and the sex-steroid binding proteins. *Endocr. Rev.* 11:65–79.

[26]   Hobkirk, R. 1993. Steroid sulfation. Current concepts. *TEM* 6:69–74.

[27]   Holmes, W. N., and J. G. Phillips. 1976. The adrenal cortex of birds. In *General, comparative and clinical endocrinology of the adrenal cortex,* vol. 1, eds. I. Chester Jones and I. W. Henderson, pp. 293–420. New York: Academic Press, Inc.

[28]   Ichikawa, I., and R. C. Harris. 1991. Angiotensin actions in the kidney: renewed insight into the old hormone. *Kidney Int.* 40:583–96.

[29]   Idelman, S. 1978. The structure of the mammalian adrenal cortex. In *General, comparative and clinical endocrinology of the adrenal cortex,* vol. 2, eds. I. Chester Jones and I. W. Henderson, pp. 1–199. New York: Academic Press, Inc.

[30]   Inagami, T., and K. Murakami. 1981. Prorenin. *Biomed. Mater. Res.* 1:456–75.

[31]   Innerarity, T. L., R. W. Mahley, K. H. Weisgraber, T. P. Bersot, R. M. Krauss, G. L. Vega, S. M. Grundy, W. Freidl, J. Davignon, and B. J. McCarthy. 1990. Familial defective apolipoprotein B-100: a mutation of apolipoprotein B that causes hypercholesterolemia. *J. Lipid Res.* 31:1337–49.

[32]   Jones, I. C., and I. W. Henderson, eds. 1976. *General, comparative and clinical endocrinology of the adrenal cortex,* vol. 1. New York: Academic Press, Inc.

[33]   ———. eds. 1978. *General, comparative and clinical endocrinology of the adrenal cortex,* vol. 2. New York: Academic Press, Inc.

[34]   Koller, K. J., D. G. Lowe, G. L. Bennett, N. Minamino, K. Kangawa, H. Matsuo, and D. V. Goeddel. 1991. Selective activation of the B natriuretic peptide receptor by C-type natriuretic peptide (CNP). *Science* 252:120–2.

[35]   Lifton, R. P. and R. G. Dluhy. 1993. The molecular basis of a hereditary form of hypertension, glucocorticoid-remediable aldosteronism. *TEM* 4:57–61.

[36] Mantero, F., and M. Boscaro. 1992. Glucocorticoid-dependent hypertension. *J. Steroid Biochem. Mol. Biol.* 43:409–13.

[37] Mason, J. I. 1993. The 3β-hydroxysteroid dehydrogenase gene family of enzymes. *TEM* 4:199–203.

[38] Müller, J. 1993. Final steps of aldosterone biosynthesis: molecular solution of a physiological problem. *J. Steroid. Biochem. Mol. Biol.* 45:153–9.

[39] Mulrow, P. J. 1992. Adrenal renin: regulation and function. *Front. Neuroendocrinol.* 13:47–60.

[40] Murray, S. R., J. Chao, F.-K. Lin, and L. Chao. 1990. Kallikrein multigene families and the regulation of their expression. *J. Cardiovascular Pharmacol.* 15:S7–16.

[41] Orchinik, M., T. F. Murray, and F. L. Moore. 1991. A corticosteroid receptor in neuronal membranes. *Science* 252:1848–50.

[42] Orti, E., L.-M. Hu, and A. Munck. 1993. Kinetics of glucocorticoid receptor phosphorylation in intact cells. *J. Biol. Chem.* 268:7779–84.

[43] Parker, K. L., and B. P. Schimmer. 1993. Transcriptional regulation of the adrenal steroidogenic enzymes. *TEM* 4:46–50.

[44] Pearce, D., and K. R. Yamamoto. 1993. Mineralocorticoid and glucocorticoid receptor activities distinguished by nonreceptor factors at a composite response element. *Science* 259:1161–5.

[45] Pepe, G. J., and E. D. Albrecht. 1990. Regulation of the primate fetal adrenal cortex. *Endocr. Rev.* 11:151–76.

[46] Phillips, M. I., E. A. Speakman, and B. Kumura. 1993. Levels of angiotensin and molecular biology of the tissue renin angiotensin systems. *Reg. Pept.* 43:1–20.

[47] Schneider, W. J. 1990. Pathogenesis and pathomechanism of coronary heart disease (atherosclerosis). Familial hypercholesterolemia: dissection of a receptor disease. *Z. Kardiol.* 79:3–7.

[48] Sealey, J. E., S. A. Atlas, and J. H. Laragh. 1978. Linking the kallikrein and renin systems via activation of inactive renin. *Amer. J. Med.* 65:994–1000.

[49] Selye, H. 1976. *The stress of life.* New York: McGraw-Hill Book Company.

[50] Shire, J. G. M. 1976. Degeneration of the adrenal X-zone in Tfm mice with inherited insensitivity to androgens, *J. Endocrinol.* 71:445–46.

[51] Simpson, E. R., and M. R. Waterman. 1988. Regulation of the synthesis of steroidogenic enzymes in adrenal cortical cells by ACTH. *Annu. Rev. Physiol.* 50:427–40.

[52] Sloviter, R. S., G. Valiquette, G. M. Abrams, E. C. Ronk, A. L. Sollas, L. A. Paul, and S. Neubort. 1989. Selective loss of hippocampal granule cells in the mature rat brain after adrenalectomy. *Science* 243:535–38.

[53] Timmermans, P. B. M. W. M., P. C. Wong, A. T. Chiu, W. F. Herblin, P. Benfield, D. J. Carini, R. J. Lee, R. R. Wexler, J. A. M. Saye, and R. D. Smith. 1993. Angiotensin II receptors and angiotensin II receptor antagonists. *Pharmacol. Res.* 45:205–51.

[54] Ulick, S. 1991. Syndrome of apparent mineralocorticoid excess. *Endocrinol. Metab. Clin. N. Amer.* 20:269–76.

[55] Veldhuis, J. D., H. E. Kulin, R. J. Santen, T. E. Wilson, and J. C. Melby. 1980. Inborn error in the terminal step of aldosterone biosynthesis. *New Engl. J. Med.* 303:117–21.

[56] Vesely, D. L. 1991. *The atrial peptides.* Prentice Hall Endocrinology Series. Englewood Cliffs, N.J.: Prentice Hall Publishing Co., Inc.

[57] Vinson, G., and B. Whitehead. 1992. *Adrenal cortical steroid hormones.* Prentice Hall Endocrinology Series. Englewood Cliffs, N.J.: Prentice Hall Publishing Co., Inc.

[58] Wong, P. C., A. T. Chiu, J. D. Duncia, W. F. Herblin, R. D. Smith, and P. B. M. W. M. Timmermans. 1992. Angiotensin II receptor antagonists and receptor subtypes. *TEM* 3:211–7.

16

Endocrinology of Sex Differentiation and Development

*No other component of the vertebrate endocrine system is as complex as the reproductive system. Although the **genetic sex** of an individual is determined by the chromosomal complement of the fertilized egg, the direction in which the gonads differentiate to produce either ovaries or testes depends on hormones secreted by the gonads. The **gonadal sex** then regulates the **phenotypic sex**. Even the development of the brain into a male or female type is dependent on early exposure to gonadal steroid hormones. The brain, in turn, affects the temporal characteristics of pituitary gonadotropin secretions which regulate further development of the gonads into functional organs capable of producing mature gametes. In addition adult behavior is dependent on both early and late effects of gonadal steroids on the brain (Fig. 16.1).*

Compared to the human female, the human adult male might be considered to possess a rather uncomplicated reproductive system. After puberty the male reproductive system is rather invariant in its structural and functional characteristics. The female, on the other hand, is cyclic in her hormonal output and gonadal function. She may become pregnant, which entails radical changes in the reproductive organs to provide an environment for fetal growth and development. Unique female hormones are involved in the maintenance of pregnancy and in the induction of parturition, and additional special hormones are required for milk synthesis and milk secretion. These sexually dimorphic female functions are regulated by a variety of hormones acting in concert or sequentially.

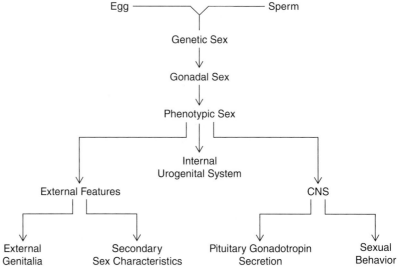

Figure 16.1   Sequential events in the determination of genetic, gonadal, and phenotypic sex.

SEX DETERMINATION, DIFFERENTIATION, AND DEVELOPMENT

Genetic sex, established at the time of conception, governs the development of the gonadal sex of the individual [9, 11]. Gonadal sex, in turn, regulates the development of phenotypic sex, that is, the differentiation of internal and external sex organs as well as attainment of adult secondary sexual characteristics [24, 41].

Chromosomal (Genetic) Basis of Sex Determination

The genetic sex of an individual is realized at the moment the egg is fertilized by a sperm. The genes specifically related to the determination of sex are grouped together on particular chromosomes. Initially, all cells of the human body contain 22 pairs of somatic chromosomes (*autosomes*) plus a pair of *sex chromosomes*. The female possesses a pair of X chromosomes (homogametic sex), whereas the cells of the male contain an X and a Y chromosome (heterogametic sex). During gametogenesis the diploid number of chromosomes is reduced through meiotic division to the haploid number. The female can normally only contribute an X chromosome, whereas the male may contribute either an X or a Y chromosome. The fertilized egg, the zygote, will normally develop in a female or male direction depending on whether a pair of XX or XY chromosomes are present, respectively. The Y chromosome in the mammal appears to be responsible mainly for sex differentiation as any embryo without a Y chromosome develops as a female. Even humans with as many as four X chromosomes and a single Y chromosome develop into males. Random union of the male gamete with the egg ensures that approximately half the progeny will be females and half will be males. Differential survival or other attributes of the X- and Y-bearing sperms may thwart the theoretical sex ratio.

The majority of vertebrates have a sex-determining scheme (XX/XY) of male heterogamety or a scheme of female heterogamety (ZW/ZZ). In birds and reptiles the W chromosome of the heterogametic female (ZW) induces differentiation of the ovary. In fishes and amphibians the male or female of certain species may be heterogametic. Some species of fishes are even *synchronous* or *asynchronous hermaphrodites*, that is, they are able to shed both eggs and sperm at the same time or, alternately, one or the other of the gametes during a particular developmental state. In reptiles all-female parthenogenic (egg development in the absence of activation by a sperm) or gynogenic (activation of the egg by a sperm without any genetic material being contributed) species have been discovered. Although the genetic sex of the species determines the direction in which the gonads initially differentiate, the exogenous administration of sex steroids at a critical time (which differs between species) can induce permanent gonadal sex reversal.

Gonadal Sex

The undifferentiated gonad has generally been considered to be composed of cortical and medullary regions [45]. In the male, sex differentiation of the gonads involves development of the medullary primordium and suppression of the cortex. In the female, on the other hand, the cortical region develops, whereas medullary differentiation is suppressed. The development of these two anatomical components was for years theorized to be controlled by hypothetical corticomedullary inductive substances, the production of which was related to whether an XX or XY chromosomal complement was present. It is now proposed that the undifferentiated primordium normally tends to develop toward the female in the mammal unless influenced by genes located on the Y chromosome [9]. Mammalian testicular organogenesis is dependent on a product (testis-determining factor, TDF) of the SRY gene (sex-determining region Y gene, denoted as Sry in the mouse and SRY in the human) localized to the short arm of the Y chromosome [16, 23, 25]. TDF is related to the DNA-binding proteins HMG1 and HMG2 and to the product of the yeast gene Mc, a possible transcription factor. This suggests a role for TDF as

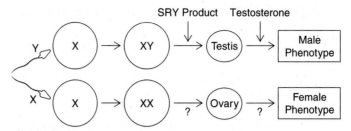

Figure 16.2   Role of the Sry/SRY antigen in the determination of gonadal sex.

the master switch for other genes downstream in the course of sexual differentiation (Fig. 16.2).

When female mice embryos carrying the normal pair of X chromosomes are injected with a small fragment of Y chromosome DNA containing the Sry gene, they grow up as males with testes and male behavior. The Y chromosome triggers the genital ridges in the embryo to develop into testes rather than ovaries. Once that happens all the other changes that make a male animal follow under the influence of hormones produced by the testes. The SRY gene is only a switch; testes can develop in XX women who have no portion of the Y chromosome. Also, in cattle some genetic females develop testes. These observations suggest that the genes needed to turn the indifferent genital ridge of the embryo into male gonads are also present in the female. However, the gene that normally triggers this change is present only in the male. One important question relates to what switches on the SRY gene. Some XY women appear to have no mutation in the SRY gene. Maybe there is a mutation "upstream" of the SRY that regulates its activation [25].

The Y chromosome is a dominant inducer of male sex determination in mammals. In the absence of the Y chromosome, fetal genital ridges develop as ovaries; in the presence of the Y chromosome, the genital ridges develop as testes. The position of the Y-located gene responsible for inducing testis formation was deduced from the study of the genomes of individuals with two X chromosomes, but who have testicular development. In four cases, the sex-reversed individuals had inherited less than 40 kb of Y chromosomal DNA, and the SRY gene was identified and cloned. SRY and the mouse homolog Sry have many of the predicted properties of the testis-determining gene [15]. By analogy with the genetic control of other developmental processes, it might be predicted that SRY/Sry is part of a course of genes that control sex-determination. The existence of this course can also be deduced directly: (1) the induction of Sry transcription at day 10.5 postcoitum implies the existence of "upstream" regulatory genes; and (2) the testicular differentiation found in some XX males, in the absence of any Y-derived sequences, can best be explained by gain-of-function mutations in "downstream" genes. Similarly, many other sex-reversing mutations in both humans and mice must be affecting genes other than SRY/Sry in the sex determination course [15, 43].

The testes differentiate under the influence of the Y chromosome during the seventh week of gestation in the human, whereas ovarian development usually does not proceed before 13 to 16 weeks [49]. Two X chromosomes appear to be essential for the development of normal ovaries as individuals with a single X chromosome develop gonads that are only partially differentiated.

The presumptive gonadal primordia are composed of coelomic epithelia, underlying mesenchyme, and primordial germ cells. The gonadal anlagen are visible in the 4-week-old human embryo as a pair of genital ridges. The primordial germ cells, the gonocytes, arise in the yolk sac endoderm, move to the mesoderm of the gut, and seed the undifferentiated gonads by migration from the hindgut. The course of migration of the gonocytes may be oriented by some chemotactic substance elaborated by the gonadal anlagen. During the migration of the primordial germ cells, the coelomic epithelium invades to varying degrees the underlying mesenchyme of the presumptive gonads to form the primary sex cords. At this stage the gonads are *indifferent,* or *bipotential,* in that, depending on the genetic sex of the individual, the gonads will develop into either testes or ovaries. An early sign of sexual differentiation is seen in the distribution pattern of the primordial germ cells. The germ cells of XX embryos remain in the periphery away from the central somatic blastema of the gonad, whereas the germ cells of the XY embryo invade the center of the blastema. Thus not only are germ cells attracted to the primordial gonads but also to the cortical or medullary regions, depending on whether they are of XX or XY genotype, respectively. Whether these primordial germ cells subsequently undergo spermatogenesis or oogenesis depends on early organizational influences of the Sry antigen on gonadal differentiation into either a testis or an ovary. In some nonmammalian vertebrates, although the germ cells normally become spermatocytes or oocytes, *sex reversal* is easily accomplished by early administration of steroids. For example, in the goldfish, presumptive male (XY) embryos can be transformed into phenotypic females by estrogens; they can be subsequently mated to normal males (XY) to produce viable male (YY) offspring [50]. In the medaka (*Oryzias latipes*), in which the presumptive female fish (XX) was converted to a phenotypic male by an androgen, subsequent mating with a normal female (XX) resulted in all-female (XX) progeny.

The primitive gonads of the male and female embryos, which appear morphologically identical, are composed of three components: the primordial germ cells, the mesenchyme of the genital ridge, and a covering layer of epithelium. In the male the primitive sex cords, which are initially solid, develop into the seminiferous tubules (Fig. 16.3). These ducts subsequently branch and their terminal endings anastomose to form the rete testis, which transports sperm to the epididymis. The seminiferous tubules are lined with epithelial cells that differentiate into *Sertoli cells*; the gonocytes become embedded within these sustentacular cells of Sertoli. The *interstitial cells of Leydig* arise from intertubular elements of the seminiferous tubules; these cells are the source of androgen necessary for development of the accessory sexual organs (e.g., prostate gland), but they disappear shortly after birth and do not become abundant until the onset of adolescence. The developing seminiferous tubules become separated by a connective tissue layer, the tunica albuginea, from the remnant of the coelomic epithelium, which atrophies into the so-called tunica vaginalis.

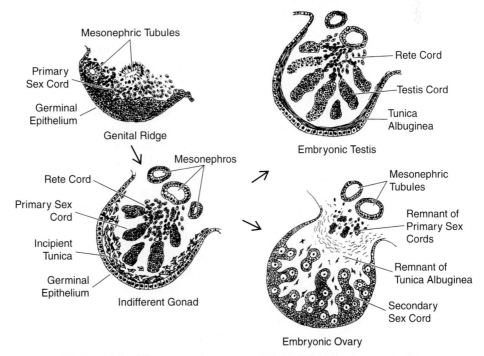

Figure 16.3 Diagrammatic representation of the development of the mammalian ovary and testis from a bipotential primordial gonad. (Prepared by Dr. R. B. Chiasson, University of Arizona.)

In the primitive ovary the coelomic epithelium undergoes proliferation, and strands of epithelial cells, the primary sex cords, move into the interior of the gonad to form a rete ovarii, which subsequently degenerates and disappears. Later in fetal development secondary sex cords extend into the underlying mesenchyme (Fig. 16.3). The primordial germ cells are carried along within the proliferating inward migration of the secondary sex (cortical) cords. Some germ cells within the sex cords become isolated and form primordial follicles at about 16 weeks of gestation in the human female.

Phenotypic Sex: Differentiation of the Genital Ducts

The definitive internal reproductive organs consist of tubular passageways for the exit of gametes produced by the gonads [13, 49]. Glands associated with these structures may contribute various secretions that aid in the dissemination and function of the gametes. During the undifferentiated stage, both Müllerian and Wolffian ducts are present. Development of the female or male accessory sex organs involves differentiation of the Müllerian or Wolffian ducts, respectively, with the concomitant loss of the other. Differentiation of the Müllerian ducts results in formation of the Fallopian tubes, with associated uterus and vagina. Differentiation of the Wolffian ducts, on the other hand, results in the development of the epididymis, ductus deferens, and seminal vesicles.

In the absence of the ovaries or testes, the Müllerian duct system develops and Wolffian ducts atrophy, suggesting that in the former these events are not dependent on any gonadal directive. Atrophy of the Wolffian ducts in the female may represent *programmed cell death (apoptosis),* a common phenomenon of developmental processes (see Chap. 12). In the male fetus, on the other hand, the testes produce a *Müllerian regression factor/inhibitor,* (MRF/MIF), also known as *antiMüllerian hormone (*AMH*)* [20], which is a glycoprotein consisting of a dimeric structure, a member of the transforming growth factor-β family of peptides (see Chap. 12). MRF acts to induce Müllerian duct atrophy. Maintenance and further development of the Wolffian ducts, however, are dependent on the presence of testicular androgen (and possibly, to some minor extent, MRF). MRF is secreted by the Sertoli cells of the fetal testes. It exerts a local effect rather than a systemic one, as unilateral castration in the fetal male rat and rabbit results in female duct development on the side where the testis was removed, and the contralateral duct develops along male lines. The MRF gene is also expressed by granulosa cells of the ovarian follicle, but its function, if any, is unknown.

Occasionally male infants are born with morphologically normal testes but an apparent inability to synthesize androgenic steroids. In these individuals the Müllerian ducts still atrophy, suggesting that MRF is nevertheless still present and not an androgen. In the *persistent Müllerian duct syndrome* genetic and phenotypic males have Fallopian tubes and a uterus together with male Wolffian duct structures. The underlying defect may be a failure to produce a functional MRF or to an inability of the tissue to respond to the hormone [20]. The development of the male or female urogenital tracts is shown schematically (Fig. 16.4).

Phenotypic Sex: Differentiation of the External Genitalia

As with the ovary and internal urogenital ducts, the external genitalia develop a female phenotype in the absence of the Y chromosome. Differentiation of the male external genitalia is dependent solely on androgen production by the testes. Development of the penis and scrotum commences shortly after onset of Wolffian duct development. The genital folds elongate and fuse to form the penis and male urethra. The urogenital swellings on each side of the urethral orifice form a bilobed scrotum into which the testes descend (Fig. 16.4). In the female embryo the genital tubercle becomes the clitoris and the adjacent genital swellings give rise to the labia majora; the genital folds become the labia minora (Fig. 16.4). Removal of the gonads from indifferent embryos of either sex results in development of a female genotype, demonstrating that the male is the induced phenotype.

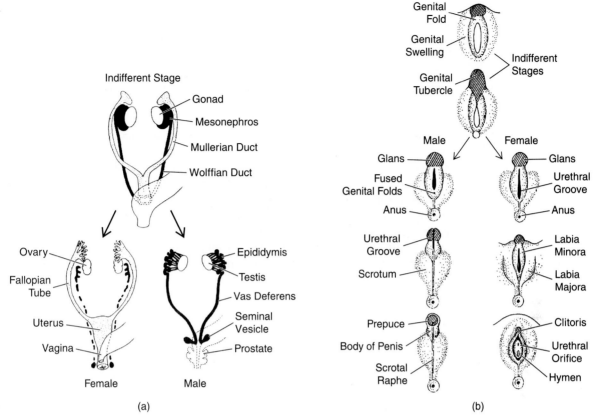

Figure 16.4 Embryogenesis of the male and female phenotypes. (a) Formation of the internal organs of accessory reproduction. (b) Formation of the external genitalia. (From Wilson et al. [49]. "The Hormonal Control of Sexual Development." *Science,* vol. 211, pp. 1278–1284, Fig. 2, March 20, 1981. © 1981 by The American Association for the Advancement of Science.)

Of critical importance in development of the external genitalia is the timing of androgen action. In the female fetus, for example, the external genitalia may become masculinized if androgen levels are elevated as in *congenital adrenal hyperplasia* (see Chap. 15). Androgens originating from the maternal circulation can also cause genital masculinization in the female fetus; except for clitoral hypertrophy, androgen excess at a later time (eleventh to twelfth week) is without effect. The role of the Y chromosome and gonadal hormones in the differentiation and development of the mammalian reproductive system is shown in Fig. 16.5.

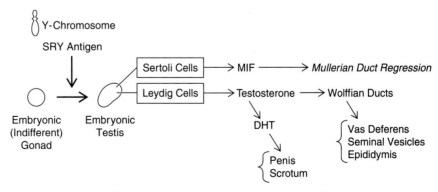

Figure 16.5 The role of the Y chromosome and gonadal hormones in the differentiation and development of the mammalian reproductive system.

GONADAL STEROID HORMONE SYNTHESIS AND CHEMISTRY

Gonadal steroids are produced by mesodermally derived tissues of the testes and ovaries. The same desmolase system as found in the adrenal is responsible for this first biosynthetic step in steroidogenesis. The nature of the stimulus that activates testosterone biosynthesis in the fetal testis is unknown. There is experimental evidence that testes or ovaries of rabbit embryos synthesize testosterone or estradiol, respectively, in media devoid of hormones. It appears, therefore, that differentiation of gonads as endocrine organs is controlled by factors intrinsic to the gonads themselves [49]. It is also possible that during early development the need for gonadotropins, which in the adult normally control conversion of cholesterol to pregnenolone, is circumvented by the presence of C-21 steroids of placental origin.

Unlike the adrenal, 17 α-hydroxylase activity is dominant and, through conversion of pregnenolone to 17 α-hydroxypregnenolone and 17 α-hydroxyprogesterone, provides substrates for androgen biosynthesis. In the testes testosterone is the major androgen secreted (Fig. 16.6). In the ovary androstenedione and testosterone serve as precursors for estrogen formation. Estradiol is the major estrogen produced by the ovaries. The key reaction in the ovary is *aromatization* of the A ring of the steroid nucleus. The first step in this

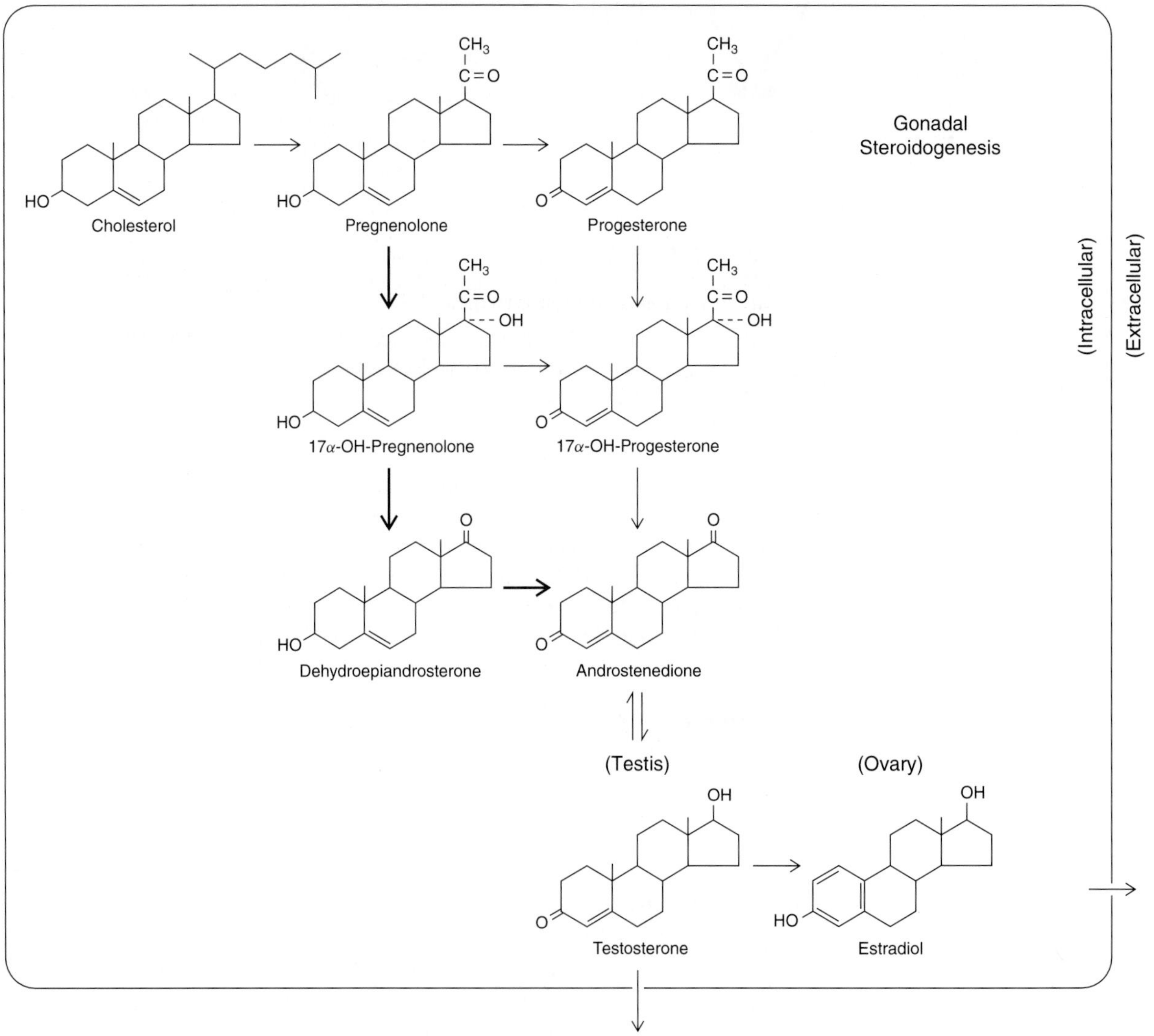

Figure 16.6 Biosynthesis of gonadal steroid hormones in the vertebrate testes and ovaries.

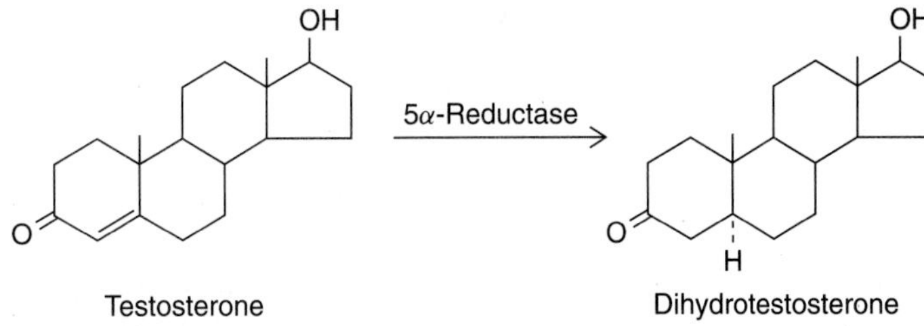

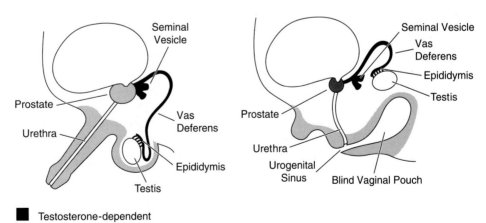

Figure 16.7 Cellular conversion of testosterone to dihydrotestosterone.

reaction involves the hydroxylation of the C-19 carbon followed by removal of the newly formed hydroxymethyl group from the steroid nucleus. The A ring is then aromatized to yield a phenolic hydroxyl group at the C-3 position (Fig. 16.6).

In some tissues testosterone is converted by 5 α-reductase activity to dihydrotestosterone (DHT) (Fig. 16.7). The rudiments of the external genitalia and prostate (the urogenital tubercle and sinus) convert testosterone to DHT, which is then responsible for the development of these organs. The importance of DHT formation in certain tissues for normal virilization is revealed in rare anomalies of male development that are due to the absence of 5 α-reductase activity (Fig. 16.8) [17, 18].

Although the ovary differentiates much later than the testes, the enzymatic machinery for estrogen synthesis is developed at the same time as the processes for androgen biosynthesis in the testes. It is unclear whether ovarian estrogen synthesis is important in the development of the human female fetus. Possibly estrogens synthesized by the ovary play a role, as does testosterone in the testes, in the maturation of the ovaries. Sexual differentiation is a sequential, ordered process. During development, the genotype of the zygote determines the nature of the gonad, which then determines the male or female phenotype (primary and secondary sex characteristics). A single treatment of chicken embryos with an aromatase inhibitor (which blocks the synthesis of estrogen from testosterone) at a stage when their gonads are biopotential causes genetic females to develop a permanent male phenotype. These sex-reversed females develop bilateral testes that are capable of complete spermatogenesis and have the physical appearance and behavior of normal males. These results identify aromatase as a key developmental switch in the sex determination of chickens [10, 46].

■ Testosterone-dependent

▨ Dihydrotestosterone-dependent

Figure 16.8 Illustration of the hypothesis for the role of testosterone and dihydrotestosterone in male sexual differentiation in utero. (From Imperato-McGinley et al., [17]. "Steroid 5 α-reductase deficiency in man: an inherited form of male pseudohermaphroditism." *Science* 186:1213–15. © 1974 by The American Association for the Advancement of Science.)

Whether the male or the female is the heterogametic sex has an important bearing on the role of hormones in gonadal and phenotypic development. In those species that bear young outside their body (e. g., egg layers) the heterogametic sex may be either male or female. Most mammals, on the other hand, grow and develop in a maternal environment characterized by elevated levels of estrogens. It is likely, therefore that to protect the genetic male from the influence of estrogens, evolution favored development of the female as the neutral sex. Rather than devising a mechanism of protecting the male from the feminine influence, differentiation toward the male gonadal and body phenotype requires the inductive actions of gonadal androgens. All aspects of human female development, ovarian as well as internal genital ducts and external genitalia, are essentially autonomous processes apparently requiring no hormonally active inductive substances. It has been said that the male mammal is "merely a female which has been subjected to induction by testosterone" [37]. This is not really true since factors other than an androgen (e.g., TDF, MRF) are necessary for normal male sexual development.

GONADAL STEROIDS AND BRAIN DIFFERENTIATION

In adult male mammals there is a tonic (generally uniform) secretion of pituitary gonadotropins, whereas in adult female mammals secretion of these pituitary hormones is cyclic in nature, that is, the amount of gonadotropins released usually follows a recurrent pattern characteristic of the species. Cyclic *estrous* behavior, the ovarian cycle of ovum maturation and ovulation, as well as the cyclic growth of the uterus, are phenomena dependent on the cyclicity of pituitary gonadotropin secretion (see Chap. 18). Questions arise as to the mechanisms controlling such cyclic or noncyclic reproductive events in mammals. Experiments have established that transplantation of the pituitary from a male or female rat to the opposite sex did not alter the normal reproductive processes in either sex. These observations revealed that the pituitaries were equivalent and could not be responsible for the cyclicity or noncyclicity of pituitary gonadotropin secretion. In contrast to the tonic uniform secretion of pituitary gonadotropins in the intact adult male rat, these hormones are released cyclically (as in the female) in adult neonatally-castrated male rats. Transplantation of an ovary into adult rats of either sex that had been neonatally castrated did not alter the function of the ovary whether or not it was transplanted into the inappropriate sex. In other words, in the adult (neonatally-castrated) male rat the ovaries cycled (ovulated) normally as in the female. Transplantation of ovaries into male rats castrated as adults produced different results. Ovaries transplanted into these rats failed to cycle. These results suggested that control of pituitary hormone secretion and subsequent gonadal function depends upon a system that was programmed early in development and was not localized to the pituitary or gonads.

It was subsequently discovered that a single injection of testosterone into a female rat during a *critical period* (a few days postnatally) resulted in adults that were acyclic. In addition these females exhibited male sexual behavior (mounting of other females). These results were consistent with earlier observations that transplanted ovaries only became functional if the transplant were into a neonatally-castrated male rat rather than into an intact adult male rat. Apparently testosterone secreted by the neonatal testes of the male conditioned the animals so that pituitary gonadotropin secretion in the adult animal was tonic rather than cyclic. Similar results were obtained by implantations of testosterone into the hypothalamus (but not other sites), suggesting that the locus of testosterone action was at the level of the hypothalamus, a postulate compatible with the emerging evidence that pituitary hormone secretion is regulated by the brain, particularly the hypothalamus (see Chap. 6).

Organizational Roles

The studies just discussed suggest that deprivation of testosterone in the male animal during his species-specific critical time of brain differentiation will result in a female pattern

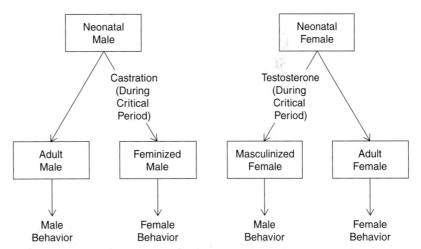

Figure 16.9   Effects of castration and testosterone administration in the neonatal rat on subsequent adult male and female behavior [30].

of sex-dimorphic behavior. Such male animals will assume the female mating posture (lordosis) when administered estrogen but will not mount females even when injected with testosterone. From these studies of androgen effects on the neonatal rodent emerged the hypothesis that testosterone was not only responsible for differentiation of the internal and external genitalia, but was of critical importance for normal differentiation of the brain into the male type (Fig. 16.9). Maximal sensitivity of the hypothalamus to testosterone may be associated with a particular stage of neuronal maturation. Thyroid hormones are known to affect maturation of the CNS, and an altered thyroid hormone status such as hyperthyroidism or hypothyroidism shortens or prolongs, respectively, the postnatal period during which the rat brain centers controlling gonadotropin secretion can be differentiated by testosterone. In species that are relatively less mature at birth (e.g., pigeons and many rodents) the critical period extends into postnatal life, whereas in animals more fully developed at birth the critical period may be predominantly prenatal.

One observation was particularly difficult to reconcile with this hypothesis: estradiol also masculinized the brain of either the male or female rodent. This dilemma was solved when it was discovered that testosterone is aromatized to E_2 within the brain. Several experimental lines of evidence support the hypothesis of androgen-to-estrogen conversion.

1. The effects of testosterone treatment in neonatal female rats are blocked by prior administration of specific estrogen (but not androgen) receptor antagonists.
2. The brain possesses the aromatase enzymes required for conversion of testosterone to E_2.
3. Dihydrotestosterone does not mimic the effect of testosterone on neonatal brain differentiation, thus revealing that the actions of testosterone are not mediated through its conversion to DHT. In addition, DHT cannot be converted to E_2.
4. [³H]-labeled testosterone is recovered from the brain mainly as [³H]-labeled estradiol.
5. Aromatase inhibitors impair brain differentiation in response to perinatal testosterone administration; and
6. In the Tfm (testicular feminization mutation) mouse, which has greatly reduced levels of androgen receptors, testosterone causes brain differentiations, as it does in normal mice.

Thus it appears that in addition to its hormonal role on a number of target tissues testosterone serves as a prohormone for DHT biosynthesis in some tissues and for E_2 production

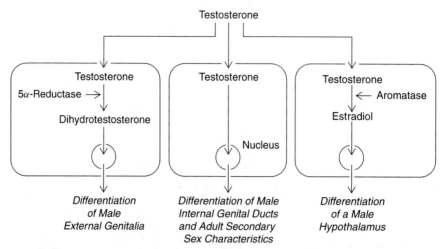

Figure 16.10 Testosterone: prohormone for dihydrotestosterone and estradiol in certain target tissues.

within the brain (Fig. 16.10). If E_2 is indeed responsible for brain differentiation in the male, why is not the brain of the female also masculinized, as E_2 is the major gonadal steroid of the female? First, E_2 production by the fetal ovaries may be minimal. Second, a circulating α-fetoprotein (fetoneonatal estrogen-binding protein, FEBP) is present in high levels within the blood of the fetus and apparently has a specific binding affinity for E_2. Theoretically, therefore, no E_2 is available to reach the brain of the female fetus. The *FEBP protection hypothesis* is supported by the observation that administration of antibodies to the protein produces effects similar to testosterone injections. Synthetic estrogens that exhibit little binding affinity for FEBP also effectively masculinize the fetal brain.

E_2 (derived from testosterone) is available in the male at a critical time in development to regulate the differentiation of the brain, but the mechanisms by which E_2 is able to alter irreversibly the brain and subsequent sexual behavior are unclear. Although the brains of males and females differ physiologically, do they also differ anatomically? It has been discovered that in the rodent there are sex-related differences in the distribution of synaptic connections of nerve cells of the preoptic area (POA) of the brain. The female pattern of synaptic contacts is established if males are castrated before the critical period of fetal development. On the other hand, the male pattern of synaptic distribution is established if newborn female animals are given testosterone. The *sexually dimorphic nucleus* of the preoptic area of the rat is actually visible with the naked eye, and is at least five times larger in the male than in the female. A sexually dimorphic nucleus has now been described for the human brain [1]. The volume of the nucleus is several times as large in men as in women and contains over twice as many cell bodies. This nucleus is located in the preoptic area of the hypothalamus, an area that is essential for gonadotropin release and sexual behavior in other animals.

The cellular mechanisms by which E_2 affects neonatal brain maturation appear similar to those controlling steroid hormone effects on other tissues. Nuclear chromatin binding and subsequent transcriptional and translational events leading to protein synthesis are involved. The ultimate effects of E_2 may involve neuronal growth and neurotransmitter synthesis. Using an in vitro system it was shown that E_2 and testosterone (but not DHT) enhanced neurite outgrowth from explants of newborn mouse preoptic tissue [44]. These steroid hormone effects are anatomically specific, as other brain regions do not respond similarly. These observations provide clear evidence that there are sex differences in the anatomy, biochemistry, and plasticity of certain regions of the brain and that some of these differences are organized perinatally by testosterone action via aromatization to E_2 [48]. In Chap. 17 we discuss whether the sexually dimorphic nucleus as an anatomical substrate for the action of steroids is responsible for homosexuality. In other words, is homosexuality biological [2]?

Activational Roles

The permanent actions of gonadal steroid hormones on differentiation and development of the brain led to the proposal that gonadal steroids can have two types of action, either organizational or activational, depending on the developmental state of the CNS. The *organizational effects* of steroids refer to the actual maturation processes leading to development of the dimorphic nuclear center of the POA and possibly other nuclear centers of the brain. The *activational effects* of steroid hormones refer to the actions on acute release of pituitary gonadotropins and to sexual behaviors associated with reproductive processes. In contrast to the organizational effects of gonadal steroids on brain differentiation and function, the activational effects of hormones are reversible, repeatable, and not limited to a critical phase of development. In adult animals steroid hormones released by the gonads play important roles in regulating behavioral events that relate to reproductive success. Gonadal steroid hormones in the fetus, as discussed, affect the organization of the brain into a sexually dimorphic adult organ. The mechanisms by which the activational effects of steroid hormones are expressed will now be considered.

Control of Pituitary Gonadotropin Secretion. There is evidence, particularly from studies in the female rat, that the preoptic area (POA), of the brain may be an important site of gonadal steroid hormone action related to the cyclic release of pituitary gonadotropins. Estradiol receptors are abundant in this area of the brain [30]. It is believed that during the estrous cycle of the female rat, for example, E_2 and progesterone (in a critical ratio) activate the POA, which in turn stimulates the arcuate-ventromedial nuclear area of the hypothalamus. This stimulation results (possibly in combination with exteroceptive stimuli in some species) in a surge of gonadotropin-releasing hormone (GnRH) secretion responsible for the midcycle surge of pituitary gonadotropin (LH) secretion, which, in turn, is then responsible for ovulation. In this model steroid hormones would interact with neuron bodies in the POA, which in turn would result in activation of neural pathways leading to the ventromedial hypothalamus where GnRH neurons would be stimulated to secrete GnRH into the hypophysial portal system to activate pituitary gonadotropin secretion. In the male rat the development of the sexually dimorphic nuclei of the POA results in a tonic stimulation of hypothalamic GnRH secretion.

Testosterone and Behavior in Humans. Although aggressive behavior is a characteristic of violent individuals, it is not consistently related to increased plasma testosterone levels. Individuals with chronic low levels of testosterone, due to genetic abnormalities in steroid biosynthesis, especially if occurring before puberty, exhibit reduced aggression and diminished sexual drive. Exogenously administered testosterone is often effective in restoring sexual interest and overt sexual behavior.

Some synthetic progestins have androgenic activity. In recent decades millions of pregnant women were treated with progestins and estrogens to prevent abortion. It has been discovered that individuals exposed to synthetic progestins during gestation show a significantly higher potential for physical aggression than their sex-matched unexposed siblings [38]. It would appear that the mechanisms controlling hormone-organized behaviors as reported in laboratory animals may also apply to human behavior.

Mood and the Menstrual Cycle. Changes in feelings and behavior can be characteristics of the menstrual cycle and are undoubtedly related to changing hormonal levels. Nevertheless, no clear correlation has been documented between gonadal steroid levels and the so-called premenstrual tension syndrome or other menstrual cycle-related behaviors.

Gonadal Steroids and Gender Identification.   Psychologists in general have argued that although sexual behavior is influenced by hormones, sexual identity is socially determined. In other words a child will identify with whatever sex he or she is brought up to be as a child. However, pubertal shifts from female to male gender identity in an interrelated group of male pseudohermaphrodites from two rural communities in the Dominican Republic have been described [18]. Feminization of the external genitalia in these males results from a defect or absence of 5 α-reductase activity. Although these individuals were brought up initially as girls, they took on male sexual identities at puberty. It was postulated on the basis of these observations that their prenatal exposure to testosterone irreversibly shaped their sexual behavior. According to these investigators, this "experiment of nature" emphasizes the importance of androgens in an organizational as well as activational role (at puberty) in the evolution of male-gender identity [18]. This interpretation has raised the argument of "nature versus nurture" relative to the basis of gender identification in humans. From other studies there is evidence that in male pseudohermaphrodites reared unambiguously as females their postpubertal gender remained consistent with their sex upbringing.

Androgens and Mathematical Ability.   A most interesting hypothesis that has been put forward is that math genius may have a hormonal basis [22, 28, 40]. It has been proposed that excess testosterone or an unusual sensitivity to testosterone during fetal life can alter brain anatomy, so that the right hemisphere of the brain becomes dominant; and it is generally thought that mathematical ability is a function of the right side of the brain. It is possible that boys who are exposed to more testosterone than normal in utero would be more likely than girls to be affected. It is also possible, however, that males might have a severe defect in mathematical ability if androgen production during gestation were affected.

Activational Roles of Gonadal Steroids in Nonmammalian Vertebrates. Castration eliminates sex behavior in the frog, *Xenopus laevis;* clasping behavior is restored by administration of exogenous testosterone, but not by estradiol. Three distinct populations of gonadal hormone-concentrating cells are present in the brain of *Xenopus;* "testosterone only" cells, "estradiol only" cells, and cells labeled after administration of either hormone. These latter cells may represent cells where testosterone is converted to estradiol [30]. The regions of hormone uptake are also known to be involved in the neural control of frog sex behavior. Sex behavior in some frogs may therefore depend on testosterone production by the testes and subsequent interaction with one or more nuclear centers within the brain where the hormone may act directly or be converted to E_2. Seasonal initiation of sex behavior would necessitate pituitary gonadotropin secretion to initiate androgen production by the testes.

In birds the homogametic sex is male, and differentiation of the female CNS phenotype occurs as a result of exposure to ovarian hormones. E_2 appears to be the ovarian product responsible for feminine differentiation. For example, embryonic exposure to an anti-estrogen masculinizes behavior in female quail; these birds exhibit the male mating pattern as adults in response to testosterone. Androgens play an important role in the control of song in male birds. Castration abolishes song in some birds; singing can be restored by exogenous testosterone administration. There are specialized brain areas concerned with the production of sound in some birds. In the zebra finch (*Poephila guttata*) all the brain nuclei of the song system are much larger in males than females. Early exposure of the chick to estradiol or dihydrotestosterone influences the establishment of the differences in functional capacity and brain architecture in the zebra finch [7]. When a neonatal female zebra finch is exposed to E_2, her system is subsequently masculinized. Testosterone or dihydrotestosterone can then induce such a female to sing when an adult. These observations suggest that the female zebra finch is the neutral sex with respect to sexual differentiation of the song system [7].

Singing is also a typical behavioral characteristic of the male canary. Ovariectomized adult canaries can be induced to sing by administration of testosterone. Some brain nuclei that compose the efferent pathway for control of song in the canary have been shown to concentrate tritiated androgen. The nucleus robustus archistriatalis (RA) of the forebrain is highly dimorphic in the adult canary, the overall volume being much greater in the male bird. Injections of testosterone into ovariectomized female canaries increase the volume of the RA as well as the length of the dendrites of this nucleus to a state resembling that of the male canary. Although steroid hormones are normally responsible for an organizational effect on the neonatal brain, results reveal that steroid hormones can induce plasticity in the adult brain [30].

In the male canary two telencephalic nuclei that control song are much larger in the spring when the birds sing than in the fall after several songless months [34]. Such fluctuations may reflect an increase and then a reduction in the numbers of synapses within the brain and may be related to the yearly ability to acquire new motor coordination. According to this hypothesis presented by Nottebohm, "The plastic substrate for vocal learning is renewed once yearly, a growing, then a shedding of synapses, much the way trees grow leaves in the spring and shed them in the fall." This species of bird truly has "a brain for all seasons" [34].

The distribution of gonadal steroid hormone receptors in the brains of members of all vertebrate classes has been determined [30]. Estrophilic neurons are localized predominantly in the medial preoptic area, the tuberal hypothalamus, and in specific limbic areas of the brain. The distribution of androgen receptors is similar, but not identical between species. Generally, the neural distribution of gonadal steroid receptors, although characteristic of the species, is independent of genetic or phenotypic sex [30]. In the zebra finch androphilic cells are found exclusively in brain regions that are the control sites of androgen-dependent song. In the spinal cord of the male rat a group of androgen-concentrating neurons are present in the lumbar region; these neurons, absent in the female, innervate striated muscles of the penis. The existence of gonadal steroid-binding sites in the members of diverse vertebrate groups suggests that binding of these hormones by nerve cells is a general vertebrate phenomenon.

PUBERTY

Although androgens produced by the fetal testes play a prominent role in the early development of the internal urogenital system and the external genital organs, as well as in brain differentiation, the Leydig cells subsequently become quiescent and remain so until activated much later by gonadotropins from the pituitary. The ovaries of the female also remain relatively inactive during preadolescence. In response to gonadotropin-induced gonadal steroidogenesis, there is a growth spurt and maturation of the gonads. The state at which the gonads come to maturity relative to their endocrine and gametogenic potential for reproductive function is referred to as *puberty*. The average age of puberty is variable between ethnic groups and individuals within any one group, but is about 12.5 to 13 years for the female and 14 years for the male. The timing of puberty in some mammals may be controlled by melatonin, a hormone synthesized and secreted by the pineal gland (Chap. 20) [8]. The adrenal glands of children begin to secrete increased amounts of androgens between 6 and 8 years of age. This change in the pre-existing pattern of adrenal steroid secretion occurs before puberty and in the absence of increased ACTH or cortisol secretion. This change in androgen secretion is termed the *adrenarche*, and it is accompanied clinically as *pubarche*, the appearance of axillary and pubic hair. There is also a transient acceleration of bone growth and maturation. The biological role and cause of adrenarche is unknown, and puberty can occur in the absence of adrenarche [36, 39, 42].

Advanced maturation of girls may be associated with an accentuation of the abdominal accumulation of subcutaneous fat. Girls with body fat that was predominantly abdominal were found to be more obese and to show increased plasma levels of total E_2 and a lower androgen/estrogen ratio in plasma, possibly due to increased aromatization, especially in abdominal adipose tissue. The findings suggest a reciprocal relationship between body fat distribution, plasma sex hormone levels, and availability of sex steroids in early female puberty.

Critical body weight or a critical amount of body fat is required for first ovulation and menarche. Body fat distribution, rather than body fat mass or body weight, appears to be related to early pubertal endocrine activity. Body fat mass and especially body fat distribution, which are affected by life-style factors such as nutritional intake and physical activities, may therefore be related to hormonal and physical parameters of early puberty [6].

Among the many physical changes occurring during puberty is a dramatic increase in the overall rate of body growth. There is considerable evidence that this pubertal growth spurt is associated with changes in endogenous GH levels. Elevated levels in IGF-I concentrations also reflect associated changes in GH concentrations. Enhanced testosterone secretion at puberty may be responsible for enhancing GH secretion, most likely after it is aromatized to E_2. GH and IGF-I levels return to prepubertal levels in early adulthood, whereas sex steroid hormone levels do not decrease [27].

Precocious and Delayed Puberty

Sexual maturity may occur earlier or later than normal; a number of possible factors determine the etiology of such divergent development [21, 33, 35]. *True precocious puberty* is defined as the attainment of sexual maturity at an earlier than normal age. This sexual precociousness may be of a constitutional (genetic) nature, or it may result from disorders of the hypothalamus that result in enhanced GnRH secretion. GnRH analogues can be used to treat precocious puberty due to enhanced gonadotropin secretion [5]. *Precocious pseudopuberty,* on the other hand, characterizes the situation where there is a development of secondary sexual characteristics without gametogenesis. The problem is that there are excessive levels of circulating steroids, either of gonadal or of adrenal origin. In *congenital adrenal hyperplasia* excessive amounts of adrenal androgens are produced and may cause early virilization and pseudohermaphroditism in the female. Interstitial cell tumors of the gonads or sex steroid-secreting tumors of the adrenal glands are also sources of excessive levels of estrogens or androgens (Table 16.1). The high levels of circulating steroids exert a negative feedback inhibition of hypothalamic release of GnRH. In the absence of pituitary gonadotropin secretion there is a failure of gametogenesis, but the secondary sexual characteristics that normally develop at puberty are well developed. The pubertal process can also be delayed possibly due to panhypopituitarism, where all pituitary hormones, including the gonadotropins, are absent. A defect at the level of the hypothalamus or an isolated deficiency in FSH or LH secretion could also be responsible for a delayed onset of puberty.

Hormonal Control of Puberty

Large fluctuations in blood and urine levels of gonadotropins, androgens, and estrogens occur during development, but lowest levels are present in the preadolescent years [8]. During the prepubertal period, the output of gonadotropins is constant, except for minor fluctuations during the day and night. Surges in gonadotropin secretion occur during sleep in the early stages of puberty, which may indicate that pubertal maturation has begun. By late puberty there are large fluctuations in gonadotropin secretion that extend throughout the day and night. Gonadotropin secretion in the postpubertal period becomes more uniform again, but at a level about double that of prepubertal individuals.

A number of theories have been put forward to account for the onset of puberty. No one theory provides all the necessary information, but it is likely that there are elements of truth in all the models. The *missing link hypothesis* suggests that some component of

TABLE 16.1   Endocrine Pathophysiology of Sexual Differentiation and Development

---

Chromosomal disorders (a few examples)
  Gonadal dysgenesis (Turners syndrome), XO karyotype
    Female phenotype but lack of secondary sexual characteristics (sexual infantilism)
  Seminiferous tubule dysgenesis (Kleinfelters syndrome) XXY karyotype
    Normal male genitalia and male characteristics but seminiferous tubules are abnormal
Hermaphroditism
  True hermaphroditism (mosaicism)
    Both ovarian and testicular components present; equivocal external genitalia
  Male pseudohermaphroditism (testes present but partial or nearly complete female
      internal and external phenotypes)
    Deficient 17-ketosteroid reductase activity
    Congenital adrenal hyperplasia (due to block in pregnenolone formation)
    Leydig cell agenesis (or hypoplasia)
    Syndromes of androgen resistance
      Testicular feminizing syndrome (absence of target tissue androgen receptors)
      Syndrome of 5 α-reductase deficiency (failure to convert testosterone to DHT)
  Female pseudohermaphroditism
    Congenital virilizing adrenal hyperplasia (due to enzyme defect in cortisol biosynthesis)
    Progestogen administration to the mother during fetal development
Sexual precocity (precocious puberty)
  Complete (increased gonadotropin secretion of pituitary or ectopic origin)
  Incomplete (precocious pseudopuberty; development of secondary sex characteristics
      but lack of gametogenesis)
    Adrenal steroid-secreting tumors (androgens or estrogens)
    Adrenal hyperplasia (e.g., 11 β-hydroxylase or 21 α-hydroxylase deficiencies;
        increased adrenal androgen production)
    Early masculinization in the male, masculinization of the female

---

the brain-pituitary-gonadal axis is missing or nonfunctional. The pituitary of immature animals is competent as it secretes normal amounts of gonadotropins when transplanted under the hypothalamus of an adult animal. The ovaries and testes of immature animals are also potentially functional, as they too become active when transplanted into adult animals or when stimulated by gonadotropins. These observations reveal that the brain, rather than the pituitary or gonads, is the site that is functionally incompetent prior to puberty.

Another hypothesis suggests that there is a decrease in hypothalamic sensitivity to feedback inhibition by gonadal steroids. Such a change would account for the higher circulating titers of gonadotropins present after puberty. This *gonadostat hypothesis* is supported by the observation that lesions of the hypothalamus often result in enhanced gonadotropin secretion. Also, castration of immature animals leads to an increase in pituitary gonadotropin secretion. Individuals lacking functional ovaries (as in Turner's syndrome) have high circulating levels of FSH and LH long before puberty, which could be evidence that the gonads depress gonadotropic hormone secretion in infancy. The administration of an estrogen elicits the discharge of FSH and LH during puberty, but not in infancy, which suggests that the mechanisms involved in such positive feedback have matured. It is even possible that an increased rate of androgen aromatization in the brain may be responsible for an alteration in hypothalamic sensitivity that results in initiation of the pubertal process.

In the primate there is convincing evidence that neither adenohypophysial nor ovarian competence is limiting in the initiation of puberty; rather, the process depends on the maturation of the neuroendocrine control system that directs the pulsatile secretion of GnRH from the hypothalamus. For example, normal ovulatory menstrual cycles have been initiated in the prepubertal female rhesus monkey by hourly infusions of GnRH [3]. These animals revert to the immature stage when administration of GnRH is discontinued [47].

The events that result in maturation of the neuroendocrine control system regulating GnRH secretion are still unclear. It has been proposed that puberty occurs in the human female at a critical weight or with a particular body fat composition. In the rat, for example, puberty is reached at a set body size rather than at a specific age [12]. Compelling support derives from the clinical observation that patients with anorexia nervosa and amenorrhea have a prepubertal or early pubertal pattern of gonadotropin secretion, which is reversed to the adult pattern in response to a weight gain. Also, leanness associated with strenuous physical activity is linked with delayed puberty, whereas the *menarche* (time of first menstruation) is usually early in obese individuals. For example, among young ballet dancers, there is a high incidence of primary amenorrhea (failure to initiate the first menstrual cycle), secondary amenorrhea (loss of previously established menstrual cycle), and irregular cycles, which are clearly correlated with excessive thinness [12]. High school and college athletes also have a statistically significant later age of menarche than do nonathletes. A change in the fat/lean ratio may affect metabolism and hormone levels, which may delay menarche and menstrual cycles. For example, obesity in humans is associated with increased peripheral aromatization of androgens to estrogens and also with a decrease in the transformation of estrogens to certain inactive metabolites. The resulting hyperestrogenicity from an extragonadal source of estrogens could be instrumental in the induction of neuroendocrine events related to the pubertal increase in pituitary gonadotropin secretion.

According to the "critical weight hypothesis" (as described above), a young female cannot ovulate for the first time until she has accumulated a critical amount of fat relative to her lean body mass. Likewise, the adult female will cease to ovulate if her fat reserves fall below this critical level. It has been suggested that the evolutionary basis for this hypothetical dependency is the need to delay pregnancy and lactation until the female has accumulated sufficient energy reserves to sustain these activities in the face of food shortage [4].

PATHOPHYSIOLOGY OF SEX DIFFERENTIATION AND DEVELOPMENT

Because of the complexity of the reproductive system, it is no surprise that there are many events that can account for abnormalities in sexual development (Table 16.1). Most defects have a genetic basis, and they may result from a failure of steroid hormone biosynthesis or a failure of steroid hormone action on target tissues [19, 32].

Hermaphroditism

In the male or female, gonadal steroid imbalance in the fetus results in *hermaphroditism.* A *true hermaphrodite,* a rare condition, is one who possesses both ovarian as well as testicular tissue. A *male pseudohermaphrodite* is one whose gonads are exclusively testes, but whose genital ducts or external genitalia or both exhibit a female phenotype or that of an incompletely differentiated male. Individuals possessing exclusively ovarian gonadal structures, but whose external genitalia exhibit some masculine characteristics, are considered *female pseudohermaphrodites.*

In those individuals in which female pseudohermaphroditism has an endocrine basis the ambiguity of the external genitalia is due to excess levels of circulating androgens. The degree of virilization depends on the amount and period (developmental time) of exposure to androgens. Female pseudohermaphroditism in most patients is due to *congenital adrenal hyperplasia.* There are several types of congenital adrenal hyperplasia, and the etiology of each relates to a specific defect in steroid biosynthesis, usually a failure in cortisol production. In the absence of cortisol biosynthesis there is a lack of negative feedback inhibition to the hypothalamus, which results in increased ACTH release and subsequently enhanced stimulation of adrenocortical steroid biosynthesis (Chap. 15). However, the metabolites that accumulate due to enzymatic failure to convert them to cortisol and aldosterone are shunted to pathways of androgen production.

The androgens that are now secreted in excess are responsible for virilization of the external genitalia, as well as development of masculine secondary sexual characteristics.

Male pseudohermaphroditism may result from sex chromosomal anomalies, mutant genes, or teratologic factors that lead to defective gonadogenesis. Only those factors whose etiology relates to endocrine dysfunction will be discussed. Testosterone is synthesized by the Leydig cells of the testes in response to LH of pituitary origin. There is evidence that male pseudohermaphroditism in some individuals may result from a defect in the LH receptors of fetal Leydig cells. A number of inborn errors of testosterone production can also account for development of hermaphroditism in the male. Three enzymes, which include the cholesterol desmolase complex, 3 β-hydroxysteroid dehydrogenase, and 17 α-hydroxylase, are present in both the adrenals and testes. Failure of their enzymatic function results in an abnormality of glucocorticoid and mineralocorticoid synthesis, as well as androgen production. These enzyme defects may be partial or complete and are caused by autosomal or X-linked recessive mutations (Table 16.1).

Syndrome of 5 α-Reductase Deficiency. Evidence from a familial group of individuals in the Dominican Republic has provided important insights into genetically based male pseudohermaphroditism [17, 18]. Failure to virilize certain androgen-dependent structures results from a lack of 5 α-reductase activity in these target tissues. The affected individuals had bilateral inguinal or labial testes and a labial-like scrotum at birth; there were no Müllerian structures, but Wolffian structures were well developed. These developmental characteristics clearly reveal the anatomically specific target tissue responses to testosterone and the near absence of DHT-dependent structures. At puberty there was striking virilization of testosterone-dependent secondary sex characteristics: axillary and pubic hair growth, deepening of the voice, increased muscle mass, and an enlargement of the phallus to a near functional size. The enhancement of the phallus mass, which is a developmentally DHT-dependent structure, may have been due to the very high circulating levels of testosterone in these individuals. Affected men had less facial and body hair and less temporal hairline recession than unaffected men from the same families. Acne was absent, and the prostate glands failed to develop. Thus it appears that the sexual characteristics absent in these individuals are those mainly regulated by DHT. Because of the extreme defect in the development of the external genitalia, male pseudohermaphrodites are usually raised as females [17, 18]. Figure 16.8 depicts the structural changes from the normal male reproductive anatomy that are a consequence of a defect in 5 α-reductase.

Syndrome of Testicular Feminization. A number of single gene mutations involve defects in production of androgen-binding protein receptors that lead to the syndrome of testicular feminization. Males with this syndrome have testes and normal (or higher) rates of testosterone secretion, but they are almost completely insensitive to exogenous or endogenous androgen action. These individuals are therefore phenotypic females, often with a truly feminine appearance. Although the external genitalia are unambiguously female and the clitoris normal, the vagina is short and blind ended and the internal genitalia are absent, except for a testis which may be in the abdomen, inguinal canal, or labia majora. Androgen resistance is due to abnormalities of the androgen receptor; the receptor protein is either absent or defective in structure (receptor-negative resistance). That the Wolffian ducts fail to differentiate and external genitalia do not develop indicates that both testosterone and DHT receptors are involved. The absence of Müllerian ducts and their derivatives in the otherwise phenotypic females indicates that the action of MRF has not been compromised. Another type of androgen resistance does not appear to involve either a defect in 5 α-reductase activity or cytosolic androgen receptors. The site of the molecular abnormality probably resides at one or more sites distal to the receptor (receptor-positive resistance, see Chap. 17).

Primary and Secondary Hypogonadism and Hypergonadism

As noted previously, hermaphroditism may result from a failure in steroid hormone biosynthesis or in end-organ resistance. Defects in the normal development of secondary sex characteristics at puberty may result from defects that reside at the level of the gonads (primary), at the level of the pituitary (secondary), or even at the level of the hypothalamus (tertiary) (Fig. 16.11a). Primary hypogonadism might relate to a failure in production of gonadal steroids due to any one of a number of causes. Failure in a negative feedback inhibition at the pituitary (or hypothalamus) by steroid hormones would lead to enhanced gonadotropin secretion in the face of hypogonadism (hypergonadotropic hypogonadism, Fig. 16.11b). Secondary hypogonadism, on the other hand, could result from a defect in pituitary gonadotropin secretion (hypogonadotropic hypogonadism, Fig. 16.11c). Hypergonadism involving overproduction of gonadal steroids could relate to a primary defect (hypogonadotropic hypergonadism) at the gonads involving a tumorous condition of the steroid-secreting cells (Leydig cells in the male or follicular thecal cells in the female, Fig. 16.11d) or to a secondary defect (hypergonadotropic hypergonadism) involving overproduction of pituitary gonadotropins (Fig. 16.11e).

Hypogonadotropic hypogonadism due to a deficiency in GnRH is common in female athletes. Strenuous physical exercise alters the integrity of various neuroendocrine systems, and in women, an exercise-induced deficiency of hypothalamic secretion of GnRH results in the syndrome of "hypothalamic amenorrhea" (Chap. 18). Highly trained male athletes, like their female counterparts, may also have a deficiency of GnRH. In habitual athletes of either sex, repeated early increases in stress hormones and gonadal steroids during prolonged periods of intense exercise may eventually cause a lasting suppression of GnRH secretion, leading to hypogonadotropic hypogonadism [26].

GnRH treatment has been used to induce puberty in children with constitutional delay of growth and puberty, and in children with hypogonadotropic hypogonadism. It is possible to mimic the endocrinology, ovarian morphology, secondary sexual characteristics, and growth acceleration of normal puberty. During induction of puberty using pulsatile GnRH treatment, larger doses of GnRH are required in boys than in girls in order to make equivalent progress through puberty. It would appear that girls secrete gonadotropin from the pituitary at a lower threshold of GnRH stimulation than do boys. This may explain why the physical signs of puberty appear slightly earlier in girls than in boys, why idiopathic central precocious puberty is more common in girls, and why constitutional delay of puberty is more common in boys [3].

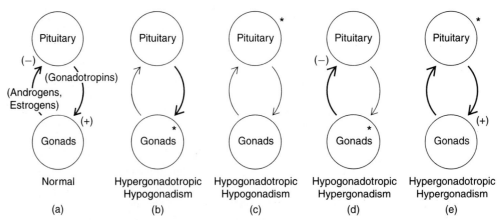

Figure 16.11 Primary (gonadal) or secondary (pituitary) defects causing underproduction or overproduction of gonadal steroids with concomitant effects on pituitary gonadotropin secretion are depicted. The site of the lesion, at either the gonads or the pituitary, is indicated (*).

Mice homozygous for the hypogonadal (*hpg*) mutation are sexually immature, and germ cell development is arrested. These mice lack detectable levels of hypothalamic gonadotropin-releasing hormone (GnRH), leading to low levels of LH and FSH. Introduction of a GnRH gene into the genome of these mutant mice resulted in a complete reversal of the hypogonadal state. Transgenic animals homozygous for the *hpg* allele developed fully their reproductive functions. Pituitary and serum levels of LH, FSH, and prolactin were restored to those of normal animals. Immunocytochemistry revealed that GnRH expression was restored in the appropriate hypothalamic neurons of the mice, indicating the neural-specific expression of the introduced gene. The use of gene replacement to rescue the *hpg* mutation illustrates the potential use of gene therapy [29].

Fertility in the hypogonadal mouse has also been restored by transplantation of normal fetal preoptic-area tissue, the major site of GnRH-containing cell bodies, into the third ventricle of adult female hypogonadal mice [14]. Immunocytochemistry revealed GnRH-containing neurons in the grafts and GnRH-containing neuron processes extending to the lateral median eminence of the host brains. These results demonstrate the plasticity of these peptidergic neurons and their functional integration within the brain.

Alcohol and Gonadal Function.   There is compelling evidence that ethanol abuse is associated with, and is the most probable cause of, Leydig cell failure in men who are chronic alcoholics. Alcohol abuse is associated with (1) induction of aromatase activity, resulting in an increased androgen-to-estrogen conversion by nonhepatic tissues (e.g., adipose tissue); (2) Leydig cell damage and subsequent diminished binding of gonadotropins to Leydig cell receptors; (3) decreased cAMP levels within Leydig cells; and (4) disturbed steroidogenic enzyme activity within microsomes of these cells. In addition, elevated levels of plasma estrogens may suppress gonadotropin secretion. Enhanced estrogen-to-androgen ratios might then lead to feminization. In rats there is evidence that prenatal alcohol exposure alters the adult expression of sexually dimorphic behavior [31].

The endocrine pathophysiology of sexual differentiation and development is summarized in Table 16.1.

REFERENCES

[1]   Allen, L. S., and R. A. Gorski. 1992. Sexual orientation and the size of the anterior commissure in the human brain. *Proc. Natl. Acad. Sci. USA* 89:7199–202.

[2]   Barinaga, M. 1991. Is homosexuality biological? *Science* 253:956–60.

[3]   Bringer, J., F. Boulet-Gibert, S. Clouet, B. Hedon, P. Mares, and C. Jaffiol. 1989. Pulsatile administration of LH-RH: diagnostic and therapeutic applications. *J. Steroid Biochem.* 33:783–8.

[4]   Bronson, F. H., and J. M. Manning. 1991. The energetic regulation of ovulation: a realistic role for body fat. 1991. *Biol. Reprod.* 44:945–50.

[5]   Couprie, C., M. Roger, and J. L. Chaussain. 1989. Treatment of precocious puberty with an LH-RH agonist (D-TRP⁶-LH-RH). *J. Steroid Biochem.* 33:805–8.

[6]   De Ridder, C. M., P. F. Brunning, M. L. Zonderland, J. H. H. Thijssen, J. M. G. Bonfrer, M. A. Blankenstein, I. A. Huisveld, and W. B. M. Erich. 1990. Body fat mass, body fat distribution, and plasma hormones in early puberty in females. *J. Clin. Endocrinol. Metab.* 70:888–93.

[7]   Devoogd, T. J. 1991. Endocrine modulation of the development and adult function of the avian song system. *Psychoneuroendocrinology* 16:41–66.

[8]   Ebling, F. J., and D. L. Foster. 1989. Pineal melatonin rhythms and the timing of puberty in mammals. *Experientia* 45:946–54.

[9]   Eicher, E. M. 1988. Autosomal genes involved in mammalian primary sex determination. *Phil. Trans. Royal Soc. Lond.* 322:109–18.

[10] Elbrecht, A., and R. G. Smith. 1992. Aromatase enzyme activity and sex determination in chickens. *Science* 255:467–70.

[11]   Fredga, K. 1988. Aberrant chromosomal sex-determining mechanisms in mammals, with spe-
       cial reference to species with XY females. *Phil. Trans. Royal Soc. Lond.* B332:83–95.

[12]   Frisch, R. E., G. Wyshak, and L. Vincent. 1980. Delayed menarche and amenorrhea in ballet
       dancers. *New Engl. J. Med.* 303:17–9.

[13]   George, F. W., and J. D. Wilson. 1986. Hormonal control of sexual development. *Vit. Horm.*
       43: 145–96.

[14]   Gibson, M. J., D. T. Krieger, H. M. Charlton, E. A. Zimmerman, A.-J. Silverman, and
       M. J. Perlow. 1984. Mating and pregnancy can occur in genetically hypogonadal mice with
       preoptic area brain grafts. *Science* 225:949–51.

[15]   Harley, V. R., D. I. Jackson, P. J. Hextall, J. R. Hawkins, G. D. Berkovitz, S. Sockanthan,
       R. Lovell-Badge, and P. N. Goodfellow. 1992. DNA binding activity of recombinant SRY
       from normal males and XY females. *Science* 255:453–6.

[16]   Hawkins, J.R. 1993. The SRY gene. *TEM* 4:328–32.

[17]   Imperato-McGinley, J., L. Guerreco, T. Gautier, and R. E. Peterson. 1974. Steroid 5 α-reduc-
       tase deficiency in man: an inherited form of male pseudohermaphroditism. *Science*
       186:1213–5.

[18]   Imperato-McGinley, J., R. E. Peterson, T. Gautier, and E. Sturla. 1979. Androgens and the
       evolution of male-gender identity among male pseudohermaphrodites with 5 α-reductase
       deficiency. *New Engl. J. Med.* 300:1233–7.

[19]   Jameson, J. I., and A. N. Hollenberg. 1992. Recent advances in studies of the molecular basis
       of endocrine disease. *Horm. Metab. Res.* 24:201–9.

[20]   Josso, N., L. Boussin, B. Knebelmann, C. Nihoul-Fekete, and J.-Y. Picard. 1991. Anti-Mül-
       lerian hormone and intersex states. *TEM* 2:227–33.

[21]   Kletter, G. B., and R. P. Kelch. 1993. Disorders of puberty in boys. *Endocrinol. Metab. Clin.
       N. Amer.* 22:455–77.

[22]   Kolata, G. 1987. Math genius may have hormonal basis. *Science* 222:1310–12.

[23]   Koopman, P., J. Gubbay, N. Vivian, P. Goodfellow, and R. Lovell-Badge. 1991. Male devel-
       opment of chromosomally female mice transgenic for Sry. *Nature* 351:117–21.

[24]   Lillie, F. R. 1916. The theory of the free-martin. *Science* 43:611–13.

[25]   Lovell-Badge, R. 1993. Sex determining gene expression during embryogenesis. *Phil. Trans.
       Royal Soc. London* B339:159–64.

[26]   MacConnie, S. E., A. Bakkan, R. M. Lampman, M. A. Schork, and I. Z. Beitins. 1986.
       Decreased hypothalamic gonadotropin-releasing hormone secretion in male marathon run-
       ners. *New Engl. J. Med.* 315:411–7.

[27]   Martha, P. M. and E. O. Reiter. 1991. Pubertal growth and growth hormone secretion.
       Endocrinol. Metab. Clin. N. Amer. 20:165–81.

[28]   Marx, J. L. 1988. Sexual responses are—almost—all in the brain. *Science* 241:903–4.

[29]   Mason, A. J., S. I. Pitts, K. Nikolics, E. Szonyi, J. N. Wilcox, P. H. Seeburg, and T. A. Stew-
       art. 1986. The hypogonadal mouse: reproductive functions restored by gene therapy. *Science*
       234: 1372–8.

[30]   McEwen, B. S. 1981. Neural gonadal steroid actions. *Science* 211:1303–12.

[31]   McGivern, R. F., A. N. Clancy, M. A. Hill, and E. P. Noble. 1984. Prenatal alcohol exposure
       alters adult expression of sexually dimorphic behavior in the rat. *Science* 224:896–8.

[32]   Mittwoch, U. 1992. Sex determination and sex reversal: genotype, phenotype, dogma and
       semantics. *Hum. Genet.* 89:467–79.

[33]   Morales, A. J., J. P. Holden, and A. A. Murphy. 1992. Pediatric and adolescent gynecologic
       endocrinology. *Curr. Opin. Obstet. Gynecol.* 4:860–6.

[34]   Nottebohm, F. 1981. A brain for all seasons: cyclical anatomical changes in song control
       nuclei of the canary brain. *Science* 214:1368–70.

[35]   Ojeda, S. R. 1991. The mystery of mammalian puberty: how much more do we know? *Persp.
       Biol. Med.* 34:365–83.

[36]   Parker, L. N. 1991. Adrenarche. *Endocrinol. Metab. Clin. N. Amer.* 20:71–83.

[37]   Price, D., J. J. P. Zaaijer, E. Ortiz, and A. O. Brinkmann. 1975. Current views on embryonic
       sex differentiation in reptiles, birds, and mammals. *Amer. Zool.* 15(Suppl. 1):173–95.

[38] Reinisch, J. M. 1981. Prenatal exposure to synthetic progestins increases potential for aggression in humans. *Science* 211:1171–3.

[39] Rosenfield, R. L. 1991. Puberty and its disorders in girls. *Endocrinol. Metab. Clin. N. Amer.* 20:15–42.

[40] Shibley Hyde, J., E. Fennema, and S. J. Lamon. 1990. Gender differences in mathematics performance: a meta-analysis. *Psychological Bull.* 2:139–55.

[41] Short, R. V. 1979. Sex determination and differentiation. *Brit. Med. Bull.* 35:121–7.

[42] Siegel, S. F., D. N. Finegold, M. D. Urban, R. McVie, and P. A. Lee. 1992. Premature pubarche: etiological heterogeneity. *J. Clin. Endocrinol. Metab.* 74:239–47.

[43] Sultan, C., J. M. Lobaccaro, C. Belon, A. Terraza, and S. Lumbroso. 1992. Molecular biology of disorders of sex differentiation. *Horm. Res.* 38:105–13.

[44] Swaab, D. F., and E. Fliers. 1985. A sexually dimorphic nucleus in the human brain. *Science* 228:1112–4.

[45] Voutilainen, R. 1992. Differentiation of the fetal gonad. *Horm. Res.* 38(Suppl. 2):66–71.

[46] Wartenberg, H., E. Lenz, and H.-A. Schweikert. 1992. Sexual differentiation and the germ cell in sex reversed gonads after aromatase inhibition in the chicken embryo. *Andrologia* 24:1–6.

[47] Wildt, L., G. Marshall, and E. Knobil. 1980. Experimental induction of puberty in the infantile female rhesus monkey. *Science* 207:1373–5.

[48] Williams, C. L., and W. H. Meck. 1991. The organizational effects of gonadal steroids on sexually dimorphic spatial ability. *Psychoneuroendocrinology* 16:155–76.

[49] Wilson, J. D., F. W. George, and J. E. Griffin. 1981. The hormonal control of sexual development. *Science* 211:1278–84.

[50] Yamamoto, T. 1975. A YY male goldfish from mating estrone-induced XY female and normal male. *J. Hered.* 66:2–4.

17

Hormones and Male Reproductive Physiology

Castration of young males to provide eunuchs was a custom of some earlier societies. Eunuchs fail to develop the secondary sex characteristics that typify postadolescent development of the normal male. The physiological basis for this atypical male development was not understood, but it was undoubtedly obvious that the testes must have provided some stimulus to normal male development. As early as 1771 Hunter was able to induce male characteristics in the hen by transplantation of testes from a rooster; spontaneous sex reversal in the hen had been noted to be associated with conversion of the ovary to a testis. In 1849 Berthold showed that transplantation of the gonads into castrated roosters prevented loss of male secondary sex characteristics and sexual behavior (Chap. 1). Brown-Séquard (1889) popularized the notion of the role of testes in the maintenance of virility by his claim that testicular extracts administered to himself restored vigor.

An active androgenic substance (androsterone) was first isolated from the urine of men by Butenandt in 1931. Testicular extracts were prepared in 1927 and the major androgenic principle was soon isolated in crystalline form. The chemical structure of this testicular androgenic principle was elucidated and synthesized by Ruzicka and Wettstein in 1935 and appropriately named **testosterone***. The role of testosterone and other hormones in the control of normal and abnormal sexual development in humans and other vertebrates is the topic of this chapter.*

ANATOMY OF THE MALE REPRODUCTIVE SYSTEM

In the human fetus the indifferent gonads of the genetic male are induced to differentiate into testes. The fetal testes, in turn, produce testosterone which is responsible for differentiation and development of the urogenital system characteristic of the male [49]. The testes become quiescent until puberty when they are activated by pituitary gonadotropins (see Chap. 16).

The development of the male phenotype involves at least two distinct sets of genes. The first comprises those genes that must be expressed for the undifferentiated gonad to form a testis and includes the gene on the Y chromosome encoding the testis-determining factor. Somatic cells of the developing testis express Müllerian-inhibiting substance, causing regression of the Müllerian ducts that would otherwise form female reproductive tract structures. Development of male reproductive tract structures and secondary sexual characteristics are, however, androgen-dependent. Thus, not only must the undifferentiated gonad form a testis but the fetal testis must begin to synthesize androgens at a critical time during testicular differentiation. Complete development of the male phenotype,

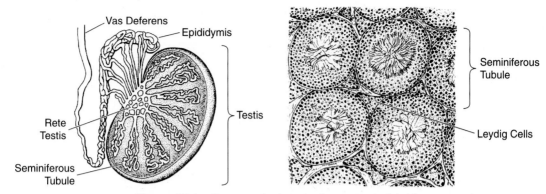

Figure 17.1   Gross and microscopic anatomy of the human testis.

therefore, requires expression of a second set of genes encoding the enzymes required for conversion of cholesterol to the male sex steroid hormones testosterone and 5 α-dihydrotestosterone [44].

The Testis

The two major functions of the adult testes are to provide an environment for spermatogenesis and to secrete testosterone to regulate a variety of bodily functions related to male reproductive function. In the human adult male the testes are located within the scrotum; each testis is ovoid in shape and is about 4 to 6 cm in length and 2 to 3 cm in diameter. A connective tissue sheath, the tunica albuginea, encapsulates each testis. The testis consists of convoluted *seminiferous tubules* within which sperms are produced. These tubules converge into the rete testis, which opens to efferential ductules to the *epididymis.* The epididymis is composed of a head (caput), body (corpus), and the tail, which connects directly with the vas deferens (Fig. 17.1) The outer sheet of the seminiferous tubules is made up of connective tissue and smooth muscle; the inner lining is composed of Sertoli cells within which are embedded the spermatogonia and various differentiated stages of immature and mature sperms. The suggestion that the Sertoli cells provide nutrients and other factors necessary for sperm maturation is compatible with the observation that the germ cells are, indeed, embedded deeply within and between the Sertoli cells. The fully matured spermatozoa, spermatids, are released into the lumen of the seminiferous tubules and subsequently advance slowly to the rete testis and epididymis, where they are stored within the tail. Between the seminiferous tubules are found the interstitial cells of Leydig, the cellular source of androgen production within the testes (Fig. 17.1).

SOURCE, SYNTHESIS, CHEMISTRY, AND METABOLISM OF ANDROGENS

As in adrenal steroidogenic tissue, cholesterol serves as the substrate for pregnenolone biosynthesis in the Leydig cells. Extracellular low-density lipoproteins are the major substrate for androgen production by Leydig cells. Unlike in the adrenal, however, conversion of pregnenolone to 17-hydroxylated steroids provides the predominant steroidogenic pathway in testicular interstitial tissue. The conversion of pregnenolone to progesterone with subsequent 17-hydroxylation appears not to provide an important pathway in humans. The 17-hydroxysteroids are converted by side-chain cleavage to 17-ketosteroids, and these, in turn, are converted to testosterone. Testosterone is the principal steroid produced by Leydig cells of the testis (Fig. 17.2). Androstenedione and dehydroepiandrosterone are also produced, but the physiological potencies of these androgens are so low

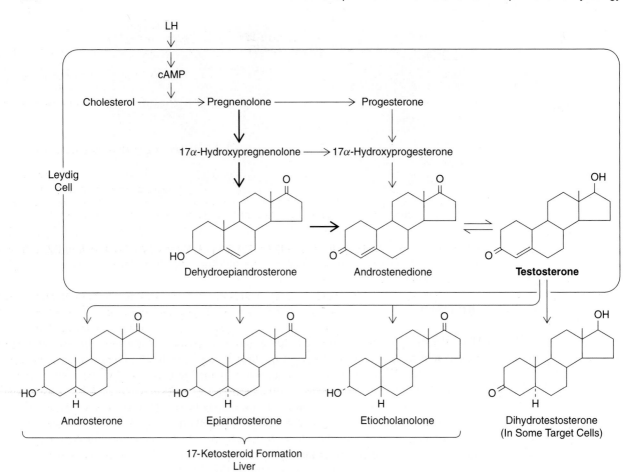

Figure 17.2   Testicular biosynthesis and hepatic metabolism of testosterone.

that they will not substitute for normal Leydig cell function. Although some androgens are
17-ketosteroids, not all 17-ketosteroids are androgens and not all androgens are 17-keto-
steroids. For example, etiocholanolone has no androgenic action and testosterone is not a
17-ketosteroid. An oxygen atom at the C-3 position and a 17-hydroxyl or keto group are
required for androgenic activity. In some tissues testosterone is converted to either dihydrotestosterone (DHT) or estradiol (E_2), which are the biologically active steroids affecting these tissues (see Fig. 16.11).

Almost 100% of the testosterone in the blood is bound to protein: about 40% is
bound to a β-globulin called gonadal steroid-binding globulin, about 40% is bound to
albumin, and 17% to other proteins. Inactivation of testosterone, which occurs primarily
in the liver, involves the following metabolism: oxidation of the 17-OH group, reduction
of the A ring, and reduction of the 3-keto group (Fig. 17.2). The primary urinary products
of androgens in humans are androsterone and etiocholanolone, which are excreted in the
form of glucuronide and sulfate conjugates.

ENDOCRINE CONTROL OF TESTICULAR FUNCTION

The testis has two major functions: androgen production and spermatogenesis. The control
of these diverse functions requires the coordinated activity of a number of pituitary hormones, which are, in turn, regulated by a complex of neurohumoral inputs from the
hypothalamus.

GnRH and Pituitary Gonadotropins

Early experiments established that hypophysectomy led to testicular atrophy (see Chap. 5). Restoration of testicular function could be affected by administration of pituitary extracts or, after further purification, of pituitary gonadotropins. Pituitary gonadotropin secretion is enhanced after orchidectomy, whereas gonadotropin secretion is diminished after administration of exogenous androgens. These observations established that testicular androgens exert a negative feedback on pituitary gonadotropin secretion. Part of this feedback is at the level of the hypothalamus, since testosterone implants into the hypothalamus are inhibitory to pituitary gonadotropin secretion. Subsequent discovery of a hypothalamic gonadotropin-releasing hormone (GnRH) provided evidence that the inhibitory feedback action of testosterone involved inhibition of GnRH secretion. Hypothalamic lesions that are inhibitory to pituitary gonadotropin secretion have provided insights into the neuronal pathways concerned with production of GnRH. By the use of a large armamentarium of drugs, the diverse neuronal circuits involved in the control of GnRH secretion have been delineated [37].

Pituitary gonadotropin secretion in the male has generally been considered to be under a tonic regulatory control. There is evidence, however, that these hormones undergo wide fluctuations in their circulating concentrations over relatively short periods of time. Apparently the release of GnRH from the hypothalamus is frequency coded, which may be necessary to prevent pituitary gonadotrophs from becoming refractory (down-regulated) to GnRH. In the adult human male there is a pulsatile release of LH about every 90 minutes. The precise pattern of this episodic release varies from day to day, suggesting that the mechanisms controlling gonadotropin secretion are not coupled to an endogenous oscillator.

In a number of mammals LH is released upon exposure of a male to a female. Successive presentation of the same female to a male mouse may lead to habituation, where LH secretion is diminished upon subsequent presentations of the female. Introduction of a novel female, on the other hand, will initiate a burst of LH secretion [8]. This adaptive neuroendocrine response may be important in providing a stimulus to courtship and copulatory behavior in some species.

The following evidence clearly establishes the individual roles of pituitary gonadotropins in regulating testicular function. Radiolabeled LH specifically binds to Leydig cells, whereas radiolabeled FSH binds only to Sertoli cells. LH increases cAMP levels in the interstitial cells of the testes, but not the seminiferous tubules. FSH, on the other hand, does not increase cAMP levels in the Leydig cells, but does stimulate production of the cyclic nucleotide in seminiferous tubules devoid of germ cells or in enriched fractions of Sertoli cells. Although the Sertoli cell is the major site of FSH action, there is evidence that FSH enhances the number of Leydig cell LH receptors (see Chap. 16). Although FSH does not by itself stimulate steroid biosynthesis within purified testis interstitial tissue, in combination with LH it causes a dramatic increase (synergism) in the action of LH on Leydig cell 3 β-hydroxysteroid dehydrogenase-isomerase activity. These latter observations are difficult to reconcile with data suggesting a lack of Leydig cell FSH receptors. The actions of FSH may be indirect.

Inhibin

The Sertoli cells of the testes produce a peptide hormone, inhibin, whose putative role is to control the secretion of pituitary FSH [13]. High levels of FSH and normal levels of LH are present in the plasma of oligospermic males and in males after testicular irradiation and cytotoxic chemotherapy. Sertoli cells alone are not capable of reducing FSH levels in the absence of spermatogenesis. It is postulated that inhibin production by Sertoli cells may be regulated by influences deriving from maturing sperms. FSH secretion from cultured anterior pituitary cells is inhibited when pituitary cells are cocultured with Sertoli cells

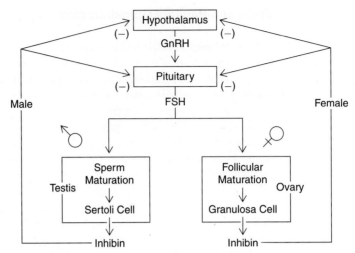

Figure 17.3 A summary scheme of the roles of FSH and inhibin in the control of testicular (and ovarian) function.

(but not spleen or kidney cells). Thus pituitary FSH secretion may normally be regulated via negative feedback by an inhibitory factor of Sertoli cell origin. This is further substantiated by the observation that prior exposure to inhibin suppresses the elevation of FSH release following GnRH administration in vitro. Other evidence suggests that inhibin also suppresses FSH by a hypothalamic site of action.

Granulosa cells from the ovarian follicle also secrete a substance during culture, presumably inhibin, that acts directly on pituitary cell cultures derived from the male or female to suppress preferentially FSH secretion. Administration of anti-inhibin antisera to rats of either sex causes a rise in serum FSH levels; LH levels, in contrast, remain unchanged. A summary scheme of the roles of FSH and inhibin in the control of testicular (and ovarian) function is provided (Fig. 17.3).

Prolactin

Hypophysectomy of the male rat results in a loss of testicular LH receptors; administration of FSH or LH does not, however, reestablish testicular LH receptor concentration. Inhibition of pituitary FSH and LH secretion from the rat pituitary by administration of anti-GnRH or by estradiol or testosterone treatment does not result in a loss of testicular LH receptors. These results suggest that one or more pituitary hormones other than the gonadotropins might be responsible for maintenance of testicular receptors. Inhibition of PRL secretion by ergot alkaloids results in a decrease in testicular LH receptors, whereas PRL treatment prevents loss of LH receptors in hypophysectomized animals. These observations suggest that PRL may play a role in the control of testicular Leydig cell LH receptor number.

PHYSIOLOGICAL ROLES OF ANDROGENS

Testicular androgens are responsible for the growth and development of those tissues and organs that characterize the male (Table 17.1) [33]. The role of gonadal androgens in the differentiation and development of the male urogenital system, the accessory sex organs, and the external genitalia has already been described (see Chap. 16). Although many target tissues respond directly to testosterone, this androgen must first be converted either to DHT or E_2 in some other tissues to mediate its actions (see Fig. 16.10). After the initial actions of testosterone in early fetal development, the gonads remain quiescent until puberty when gonadal activity is increased in response to secretion of pituitary gonad-

TABLE 17.1   Biological Effects and Roles of Testicular Androgens in the Human Male

Primary locus of action	Physiological response
Prepubertal	
Accessory sex glands	Wolffian duct differentiation and growth
External genitalia	Growth and differentiation (scrotum and penis)
Pubertal	
Skeletal muscle (enhanced protein synthesis)	Masculine body growth and physique (Na^+, K^+, H_2O retention)
Bone (bone formation)	Epiphysial closure (Ca^{2+}, SO_4^{-2}, PO_4^{-3} retention)
Vocal cords	Voice change
Skin	Hair growth (beard, axilla, chest, pubic, and general body surface)
	Hair loss (e.g., forehead)
	Sebaceous gland growth and sebum production
Testis	Sertoli cell maturation and androgen-binding protein synthesis
	Spermatogenesis
External genitalia	Penile and scrotal growth
Accessory sex glands	Prostate gland, seminal vesicle, bulbourethral gland growth and secretion
Central nervous system	Sexual activity (libido increased)
Hypothalamo-pituitary axis	Inhibition of LH secretion

otropins. The elevated circulating levels of androgens that ensue are responsible for initiating spermatogenesis (gametogenesis) and for growth and development of the secondary sex characteristics that first become evident during the pubertal process. Some of the established roles of androgens in the male are discussed below.

Spermatogenesis

FSH and testosterone are required for the initiation of spermatogenesis during sexual maturation [42]. Administration of FSH to immature or mature hypophysectomized rats markedly increases the size of the testes but does not accelerate the appearance of mature sperm or increase the secretory activity of the Leydig cells. For completion of spermatogenesis, an androgenic influence is needed, which can be provided by the administration of testosterone. Spermatogenesis can be maintained in hypophysectomized adult animals by testosterone in the absence of gonadotropins, but its initiation at puberty requires FSH. Resumption of spermatogenesis in regressed testes following hypophysectomy also requires administration of FSH. In immature animals FSH increases the number of Sertoli cells, which accounts for the testicular hypertrophy that follows hemicastration. FSH is required for the normal reinitiation of sperm production during the breeding season of monkeys. Although LH alone stimulates sperm production in some patients with deficiencies in LH and FSH production, others have required a combination of FSH and LH to initiate spermatogenesis. FSH alone has never been reported to initiate or maintain spermatogenesis in males.

Although the details of the individual roles of FSH and testosterone in spermatogenesis remain unresolved, the following model has been proposed. FSH interaction with Sertoli cell plasmalemmal receptors results in cAMP production and the synthesis of an androgen-binding protein (ABP). Presumably, cAMP activates a protein kinase that leads to the genomic production of a mRNA coding for ABP. The ABP is then secreted into the lumen of the seminiferous tubules. Testicular receptors for LH are specifically localized to the Leydig cells. In response to LH, cAMP is produced that causes Leydig cell testosterone production (Fig. 17.4). Testosterone is released from the Leydig cells and finds its way into the systemic circulation and to the adjacent seminiferous tubules. Because Sertoli cells are connected by tight junctions, they apparently provide a barrier (blood-testis) to most large molecules. Testosterone may be taken up by the Sertoli cells by an active transport

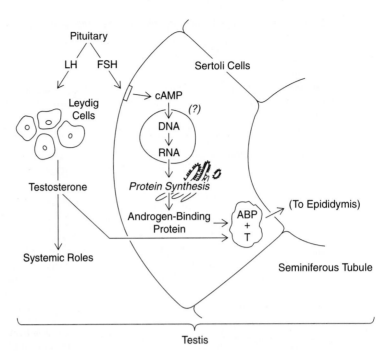

Figure 17.4 Model of FSH and LH action on Sertoli and Leydig cells.

mechanism or by facilitated diffusion [40]. The blood-testis barrier first appears at puberty and may function to create some special environment for spermatogenesis. The barrier may also protect the germ cells from the immunological system. Within the Sertoli cells testosterone is bound to ABP. This binding protein may provide a mechanism for testosterone sequestration close to the spermatocytes whose maturation is androgen dependent. Because germ cells lacking androgen receptors develop into fertile spermatozoa in the presence of normal Sertoli cells, it is presumed that the hormonal effects of testosterone on spermatogenesis are mediated via the Sertoli cells.

Androgen-binding protein may also provide a mechanism for the accumulation of androgen within Sertoli cells, which can then be released (via vesicular exocytosis) into the lumen of the seminiferous tubules. Within the lumen, ABP may function to transport testosterone to the epididymis. The spermatozoa mature in the caput and corpus regions of the epididymis where they develop the potential for fertilization and motility. These characteristics of mature sperm within the epididymis are soon lost in castrated animals, but can be maintained by testosterone administration.

Nervous System

Unlike in the female, gonadal steroids do not feed back to the pituitary or hypothalamus of the male to regulate the cyclic release of pituitary hormones. Nevertheless, pituitary gonadotropin secretion is increased after gonadectomy, and exogenous androgens depress the elevation of gonadotropin secretion in the castrated animal. Therefore, testicular androgens exert a tonic inhibitory feedback action on pituitary gonadotropin secretion. Nuclear androgen-binding sites are present in the brain of vertebrates, and they represent loci of androgen activation of sexually related behavior (see Chap. 16). For example, implantation of androgen within specific areas of the brain can induce copulatory behavior in fowl [48].

In the dove, *Streptopelia risoria,* male courtship depends on the action of androgen on the preoptic-anterior hypothalamus (AHPOA) of the brain. The aggressive components of courtship, as well as perch calling, are specifically testosterone dependent, whereas nest-oriented courtship activity and nest soliciting appear to be mediated by estrogens (derived from testosterone) acting on the AHPOA.

A sexually dimorphic nucleus is present in the fifth and sixth lumbar segments of the male rat spinal cord [4]. This nucleus contains motoneurons that innervate the perineal striated muscle of the penis. This nucleus is diminished or absent in the normal female and in males who are genetically insensitive to androgens. The cell bodies of these motoneurons accumulate androgens but not E_2. These motoneurons probably represent a site of androgen action modifying penile reflexes during copulatory behavior.

The spinal nucleus of the bulbocavernosus (SNB) contains many more motor neurons in adult male rats than in females. Androgens establish this sex difference during a critical prenatal period that coincides with normally occurring cell death in the SNB region. The sex difference in SNB motoneuron number arises primarily because motor neuron loss is greater in females than in males during the early postnatal period. Prenatal androgen treatment in females attenuates cell death in the SNB region, reducing motor neuron loss to levels typical of males. These observations suggest that steroid hormones determine sex differences in neuron numbers by regulating normally occurring cell death (apoptosis) and that the timing of this cell death may therefore define critical periods for steroid hormone effects on neuron number [34].

In androgen-sensitive motor neurons that mediate male copulatory functions, decreases in androgen levels after castration of adult rats resulted in a decrease in both the dendritic length and soma size of the neurons. The changes could be reversed by androgen replacement. These results indicate a high degree of synaptic plasticity in adult motor neurons and suggest that normal changes in androgen levels in adulthood are associated with significant alterations in the structure and function of these neurons [28].

In the male frog, *Xenopus laevis*, spinal neurons projecting to muscles primarily involved in the clasp reflex during amplexus accumulate [^{3}H]dihydrotestosterone. DHT added to an isolated spinal cord preparation containing these neurons changes the firing patterns of the neurons. Androgens or their metabolites may therefore regulate mating behavior in these animals by an initial action within specific spinal neurons that control muscle activity during mating.

Gonadal hormones alter the level of spontaneous electrical activity of anatomically defined populations of neurons within the brain and change the responses of peripheral and central neuronal pathways to sensory stimulation in some vertebrate species. For example, testosterone alters preoptic neuron responses to electrical stimulation of the olfactory bulb and to natural sexual odors. Therefore, in the adult animal, androgens may be significant in the interception and interpretation of olfactory cues important to reproductive success.

Gonadal androgens are essential for establishment and maintenance of male dominance and aggressive behavior in most birds (e.g., domestic fowl, mallards) [48]. Sexual aggressiveness is diminished after castration but can be re-established by administration of androgens. In phalaropes (*Steganopes tricolor*), however, the female is more active than the male in courtship behavior. During the breeding cycle, female phalaropes produce more gonadal androgens than males [19]. In females the nuptial plumage is also more brilliant than that of males. Administration of testosterone (but not E_2 or PRL) to phalaropes of either sex in the dull juvenile or adult nonbreeding plumage results in formation of the full plumage pattern that normally develops only in the female [23]. These results clearly establish that androgens in the female phalarope are responsible for inducing nuptial plumage and dominant mating behavior during the breeding season.

Hormones and Homosexuality

The anterior hypothalamus of the brain participates in the regulation of male-typical sexual behavior [2, 6, 14, 17]. The volumes of four cell groups in this region (interstitial nuclei of the anterior hypothalamus (INAH) 1, 2, 3, and 4) were measured in postmortem tissue from three subject groups: women, men who were presumed to be heterosexual, and homosexual men. No differences were found between the groups in the volumes of INAH

1, 2, or 4. As has been reported previously, INAH 3 was more than twice as large in the heterosexual men as in the women. It was also, however, more than twice as large in the heterosexual men as in the homosexual men. This finding indicates that INAH 3 is dimorphic with sexual orientation, at least in men, and suggests that sexual orientation has a biological substrate. Further interpretation of the results of this study must be considered speculative. In particular, the results do not allow one to decide if the size of INAH 3 in an individual is the cause or consequence of that individual's sexual orientation, or if the size of INAH 3 and sexual orientation covary under the influence of some third, unidentified variable. Although the validity of the comparison between species is uncertain, it seems more likely that in humans, too, the size of INAH 3 is established early in life and later influences sexual behavior, rather than the reverse [3, 30, 36, 38].

Secondary Sex Characteristics

Puberty is the last phase of the complex process of sexual maturation, a process by which an individual acquires reproductive competency. The dramatic developmental and behavioral changes in the male at puberty result from enhanced testosterone secretion by the testes and the actions of testosterone or one of its metabolites on specific target tissues. Dimorphic secondary sex characteristics are typical of all vertebrates. These differences are most often modifications of the integument or underlying tissues: skin coloration; hair color, distribution, and coarseness; development of specialized integumental structures such as horns, antlers, beaks, claws, and spines [11]. In the male, androgens profoundly affect such courtship behaviors as aggression, bodily movements and display, and even vocalization. Only a few representative examples of the role of androgens among the major groups of vertebrates are discussed here.

Sex Organs. The accessory reproductive glands are dependent on testosterone to enable them to contribute secretory products to the semen. Androgens increase the content of endoplasmic reticulum within the cells of the prostate, seminal vesicles, and bulbourethral glands. The spermatozoa contain only a relatively small amount of cytoplasm and apparently must be nourished by constituents of the seminal fluid. Fructose, a source of metabolic energy for the spermatozoa, is secreted by the seminal vesicles. The effects of testosterone on the prostate gland are greatly augmented by PRL, which is without effect on this gland in the castrated animal. The penis and scrotum also enlarge in response to testosterone or DHT.

Skin. Sebaceous gland activity is stimulated by androgens most likely derived from testosterone. The acne often present in the male during the pubertal process is due to the increased activity of these glands in response to elevated plasma levels of androgens. The coarseness of hair in some animals is increased by androgens, and the pattern of hair growth is also affected. Androgens are stimulatory to hair growth in the axilla, the pubic area, and on the chin. In contrast, androgens cause recession of the male hairline. Androgens may even cause baldness (alopecia) in individuals with such a genetic predisposition. Castration of males who are becoming alopecic prevents further extension of the bald areas but does not promote general regrowth of hair. In females with adrenal virilism the excessive levels of androgens may induce baldness; loss of hair ceases when the abnormal masculinization ends [18].

Androgenic response of a tissue depends on the presence of a specific androgen-binding protein. In addition, enzymes of steroid metabolism alter the chemical structure of steroids and also their hormonal potency. A recent study demonstrated the conversion of dehydroepiandrosterone into androstenedione, testosterone, and DHT in human sebaceous glands, and the greater enzymic activity of Δ^5-3 β-hydroxy steroid dehydrogenase (3 βHSD) activity in sebaceous glands of bald scalp than in hairy scalp. Taken together, greater 3 βHSD activity and increased androgen-binding capacity may provide a biochemical explanation for the disease mechanism of androgenic alopecia. Furthermore such studies may provide new insight into the mechanism of skin diseases caused by hyperandrogenization, such as acne, hirsutism, and seborrhea, besides male pattern baldness [39].

In most vertebrates, skin, hair, and feather coloration differ between the sexes and can be striking in some teleosts and birds [19, 23]. Often the color of the skin changes during the breeding season. These pigmentary changes are usually androgen dependent and involve increases or decreases in the number of pigment cells and the amount and kind of pigment within integumental chromatophores. In some birds, such as the weaver finch, the bill becomes melanized in response to androgens during the breeding season.

The Sexually Dimorphic Kidney.   In Chap. 16, it was noted that gonadal steroids affect sexual dimorphic differentiation and development of nuclear centers within the vertebrate central nervous system. Other organs and tissues are also differentially affected by gonadal steroids. The proximal tubules of the kidneys of male mice, for example, contain mitochondria and lysosomes that are ultrastructurally different from those of females. Males also have higher kidney activities of mitochondrial cytochrome C oxidase and lysosomal hydroxylases. The female pattern of organellar structure develops after orchidectomy. Testosterone administration induces the male pattern of cellular structure and function in castrated male mice or in female mice [27]. Sex differences in kidney function and metabolism, as well as pathophysiology, have been documented and may relate to differences in the hormonal milieu between the two sexes.

Submaxillary Glands of Mice.   As noted in Chap. 12, submaxillary gland production of nerve growth factor (NGF) and epidermal growth factor (EGF) in the mouse is acutely controlled by androgens. Several enzymes are more abundant in the male submaxillary gland than in the female. The cellular synthesis of these enzymes is androgen dependent and can be induced in the female by administration of an androgen. In boars, salivary glands use nonandrogenic steroids of testicular origin and secrete them into the saliva where they may function as sex attractants (e.g., musk).

Brood Patches.   Some birds develop a brood patch on the abdomen during the breeding season. Feathers are lost from this area and the skin becomes thick and hypervascularized so that warmth can be imparted to the incubating eggs. In female passerine birds, where the female develops a patch, estrogen and PRL synergize to cause brood patch development [24]. In those species in which both sexes develop a patch (e.g., quail), estrogens or androgens synergize with PRL to initiate patch development. In the phalarope, in which only the male develops a patch, patch development is regulated by the synergistic actions of PRL and androgens.

Epidermal Cornifications.   In many amphibians black, cornified structures may occur on the forelimbs or hindlimbs. These nuptial pads, as they are designated, assist the male in grasping the female during amplexus. These are androgen-dependent structures that regress after castration and can be reinstated following androgen replacement therapy. In the newt, nuptial pads develop in response to androgens, but only if prolactin and thyroid hormone are also present [11].

Antlers.   A vast array of morphological outgrowths of the integument characterize the male of the species and are often enlarged or otherwise exaggerated during the breeding season. The growth of antlers in some species of deer might be considered the most conspicuous of integumental growths. The antlers are solid bony outgrowths that arise from the frontal bones and are borne usually by the male. The growth and shedding of antlers is under the control of androgens, except in caribou where both the male and female possess antlers. In the red deer stag (*Cervus elaphus*) the cycle of testosterone secretion is responsible for the redevelopment of the secondary sexual characteristics each year; the animal undergoes a type of "annual puberty and senescence" [31]. Testosterone stimulates development of the neck mane and rutting odor and is responsible for loss of velvet from the antlers. Changes in photoperiod affect testicular androgenesis. Increasing day length is inhibitory to testicular androgenic activity in the Sitka deer (*Cervus nippon*) [15]. Testicular activity resumes at the summer solstice when the hours of daylight stabilize.

Breeding Tubercles.   Androgens increase the skin thickness of the salmon and also increase integumental mucous production. In some fishes breeding tubercles develop on the head of the male. These structures apparently evolved to enable breeding individuals to maintain close contact during spawning and may be particularly important in fishes that spawn in fast-moving water [41, 47].

Anabolic Actions

The major extragenital site of androgen action is skeletal muscle, which may account for part of the body weight difference between males and females of many species. Growth of the musculature and cartilage of the larynx of the human causes a permanent deepening of the voice. Because skeletal muscle cannot convert testosterone to DHT, it is likely that testosterone has a direct anabolic action on muscle. The myotropic actions of androgens result from their ability to increase retention of dietary nitrogen through protein synthesis. A great many derivatives of testosterone have been prepared with the hope that they might be of practical use in promoting general body growth without concomitantly producing masculinizing effects. These compounds are referred to as *anabolic steroids*.

Anabolic steroids are synthetic molecules developed in the hope of obtaining a complete separation of the androgenic and myotropic (anabolic) actions of testosterone. Such a goal has never been fully achieved. However, some synthetic steroids present a partial dissociation between these two activities. Since a single hormonal receptor apparently mediates the androgenic as well as the anabolic actions of testosterone, differences in patterns of androgen metabolization in the muscles and the sex accessory organs have been proposed as a possible cause of the phenomenon.

Most unusual, however, is the observation that skeletal muscle does not contain specific receptors for androgens; nevertheless, androgens have anabolic actions in a variety of skeletal muscles. It has been proposed that the anabolic actions of androgens (at least in pharmacological doses) in skeletal muscle may derive from androgen competition for cytosolic glucocorticoid receptors (which enhance protein catabolism).

Undoubtedly, androgens are able to exert a trophic effect on skeletal and cardiac muscle fibers in subjects with low circulating levels of testosterone such as prepubertal or hypogonadal males and females; however, with the widespread use of anabolic steroids by male athletes to increase their physical performances one poses the question of whether these compounds are active in the presence of normal circulating levels of testosterone. Most experimental animal studies indicate that anabolic steroids are ineffective in this situation. Since the results of the experiments performed in humans are largely contradictory, it is still not clear whether anabolic steroids are able to improve athletic performances. Clearly, the literature shows that the continuous administration of high doses of anabolic steroids produces a large number of side-effects, some of which are serious, irreversible, and possibly life-threatening [7].

MECHANISMS OF ANDROGEN ACTION

Androgens mediate their actions through the classical scheme of steroid hormone action (see Fig. 13.10): they interact with cytoplasmic and nuclear receptors, a two-step mechanism, to stimulate transcriptional and translational processes related to protein synthesis. For example, $\alpha_2\mu$-globulin is a protein synthesized by the liver of the male but not the

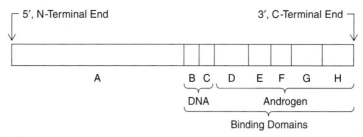

Figure 17.5 Schematic structure of the androgen receptor. The steroid hormone receptor is comprised of eight exons. The role of the amino terminal exon (A) is undetermined but like similar receptors provides specificity for binding the receptor to its substrate, DNA. The DNA-binding domain (66 amino acids in length), encoded by exons B and C, interacts with the hormone responsive element of the DNA. The androgen-binding domain (about 252 amino acids) at the C-terminal end is encoded by exons D–H [21].

female rat. Androgen treatment of spayed female rats or castrated male rats induces the appearance of both $\alpha_2\mu$-globulin and its corresponding messenger RNA. Glucocorticoids, thyroid hormones, and STH are required for the action of androgens on $\alpha_2\mu$-globulin production.

Androgen Receptors. The androgen receptor belongs to the subfamily of steroid hormone receptors within a larger family of nuclear proteins that likely evolved from a common ancestral gene. The androgen receptor has been cloned and its sequence determined. The receptor has highest sequence identity with the progesterone receptor. The gene for the receptor is localized on the human X chromosome [32]. The androgen receptor gene is comprised of eight exons (A–H), coding for three specific functionalities of the receptor (Fig. 17.5). The N-terminal segment is coded by exon A. The function of this "transactivator segment" at present is not clearly defined, but may (1) optimize the transactivation capability of the receptor and (2) specify gene recognition in the transcriptional regulation. The DNA-binding domain, a 66–68 amino acid sequence, is encoded by exons B and C, which code the first and second (C-terminal) zinc finger motifs, respectively. The first zinc finger specifies the receptor's DNA recognition, while the second is mainly responsible for dimerization of two receptor molecules during their association with DNA [21, 22]. The androgen-binding C-terminal domain consists of about 252 amino acids and is encoded by exons D–H (Fig. 17.5). A model for androgen activation of the cognate receptors is depicted in Fig. 17.6.

Antiandrogens

Some of the most potent antiandrogens are derivatives of progesterone. Although they may possess weak androgenic activity, they are inhibitory to the actions of testosterone because of their receptor occupancy. Cyproterone acetate is one of the most potent antiandrogens (Fig. 17.7). For example, treatment of the pregnant rat with cyproterone acetate results in male fetuses that are morphologically feminized, and the adult male rat behavior is that of the female. Administration of the antiandrogen in the mature male causes atrophy of the seminal vesicles, prostate, and other androgen-responsive target organs. Pituitary gonadotropin secretion is enhanced after antiandrogen treatment, as after castration, and in the human male cyproterone acetate causes a loss of libido. In the female, on the other hand, this antiandrogen has been used successfully to treat hirsutism and virilization. In the male, acne and the development of baldness are reversed by antiandrogen treatment. Although cyproterone acetate has been used with some success to treat (delay) precocious puberty, its inhibition of the anabolic actions of androgens may preclude its use in the treatment of sexual precocity.

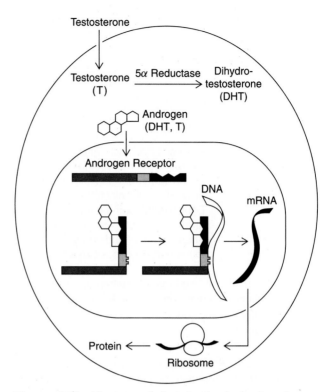

Figure 17.6 Diagram of the mechanism of androgen action at the cellular level. The androgen enters the cell by passive diffusion. It binds to the androgen-binding domain of the receptor. This binding is hypothesized to result in a conformational change exposing the receptor's DNA-binding domain and enabling it to bind to the nuclear chromatin. This binding to DNA initiates transcription of mRNA and, ultimately, translation into androgen-specific proteins. (From Imperato-McGinley and Canovatchel [21]. Reprinted by permission of the publisher from *Trends in Endocrinology and Metabolism* 3:75–81, 1992. ©1992 by Elsevier Science Inc.)

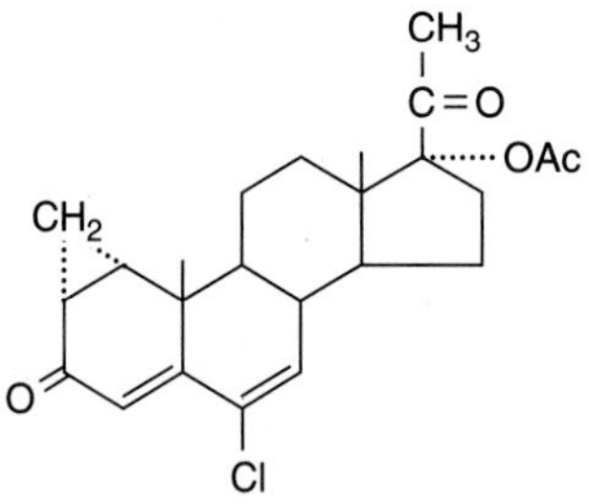

Cyproterone Acetate

Figure 17.7 Structure of cyproterone acetate, an antiandrogen.

PATHOPHYSIOLOGY

Mutations that impair male reproductive function (e.g., androgen action) appear to be relatively common. The comparative frequency may stem in part from the fact that sexual development is essential for reproduction, but not for the life of an individual. Mutations that block androgen action completely do not affect life span, whereas mutations that severely impair the action of hormones essential for life (e.g., insulin, cortisol, thyroxine) are probably lethal in utero [16].

TABLE 17.2   Endocrine Pathophysiology of the Human Male Reproductive System

---

Hypogonadism
  Primary
    Leydig cell deficiency (Leydig cell agenesis)
    Adult Leydig cell failure (male climacteric phase)
    Germinal cell aplasia (Sertoli-cell-only syndrome)
  Secondary
    Gonadotropin deficiency (hypogonadotropic hypogonadism)
    Hypothalamic hypogonadism (defect in GnRH secretion)
Hypergonadism
  Primary (steroid-secreting testicular tumors)
    Virilizing (androgen-secreting) Leydig (interstitial) cell tumors (macrogenitosomia
      in the prepubertal male)
    Feminizing (estrogen-secreting) Leydig (interstitial) cell tumors
  Secondary
    Hypothalamic origin (enhanced GnRH secretion)
    Pituitary origin (hypergonadotropic hypergonadism)
Syndromes of androgen resistance
  Testicular feminizing syndrome (absence of target tissue androgen receptors)
  Syndrome of 5 α-reductase deficiency (failure to convert testosterone to DHT)
Gynecomastia (breast enlargement)

Hypogonadism/Hypergonadism.   Hypogonadism may result from a failure in pituitary gonadotropin secretion because of an isolated defect in one or the other of the gonadotrophs or to some defect in the hypothalamus resulting in a failure to secrete GnRH [45, 46]. Leydig cell agenesis due to a congenital defect would lead to male pseudohermaphroditism, whereas adult Leydig cell dysfunction may be responsible for the climacteric experienced by some men.

Primary hypergonadism may derive from tumors that secrete excess androgens. Feminizing tumors that secrete estrogens have even been documented in the male. Secondary hypergonadism may result from any factors leading to excessive pituitary gonadotropin secretion. Gonadal dysfunction in hyperprolactinemia is now widely recognized [1]. In males, impotence, loss of libido, reduced androgen secretion with testes and prostate involution and oligospermia are not commonly involved with galactorrhea and/or gynecomastia. The pathogenic role of hyperprolactinemia in hypogonadism is confirmed in men and women by its reversal when PRL is lowered either by surgically ablating a prolactinoma or by the use of drugs [9]. Some examples of endocrine disorders are outlined in Table 17.2 and discussed below.

Syndromes of Androgen Resistance.   Various genetic defects can result in the synthesis of an abnormal androgen receptor with loss or impairment of its ability to function. In general, mutations in the androgen-binding domain result in an androgen receptor that is unable to bind androgen, that is, the "receptor-negative" androgen insensitivity syndrome, or one that has altered or impaired binding affinity (Fig. 17.8). In the "receptor-positive" form of complete androgen insensitivity, there is normal binding to the androgen receptor. However, the androgen-receptor complex is incapable of interacting with androgen-responsive DNA sequences. A single nucleotide substitution in exon C of the DNA-binding domain of the androgen receptor (Fig. 17.9) has been determined to cause at least one form of receptor-positive complete androgen insensitivity [22]. It is expected that other deletions, substitutions, and so on, will be found in other subjects with the syndrome [21, 43].

Male Pseudohermaphroditism.   Male pseudohermaphroditism traditionally implies female or intersexual genital development in individuals with histologically normal or almost normal testes [49]. As noted in Chap. 16, male pseudohermaphroditism may be classified into three broad categories related to defects in the following: (1) testosterone

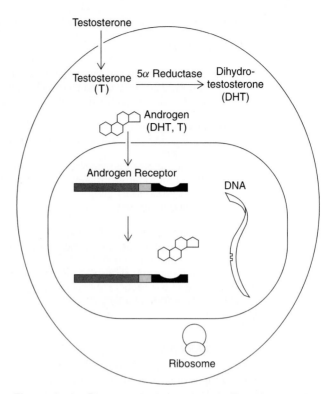

Figure 17.8 Diagram depicting the inability of the androgen receptor to bind to the ligand owing to mutations in the androgen-binding domain of the androgen-receptor genome (receptor-negative resistance). Consequently, no binding to nuclear chromatin occurs. (From Imperato-McGinley and Canovatchel [21]. Reprinted by permission of the publisher from *Trends in Endocrinology and Metabolism* 3:75–81, 1992. ©1992 by Elsevier Science Inc.)

synthesis, (2) androgen receptor synthesis or function, and (3) absent or defective activity of Müllerian regression factor. In addition an isolated deficiency of Leydig cells and a defect in any one of the five or more enzymes required for testosterone biosynthesis will individually lead to male pseudohermaphroditism [25, 26].

A lack of LH production and secretion or a LH receptor defect would also result in failure of testosterone production and, therefore, defects in normal genital development. In sex-reversed XY females, several de novo mutations or deletions in the SRY gene have been described. Testis determination depends on the inheritance of the Y chromosome-encoded testis-determining factor (TDF). In the absence of the Y chromosome, the testis-determining pathway fails to be initiated or is blocked so that the gonads follow the pathway of ovarian development [43]. Dihydrotestosterone (DHT), the product of testosterone metabolism by the testicular enzyme, 5 α-reductase, virilizes the urogenital sinus and external genitalia. Both steroids exert their androgenic effects by interacting with an androgen receptor protein, whose affinity for DHT is much greater than for testosterone, hence the poor virilization of patients who lack 5 α-reductase [26] (see Fig. 16.8).

Gynecomastia. Growth of the mammary tissue of the male, gynecomastia, may be common during the neonatal period. This enlargement of the breasts is generally attributed to maternal hormones reaching the fetus during gestation. Prepubertal gynecomastia may result from a peripheral conversion of androgens produced by the testes and adrenals to estrogens. Adolescent gynecomastia may be associated with a decreased testosterone/estradiol ratio of unknown etiology. The slow increase in the prevalence of

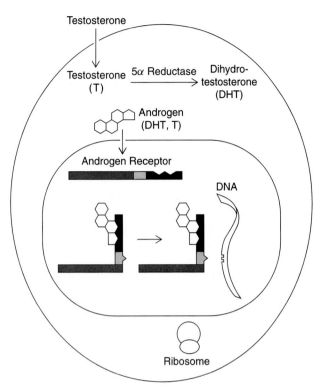

Figure 17.9 Diagram showing the inability of the androgen-receptor complex to bind to nuclear DNA (receptor-positive resistance), secondary to mutations in the DNA-binding domain of the androgen-receptor genome. (From Imperato-McGinley and Canovatchel [21]. Reprinted by permission of the publisher from *Trends in Endocrinology and Metabolism* 3:75–81, 1992. ©1992 by Elsevier Science Inc.)

gynecomastia in adult males, which is accentuated over the age of 45, may also be accounted for by the age-related increase of estrogen/testosterone levels. Although uncommon, gynecomastia may occur unilaterally rather than bilaterally. If gynecomastia is accompanied by galactorrhea, the possibility of a PRL-secreting tumor should be considered.

Congenital adrenal hyperplasia due to 11 β-hydroxylase deficiency has a high incidence among Jews of North African origin and results in the development of gynecomastia in untreated patients. Estrogen production is high as a result of increased steroidal substrates for aromatization. Estrogens are formed predominantly from extraglandular aromatization of adrenal androgens (e.g., androstenedione) [29].

An interesting clinical report described how a 70-year-old man developed gynecomastia. The etiology of the breast enlargement could not be immediately determined. It was then realized that his wife had been using a vaginal cream containing an estrogen. In fact, the cream was also used as a lubricant to facilitate intercourse two to three times a week. When the exposure to estrogen was terminated, gynecomastia disappeared over the subsequent three months [12]. Gynecomastia in males exposed to other sources of estrogens (as well as marihuana smoke) has been reported.

Premature Adrenarche/Pubarche.   Premature pubarche refers to the isolated development of sexual hair at an early age due to increased levels of adrenal androgens (adrenarche). In the female it is known that adrenal androgens are responsible for growth of sexual hair. In the male the penis is of normal size, therefore it is believed that adrenal androgens, rather than testosterone, are responsible for early sexual hair growth.

Adult Leydig Cell Failure (Male Climacteric Phase). In some men Leydig cell function may decline with age; the fall in serum testosterone levels may produce symptoms similar to those of the postmenopausal woman. The age of onset is variable and may be caused by a variety of factors (e.g., as a result of mumps). Although androgen therapy may not improve sexual function, muscle function may be restored, thus counteracting the negative nitrogen balance that is a sequel of androgen deficiency.

Feminizing Adrenocortical Carcinoma. Increased estrogen production by an adrenal tumor may inhibit pituitary-hypothalamic function, resulting in decreased pituitary gonadotropin secretion, which, as expected, leads to testicular atrophy.

Sertoli-Cell-Only Syndrome (Germinal Cell Aplasia). This syndrome may arise from a congenital absence of germ cells. The seminiferous tubules are therefore populated only by Sertoli cells. FSH levels may be preferentially elevated (absence of inhibin?) in this syndrome.

Benign Prostatic Hyperplasia. Prostatic hyperplasia is a common occurrence in aging men. Dihydrotestosterone accumulation within the prostate serves as the humoral mediator of hyperplasia of the gland. An enhanced uptake of DHT in the gland may be due in part to enhanced intracellular binding of the androgen. The process is accelerated, however, by estrogens, which enhance the level of androgen receptors in the gland. Thus an increase in androgen receptors allows for androgen-mediated growth even in the face of declining androgen production in advanced age. Both gynecomastia, as discussed above, and prostate hyperplasia may relate to the declining ratio of androgens to estrogens, which is common in the aging process of men.

Prostate Carcinoma. About seventy thousand new cases of prostatic carcinoma, of which about 80% are androgen dependent, are diagnosed each year in the United States. Surgical castration and administration of pharmacological amounts of estrogen are treatments that have been employed to lower androgen levels in the management of the cancer. Castration is generally not acceptable to many men, and cardiovascular disease may ensue from the use of high doses of estrogens. "Medical castration" using analogues of gonadotropin-releasing hormone (GnRH) now appear to be useful in the clinical treatment of the cancer. Inhibitors of 5 α-reductase also show some success in the treatment of prostate neoplasia.

Impotence. The physiologic basis for the control of penile erection is not totally understood. Relaxation of the vascular and cavernous smooth muscle is not mediated by adrenergic or cholinergic mechanisms. Vasoactive intestinal peptide (VIP, see Chap. 10) has now been implicated as a mediator of penile erection [35]. Erection induced by visual erotic stimulation in normal subjects and induced pharmacologically in patients under evaluation for erectile dysfunction was accompanied by very significant elevations of VIP in blood taken from the corpus cavernosum, whereas concentrations of VIP in peripheral blood remained stable. Infusions of VIP into the cavernous bodies of normal individuals induced varying degrees of tumescence in all subjects. VIP is present in nerve fibers within nerve endings in cavernous smooth muscle and blood vessels. Since VIP is released when erection is induced and stimulates erection when administered, it appears likely that VIP regulates penile erection. Injections of VIP directly into the penis are ineffective in establishing full erectile response and, hence, are inadequate for the treatment of impotency.

Nitric oxide (NO) is a cytotoxic agent of macrophages, a messenger molecule of neurons, and a vasodilator produced by endothelial cells (see Chap. 21). NO synthase was localized to rat penile neurons innervating the corporal cavernosa and to neuronal plexuses in the adventitial layer of penile arteries. Small doses of NO synthase inhibitors abolished electrophysiologically induced penile erections. These results establish NO as a physiologic mediator of erectile function [5, 20].

Pharmacological Considerations

Cannabinoids (substances present in marihuana, e.g., Δ^9-tetrahydrocannabinol, Δ^9-THC) inhibit testicular function in all vertebrate species studied. Testicular testosterone synthesis is decreased, which is correlated with lowered plasma levels of testosterone and involution of the prostate, seminal vesicles, and epididymis. Prolonged cannabinoid intake also leads to diminished spermatogenesis. The immediate effects of cannabinoids on the male reproductive system appear to be reversible. In humans marihuana smoking decreases plasma testosterone levels and the sperm count. In mice cannabinoids reduce fertility and increase the incidence of chromosomal abnormalities, not only in the treated mice but also in their untreated male offspring. The occurrence of congenital birth defects indicates that cannabinoids are capable of inducing genetic mutations that are transmissible to offspring [10]. Alcoholism may also lead to gonadal dysfunction, possibly by diminishing the number of gonadotropin receptors possessed by Leydig cells.

REFERENCES

[1]   Abramsson, L., and M. Duchek. 1989. Gonadotropins, testosterone and prolactin in men with abnormal semen findings and an evaluation of the hormone profile. *Int. Urol. Nephrol.* 21: 499–510.

[2]   Allen, L. S., and R. A. Gorski. 1992. Sexual orientation and the size of the anterior commissure in the human brain. *Proc. Natl. Acad. Sci. USA* 89:7199–202.

[3]   Barinaga, M. 1991. Is homosexuality biological? *Science* 253:956–60.

[4]   Breedlove, S. M., and A. P. Arnold. 1980. Hormone accumulation in a sexually dimorphic motor nucleus of the rat spinal cord. *Science* 210:564–6.

[5]   Burnett, A. L., C. J. Lwenstein, D. S. Bredt, T. S. K. Chang, and S. H. Snyder. 1992. Nitric oxide: a physiologic mediator of penile erection. *Science* 257:401–3.

[6]   Byne, W., and B. Parsons. 1993. Human sexual orientation. The biological theories reappraised. *Arch. Gen. Psychiatry* 50:228–39.

[7]   Celotti, F., and N. Cesi. 1992. Anabolic steroids: a review of their effects on the muscles, of their possible mechanisms of action and of their use in athletics. *J. Steroid. Biochem. and Mol. Biol.* 43:469–77.

[8]   Coquelin, A., and F. H. Bronson. 1979. Release of luteinizing hormone in male mice during exposure to females: habituation of the response. *Science* 206:1099–1100.

[9]   Crosignani, P. G., and C. Ferrari. 1987. Synthesis, release and biological actions of human prolactin. *Res. Reprod.* 19:2–3.

[10] Dalterio, S., F. Badr, A. Bartke, and D. Mayfield. 1982. Cannabinoids in male mice: effects on fertility and spermatogenesis. *Science* 216:315–6.

[11] Dent, J. N. 1975. Integumentary effects of prolactin in the lower vertebrates. *Amer. Zool.* 15: 923–35.

[12] DiRaimondo, C. V., A. C. Roach, and C. K. Meador. 1980. Gynecomastia from exposure to vaginal estrogen cream. *New Engl. J. Med.* 302:1089–90.

[13] Fingscheidt, U., G. F. Weinbauer, S. A. Khan, and E. Nieschlag. 1990. Follicle-stimulating hormone stimulates inhibin in the serum of male monkeys (*Macaca mulatta*). *Acta Endocrinol.* 122:96–100.

[14] Friedman, R. C., and J. Downey. 1993. Neurobiology and sexual orientation: current considerations. *J. Neuropsychiatry Clin. Neurosci.* 5:131–53.

[15] Goss, R. J. 1968. Inhibition of growth and shedding of antlers by sex hormones. *Nature* 220: 83–5.

[16] Griffin, J. E., and J. D. Wilson. 1987. Syndromes of androgen resistance. *Hosp. Pract.* 22:69–74.

[17] Hamer, D. H., S. Hu, V. L. Magnuson, N. Hu, and A. M. L. Pattatucci. 1993. A linkage between DNA markers on the X chromosome and male sexual orientation. *Science* 261:321–7.

[18] Hamilton, J. B. 1942. Male hormone stimulation is prerequisite and incident in common baldness. *Amer. J. Anat.* 71:451–80.

[19] Höhn, E. O., and S. C. Cheng. 1967. Gonadal hormones on Wilson's phalarope (*Steganopus tricolor*) and other birds in relation to plumage and sex behavior. *Gen. Comp. Endocrinol.* 8:1–11.

[20] Ignarro, L. J. 1992. Nitric oxide as the physiological mediator of penile erection. *J. NIH Res.* 4:59–62.

[21] Imperato-McGinley, J., and W. J. Canovatchel. 1992. Complete androgen insensitivity. Pathophysiology, diagnosis, and management. *TEM* 3:75–81.

[22] Janne, O. A., J. J. Palvimo, P. Kallio, and M. Mehto. 1993. Androgen receptor and mechanism of androgen action. *Ann. Med.* 25:83–9.

[23] Johns, J. E. 1964. Testosterone induced nuptial feathers in phalaropes. *Condor* 66:449–54.

[24] Jones, R. E. 1971. The incubation patch of birds. *Biol. Rev.* 46:315–39.

[25] Josso, N. 1992. Anti-Müllerian hormone and Sertoli cell function. *Horm. Res.* 38:72–6.

[26] Josso, N., L. Boussin, B. Knebelmann, C. Nihoul-Fekete, and J.-Y. Picard. 1991. Anti-Müllerian hormone and intersex states. *TEM* 2:227–33.

[27] Koenig, H., A. Goldstone, G. Blume, and C. Y. Lee. 1980. Testosterone-mediated sexual dimorphism of mitochondria and lysosomes in mouse kidney proximal tubules. *Science* 209:1023–6.

[28] Kurz, E. M., D. R. Sengelaub, and A. P. Arnold. 1986. Androgens regulate the dendritic length of mammalian motoneurons in adulthood. *Science* 232:395–98.

[29] Leiberman, E., and M. Zachmann. 1992. Familial adrenal feminization probably due to increased steroid aromatization. *Horm. Res.* 37:96–102.

[30] Levay, S. 1991. A difference in hypothalamic structure between heterosexual and homosexual men. *Science* 253:1034–7.

[31] Lincoln, G. A. 1971. The seasonal reproductive changes in the Red Deer stag (*Cervus elaphus*). *J. Zool. Lond.* 163:105–23.

[32] Lubahn, D. B., D. R. Joseph, P. M. Sullivan, H. F. Willard, F. S. French, and E. M. Wilson. Cloning of human androgen receptor complementary DNA and localization to the X chromosome. *Science* 240:327–30.

[33] Mooradian, A. D., J. E. Morley, and S. G. Korenman. 1987. Biological actions of androgens. *Endocr. Rev.* 8:1–28.

[34] Nordeen, E. J., K. W. Nordeen, D. R. Sengelaub, and A. P. Arnold. 1985. Androgens prevent normally occurring cell death in a sexually dimorphic spinal nucleus. *Science* 229:671.

[35] Ottesen, B., G. Wagner, R. Virag, and J. Fahrenkrug. 1984. Penile erection: possible role for vasoactive intestinal polypeptide as a neurotransmitter. *Br. Med. J.* 288:9–11.

[36] Pool, R. 1993. Evidence for homosexuality gene. *Science* 26:291–2.

[37] Reyes-Fuentes, A., and J. D. Vedhuis. 1993. Neuroendocrine physiology of the normal male gonadal axis. *Endocrinol. Metab. Clin. N. Amer.* 22:93–124.

[38] Risch, N., E. Swuires-Wheeler, and B. J. B. Keats. 1993. Male sexual orientation and genetic evidence. *Science* 262:2063–5.

[39] Sawaya, M. E., L. S. Honig, and S. L. Hsia. 1989. Increased androgen binding capacity in sebaceous glands in scalp of male-pattern baldness. *J. Invest. Dermatol.* 92:91–95.

[40] Setchell, B. P. 1980. The functional significance of the blood-testis barrier. *J. Androl.* 1:3–10.

[41] Smith, R. J. F. 1974. Effects of 17 β-methyltestosterone on the dorsal pad and tubercles of flathead minnows (*Pimephales promelas*). *Can. J. Zool.* 52:1031–38.

[42] Spiteri-Grech, J., and E. Nieschlag. 1993. Paracrine factors relevant to the regulation of spermatogenesis—a review. *J. Reprod. Fert.* 98:1–14.

[43]   Sultan, C., J. M. Lobaccaro, C. Belon, A. Terraza, and S. Lumbroso. 1992. Molecular biology of disorders of sex differentiation. *Horm. Res.* 38:105–13.

[44]   Waterman, M. R., and D. S. Keeney. 1992. Genes involved in androgen biosynthesis and the male phenotype. *Horm. Res.* 38:217–21.

[45]   Whitcomb, R. W., and W. F. Crowley, Jr. 1990. Diagnosis and treatment of isolated gonadotropin-releasing hormone deficiency in men. *J. Clin. Endocrinol. Metab.* 70:3–7.

[46]   ———1993. Male hypogonadotropic hypogonadism. *Endocrinol. Metab. Clin. N. Amer.* 22:125–43.

[47]   Wiley, M. L., and B. B. Collette. 1970. Breeding tubercles and contact organs in fishes, their occurrence, structure and significance. *Amer. Mus. Natur. Hist. Bull.* 143:147–53.

[48]   Wingfield, J. C., G. F. Ball, A. M. Duffy, Jr., R. E. Hegner, and M. Ramenofsky. 1987. Testosterone and aggression in birds. *Amer. Sci.* 75:602–8.

[49]   Zachmann, M. 1992. Recent aspects of steroid biosynthesis in male sex differentiation. Clinical studies. *Horm. Res.* 38:211–6.

18

Hormones and Female Reproductive Physiology

It was noted earlier that in mammals the female phenotype develops spontaneously, apparently in the absence of any gonadal hormone directive. At puberty, however, ovarian steroid hormone secretion is essential for development of female secondary sex characteristics. In addition gonadal hormone production regulates the cyclic pattern of pituitary gonadotropin secretion characteristic of the female and is responsible for other cyclic phenomena as egg maturation, ovulation, and the menstrual cycle.

*It has long been known that ovariectomy results in uterine atrophy and the loss of sexual activity and reproductive function. The role of the ovaries in the control of reproductive function was established in 1900 by Knauer who found that ovarian transplants prevented the atrophic symptoms of gonadectomy. Ovarian extracts were then found to maintain the integrity of reproductive structures following ovariectomy. Allen and Doisy identified the Graafian follicle as a major source of estrogenic activity [1]. A putative female sex hormone was then discovered in the blood of a number of animals, and it was further observed that the concentration of the substance varied with the phase of the menstrual cycle in the human female. An important discovery was the finding that this substance, a steroid, was present in the urine in large amounts during pregnancy. Chemists were able to isolate the active substance from urine in crystalline form and to determine its chemical structure. This steroid hormone, **estradiol**, plays an essential role in the control of secondary sex characteristics in the female of most vertebrate species. It was also established that the corpus luteum of the ovary secreted a steroid hormone that is necessary for normal reproductive function during pregnancy. This hormone, **progesterone**, was isolated and subsequently synthesized in 1934.*

Although ovarian estrogens and progestins play pivotal roles in the regulation of female reproductive function, it is now realized that many other hormones of neural, placental-uterine, and adrenal origin are also essential for normal reproductive function in the female.

ANATOMY OF THE FEMALE REPRODUCTIVE SYSTEM

Like the testes in the male, the ovaries serve both a gametogenic and an endocrine function (Fig. 18.1). The female gametes, ova, are released (ovulated) from the ovary into the abdominal cavity where they find their way into the closely adherent uterine tubes (Fallopian tubes, oviducts). The eggs may become fertilized en route down the oviducts

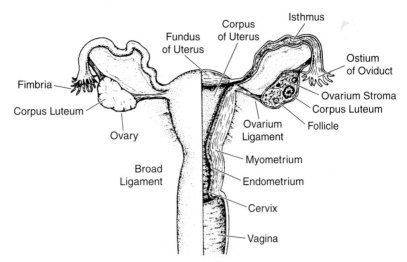

Figure 18.1   Reproductive organs of the human female.

by spermatozoa previously introduced into the vagina by the male ejaculate. If fertilization occurs, the fertilized egg, the *zygote,* may then become embedded within the lining of the uterus and through embryogenesis develop into a fetus. The general morphological and functional features of the human female reproductive system will be described.

Ovary

The ovary has two functional roles that are distinct but intertwined. The first is hormonogenesis, and the second is gametogenesis [21]. The gonad in the homogametic species develops in the absence of any apparent endocrine influence (see Chap. 16). In the human female the gametogenic potential of the ovary is established early in fetal development, but the endocrine role of the ovary is not realized until puberty. Each of the embryonic ovaries is initially populated by about one thousand to two thousand *primordial germ cells,* which, through rapid proliferation, give rise in each ovary to about 3 million oocytes. At birth this number is reduced through cell death to about 1 million oocytes in each ovary, and by puberty each ovary may only be populated by about 250,000 oocytes. Only an exceedingly small fraction of these viable oocytes will develop fully into mature egg cells. Indeed, because a single ovum is usually ovulated during each human reproductive cycle, a total of only 400 to 500 oocytes are released from the ovaries; the remaining 99.9% are destined for atresia during the years of ovarian activity (puberty to menopause) [16].

   The ovary consists of both epithelial and mesenchymal components. The mesenchymal tissue differentiates into interstitial tissue, which will be the primary source of estrogen production by the ovary. The epithelial tissue will become closely associated with the germinal elements of the ovary and, in addition to providing a nutritive environment for the oocytes, will also provide an important source of hormones during particular phases of the female cycle.

   At birth each oocyte is surrounded by a single layer of flattened epithelial-derived *granulosa cells*; the combined structure is termed a *primordial follicle* (Fig. 18.2). These primordial follicles lie mostly near the periphery (cortex) of the ovary but are separated from each other by stromal (connective) and interstitial tissue. Most primordial follicles remain in an arrested state, which may last until puberty or even menopause, if they are not selected for further differentiation and development. Within the embryonic ovary the primordial follicles begin the reduction division of meiosis, but when meiotic division is delayed in the late prophase, the follicles and their primary oocytes may continue to increase greatly in size. Further development of a primordial follicle involves

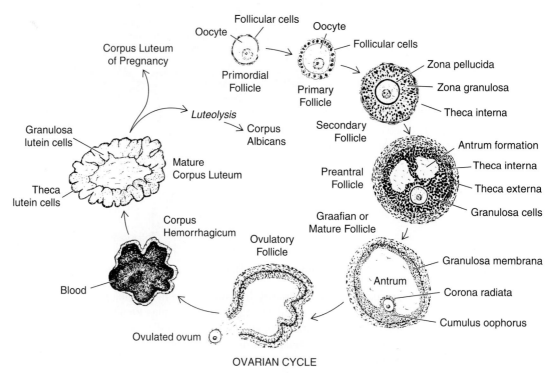

OVARIAN CYCLE

Figure 18.2   The primate ovarian follicular cycle.

transformation of the follicular epithelial cells into a single layer of cuboidal cells surrounding the oocyte; the composite structure is referred to as a *primary follicle* (Fig. 18.2).

Under endocrine stimulation once during each ovarian cycle after puberty, 6 to 12 primary follicles develop into *secondary follicles.* This process involves an increase in the size of the oocyte and in the number of granulosa cell layers that surround each oocyte (Fig. 18.2). During the development of these secondary follicles, the granulosa cells secrete a mucoid material that forms the *zona pellucida* around the oocyte (Fig. 18.2). The granulosa cells develop protoplasmic processes that penetrate the zona pellucida and make contact with the plasmalemma of the oocyte. Although a number of primary follicles may be selected for further development into secondary follicles during each menstrual cycle, usually only one is destined to develop into a mature follicle. The others, by some unknown process, become atretic and disappear with time.

During each ovarian cycle selected primary oocytes complete first meiotic division with resulting extrusion of the first polar body and formation of the *secondary oocyte,* which contains most of the cytoplasm. The first meiotic division is completed shortly before ovulation. The secondary oocyte immediately enters the second reduction division of meiosis, a process that is arrested in metaphase unless fertilization occurs subsequent to ovulation. The second polar body is extruded if the oocyte is penetrated by a sperm. The diploid state of the transiently haploid oocyte is therefore reconstituted by the haploid chromosomal contribution of the sperm to the zygote.

The granulosa cells of follicles destined for further maturation continue to increase in number. At the same time interstitial tissue adjacent to the follicle becomes arranged concentrically around it to form the *theca* (theca folliculi). Those thecal cells adjacent to the follicle, the *theca interna,* are surrounded by an additional outer layer of interstitial cells, the *theca externa,* which merges imperceptibly with the ovarian stroma. The theca interna remains separated from the granulosa cells by a basement lamella. Although the theca is penetrated by vascular elements, no capillaries penetrate into the granulosa.

Continued proliferation of granulosa cells and the incorporation of surrounding interstitial cells into the theca are accompanied by the accumulation of fluid in spaces or

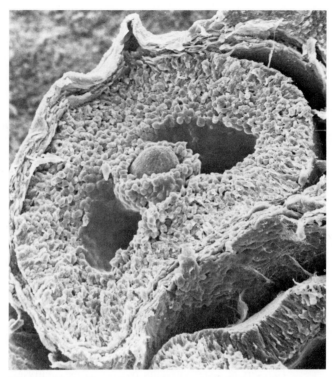

Figure 18.3 Scanning electron micrograph of the human Graafian follicle. (From P. Bagavadoss. The Reproductive Endocrinology Program, Department of Anatomy, The University of Michigan.)

clefts within the granulosa cells. As the follicle enlarges, a single large vesicle or antrum is formed. Those granulosa cells that remain adherent to the ovum comprise the coronal granulosa cells; those granulosa cells that remain in contact with the surrounding theca constitute the *membrana granulosa.* A bridge of granulosa cells connects those cells adherent to the ovum with the membrana granulosa and constitutes the *cumulus oophorus.* During ovulation this connection is severed and the ovum is ejected with its surrounding layer of granulosa cells, the *corona radiata.* The fully developed mature follicle, shown in Fig. 18.3, is known as a *Graafian follicle.*

The mechanisms controlling rupture of the mature ovarian follicle during ovulation have been debated and many hypotheses provided. In the hamster, for example, smooth muscle cells (SMC) are present within the theca externa at the base of the follicle. Contraction of these muscle cells is believed to squeeze the cumulus mass toward the apex of the follicle. Tension within the follicle wall then results in a thinning of the apical layers leading to rupture of the follicle. Although it might be assumed that high levels of LH are responsible for follicular SMC contraction, it is not known whether the hormone directly or indirectly stimulates the cells. Local changes in the environment of the SMC could lead to their contraction. Whatever the stimulus may be, it appears to be mediated through the production of $PGF_{2\alpha}$, probably generated in response to an inward Ca^{2+} ion flux. Other models have suggested that production or activation of follicular proteases (collagenases) may be essential to the mechanism of ovulation. Bradykinin released at localized sites by cleavage of a kininogen by a serine protease (kallikrein) may also modulate ovulation by stimulation of prostaglandin synthesis, resulting in ovarian contractility and possibly activation of a collagenase [21].

The Dominant Ovarian Follicle. Although many follicles may begin to maturate during each ovarian/menstrual cycle, typically only a single follicle sustains its inherent

Folliculogenesis

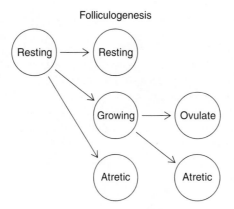

Figure 18.4 Ovarian follicles may be found in four basic conditions: at rest, growing, atretic, or ready to ovulate. (From Irianni and Hogden [21], with permission. *Endocrinology and Metabolism Clinics of North America* 21:19–38, 1992.)

gametogenic potential, whereas the others become atretic. Any ovarian follicle destined to ovulate is derived from a group of growing follicles drawn, in turn, from a pool of non-proliferating primordial follicles formed during fetal development (Fig. 18.4). Pituitary gonadotropins support this progression of follicular maturation, and about 99.9% of all ovarian follicles are lost spontaneously to atresia; only a few achieve ovulation. Depending on the species, usually only a few, or even just one, of these follicles of a given group escapes atresia at various stages of development and finally reaches maturity, culminating in ovulation of a fertilizable oocyte. This successive reduction of potentially ovulatory follicles during each ovarian cycle to a number characteristic of the species suggests some sort of selection. This process is especially evident in the higher primates, including women, where typically the process of folliculogenesis leading to the elaboration of a single mature gamete in each menstrual cycle is regulated with a high degree of precision [21].

The follicle that eventually matures and ovulates is thought to be the one whose granulosa cells most rapidly acquire high levels of aromatase and LH receptor in response to the intercycle FSH rise, that is, the one with the lowest FSH "threshold." During the mid-follicular phase, this follicle begins to increase E_2 secretion and the steroid feeds back to regulate pituitary FSH secretion negatively. This causes a progressive reduction in the circulating FSH level and thereby limits FSH-dependent development of other follicles with relatively high FSH thresholds. Thus only one follicle becomes fully mature, being protected against the fall in circulating FSH by the relatively high responsiveness of its granulosa cells to both FSH and LH [19].

It has been stated that "The purposes of the ovarian follicle are to (1) preserve the resident oocyte; (2) mature the oocyte at the optimal time; (3) produce a hormonal milieu that will develop a lush proliferative endometrium; (4) yield well-timed release of the oocyte; (5) provide for a high quality corpus luteum function, leading to implantation; and (6) preserve the hormonal conditions required for gestation until the fetoplacental metabolism is adequate—a formidable sequence designed by nature" [21].

The Corpus Luteum.   After rupture of the mature follicle and liberation of the ovum during ovulation, the follicle promptly fills up with blood, forming what is called a *corpus hemorrhagicum.* The granulosa and thecal cells rapidly increase in number and the clotted blood is absorbed. Vascular elements from the theca now penetrate the granulosa cells. The granulosa cells begin to accumulate large quantities of cholesterol; this luteinization process leads to formation of the *corpus luteum* [40]. The mature corpus luteum of some species appears to contain a number of distinct cell types. Cells derived from the theca interna migrate into granulosa-derived areas of the luteal tissue soon after ovulation to give rise to small luteal cells, theca lutein cells, and fibroblasts. The large luteal cells apparently differentiate from the membrana granulosa. Although luteal cell heterogeneity is commonly accepted, the definitive origin of each cell type and its individual functions within the corpus luteum of pregnancy remain unclear.

Fallopian Tubes

In the human female these paired oviducts are about 10 cm long and are closely adherent to the superiolateral aspects of the uterus (see Fig. 18.1). The ostium tubae, the fimbriated ovarian extremity of the oviduct, spread over most of the medial surface of the ovary, and the undulatory movements of the fimbriae assist ova transport into the lumen of the Fallopian tubes. The oviducts proper are composed of longitudinal and circular muscular layers covered by a simple columnar epithelium that comprises the mucosa. The ciliated mucosal cells beat toward the uterus and thus rapidly convey the ova toward the uterus. Fertilization of the egg takes place within the oviducts.

Uterus

The uterus, connected to the oviducts at superiolateral angles, is a thick-walled, muscular organ that serves as a site for fetal development and as an endocrine organ during pregnancy. The bulk of the uterus is composed of smooth muscle, the *myometrium* (Fig. 18.1). An *endometrium* covers the mucosal aspect of the myometrium and is composed of connective tissue and an extensive vascular network. The endometrium, in turn, is covered by a simple epithelium. The thickness of the endometrium varies dramatically throughout the menstrual cycle in response to ovarian hormones. The myometrium is also similarly variable in thickness, most profoundly during pregnancy.

OVARIAN STEROID HORMONES

The ovarian follicle is the source of three types of steroid hormones: progestogens (progestins), androgens, and estrogens. The relative amounts of each class of steroid vary throughout the menstrual cycle and drastically change in the pregnant state. During the follicular phase of the menstrual cycle estradiol is the major steroid hormone secreted by the ovary, whereas during the luteal phase and during pregnancy progesterone is the major steroid hormone secreted.

Estrogen Biosynthesis

It is believed that the thecal cells are the source of estrogen production that predominates during the follicular phase of the cycle. The *two-cell theory* of estrogen production states, however, that the thecal cells produce C-19 androgens that are delivered to the granulosa cells wherein they are aromatized to estrogens (Fig. 18.5). This theory is supported by the observation that granulosa cells from several species secrete estrogens if given an androgen substrate. In addition, thecal cells produce large amounts of androgens. Granulosa cells, on the other hand, have little or no capacity for producing C-19 androgens from C-21

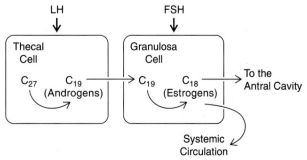

Figure 18.5 Two-cell, two-gonadotropin hypothesis of estrogen synthesis.

steroids but do have an active aromatase system. There is evidence that as follicular maturation progresses the ability of granulosa cells to aromatize androgens increases. Estrogen production increases within the follicle during the preovulatory phase and is highest at the time of the LH/FSH surge. Before exposure to a high level of LH, androgen and estrogen levels predominate; after the LH surge and during the luteal phase of the cycle, however, progesterone is the major steroid produced. A complex number of interactions involving LH, FSH, androgens, progesterone, and estrogens are undoubtedly involved in the shift from estrogen to progesterone synthesis [43].

A modified version of the two-cell theory suggests that LH stimulates androgen production within the thecal cells. The androgens are then aromatized within the thecal cells but are also made available to the granulosa cells for aromatization to estrogens. The estrogens produced by the thecal cells would be the major source of circulating levels of the steroid, whereas estrogens synthesized by the granulosa cells would serve a local role, possibly related to ovum maturation. The granulosa cells are regulated through FSH stimulation of cAMP production and subsequent induction and activation of aromatase activity.

Estradiol (E_2) is readily oxidized to *estrone* within the liver (Fig. 18.6); estrone may be further hydrated to *estriol* (E_3). These three estrogens are excreted in the urine as glucuronides and sulfates. During pregnancy the placenta is an additional source of estrogens. Indeed, the formation of estrogens is not limited to the ovaries, placenta, or adrenals, as some peripheral tissues (e.g., adipose tissue) can produce significant quantities of estro-

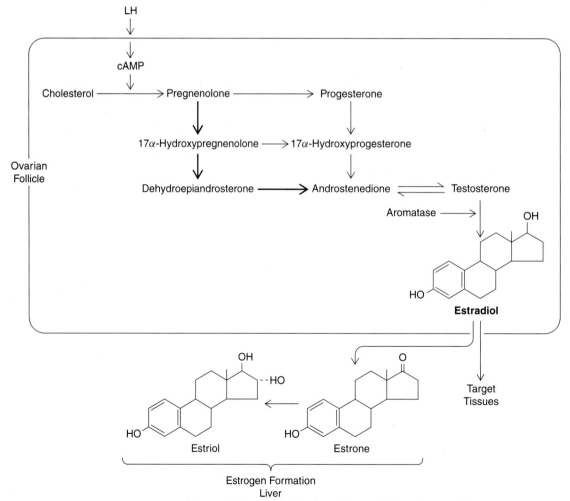

Figure 18.6   Biosynthesis and metabolism of estradiol.

gens from steroid precursors. Aromatization of androstenedione and testosterone within tissues is a major source of estrogens in the male and postmenopausal female.

Progesterone Biosynthesis

The growth of the preovulatory follicles in the ovary is dependent on both FSH and LH acting in concert. FSH promotes the growth of the follicle by acting through receptors on the granulosa cells and inducing the aromatase enzyme required to convert androgens to estrogens, the action of FSH being enhanced initially by androgens. The androgens originate from the theca under the control of LH (Fig. 18.5). While FSH receptors are only present on granulosa cells, in the latter stages of preovulatory development, LH receptors, present initially only in the theca, appear in the granulosa cells and are probably coupled to the same second-messenger (cAMP) system as FSH receptors. During the preovulatory surge, LH acting directly on the granulosa cells initiates luteinization, resulting in a reduction or abolition of aromatase enzyme activity, depending on the species, and the enhancement of progesterone synthesis and secretion as the luteinized granulosa cells transform to become the corpus luteum [38].

Progesterone synthesis is an early step in the biosynthesis of androgen and estrogen production within the thecal cell. Thecal cell progesterone production is not, however, considered an important source of vascular levels of progesterone. The corpus luteum is the major source of circulating progesterone. During the follicular phase of the cycle these cells, which are essentially devoid of a smooth endoplasmic reticulum characteristic of steroid-secreting cells, may use an androgen substrate for aromatization to estrogens as discussed above. Just prior to the LH/FSH surge in some species, progesterone biosynthesis is initiated within the granulosa cells. The fact that granulosa cells from large follicles spontaneously luteinize in culture, but fail to do so in the presence of follicular fluid obtained from small follicles, suggests that a luteinization inhibitor may be present and may function to keep granulosa cells from secreting prematurely. Luteinized cells contain large quantities of cholesterol; it has been shown that rat luteal cells preferentially use, and are acutely dependent on, plasma low-density lipoprotein complexes (see Chap. 15). Luteal cells are the major source of circulating progesterone following the luteinization process.

Androgens

With the commencement of ovarian estrogen synthesis at puberty, androstenedione and testosterone, precursors of estrogens, are secreted by the ovaries [43]. The development of secondary sex characteristics during the pubertal process appears to be almost totally accounted for by the actions of estrogens. Nevertheless, it is possible that the growth spurt that occurs at puberty may, in part, be influenced by androgens of ovarian origin. In addition, acne, common to many females at puberty, results from sebaceous gland activation by ovarian androgens. Pubic and axillary hair growth are also attributed to androgens of ovarian and/or adrenal origin.

Adrenarche leads to the development of sexual (pubic or axillary) hair (pubarche). It is associated with an increase in serum levels of dehydroepianodrosterone sulfate (DHEA-S) and changes in the adrenal response to ACTH. These changes in adrenal androgen production are referred to as biochemical adrenarche and result from maturational changes in the activities of the adrenal enzymes 3 β-hydroxysteroid dehydrogenase (3 βHSD), 17-hydroxylase, and 17,20-desmolase. The consequence of these changes in enzyme activity is increased production of adrenal androgens [17].

Somatomedin Regulation of Gonadal Steroidogenesis

The roles of insulinlike growth factors (IGFs), especially IGF-I, in regulating the ovarian cycle and granulosa cell steroidogenesis have been documented. Studies from several

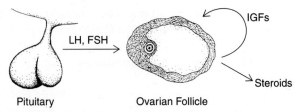

Pituitary   Ovarian Follicle

Figure 18.7   Role of IGFs in ovarian steroidogenesis.

laboratories demonstrated that IGFs promote both replication and differentiation of cultured granulosa cells. IGFs affect FSH-induced enhancement of progesterone, estrogen, and cAMP production, as well as LH receptor induction. In porcine thecal cells, IGFs increase basal and gonadotropin-induced progesterone secretion. In addition, hCG-induced synthesis of thecal androstenedione and testosterone are enhanced when estradiol synthesis is decreased. Porcine theca and granulosa cells contain receptors for IGF-I. The possible involvement of ovarian IGFs in follicular development in vivo was also suggested by measurements of IGF-I in porcine follicular fluid and culture media from porcine granulosa cells. Indeed, gonadotropin, estrogen, as well as cAMP (the presumed mediator of gonadotropin action), enhance the secretion of immunoreactive IGF-I by porcine granulosa cells. Thus the hormone-induced secretion of growth factors appears to serve an important autocrine mechanism by which follicular growth and differentiation occur (Fig. 18.7) [38].

PHYSIOLOGICAL ROLES OF OVARIAN STEROID HORMONES

There is no evidence that the fetal or preadolescent human ovary produces significant quantities of estrogens or other gonadal steroids. At puberty, however, ovarian steroidogenesis is activated by pituitary gonadotropins. During the follicular phase of the ensuing menstrual cycles estrogens are the main steroidal products of the ovary, whereas during the luteal phase of each cycle progesterone is the hormonally important steroidal product of the postovulatory follicle.

Estrogens

Estrogens produced during pubertal maturation in the human female are responsible for growth and development of the vagina, uterus, and oviducts, organs essential to ovum transport, zygote maturation, and implantation of the conceptus. Estrogens affect the distribution of fat deposition, a process that occurs in the postadolescent female. Mammary growth and development is also initiated by the actions of estrogens in concert with other hormones. Other physiological actions of estrogens are summarized in Table 18.1.

Progesterone

Progesterone is the ovarian hormone of pregnancy and is responsible for preparing the reproductive tract for zygote implantation and the subsequent maintenance of the pregnant state. It has been speculated that preovulatory plasma levels of progesterone may trigger sexual behavior in some species. In some rodents, for example, progesterone appears necessary for induction of sexual receptivity. Progesterone may also play a role in the initiation of nest-building activity and brooding behavior in some avian species. It must be emphasized that many actions of progesterone are usually, if not exclusively, on estrogen-primed tissues. Table 18.1 summarizes the known physiological roles of progesterone in the human female.

TABLE 18.1 Some Physiological Effects and Roles of Ovarian Steroid Hormones in Mammals

Primary site of action	Physiological action
Estradiol	
CNS	Maintains libido and sexual behavior [41]
Pituitary	Has negative and positive feedback effects on gonadotropin secretion
	Increases pituitary TRH receptor number
	Increases pituitary GnRH receptor number
	Increases oxytocin production
Ovary	Is required for ovum maturation (is luteolytic in some mammalian species)
Vagina	Causes proliferation and cornification of the mucosa
Oviducts	Causes growth and development in preparation for gamete transport
Uterus	
Cervix	Increases mucus secretion
Endometrium	Increases blood flow
	Increases prostaglandin biosynthesis at term
	Increases number of oxytocin receptors at term
	Causes decidualization response (increases the number of estrogen receptors in the decidua)
Myometrium	Synthesizes contractile proteins of smooth muscle cells
	Increases membrane excitability (increases sensitivity to oxytocin)
Mammary glands	Causes ductule and stromal growth and development, fat accretion
Skin	Induces sebaceous gland secretion (thinner fluid)
	Stimulates axillary and pubic hair growth (possibly in concert with gonadal and adrenal androgens)
General body effects	Causes H_2O and Na^+ retention, weight gain (anabolic action), and female type of fat distribution
	Maintains bone mineral deposition
Liver	Causes hepatic angiotensinogen production
	Causes hepatic production of thyroid-binding globulin
Blood	Decreases plasma cholesterol formation
Progesterone	
CNS	Increases sexual receptivity (at least in some mammalian species)
	Inhibits pituitary gonadotropin secretion by an action on the hypothalamus during the ovarian luteal phase
Oviducts	Causes growth and development for gamete transport
Uterus	
Endometrium	Stimulates growth and development in preparation for blastocyst implantation
	Decreases estrogen receptor number (at least, in the rat)
Cervix	Increases mucus consistency
Myometrium	Causes antiestrogen effects (myometrial hyperpolarization, decreased sensitivity to oxytocin, decreased estrogen receptor number, "maintenance of pregnancy)
Vagina	Inhibits estrogen-induced vaginal cornification
Mammary glands	Is necessary for lobular-alveolar development (in some species)
	Inhibits prepartum prolactin-induced lactogenesis by decreasing PRL receptor number
General body effects	Causes thermogenic action (rise in basal metabolic rate)

Hormones and Sexual Desire in Women

In most subprimates, sexual behavior is closely linked to ovulation and is dependent on the activating effect of E_2 and, sometimes, on the inhibiting effect of progesterone. Only in this phase of the estrous cycle is the female sexually receptive and attractive to the male. In most species of subhuman primates sexual activity becomes less confined to any one phase of the menstrual cycle, although peaks still are observed at midcycle. A number of studies have verified a direct hormonal effect on the sexual receptivity and proceptivity of female primates.

In human females, however, problems in operationally defining and measuring sexual motivation, designating menstrual cycle phases, and sampling reproductive hormones have limited most investigations. The role of gonadal hormones in modulating human female sexual interest therefore remains a controversial subject. Results have indicated that in the hypoactive sexual desire disorder (HSD), women's gonadal hormones fluctuated normally over the menstrual cycle, were within normal limits for each cycle phase, and were never significantly different from those of controls. Testosterone, non-SHBG-bound testosterone, and PRL did not differ between the HSD women with the most and least severe HSD parameters (e.g., frequency of fantasy, masturbation, or female-initiated coitus), or between women with lifelong and acquired HSD. These findings provide no evidence that reproductive hormones are important determinants of individual differences in the sexual desire of these eugonadal women [42].

MECHANISMS OF ACTION OF OVARIAN STEROID HORMONES

Ovarian steroid hormones, E_2 and progesterone, manifest their actions as described for the general actions of steroid hormones (see Chaps. 4, 17). Steroids interact with cytoplasmic and/or nuclear protein receptors. This results in the release of the two receptor subunits with attached steroid hormones from association with a heat-shock protein. Either identical subunits, singly or possibly together, can now interact directly with the DNA hormone responsive element to activate transcriptional events leading to the translation of a cell-specific protein (e.g., ovalbumin).

Nonsteroidal Estrogens and Antiestrogens

A number of nonsteroidal compounds possess estrogenic activity, the most potent of which is diethylstilbestrol (DES). The similarity between the structures of DES and the natural steroids is illustrated (Fig. 18.8). DES is highly active when given orally, apparently because it is degraded more slowly in the GI tract. Antiestrogens, such as clomiphene and tamoxifen (Fig. 18.8), are nonsteroidal compounds that, through competition with estrogen receptors, prevent actions of endogenous estrogens from expressing their full effects on their target tissues. By this action they antagonize a variety of estrogen-dependent processes, such as uterine growth and negative feedback to the hypothalamus. Interest in these drugs derives from the hope that they might prove useful in preventing the growth of estrogen-dependent mammary tumors (see Chap. 19).

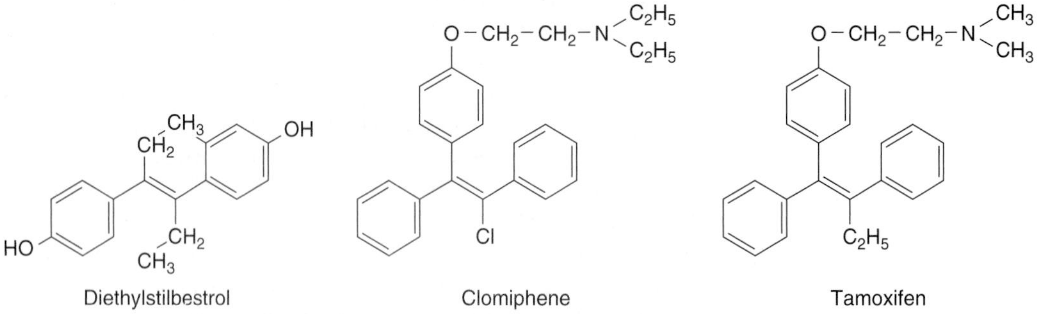

Diethylstilbestrol   Clomiphene   Tamoxifen

Figure 18.8   Diethylstilbestrol (DES) is an example of a synthetic nonsteroidal estrogen. Note the partial structural similarity of two antiestrogens, clomiphene and tamoxifen, to DES.

NEUROENDOCRINE CONTROL OF OVARIAN FUNCTION

Activation and maintenance of normal follicular function is dependent on gonadotropins secreted by the adenohypophysis (see Chap. 5). Both follicle-stimulating hormone (FSH) and luteinizing hormone (LH) are required to stimulate ovarian changes leading to ovulation [23, 25, 28]. Treatment of hypophysectomized, immature, female animals with purified LH causes thecal and interstitial cell stimulation, but no follicular growth and, depending on the species, no significant estrogen production [28]. When injections of purified FSH are given, follicular development proceeds only to antrum formation and only minimal amounts of estrogens are produced. Normal follicular development occurs only when both FSH and LH are administered to an animal. These observations support the two-cell, two-gonadotropin scheme of follicular development and steroid hormone production.

Pituitary gonadotropin secretion is initiated during pubertal development and, indeed, secretion of gonadotropins at this time is responsible for the development of secondary sex characteristics typical of the adult female. The CNS organizational basis for cyclic release of pituitary gonadotropins in the adult female is established early in fetal development (see Chap. 16). The detailed mechanisms controlling pituitary gonadotropin secretion are best understood in the primate and rodent [23, 28]; this text will discuss only the former.

Elegant studies on the rhesus monkey have established the role of the brain and pituitary in the control of ovarian function in the primate [23]. Pituitary gonadotropin secretion is critically dependent on hypothalamic GnRH release. Administration of antisera to GnRH causes an abrupt reduction in plasma gonadotropin concentrations. Discrete lesions within the medial basal hypothalamus of the female monkey result in a sudden decrease in plasma gonadotropin levels. There is a pulsatile pattern of gonadotropin secretion with a frequency of approximately one pulse per hour (circhoral) [23]. The concentration of GnRH in pituitary stalk blood of ovariectomized monkeys fluctuates with a frequency similar to that of pituitary gonadotropin secretion. The circhoral rhythm of gonadotropin secretion is abolished by α-adrenoceptor antagonists, suggesting that pulsatile GnRH release is regulated by neural elements, most specifically, neurons of the arcuate nucleus. The neuroendocrine elements responsible for the regulation of gonadotropin secretion appear to be restricted to the medial basal hypothalamus.

Clinical trials involving pulsatile GnRH delivery have demonstrated that pulses of unchanging doses and frequency resulted in normal pituitary and ovarian function in women with hypothalamic amenorrhea. The first pregnancies were reported later that year. Subsequent clinical trials have now established pulsatile GnRH as the treatment of choice for ovulation induction in hypogonadotropic hypogonadism [4].

Although GnRH of hypothalamic origin is an obligatory requirement for gonadotropin secretion, its stimulatory action on the pituitary appears to be dependent on the permissive actions of E_2. There is compelling evidence that the duration of the primate menstrual cycle is determined not by the brain, but rather by the ovary itself, through estrogens acting directly on the pituitary. If the hypothalamic source of GnRH is removed by discrete lesions and GnRH is administered by chronic, intermittent intravenous infusion, the pituitary responds by pulsatile release of gonadotropins. These animals go through "normal" menstrual cycles, including a preovulatory surge of LH/FSH and typical follicular and luteal phase levels of plasma E_2 and progesterone. The preovulatory gonadotropin surge does not require an increase of GnRH by the hypothalamus. The initial levels of estrogens during the early follicular phase of the menstrual cycle exert a negative feedback action directly on pituitary gonadotropin secretion. After estrogen levels rise and remain above a critical level for at least 36 hours, the negative feedback effect is reversed and a positive feedback ensues, which results in the preovulatory gonadotropin surge. The positive effect of estrogens on LH and FSH secretion may be due to an increase in pituitary GnRH receptors [22].

Apparently the duration of the ovarian cycle, at least in the rhesus monkey, is determined by the characteristic (genetically programmed) duration of follicular development, as well as the functional life span of the corpus luteum. The sum of both processes is approximately 28 days [23]. Evidently there is activation of a hypothalamic arcuate (nucleus) oscillator from almost total inactivity before puberty to an adult frequency of

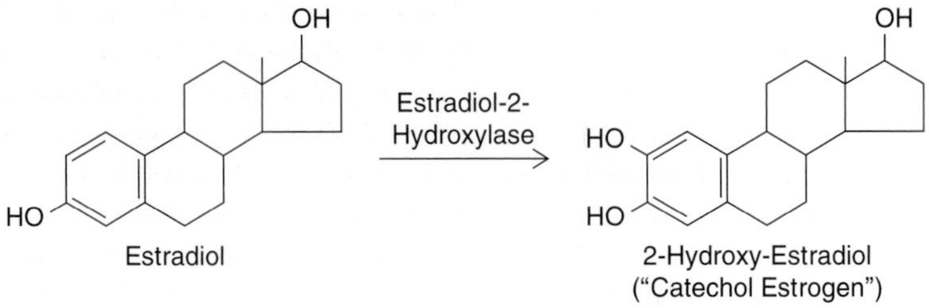

Figure 18.9 Biosynthesis of a catecholestrogen.

about one pulse of GnRH secretion per hour. During the luteal phase of the cycle, ovarian progesterone inhibits estrogen-induced gonadotropin surges by an action on the central nervous system. This neuronal mechanism is inhibited again during pregnancy and lactation as a result of suckling-induced PRL secretion. This inhibitory action may involve a reduction of the frequency of the arcuate oscillator [23].

Catecholestrogens

The first step in the metabolism of E_2 is oxidation to estrone, which may be further metabolized through hydroxylation of the A and D rings. The principal product of A-ring hydroxylation is 2-hydroxyestrone, referred to as a *catecholestrogen* because of the structural similarity of the hydroxylated A ring to the catechol nucleus (Fig. 18.9; see also Fig. 14.1). There is evidence that 2-hydroxyestrone may play a role in the control of pituitary gonadotropin secretion [12]. This catecholestrogen is reported to affect both LH and PRL secretion in humans. 2-hydroxyestrone could act as a competitive inhibitor of estradiol on hypothalamic and pituitary estrogen receptors. Because catecholestrogens are competitive inhibitors of catechol-O-methyltransferase, they could also cause a decrease in the turnover of CNS catecholamine neurotransmitters. Catecholestrogens also inhibit tyrosine hydroxylase, the rate-limiting enzyme in catecholamine biosynthesis, and therefore decrease the catecholamine content of the CNS. Evidence that E_2 metabolism in the rat brain changes during the estrous cycle indicates that 2-hydroxylation of E_2 in the brain may be involved in the negative feedback control of estrogens on pituitary gonadotropin secretion [12].

Throughout life estradiol provides physiological signals to the brain that are necessary for the development and regulation of reproductive function. In addition to its multiple physiological actions, E_2 is also selectively cytotoxic to β-endorphin neurons in the hypothalamic arcuate nucleus (see Chap. 21). The mechanism underlying this neurotoxic action appears to involve the conversion of estradiol to catecholestrogen (Fig. 18.9) and subsequent oxidation to *o*-semiquinone free radicals. The estradiol-induced loss of β-endorphin neurons engendered by compensatory increment in μ opioid binding in the medial preoptic area rendering this region supersensitive to residual β-endorphin or to other endogenous opioids (see Chap. 21). The consequent persistent opioid inhibition results in a cascade of neuroendocrine deficits that are ultimately expressed as a chronically attenuated plasma LH pattern to which the ovaries respond by becoming anovulatory and polycystic. This neurotoxic action of E_2 may contribute to a number of reproductive disorders in humans and in animals in which aberrant hypothalamic function is a major component [5].

Intrafollicular Polypeptide Regulatory Factors

Several peptides have been isolated from ovarian follicles and have been claimed to function as putative hormones in the regulation of oocyte maturation [15, 46].

Oocyte Maturation Factor.   Oocytes obtained from middle and late antral follicles of mice resume meiosis when removed from the follicle and cultured in vitro. In contrast, oocytes cultured with granulosa cells do not mature, and antral follicular fluid from a number of species is also inhibitory to oocyte maturation in culture. The putative oocyte maturation inhibitor (OMI) appears to be a low molecular weight peptide whose concentration in antral fluid decreases as the follicle matures. The inhibitory action of granulosa cells on oocyte maturation is reversed by addition of LH to the medium. LH is not effective, however, in overcoming the inhibitory activity of granulosa cell-conditioned medium on oocyte maturation. These results suggest that LH may mediate its effect through an action on the granulosa cells. Gap junctions, present between cells of the corona radiata and the oocyte, may provide a structural pathway for cell-to-cell communication between these two cell types. In addition cumulus cell extensions project through the zona pellucida to the oocyte. Because follicular fluid extracts inhibit maturation of oocytes cultured with their intact cumuli, but not maturation of denuded oocytes, the OMI may exert its action indirectly through an action on cumulus cells. It might be postulated that LH-induced oocyte maturation results from an uncoupling between the cumulus cells and the oocyte.

Ovarian Growth Factors. Induction of LH receptors is a critical aspect of granulosa cell differentiation and ovarian follicular development. By this process the follicle acquires the responsiveness to LH and the subsequent capacity to ovulate and luteinize. Pituitary FSH functions as the inducer of granulosa cell LH receptor acquisition. This FSH-dependent LH receptor induction is inhibited by epidermal and fibroblast growth factors (see Chap. 12). These and other growth factors may represent physiological effectors that regulate follicle development [46].

Inhibins. Evidence supporting the existence of a gonadal peptide inhibitory to pituitary FSH secretion in the male was reviewed (see Chap. 17) [11, 14, 15, 20]. Equally compelling evidence for a granulosa-derived peptide in the female has been marshaled. A follicular inhibin has been shown in follicular fluid, ovarian and granulosa cell extracts, granulosa cell conditioned media, and ovarian venous plasma [9]. This peptide substance exerts a suppressive action on both basal and GnRH-stimulated pituitary FSH secretion. The precise cellular localization and factors that may regulate the synthesis and secretion of this peptide remain to be clarified. A model for the role of inhibin in the control of pituitary FSH secretion was shown (see Fig. 17.3).

Inhibin has been isolated from follicular fluid from several species of animals. The peptide is composed of two subunits that are linked by disulfide bridges. The two subunits are, however, encoded by separate genes (Fig. 18.10). Antibodies to the peptide confirm

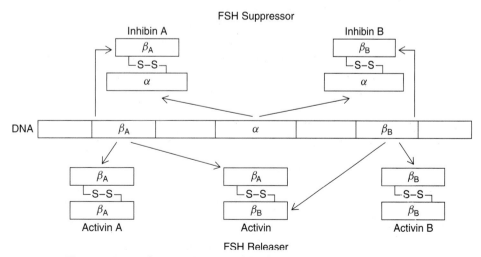

Figure 18.10   Structural relationships between inhibins and activins.

the presence of inhibin in the plasma of men and women. The half-lives of the inhibin mRNAs in the rat are very short. This is consistent with inhibin production being tightly regulated in response to transient conditions during the estrous cycle and suggests that the major control site of inhibin biosynthesis is at the level of transcription.

There are reports that circulating levels of inhibin are inversely related to plasma FSH levels. For example, inhibin can be detected in the plasma of women given FSH, but not in castrated subjects. Cultured granulosa cells secrete inhibin when exposed to FSH. Inhibin levels in the plasma of women undergoing induced ovulation by FSH rise and are correlated with E_2 levels. Similarly, in the male, inhibin is decreased in the testis following hypophysectomy and becomes elevated in response to FSH. These observations support the view of a feedback loop between the release of ovarian inhibin and FSH secretion.

Activins.   During the initial steps of inhibin purification, purified fractions of follicular fluid exhibited stimulatory rather than inhibitory effects on FSH release from pituicytes in vitro [29]. When the amino acid sequence of inhibin was identified, it was found that the β subunits of inhibin and transforming growth factor β (TGFβ) were similar. As TGFβ can enhance FSH release in vitro, it was initially suggested that this stimulatory effect might be due to TGFβ or a protein similar to TGFβ. It was then discovered that the stimulatory activity was due to dimers of the β subunits of inhibin, $\beta_A\beta_B$, $\beta_A\beta_A$, and $\beta_B\beta_B$. These peptides were named activin, activin-A, and activin-B, respectively (Fig. 18.10). Activins can enhance basal secretion of FSH in a dose-dependent manner in vitro without affecting the secretion of LH [29].

Follistatin.   Follistatin is a single peptide chain of molecular weight 32,000–35,000 isolated from porcine follicular fluid, which is distinct from inhibin and can inhibit the release of FSH, but not LH, from cultures of pituitary cells. Incubation of pituicytes with both inhibin and follistatin results in an additive inhibition of FSH release. After pituitary cells are exposed to follistatin, there is a decrease in intracellular FSH, but not to the extent of that with inhibin; this suggests that follistatin is involved in the suppression of release as opposed to synthesis of FSH. Therefore, regulation of synthesis and secretion of FSH from the pituitary is regulated by GnRH from the hypothalamus, as well as by steroidal and nonsteroidal factors from the ovary [26].

MAMMALIAN REPRODUCTIVE CYCLES

Females of most vertebrate species are subject to cyclic changes in reproductive activity [3]. Most often these changes are integrated with seasonal environmental changes so that the young are born under more favorable conditions of climate and food availability. In many mammals other than primates, females experience recurring periods of sexual excitement referred to as *estrus* (from the Greek, *oistros,* meaning mad desire or heat), during which time they are psychologically as well as physically receptive to the male. The female primate does not go through an *estrous cycle,* but eggs are nevertheless matured within the ovaries during a precise follicular cycle of events, and the genital tract is also cyclically prepared for passage and implantation of the zygote. The monthly cycle of uterine maturation and sloughing is therefore a characteristic feature of the primate *menstrual cycle.*

Primate Menstrual Cycle

Ovarian Cycle.   The production and secretion of pituitary gonadotropins in the primate are controlled by cyclic ovarian follicular events; the duration of the cycle appears to be dependent on the genetic program that is read out to completion once follicular maturation is initiated. FSH levels are elevated at the beginning of the cycle, but they become diminished through most of the early and middle follicular phases. Follicular selection and early maturation may be dependent on the initially elevated plasma levels of FSH. Increased estrogen (and inhibin) secretion by the maturing follicles exerts a negative feedback inhibition of pituitary gonadotroph FSH secretion. Luteinizing hormone levels also remain low during most of this follicular phase due to the negative feedback action of estrogens on the pituitary. With continued follicular maturation, estrogen levels become increasingly elevated to a peak at midcycle. The prolonged action of the higher concentrations of estrogens is the stimulus to the midcycle FSH/LH surge (through enhancement of pituitary gonadotroph GnRH receptor number). The subsequently elevated plasma levels of LH provide the stimulus to ovum release from the mature Graafian follicle. The granulosa cells, which have now become responsive to LH, initiate progesterone biosynthesis and secretion. At this stage, the postovulatory follicle has become an endocrine gland in the classical sense. During the follicular phase plasma progesterone levels are low, but with commencement of the luteal phase they become elevated.

Progesterone levels are elevated just prior to the LH/FSH surge, apparently in response to increasing levels of LH, which is also secreted at that time. The action of progesterone on the hypothalamus results in postovulatory decreases in both LH and FSH secretion. Under conditions of low circulating levels of these gonadotropins, there is no stimulus to folliculogenesis, and estrogen levels therefore remain only minimally elevated during the luteal phase. As the corpus luteum matures during the subsequent week following ovulation, progesterone levels become increasingly elevated to a midluteal peak. Afterward they level off and decline unless the ovulated ovum is fertilized and takes up residence within the uterine lining. With the demise of the corpus luteum in the nonpregnant female and the sharp decline in plasma progesterone levels, pituitary gonadotropins are again secreted, which leads to the initiation of the next round of ovarian folliculogenesis and steroid hormone production. The cyclic pattern of pituitary gonadotropin and gonadal steroid hormone secretion in the rhesus monkey is illustrated in Fig. 18.11 [8].

Uterine Cycle.   The menstrual cycle of the human female is approximately 28 days long and is numbered from the first day of the menses. Menstruation is the process where the lining of the uterus is shed once during each cycle, a process that in most women takes 4 to 5 days. Under the influence of increasing titers of plasma estrogens, the endometrium of the uterus increases in thickness, reaching a maximal width of 3 to 5 mm just prior to ovulation (Fig. 18.12). Stromal connective tissue cells proliferate and extracellular collagen deposits are increased. In response to luteal phase progesterone levels, uterine glands increase in complexity from simple tubular elements during the follicular phase of the cycle to thick-coiled structures with a glandular lumen containing abundant secretory material. Spiral arteries within the endometrium become thickened and engorged with blood, particularly in response to luteal levels of progesterone. If implantation of a zygote fails to occur, by about 11 days following ovulation lymphocytes begin to invade the endometrium, and by day 14 (day 1 of the cycle) sloughing of the endometrium occurs due to loss of ovarian steroid hormone support. In the absence of a hormonal directive the spiral arteries become constricted and the blood lost from these arteries along with stromal debris composes the bulk of the menstrual flow [10].

The nature of the cervical mucus is also characteristically altered during the menstrual cycle. During the follicular phase the mucus is rather thin and watery. In response to periovulatory levels of progesterone the mucus becomes thickened and is composed of innumerable tiny channels that apparently provide access for the sperm through the cervical os.

Vaginal Cycle.   In prepubertal and postmenopausal females the vaginal epithelium is thin, being composed of a few layers of epithelial cells. In response to estrogens this epithelium proliferates and subsequently consists of many more layers of epithelial cells.

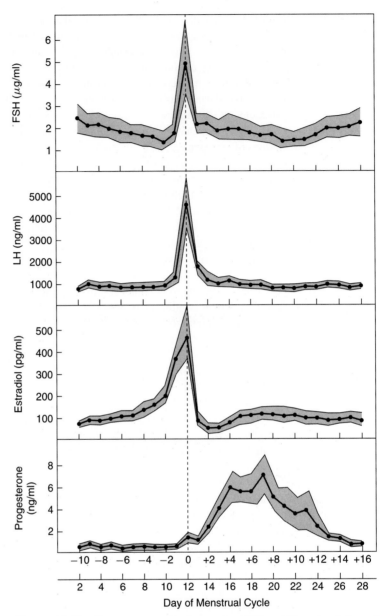

Figure 18.11   Serum concentrations of mFSH, mLH, estradiol, and progesterone in 20 rhesus monkeys during ovulatory menstrual cycles. (From DiZerega and Hodgen [8], with permission.)

The histological features of the vaginal epithelium change in a characteristic manner during the menstrual cycle. Early in the cycle the epithelium consists mainly of rounded basal cells that stain intensely with certain dyes. Maximal growth of the epithelium occurs during the periovulatory period. At this time the basal cells are overlain with layers of more flattened cells; the outermost cells are very flat and keratinized (cornified), and they fail to stain, thus indicating that they are dead. Toward the end of the luteal phase the vaginal epithelium becomes invaded with leukocytes, and by the initiation of the next cycle cells of the outer layers of the epithelium are lost.

Induced and Spontaneous Ovulators

Most mammals (e.g., primates, hamsters, mice, rats) ovulate at the end of a follicular phase and then initiate development of corpora lutea. In contrast to these *spontaneous*

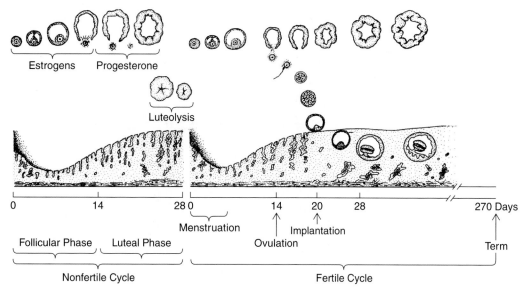

Figure 18.12 Cycle of uterine endometrial growth and development during nonfertile and fertile cycles in the human female.

ovulators, certain animals (domestic cats, rabbits, minks) go through a follicular phase, but then remain in a state of sexual receptivity where the follicles mature and are usually released after copulation. These *induced* or *reflex ovulators* generally mate during estrus. Some animals may exhibit a *constant estrus* (e.g., rabbits), whereas estrus in other species may be a seasonal phenomenon with a long anestrous period between cycles, where ovaries and follicles remain small.

During mating there is a reflex release of LH from the pituitary that leads to ovulation usually 12 to 48 hours later (Table 18.2). Although spontaneous ovulators are characterized by ovarian cycles that do not normally exhibit an estrous component, coitus can affect the time of ovulation in some of these species. These spontaneous ovulators can be divided into two major groups: (1) animals with nonfunctional corpora lutea and short (4- to 5-day) ovarian cycles (e.g., rats, mice, hamsters); and (2) animals with functional corpora lutea and long estrous cycles (e.g., pigs, cows, horses). The spontaneous ovulators with long cycles can be further subdivided into two groups: (1) animals with but one estrous cycle (monestrous) in a mating season; and (2) animals that have two or more estrous cycles (polyestrous) in the mating season.

Delayed Implantation

In some species the fertilized egg, the zygote, may reside within the uterine cavity for a considerable time. This *delayed implantation* allows flexibility between mating and birth. Most often, all reproductive events must be crowded into a short time interval. Of fundamental importance is that the young be born at the optimum season of the year for survival and growth [47]. In colonial animals, such as certain seals, the sexes are usually together only for a short time each year and must breed, give birth, and rear their young during this critical interval. In certain marsupials the suckling young may be lost due to harsh environmental conditions. The loss of the suckling stimulus (absence of prolactin) causes an unimplanted blastocyst to break diapause (from the Greek, *dia,* through, completely, and *pausa,* pause; arrested embryonic development). Within each species the length of the implanted gestation period is rigidly fixed, but in some species of bats the young may experience a delayed development. The hormonal requirements for implantation of a delayed blastocyst are poorly understood. In the European badger there is a fertile postpartum coitus in February, but the fertilized eggs remain in the blastocyst stage until December when implantation occurs [47].

TABLE 18.2 The Estrous Cycle of Various Mammalian Species[a]

Species	Length of cycle (days)	Duration of estrus	Ovulation Type	Ovulation Time
Cow (*Bos taurus*)	21	13—14 hours	Spontaneous	12—16 hours after end of estrus
Goat (*Capra hircus*)	20—21	1—3 days	Spontaneous	30—36 hours after onset of estrus
Sheep (*Ovis aries*)	16	20—48 hours	Spontaneous	12—24 hours before end of estrus
Pig (*Sus scrofa*)	21	2—3 days	Spontaneous	35 hours after onset of estrus
Horse (*Equus caballus*)	19—23	4—7 days	Spontaneous	1—2 days before end of estrus
Dog (*Canis familiaris*)	60	7—9 days	Spontaneous	1—3 days after start of estrus
Cat (*Felis catus*)	—	4 days with male; 9—10 days without male	Induced	20—30 hours after mating
Ferret (*Mustela furo*)	—	Continuous	Induced	30 hours after mating
Mink (*Mustela vison*)	8—9	2 days	Induced	40—50 hours after mating
Fox (*Vulpes vulpes*)	90	1—5 days	Spontaneous	1—2 days after onset of estrus
Ground squirrel (*Citellus tridecemlineatus*)	16	6—11 hours	Induced	8—12 hours after mating
Guinea pig (*Cavia porcellus*)	16	6—11 hours	Spontaneous	10 hours after start of estrus
Golden hamster (*Mesocricetus auratus*)	4	20 hours	Spontaneous	8—12 hours after start of estrus
Mouse (*Mus musculus*)	4	10 hours	Spontaneous	2—3 hours after start of estrus
Rat (*Rattus norvegicus*)	4—5	13—15 hours	Spontaneous	8—10 hours after start of estrus
Rabbit (*Oryctolagus cuniculus*)	No cycle	Continuous	Induced	10 hours after mating
Rhesus monkey (*Macaca mulatta*)	28[b]	None	Spontaneous	14 days prior to onset of menstrual bleeding
Human (*Homo sapiens*)	28[b]	None	Spontaneous	14 days prior to onset of menstrual bleeding

[a] From van Tienhoven [47], with permission.
[b] Menstrual cycle.

Environment and Reproduction

Reproductive success depends on successful mating, fetal growth and development, and the birth and rearing of young under appropriate environmental conditions. Success in these sequential events requires that eggs be ovulated at the right time, eggs become fertilized, and the nutritional state of the mother be adequate to provide for the needs of the growing offspring, whether in utero or postpartum. Environmental cues play important roles in synchronizing mating behavior in animals and provide signals indicative of when food sources may become available. For example, some desert species are opportunistic breeders and mate following rainfall. In many small rodents reproductive activity is restricted to the spring and the fall; within the confines of the laboratory, however, these animals become continuous breeders.

A variety of exogenous factors—auditory, visual, tactile, and odoriferous—serve as signals to initiate reproductive behavior in some species. Lighting conditions as well as species-specific odors play particularly important roles.

Light. The most universal environmental synchronizing cue is light. Seasonal and daily changes in light duration and intensity are cyclic phenomena that usually directly or indirectly relate to other environmental factors such as the abundance of water and food. Light information must be received (sensed), transcribed (a neural processing mechanism), and translated into a physiological response. In vertebrates a neural sensory system, or "eye" must monitor the presence or absence of light and transmit this information by neural afferents to the central nervous system, which then directly or indirectly affects pituitary gonadotropin secretion. In either case neurohormones released from the hypothalamus provide the initial input to pituitary hormone secretion. The important role of the pineal gland in the control of reproductive processes in vertebrates is discussed in Chap. 20.

Olfaction. Smell is particularly crucial in eliciting mating behavior in many animals [36]. Chemical messengers released by one member of a species may be received by a second member of the same species and produce a physiological response. These *pheromones* are volatile hydrocarbons (see Fig. 2.5) which, in mammals at least, interact with receptors of olfactory epithelial cells of the recipient animal. Nervous afferents to the CNS then cause either a rapid behavioral response or slower physiological response involving the release of pituitary gonadotropins. Again, as for light stimuli, hypothalamic neurosecretory neurons provide the final common pathway linking sensory perception to pituitary-gonadal activation.

In the mouse a number of effects ascribed to pheromones have been noted [45]. Female mice housed with four or more other female mice may become *pseudopregnant;* that is, the corpora lutea are maintained in the absence of mating (Lee-Boot effect). If female mice are housed in very large groups, the incidence of anestrus increases. These observations suggest that female mice secrete one or more pheromones that affect the estrous cycle. The presence of a male mouse may cause shortening and synchronization of the estrous cycle of grouped female mice (*Whitten effect*). Bedding or urine from a male mouse is equally effective, suggesting that odor is the stimulus to synchronization and shortening of the estrous cycle. When prepubertal female mice are reared in the presence of a male (or his urine), they attain first estrus several weeks earlier than if reared in the absence of the male (*Vandenbergh effect*). An additional observation made by Vandenbergh was that the odor of an adult female caused precocious testicular development of young males. In contrast, testes development is markedly retarded when young males are reared with adult males. If a recently impregnated female mouse is exposed to a strange male, pregnancy may be blocked; she will return to estrus within one week. The bedding or urine of the strange male is equally effective in terminating pregnancy (*Bruce effect*). Females made anosmic by destruction of the olfactory bulbs are unaffected by the presence of the "strange" male. The source of the male odor is unknown but may be derived from the preputial glands.

Pheromones and other stimuli that activate reproductive behavior fall into two broad categories: *releaser effects* and *primer effects*. Releaser effects resulting from a visual or odoriferous signal involve an immediate behavioral response on the part of the recipient. This often involves activation of a stereotyped mating behavior in the female, such as assuming a posture (lordosis) conducive to copulatory activity by the male. Primer effects also involve activation of central nervous system afferents, but in addition pituitary gonadotropin secretion is enhanced or inhibited, most likely due to increases or decreases in hypothalamic secretion of GnRH. The Bruce effect appears to involve an inhibition of pituitary PRL secretion as the hormone is required for maintenance of the corpus luteum and can repair the block to pregnancy induced by the strange male if administered to the female. It has been speculated that the block to pregnancy involves the re-establishment of PRL-inhibiting factor (dopamine) secretion by the hypothalamus.

A study was made of the female stimuli that induce male gonadotropin (GtH) surge during spawning in the goldfish. In the presence of ovulatory females, olfactory tract sectioned (OTX) males failed to show sexual behavior or the GtH surge, while sham-operated (sham) males spawned and showed a GtH surge. When OTX and sham males were separated from ovulatory females with an opaque partition, but with water circulating between male and female compartments, the GtH surge occurred only in sham males, although they could not court with the females. These results indicate that an olfactory stimulus (pheromone) from ovulatory females is essential for the occurrence of male GtH surge. Pheromone(s) from ovulatory female goldfish thus function both as a releaser stimulating sexual behavior and as a primer inducing GtH surge in males [24].

Scientists have obtained data suggesting that human beings produce pheromones, aromatic chemical substances produced by one individual that affect the sexual physiology of another [7]. Animals have long been known to secrete pheromones that typically function as sex attractants, but the existence of such substances in humans has only been speculated. However, recent research suggests their existence in humans. Women who had sex with men at least once a week were found to be more likely to have normal-length menstrual cycles, fewer infertility problems, and a milder menopause than women who were celibate or who had sex in a sporadic "feast-or-famine" pattern [7].

The pheromone findings indicate that an essential factor, aside from sexual intercourse itself, is exposure to specific aromatic chemicals exuded in a man's normal body odors. When a women receives these chemicals, by smell or skin absorption, even though she may not consciously notice them, they automatically improve her physiological functioning. The evidence suggests that the male chemicals, which are secreted in special sweat glands in the armpits and possibly around the nipples and in the genital region, are not effectively transmitted except in the intimate contact ordinarily associated with sex. Researchers have been able to duplicate some of the male pheromone's effects by exposing women who had no current sexual relationship to male pheromones in the form of what they dubbed "male essence." This contained substances extracted with alcohol from absorbent pads that male volunteers wore under their arms. The study was done with female volunteers whose menstrual cycles were longer than 33 days or shorter than 26 days, deviations from the normal average of 29.5 days. Three times a week the women came to the clinic to have male essence rubbed under their noses. The women said they could smell only the alcohol. After about 12 to 14 weeks, their menstrual cycles changed, slowing in some cases and speeding up in others, to approximately 29.5 days. A control group of similar women who were dosed with plain alcohol only showed no significant change in cycle length [7].

In a related experiment, scientists found that women produce another pheromone that can cause other women's menstrual cycles to shift into synchrony. The researchers used a similarly obtained "female essence," which was collected at measured intervals during the donor's menstrual cycle and administered in the same sequence. Within a few menstrual cycles, the recipients shifted their cycles to synchronize with those of the donor. This finding confirms widely reported anecdotes that women who live (e.g., dormitories) or work together eventually develop synchronized menstrual cycles [7].

PATHOPHYSIOLOGY

Amenorrhea. The term designates a relatively common disturbance in the human female characterized by an absence of the monthly menstrual flow. The etiology relates to a deficiency in estrogen production and a failure, therefore, in the monthly proliferative growth of the endometrium resulting in an absence of monthly sloughing of the uterine lining. The failure of the menses to be initiated at puberty is referred to as *primary amenorrhea*. The etiology may relate to a genetic defect, resulting in a failure of gonadal maturation (or total gonadal dysgenesis), or more specifically to a defect in estrogen biosynthesis. *Secondary amenorrhea* refers to a failure to menstruate after regular menses have been initiated. Pregnancy and the menopause are, of course, examples of normal physiological bases for failure to resume the menses. Failure of pituitary gonadotropin secretion or hyperprolactinemia are defects that result in amenorrhea.

Disturbances of the menstrual cycle are a frequent symptom in patients with eating disorders. Amenorrhea develops early in anorexia nervosa. A disturbed hypothalamic regulation of gonadotropin secretion causes amenorrhea and anorexia. In bulimia (binge eating), amenorrhea is less frequent, occurring in about half the patients [35]. The pulsatile, intravenous administration of GnRH is a highly successful method of inducing ovulation in patients suffering from amenorrhea secondary to hypothalamic dysfunction [4].

Altered Gonadotropin Secretion in Female Athletes. Secondary amenorrhea may be a consequence of strenuous exercise in some female athletes. Menstrual alterations have been noted in women participating in a variety of athletic endeavors. Studies have linked menstrual disturbances to weight loss and decreased body fat-to-lean ratios (see Chap. 16), but the discrete disturbances in the brain pituitary-ovarian axis have not been pinpointed. Pulsatile gonadotropin secretion is critical to maintaining normal cyclical function of the pituitary-gonadal axis. It has now been shown that some long-distance runners with secondary amenorrhea or severe oligomenorrhea have unambiguously decreased spontaneous LH pulse frequencies [48]. Generally the effect is reversible with weight gain.

Isolated Gonadotropin Deficiency. This defect is characterized by a bihormonal deficiency of FSH and LH. In patients with isolated gonadotropin deficiency (IGD) administration of GnRH enhances FSH and LH secretion, thus restoring normal gonadal function [18, 33]. It is likely that IGD may relate to a suprapituitary etiology involving an impaired synthesis and secretion of endogenous GnRH [50].

Premature Ovarian Failure. Premature ovarian failure has usually been assumed to represent one extreme of the temporal spectrum of menopause and has been a subject of neglect. Premature ovarian failure may be secondary to hypothalamic or pituitary failure (hypogonadotropic hypogonadism) or to a primary ovarian unresponsiveness to gonadotropins (hypergonadotrophic hypogonadism). The latter condition has been defined as secondary amenorrhea with persistently elevated gonadotropin levels before the age of 35 years [13]. Within this definition there are two subsets of patients. In one there has been a true premature menopause with a total depletion of ovarian follicles and therefore a permanent loss of ovarian function. In the other group, follicles are still present but apparently unresponsive to circulatory gonadotropins. In the case of "follicular ovarian failure" there are numerous primordial follicles, and gonadotropin levels are elevated. A follicular ovarian failure may be due to genetic abnormalities, radiation injury, or chemotherapy. The defect could also relate to an FSH receptor defect, or to an autoimmune disease with production of anti-FSH receptor antibodies. The etiology of this condition is clearly speculative [13].

Polycystic Ovarian Disease.   Deficient ovarian estrogen production and excessive ovarian androgen secretion are the major abnormal hormonal features of the polycystic ovary syndrome. Women with this syndrome ovulate infrequently or not at all. The defect appears to relate to a failure of follicular maturation. Excess adrenal androgen production may be the etiological factor involved. Estrone levels are elevated relative to E_2 and may derive from excessive conversion of androstenedione to estrone. Elevated estrone may be inhibitory to pituitary FSH secretion, but stimulatory to LH secretion, thus leading to failure of follicular development and ovulation.

Premenstrual Syndrome.   Premenstrual syndrome (PMS) is one of the most common disorders of the reproductive-aged woman. PMS has been defined as "the cyclic recurrence, in the luteal phase of the menstrual cycle, of a combination of distressing physical, psychologic, and/or behavioral changes of sufficient severity to result in deterioration of interpersonal relationships and/or interference with normal activities" [34]. There is a specific temporal relationship of symptoms to menstruation; symptoms present during the luteal phase are absent during the follicular phase of the cycle. PMS is a repetitive phenomena; symptoms are present month after month, to some degree or another [44]. No diagnosis-related differences in gonadal steroids, gonadotropins, or sex hormone-binding globulin have been consistently observed in patients with PMS, compared with controls. Thus, both the levels of reproductive hormones (including estradiol, progesterone, follicle-stimulating hormone, luteinizing hormone, and ovarian and adrenal androgens) and their pattern of secretion over the menstrual cycle do not appear to be disturbed in PMS [41].

Mood and the Menstrual Cycle.   Changes in feelings and behavior can be characteristics of the menstrual cycle and are undoubtedly related to changing hormonal levels [49]. Nevertheless, no clear correlation has been documented between gonadal steroid levels and the so-called premenstrual tension syndrome or other mensural cycle-related behaviors [39].

Hirsutism and Virilization.   Hirsutism is defined as the presence of hair in women on areas of the body where hair usually is not present [31]. Chief locations include the face, chest, areola of the breasts, or the abdomen above the symphysis pubis (male escutcheon). The underlying endocrine etiology of hirsutism is increased androgen production by the ovary and/or the adrenal gland. The presence of excess unbound testosterone leads to the development of hirsutism. Approximately 10% of women in the United States exhibit hirsutism during their reproductive years, and the incidence is even greater in menopausal women. Measurement of circulating androgens in these women has revealed that 80% to 90% are hyperandrogenic. Enzymatic defects in adrenal cortisol metabolism that lead to excess androgen secretion (see Chap. 15) or excess androgen production by an adrenal or ovarian tumor may cause hirsutism. Increased facial and body hair growth, increased muscle mass, and clitoral enlargement are manifestations of excessive adrenal or gonadal androgen production (adult adrenogenital syndrome). Cyproterone acetate (see Fig. 17.7), an androgen antagonist, has been used successfully in the treatment of hirsutism and masculinization.

Hirsutism is only one manifestation of hyperandrogenic conditions. The degree of hirsutism does not correlate with the degree of androgen production or the circulating levels of serum testosterone; rather, the severity of hirsutism depends on the availability and metabolism of testosterone by the skin and its appendages. The skin of hirsute women is highly sensitive to available testosterone owing to increased activity of 5 α-reductase, as compared with nonhirsute women. The peripheral effects of testosterone, in addition to hirsutism, include increased sebum secretion from sebaceous glands. This leads to oily skin. Infection of these active sebaceous glands with resident microorganisms leads to the aciniform eruptions, which are a common feature of this condition.

The effect of excess androgen production on the hypothalamic-pituitary-gonadal system depends on the sensitivity of that system to testosterone. Thus some women may be hirsute but have regular menstrual cycles. In contrast, others will have bleeding irregularities, such as oligomenorrhea, amenorrhea, and/or irregular menstrual cycles. In these women, testosterone is aromatized to E_2 in the hypothalamus. This in turn leads to disturbed gonadotropin secretion, which subsequently interferes with follicular growth and maturation. Furthermore, testosterone excess inhibits gonadotropin receptor formation in the ovary. The end result is anovulation manifested by the amenorrhea and oligomenorrhea syndrome [2, 31].

Hyperestrogenemia, Diet, and Disorders of Western Societies

There is a striking difference in the incidence of certain disorders between Western societies and the so-called less-developed countries. The prevalent disorders are coronary heart disease, diabetes, obesity, deep-vein thrombosis and pulmonary embolism, gallstones, and cancer, including the four most common forms of cancer (i.e., lung, colon, breast, and prostate) [37]. The factor most commonly implicated in epidemiologic studies is diet. There is evidence suggesting that each of these disorders, as well as diet, may be related to hyperestrogenemia and that the elevated estrogen levels may be an underlying factor in their development. One way in which the Western diet may be responsible is by causing obesity. There is a general correlation between body weight and estrogen levels. But whether it is the obesity itself, or the diet eaten by the obese, or both, that raises the estrogen level is not clear. Estrogen levels in obese individuals appear to correlate better with change in diet than with change in weight. Diet appears to have a profound effect on serum estrogen levels. Therefore, if hyperestrogenemia is a common underlying factor in the development of these disorders, hyperestrogenemia induced by diet could explain, at least in part, the prevalence of these disorders in Western societies [37].

REFERENCES

[1]   Allen, E., and E. A. Doisy. 1923. An ovarian hormone: preliminary report on its localization, extraction, and partial purification and action in test animals. *JAMA* 81:819–21.

[2]   Bailey-Pridham, D. D., and J. S. Sanfilippo. 1989. Hirsutism in the adolescent female. *Pediat. Clinics N. Amer.* 36:581–99.

[3]   Bennett, L. L. 1991. The Long and Evans monograph on the estrous cycle in the rat. *Endocrinology* 129:2812–4.

[4]   Blunt, S. M., and W. R. Butt. 1988. Pulsatile GnRH therapy for the induction of ovulation in hypogonadotropic hypogonadism. *Acta Endocrinol.* 288:58–65.

[5]   Brawer, J. R., A. Beaudet, G. C. Desjardins, and H. M. Schipper. 1993. Pathologic effect of estradiol on the hypothalamus. *Biol. Reprod.* 49:647–52.

[6]   Chen, F., and D. Puett. 1992. A single amino acid residue replacement in the β-subunit of human chorionic gonadotropin results in a loss of biological activity. *J. Mol. Endocrinol.* 8:87–9.

[7]   Cutler, W. B., G. Preti, A. Drieger, G. R. Huggins, C. R. Carcia and H. J. Lawley. 1986. Human axillary secretions influence women's menstrual cycles: The role of donor extract from men. *Horm. Behav.* 20:463–73.

[8]   DiZerega, G. S., and G. D. Hodgen. 1980. Changing functional status of the monkey corpus luteum. *Biol. Reprod.* 23:253–63.

[9]   Eramada, M., K. Heikinheimo, T. Touri, K. Hilden, and O. Ritous. 1993. Inhibin/activin sub-unit mRNA expression in human granulosa-luteal cells. *Mol. Cell. Endocrinol.* 92:R15–20.

[10] Ferenczy, A. 1993. Ultrastructure of the normal menstrual cycle: A review. *Microscop. Res. Tech.* 25:91–105.

[11] Findlay, J. K. 1993. An update on the roles of inhibin, activin, and follistatin as local regulators of folliculogenesis. *Biol. Reprod.* 48:15–23.

[12] Fishman, J. 1981. Biological action of catechol oestrogens. *J. Endocrinol.* 89:59P–65.

[13] Fox, H. 1992. The pathology of premature ovarian failure. *J. Pathol.* 167:357–63.

[14] Fraser, H. M., and S. F. Lunn. 1993. Does inhibin have an endocrine function during the menstrual cycle? *TEM* 4:187–94.

[15] Giordano, G., A. Barreca, and F. Minuto. 1992. Growth factors in the ovary. *J. Endocrinol. Invest.* 15:689–707.

[16] Gosden, R. G. 1987. Ovarian follicles at the menopause in women. *Human Reprod.* 2:617.

[17] Hawkins, L. A., F. I. Chasalow, and S. L. Blethen. 1992. The role of adrenocorticotropin testing in evaluating girls with premature adrenarche and hirsutism/oligomenorrhea. *J. Clin. Endocrinol. Metab.* 74:248–53.

[18] Henzl, M. R. 1993. Gonadotropin-releasing hormone and its analogues: from laboratory to bedside. *Clin. Obstet. Gynecol.* 36:617–35.

[19] Hillier, S. G. 1990. Ovarian manipulation with pure gonadotrophins. *J. Endocrinol* 127:1–4.

[20] Hillier, S. G., and F. Miro. 1993. Inhibin, activin, and follistatin. Potential roles in ovarian physiology. *Ann. New York Acad. Sci.* 687:29–38.

[21] Irianni, F., and G. D. Hodgen. 1992. Mechanism of ovulation. *Reprod. Endocrinol.* 21:19–38.

[22] Karsch, F. J. 1987. Central actions of ovarian steroids in the feedback regulation of pulsatile secretion of luteinizing hormone. *Annu. Rev. Physiol.* 49:365–82.

[23] Konbil, E. 1980. Neuroendocrine control of the menstrual cycle. *Rec. Prog. Horm. Res.* 36:53–88.

[24] Kobayashi, M., K. Aida, and I. Hanyu. 1986. Pheromone from ovulatory female goldfish induces gonadotropin surge during spawning in male goldfish. *Gen. Comp. Endocrinol.* 62:70–9.

[25] Kordon, C., and S. V. Drouva. 1992. Gonadotropin regulation, oestrogens and the immune system. *Horm. Res.* 37 (Suppl 3):11–5.

[26] Lee, B. L., G. Unabia, and G. Childs. 1993. Expression of follistatin mRNA by somatotropes and mammotropes early in the rat estrous cycle. *J. Histochem. Cytochem.* 41:955–60.

[27] Leiberman, E., and M. Zachmann. 1992. Familial adrenal feminization probably due to increased steroid aromatization. *Horm. Res.* 37:96–102.

[28] Martin, M. C. 1989. Gonadotropin releasing hormone agonists and the induction or augmentation of ovulation. *J. Reprod. Med.* 34:1034–8.

[29] Mather, J. P., T. K. Woodruff, and L. A. Krummen. 1992. Paracrine regulation of reproductive function by inhibin and activin. *Proc. Soc. Exp. Biol. Med.* 201:1–15.

[30] McFarland, K. C., R. Sprengel, H. S. Phillips, M. Kohler, N. Rosemblit, K. Nikolics, D. L. Segaloff, and P. H. Seeburg. 1989. Lutropin-choriogonadotropin receptor: an unusual member of the G-protein coupled receptor family. *Science* 245:494–9.

[31] Mckenna, T. J., S. K. Cunningham, and T. Loughlin. 1985. The adrenal cortex and virilization. *Clin. Endocrinol. Metab.* 14:997–1020.

[32] McNeilly, A. S. 1990. The ovarian follicle and fertility. *J. Steroid Biochem. and Mol. Biol.* 40:29–33.

[33] Moghissi, K. S. 1992. Clinical applications of gonadotropin-releasing hormones in reproductive disorders. *Endocrinol. Metab. Clin. N. Amer.* 21:125–40.

[34] Muse, K. 1992. Hormonal manipulation in the treatment of premenstrual syndrome. *Clin. Obstet. Gynecol.* 35:658–66.

[35] Newman, M. M., and K. A. Halmi. 1988. The endocrinology of anorexia nervosa and bulimia nervosa. *Endocrinol. Metab. Clin. N. Amer.* 17:195–212.

[36] Parkes, A. S., and H. M. Bruce. 1961. Olfactory stimuli in mammalian reproduction. *Science* 134:1049–54.

[37]   Phillips, G. B. 1985. Hyperestrogenemia, diet, and disorders of Western societies. *Amer. J. Med.* 78:363–6.

[38]   Richards, J. S., and L. Hedin. 1988. Some molecular aspects of hormone action in ovarian follicular development, ovulation, and luteinization. *Annu. Rev. Physiol.* 50:441–63.

[39]   Rosenfield, R. L. and R. B. Barnes. 1993. Menstrual disorders in adolescence. *Endocrinol. Metab. Clin. N. Amer.* 22:491–505.

[40]   Rossmanith, W. G. 1993. Contemporary insights into the control of the corpus luteum function. *Horm. Metab. Res.* 25:192–8.

[41]   Rubinow, D. R. 1992. The premenstrual syndrome. *JAMA* 268:1908–12.

[42]   Schreiner-Engel, P., R. C. Schiavi, D. White, and A. Ghizzani. 1989. Low sexual desire in women: the role of reproductive hormones. *Horm. Behav.* 23:221–34.

[43]   Simone, D. A., and V. B. Mahesh. 1993. An autoregulatory process for androgen production in rat thecal-interstitial cells. *Biol. Reprod.* 48:46–56.

[44]   Smith, S., and I. Schiff. 1989. The premenstrual syndrome—diagnosis and management. *Fertil. Steril.* 52:527–43.

[45]   Stoddart, D. M. 1976. *Mammalian odours and pheromones.* London: Edward Arnold, Ltd.

[46]   Tonetta, S. A., and G. S. DiZerega 1989. Intragonadal regulation of follicular maturation. *Endocr. Rev.* 10:205–29.

[47]   Van Tienhoven, A. 1968. *Reproductive physiology.* Philadelphia: W. B. Saunders Company.

[48]   Veldhuis, J. D., W. S. Evans, L. M. Demers, M. O. Thorner, D. Wakat, and A. D. Rogol. 1985. Altered neuroendocrine regulation of gonadotropin secretion in women distance runners. *J. Clin. Endocrinol. Metab.* 61:557–62.

[49]   Warren, M. P., and J. Brooks-Gunn. 1989. Mood and behavior at adolescence: evidence for hormonal factors. *J. Clin. Endocrinol. Metab.* 69:77–83.

[50]   Yen, S. S. 1993. Female hypogonadotropic hypogonadism. Hypothalamic amenorrhea syndrome. *Endocrinol. Metab. Clin. N. Amer.* 22:29–58.

19

Endocrinology of Pregnancy, Parturition, and Lactation

The ovulated egg has two possible fates: (1) if it fails to become fertilized, it undergoes lysis; (2) if, on the other hand, the ovum becomes fertilized, it (the zygote) may develop into an offspring of the species. If such an event is to be successful, a complex number of integrated neuroendocrine events between both conceptus and mother must transpire.

OVIPARITY, OVOVIPARITY, AND VIVIPARITY

*After fertilization embryonic development in **oviparous** species (all birds) takes place outside the body in eggs that are covered with one or more protective membranes (shell, jelly). In **ovoviparous** species (e.g., reptiles) the mother gives birth to live young, which are nevertheless developed within a protective egg retained within the oviduct but receive no nutrition from the mother. In **viviparous** animals the young develop within the mother and receive nourishment through vascular connections between embryo and mother. Except for the duckbilled platypus and spiny anteater, all mammals are viviparous.*

Hormones play essential roles in the processes of fetal growth and development, parturition at term, and, in most mammals, the control of lactation [47]. Due to the introductory nature of this book, only a few details of this complex topic can be discussed and these are limited mostly to the primate.

PREGNANCY

Fertilization and Implantation

In the primate usually a single egg is ovulated approximately midway through the menstrual cycle. During coitus spermatozoa released by the male into the vagina travel via the uterus to the oviducts where the ovum may become fertilized. Many spermatozoa may penetrate the corona radiata surrounding the ovum and, although more than one sperm can penetrate the zona pellucida, usually only one enters the ovum. In response to the sperm the oocyte completes the second meiotic division and expels the second polar body. The resulting female pronucleus comes in contact with the male pronucleus that has been formed after loss of the sperm tail. Fusion of the male and female pronuclei, to form the zygote, re-establishes the diploid chromosomal number of the egg. During passage down the uterine tube, which takes about 2 days, the zygote undergoes rapid mitotic divisions, and the resulting cells are referred to as *blastomeres*. By about 3 days a compact mass of

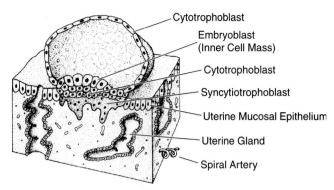

Figure 19.1 Implantation of the blastocyst within the uterus.

cells, the *morula,* enters the uterus. Continued cell division produces a hollow sphere, the early *blastocyst,* which is composed of a single layer of cells, the *trophoblast,* and an inner cell mass, the *embryoblast,* which is attached to the trophoblastic wall at the embryonic pole of the blastocyst. The inner cell mass, through differentiation and growth, will form the embryo, whereas the trophoblast will establish contact with the maternal circulation to provide the initial mechanism for the exchange of nutrients, oxygen, and waste products between fetus and mother. After residing within the uterus for about 2 days, the embryonic pole of the blastocyst becomes implanted in the endometrial epithelium on about day 6 (Fig. 19.1). In response to the blastocyst the underlying epithelium and endometrium undergo cellular changes, a so-called *decidualization* process. As a result, the endometrial tissue enlarges to form an implantation chamber, the *decidua,* to accommodate the growing embryo. The trophoblastic cells in contact with the uterine epithelium proliferate into an invasive *syncytiotrophoblast,* which consists of a multinucleated protoplasmic mass (Fig. 19.1). By 10 days the conceptus is completely embedded within the endometrium. The syncytiotrophoblast forms lacunar networks that establish contact with the endometrial capillaries to form the primitive uteroplacental circulation.

Gonadal steroids may be required for implantation. There is evidence that the blastocyst synthesizes estrogens, and it has been proposed that steroids synthesized or accumulated by the blastocyst may play a role in implantation through a local action on the adjacent endometrium. Indeed, in the rat uterus the concentrations of nuclear receptors for both E_2 and progesterone are higher in implantation sites than in nonimplantation regions of the endometrium.

The Corpus Luteum

The corpus luteum normally regresses about 12 days after ovulation during an infertile cycle in the primate [22]. If, however, the ovum is fertilized and subsequently implants within the uterus, by 10 days after ovulation a glycoprotein molecule unique to pregnancy is now present within the blood. This protein is secreted by the syncytiotrophoblast and, in humans, is referred to as *human chorionic gonadotropin* (hCG) or choriogonadotropin [6, 21]. Detection of this protein in the urine provides the basis for the most common test for pregnancy.

The role of hCG is to stimulate progesterone biosynthesis by the luteal cells of the corpus luteum. Initially, LH of pituitary origin is stimulatory to progesterone production by the corpus luteum. But LH levels drop precipitously after the midcycle LH/FSH surge. During the menstrual cycle progesterone secretion by the corpus luteum reaches a peak about 8 days after its formation. If the egg is not fertilized, progesterone levels decline rapidly and menstruation follows. The role of hCG is to rescue the corpus luteum, thereby prolonging its life span by converting it into a corpus luteum of pregnancy. Plasma levels of hCG rise to their highest between about the ninth and fourteenth weeks of pregnancy and then begin to decline gradually, reaching a nadir at approximately

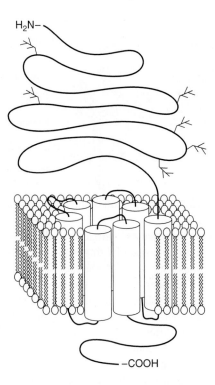

Figure 19.2 Hypothetical structural features of the LH/CG receptor. (From McFarland et al. [27], with permission. Copyright 1989 by the American Association for the Advancement of Science.)

twenty weeks of gestation. Luteal function begins to decline while circulating levels of hCG are at their peak, suggesting that failure of luteal activity is not related to declining levels of hCG.

There is evidence that luteal cell hCG receptors are identical to LH receptors; therefore they are often referred to as LH/hCG receptors, and either hormone may be used to study activation of cAMP formation and progesterone synthesis by luteal cells [9]. The β subunits of LH and hCG are closely related in sequence, and these two hormones bind to the same receptor and elicit identical biological responses [9, 36]. The immediate response of target cells to the binding of LH or hCG is an increase in adenylate cyclase activity mediated by intracellular, membrane-associated G proteins. The receptor protein displays the structural features of both a leucine-rich proteoglycan (extracellular domain) and of a G protein-coupled receptor. The other members of the G protein-coupled receptor family bind small ligands (such as serotonin or acetylcholine). Whereas binding of such ligands is thought to occur at sites formed by the assembly of the seven transmembrane helices, LH and hCG are thought to bind to a site on the extracellular part of this receptor. Thus the large extracellular domain and the specific mechanism of hormone-mediated signal transduction set the LH/CG-R apart from other G protein-coupled receptors. This receptor may have originated by recombination of genes encoding a hormone-binding glycoprotein and a seven-transmembrane protoreceptor [27] (Fig. 19.2).

In many mammals (e.g., rats, rabbits, but not primates) the pituitary gland is essential for the initial development as well as the survival of the corpora lutea in the pregnant female. Hypophysectomy in these animals results in atrophy of the corpus lutea, which can, however, be maintained by administration of pituitary extracts. The pituitary hormone responsible for luteotropic action in these species is PRL. In the rat, transplantation of the adenohypophysis to an ectopic site, such as the kidney, shortly after ovulation will allow development of the corpora lutea to an active state and at the same time keep the female in a state of pseudopregnancy. In the absence of an inhibitory hypothalamic control the ectopically transplanted adenohypophysis autonomously secretes PRL [31]. Implantation of fertilized ova within the uterus is apparently perceived by sensory neural elements, which, through spinal afferents, convey this information to the hypothalamus. This is believed to result in an inhibition of hypothalamic dopaminergic neurons and, in the

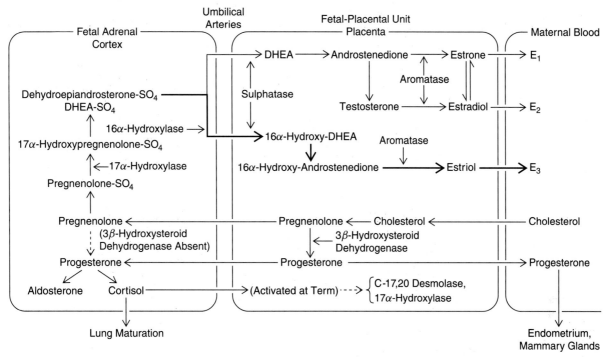

Figure 19.3 The fetal-placental unit.

absence of dopamine secretion into the hypophysial portal system, PRL is secreted autonomously.

The Fetal-Placental Unit

With the demise of the corpus luteum in the primate, E_2 and progesterone production is taken over by the placenta. However, the placenta is not capable of producing these steroid hormones without a supply of precursors from both the fetus and the maternal compartment.

Progesterone. The placenta, incapable of de novo progesterone biosynthesis, is dependent on cholesterol derived from the maternal blood supply (Fig. 19.3). The progesterone produced by the placenta is released into the maternal circulation to serve a multitude of functions related to pregnancy: maintenance of uterine structure and function, mammary growth and development, and inhibition of pituitary gonadotropin secretion. In addition placental progesterone is used as a substrate for corticoid production by the fetal adrenals that lack an active 3 β-hydroxysteroid-dehydrogenase.

Estrogens. Pregnenolone of placental origin is also used by the fetal adrenals in the production of precursors for estrogen production within the placenta. The placenta itself has only a limited capability for estrogen synthesis due to minimal 17 α-hydroxylase activity. Within the fetal adrenal cortex, however, this enzyme is responsible for production of dehydroepiandrosterone sulfate (DHEA-SO$_4$). This steroid metabolite serves as a precursor substrate for estrone (E_1) and E_2 synthesis by the placenta. Much of the substrate is, however, converted by a fetal adrenal 16 α-hydroxylase to precursors that lead to copious estriol (E_3) production. Measurements of E_3 levels in the maternal plasma or urine as a means of evaluating fetal well-being have been undertaken, but their usefulness is questionable. It is obvious from the preceding discussion that the fetal adrenals and the placenta, with respect to steroid hormone production, are incomplete endocrine organs. There is a circular flow of steroid metabolites that passes from the maternal compartment to the placenta, to the fetal adrenals, and then back through the placental compartment to the maternal bloodstream (Fig. 19.3). The evolution of this complex system and the intricate signals between these compartments, which must exist to ensure maintenance of pregnancy and yet provide the means for the eventual process of parturition, are still ambiguous.

PARTURITION

A functional corpus luteum is required for maintenance of pregnancy in many mammalian species (e.g., goat, sow); its demise in these species initiates the process of parturition. In other placenta-dependent species (e.g., sheep, primates) in which the corpus luteum regresses well before term, a decrease in particular placental steroids may be the key to the parturition process. The factors regulating placental hormone production probably vary considerably among these latter species. Prostaglandins of uterine origin participate in the initiation of delivery of the fetus at term by actions at a number of target sites. One or more pituitary hormones of maternal and fetal origin may also be instrumental in activating processes leading to parturition. The particular roles of neural and endocrine factors in parturition vary considerably among species and, therefore, no single model adequately describes the process in any one species.

Neuroendocrine Control of Parturition

Progesterone.   In most mammalian species a drop in circulating levels of progesterone occurs prior to labor. In corpus luteum-dependent species this may be accomplished by uterine luteolytic factors (PGs in some species). In other placenta-dependent species changes in enzyme activities that increase estrogen production may lower progesterone levels. Progesterone is directly antagonistic to uterine smooth muscle contraction induced either by oxytocin or PGs. The *progesterone block hypothesis* was formulated to provide a theoretically relevant mechanism by which the uterus might be protected from premature contraction and expulsion of the fetus. In this model a lowering of progesterone levels at term would be the stimulus to parturition.

Estrogens.   Estrogens increase myometrial excitability, possibly by lowering the membrane potential of uterine smooth muscle. The actions of estrogens on the myometrium are, however, antagonized by the action of progesterone. In the rat the number of uterine estrogen receptors increases as progesterone levels decline. Estrogens enhance uterine excitability by a number of mechanisms: increasing endometrial PG synthetase activity, increasing myometrial and endometrial oxytocin receptors, and increasing oxytocin production and secretion by the neurohypophysis (see Chap. 7).

Prostaglandins.   There is evidence that in most species studied PGs play an important role in parturition. In many species increased synthesis and release of PGs precede labor. In some large animals (e.g., goat, sow) that depend on the corpus luteum as a source of progesterone, $PGF_{2\alpha}$ released from the endometrium may be the luteolytic factor responsible for luteal regression. The resulting drop in luteal progesterone production is followed by uterine contractions and parturition. As noted, uterine PG synthesis may be dependent on stimulation by placental estrogens.

Placental Prolactin.   Levels of PRL increase in the human fetus during late gestation. PRL levels are very high in amniotic fluid, and synthesis of PRL by chorion-decidual tissue has been demonstrated. This placental PRL is immunologically similar to pituitary PRL and should not be confused with placental lactogen (PL), which differs considerably in primary structure. Increased levels of PRL coincide with a stage in development during which major changes in organ growth occur in the fetus and may be responsible for increased growth and function of the fetal adrenal cortex (see Chap. 12).

Autonomic Motor Innervation.   The female reproductive tract is richly innervated by adrenergic neurons. The role, if any, of such innervation in parturition is unresolved. Both estrogens and progestins affect the norepinephrine content of these nerves, as well as the turnover of NE, the activity of enzymes related to catecholamine biosynthesis, and the release of NE from nerve terminals. In the progesterone-dominated uterus catecholamine stimulation of myometrial smooth muscle β-adrenoceptors causes relaxation of the uterus. During the latter stages of pregnancy in some species, stretch-induced hypertrophy of the uterus causes degeneration of the nerves in the uterine corpus. Withdrawal of this neural inhibitory influence to the corpus may allow spontaneous myogenic contractions to intensify [26].

It has been noted that gap junctions (nexuses, low-resistance electrical pathways) are present between the uterine muscle cells of a number of species (including the human) immediately before, during, and immediately after delivery [14]. These junctions are absent at all other times during pregnancy and are also lacking in immature or nonpregnant animals. Ovariectomy of pregnant animals at midterm causes the rapid appearance of gap junctions, and the appearance of gap junctions at term is prevented by progesterone administration. The absence of gap junctions throughout the gestation period may be important in preventing electrical communication between uterine muscle cells. The acquisition of gap junctions at term may be an essential element in synchronizing uterine contractility for effective expulsion of the fetus [14]. Because gap junction formation may be initiated by progesterone withdrawal, this could provide the morphological and functional bases for the progesterone block hypothesis formulated much earlier by Csapo.

Oxytocin.   Oxytocin, a neurohypophysial hormone, has a direct uterine-contracting (oxytocic) action (see Chap. 7). Fetal movements monitored by the uterine cervix and relayed by spinal afferents are stimulatory to OT release during labor in the human. The sensitivity of the myometrium to OT is enhanced by estrogens and depressed by progesterone. In the human female maternal plasma OT levels increase with advancing gestation. It is not clear, however, whether OT is an initiating factor or only facilitative to human labor. Plasma estrogen concentrations increase during gestation and in the rat are known to increase the affinity and number of uterine OT receptors. The actions of OT on the uterus could be mediated indirectly through stimulation of endometrial and myometrial $PGF_{2\alpha}$ production. $PGF_{2\alpha}$ might then stimulate uterine smooth muscle cells, leading to contraction of the uterus and expulsion of the fetus.

The Fetal Adrenal Cortex.   There is compelling evidence, particularly in sheep but also in other large mammals, that the onset of parturition is initiated by the activation of the fetal pituitary-adrenal axis. The fetal adrenal gland increases in weight rapidly during the last 2 weeks of gestation. This growth is primarily due to hypertrophy and hyperplasia of adrenal cortical cells. Premature delivery can be induced in the pregnant ewe by infusion of ACTH or glucocorticoids (but not mineralocorticoids) and can be prevented by fetal adrenalectomy or hypophysectomy. There is evidence that the fetal brain signals the precise "time for birth." The paraventricular nucleus (in sheep) apparently acts as a computer assessing signals from various organs. When the organs have reached the proper degree of development, the PVN sends a hormonal signal (CRH?) to the pituitary to start producing ACTH, thereby initiating labor [30, 45].

Increased fetal glucocorticoid production in sheep is stimulatory to placental production of estrogen from progesterone; this, therefore, leads to a subsequent fall in maternal plasma and tissue progesterone concentrations and a consequent rise in estrogen concentrations. The actions of fetal adrenal glucocorticoids may be to induce synthesis of

17,20 desmolase and 17 α-hydroxylase within the placenta (Fig. 19.3). The resulting change in estrogen-progesterone levels may provide the stimulus to uterine production of PGs or related hormones (prostacyclins) and to an increase in uterine OT receptor number.

Relaxin. In 1926 Hisaw reported that an aqueous extract of the corpora lutea of the pregnant sow "relaxes" the pubic symphysis of the guinea pig. This biologically active substance was purified and named *relaxin* [12]. Because of difficulties in isolating this factor, the chemical structure was not determined until much later. The development of a reliable radioimmunoassay made possible the determination of the blood levels of the peptide throughout pregnancy, the production sites of the hormone, and the factors that may regulate relaxin secretion. Most interesting was the discovery that the primary structures of relaxin and insulin are similar. Although there is only about 40% homology between the residues, the conformations of the two peptides are comparable. The cross-linking pattern of the two hormones strongly suggests that they have come into existence by gene duplication. It has been concluded, a posteriori, that relaxin, like insulin, is synthesized as a prohormone in a single chain to facilitate the correct folding of the protein.

Studies on a variety of species, including humans, leave little doubt that the corpus luteum is the source of relaxin [8]. The source of luteal relaxin may be the granules observed in the granulosa lutein cells. Relaxin may also be produced and stored within granulocytes localized to the endometrium of rhesus monkeys and adult human females. In other species, such as the guinea pig, cat, rabbit, and horse, immunoreactive or bioactive relaxin levels in plasma or serum appear to be derived primarily from the placenta or uterus. Relaxin concentrations in luteal and other tissues are highest during pregnancy (Fig. 19.4). In the human, relaxin concentrations are four times higher in the ovarian vein draining the ovary containing the corpus luteum of pregnancy, than in either peripheral plasma or the contralateral ovarian vein. Immunoreactive relaxin is present in the serum as early as the fourth week of pregnancy; it is detectable throughout the course of gestation but is only rarely detected in the plasma of nonpregnant women. Plasma levels of immunoreactive relaxin rise to a peak shortly before parturition in rodents and pigs, which

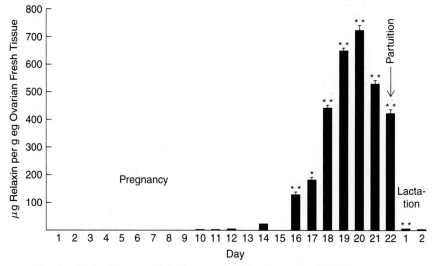

Figure 19.4 Mean relaxin immunoactivity levels (± SEM) in ovarian extracts from pregnant and lactating rats. Ovaries obtained from two animals were pooled for each day shown. Multiple volumes of extract, containing 0.2 to 5 ngeq ovarian fresh tissue, were employed. Asterisks denote those mean relaxin concentrations that differ significantly from those of the preceding observation (*P < 0.05; **P < 0.01). (From Sherwood and Crnekovic [37], with permission).

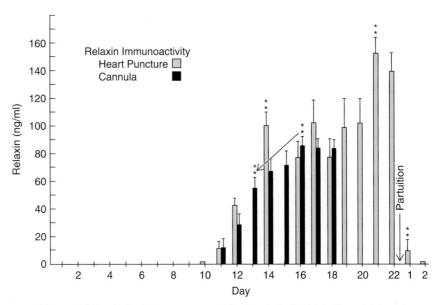

Figure 19.5 Relaxin immunoreactivity levels (± SEM) in the peripheral sera of anesthetized (heart puncture) and unanesthetized (cannula) rats. Asterisks denote those mean values that differ significantly (*P < 0.05; **P < 0.01) from those using the same end point that precede or are indicated with an arrow. (From Sherwood et al. [38], with permission).

is correlated with the increase in cervical dilatability and the formation of an interpubic ligament (Fig 19.5). Plasma RIA relaxin is also markedly elevated in late pregnancy in the dog, rhesus and Java monkeys, and humans. Immunoreactive relaxin was found in the decidua, the placenta, and the myometrium of a pregnant baboon in which the corpus luteum had been removed much earlier. This observation suggests that these tissues have the ability to synthesize relaxin and may function in primate pregnancy during late gestation. Relaxin has also been found in the testes of armadillos and roosters, but is undetectable in the testis and serum of a number of male mammals, including humans. The role, if any, of relaxin in the male is therefore unknown.

The biological effects of relaxin are associated with pregnancy and parturition [39]. Relaxin acts on the pubic symphysis to transform the connective tissues from a compact cartilaginous type to a more fluid, flexible structure. This results, in some species, in the formation of a ligament between the pubic bones. This increased flexibility and enlargement of the birth canal is important to successful parturition in a number of species.

Relaxin may be present within the endometrium of the uterus; in the rhesus monkey the peptide may function as a local hormone to control endothelioid cytomorphosis. This response involves hypertrophy and proliferation of the endothelial cells of the blood vessels just below the implanted embryo. This vascular response to relaxin could provide increased blood flow to the fetus. Relaxin also inhibits uterine motility by relaxing the myometrium. It has been speculated that because of its myometrium-inhibiting activity, relaxin may play a role in maintenance of pregnancy. Other effects of relaxin on the collagen framework and distensibility of the uterus, as well as similar effects on the uterine cervix, have been described.

Relaxin increases the secretion of two key collagenolytic enzymes, collagenase and plasminogen activator, from dispersed amnion and chorion cell cultures in vitro. These results support a possible localized action of relaxin on collagen degradation in fetal membranes, leading to their eventual rupture at the time of parturition. Relaxin and somatotropin may act synergistically in stimulating mammary gland growth. The evidence is convincing that relaxin subserves a multifunctional role in preparing the female for parturition and possibly other roles related to pregnancy.

Parturition in Humans

A model for the initiation of labor in the human suggests that, as a result of the rising estrogen levels during gestation, the concentration of uterine OT receptors increases [13]. Rapid fetal growth near term increases uterine distension, which may also contribute to the increase in uterine OT receptors near term, as shown in rats (see Chap. 7). The increased numbers of OT receptors probably lower the threshold of the uterus to a level where myometrial contractions are initiated. Oxytocin may bind to decidual receptors and stimulate PG biosynthesis. The coupling of OT receptor activation and PG biosynthesis may be the crucial event in the initiation of labor. During spontaneous labor there is an increase in plasma OT levels in the fetal umbilical artery compared to the umbilical vein, indicating a flow of OT from the fetus toward the maternal compartment. Oxytocin derived from the fetus may provide the stimulus for the increased production of PGs at the onset of labor. Hypothalamoneurohypophysial maturation within the fetus, leading to fetal-adrenal activation and a decline in progesterone biosynthesis, as well as increased neurohypophysial hormone secretion (by the neurohypophysis as well as the uterus), may provide the final essential directive for the induction of parturition.

LACTATION

In mammals two ectodermal ridges (so-called milk lines) appear on either side of the ventral midline early in fetal life. Localized thickenings become the mammary buds, which, in the female, grow into the underlying dermis to form the primary mammary cords, the precursors of the duct systems. In the human male early mammary gland development is suppressed by gonadal androgens and, although there is an initial hypertrophy of the primary ducts and the secretion of a colostrumlike "witch's milk," caused by the maternal hormones of pregnancy, these glands soon become inactive. Further growth of the undeveloped mammae in the human female is not initiated until ovarian cycles begin. At puberty, further growth and branching of the ducts occurs and a lobular system is developed. Most of the size increase of the mammary glands is due to interlobular fat deposition. Mammary growth and development at puberty is mainly in response to gonadal estrogens, but adrenal glucocorticoids and GH may also be involved (Fig. 19.6).

Proliferation of a lobular-alveolar system is initiated at pregnancy. Besides the requirement for estrogens and possibly glucocorticoids and GH for continued duct growth, progesterone and prolactin are required for full development of the ductule system (Fig. 19.6). Placental lactogen may also be required for full development of the breasts in the pregnant human female. Milk production in the mature mammary gland occurs near parturition. The following hormones have been implicated as essential to

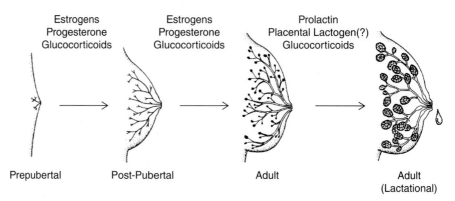

Figure 19.6 Hormonal regulation of mammary gland growth and development.

mammary growth and lactogenesis in some species: estrogen, progesterone, glucocorticoids, GH, insulin, placental lactogen, relaxin, and PRL [34].

Although milk constituents begin to appear before parturition in most species, high rates of synthesis do not usually occur until after birth. Milk is synthesized within the cells lining the mammary gland alveoli. Milk is a complex nutrient consisting mainly of milk sugar (lactose) lipids, milk proteins (casein and whey), as well as monovalent and divalent cations, and most interesting, immune antibodies. These products are released by macrovesicular exocytosis into the alveolar lumen, where they are stored until ejected by the action of OT on the myoepithelial cells covering the contraluminal surface of the alveolus (see Fig. 7.4). Many hormones of unknown function are found in milk [24].

Milk secretion is regulated by PRL through an action on plasmalemmal receptors of mammary gland alveolar secretory cells [32]. In the rabbit an increase in PRL receptors, synchronous with the onset of lactation, occurs at the same time as the major rise in serum PRL levels at parturition. Estradiol increases the number of mammary gland PRL receptors, whereas progesterone suppresses this increase. PRL also upregulates its own receptors. The dramatic increase in lactogenesis that follows parturition can be partly explained, therefore, by the removal of the inhibitory action of progesterone on the mammary gland coupled to the positive actions of PRL on the stimulation and production of its own receptors. Suckling-induced PRL secretion is required for maintenance of postpartum lactogenesis in some animals, such as the human, but not in others, such as the cow.

Fatty acids derived from dietary fat intake are converted within mammary gland epithelial cells to triglycerides (milk fats). These fatty acids are made available to mammary gland epithelial cells by activation of membrane-bound lipoprotein lipase. The activity of this enzyme is negligible in nonlactating animals but is enhanced 2 to 3 days before parturition, apparently in response to rising levels of PRL. Prolactin activation of lipoprotein lipase is blocked by simultaneous administration of actinomycin D, indicating that synthesis or activation of the enzyme requires mRNA-directed protein synthesis. Fatty acids are also synthesized within mammary gland epithelial cells in response to PRL.

In certain fishes PRL stimulates renal Na^+/K^+-activated ATPase and controls salt excretion by the nasal salt gland of some marine birds. Prolactin also activates the transport of Na^+ and K^+ in mammary tissue apparently through an action on a Na^+/K^+ pump, which is localized almost exclusively to the basolateral membranes of mammary epithelial cells. Control of transepithelial Na^+ transport may be the underlying and most basic action of PRL on mammary gland milk production.

The secretion of PRL from the pituitary is under an inhibitory control by the hypothalamus (see Chap. 6). A PRL release-inhibiting hormone, most probably dopamine, is released from hypothalamic dopaminergic neurons into the hypophysial portal system where the catecholamine is carried to the lactotrophs of the pars distalis. Inhibition of hypothalamic dopamine release or inhibition of dopamine interaction with lactotroph receptors (by ergot alkaloids, e.g., ergocryptine) results in PRL secretion.

Lactotroph hyperplasia is a prominent finding in the adenohypophyses of pregnant women. The increase in the amount of PRL mRNA is paralleled by lactotroph hyperplasia. The presence of mitoses in PRL-immunoreactive cells provides evidence that proliferation of pre-existing lactotrophs contribute to lactotroph accumulation. Growth hormone (GH) immunoreactive cells show a marked reduction in GH mRNA, indicating that GH synthesis is inhibited. In many GH-immunoreactive cells, PRL mRNA becomes apparent. These findings demonstrate that GH is stored following discontinuation of GH synthesis. It appears that, when PRL is secreted in excess during pregnancy, somatotrophs are recruited to produce PRL. These somatotrophs begin to express PRL mRNA, transform to bihormonal mammosomatotrophs, and possibly later to lactotrophs, contributing to PRL production. Mature somatotrophs may be regarded as reserve cells in the adenohypophysis, having the potential to switch hormone synthesis and to convert to mammosomatotrophs and possibly lactotrophs [42].

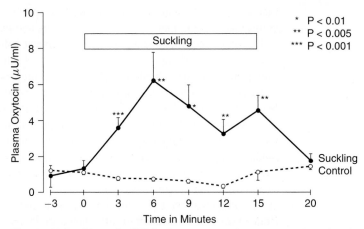

Figure 19.7 Mean (± SEM) plasma oxytocin concentrations for six nursing and six control subjects. Asterisks indicate significance relative to control subjects. (©1979 *The Endocrine Society*. Baltimore: The Williams & Wilkins Company.)

The stimulus to PRL secretion is a neuroendocrine reflex involving neural afferents from the teats to the hypothalamus. A suckling-induced neuroendocrine reflex mechanism is also responsible for secretion of OT from the neurohypophysis (Fig. 19.7) [13]. Blood concentrations of PRL increase progressively throughout pregnancy; apparently due to the influence of increasing concentrations of placental steroids, particularly estrogens. Nevertheless, milk secretion is inhibited by a direct action of progesterone on the mammary glands. At parturition, blood levels of PRL are about 20 times greater than normal, but the level of the hormone remains elevated for only about a week postpartum in the absence of suckling. Blood concentrations of PRL remain high for the duration of lactation in breast-feeding women, and PRL is also released during each suckling episode in response to tactile stimulation of the nipple. Estrogens exert a profound action on pituitary mammotroph PRL production. The elevated plasma levels of estrogens just prior to parturition may, indeed, be important in stimulating lactogenesis through stimulation of

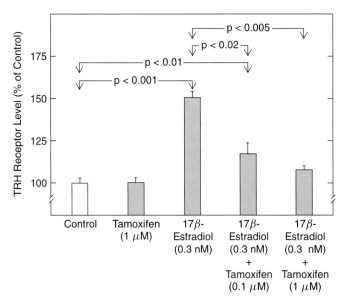

Figure 19.8 Effect of tamoxifen, an estrogen antagonist, on pituitary TRH receptor number. (From Gershengorn, Marcus-Samuels, and Geras [15], with permission.)

PRL secretion. Estrogens appear to enhance lactotroph PRL secretion (at least in rats) by increasing the number of TRH receptors (TRH stimulates PRL secretion) present in these cells, an action that is blocked by the estrogen receptor antagonist, tamoxifen (Fig. 19.8) [15].

The placenta secretes large amounts of estrogens and progesterone, hormones inhibitory to FSH secretion during pregnancy. Therefore, plasma FSH levels are normally suppressed during pregnancy and, at term, are low or undetectable. Blood levels of FSH increase postpartum to normal follicular phase levels. Both pituitary and plasma levels of LH are also extremely low during pregnancy, apparently also due to a negative feedback inhibition by placental steroid hormones. Inhibition of pituitary gonadotropin production during pregnancy may provide an adaptive mechanism whereby further egg maturation and release is inhibited so that the nutritive needs of the nursing infant are sustained. In nonlactating women LH concentrations may remain low during the early puerperium (state of the woman after childbirth) but return to normal cyclic levels within 3 to 5 weeks, when the PRL concentration returns to its normal low levels.

In lactating women, blood E_2 concentrations are significantly lower than those of nonlactating women, and no ovarian follicular development occurs during the period of lactation as long as PRL levels remain high. Plasma levels of LH and E_2 increase soon after weaning, concomitant with a drop in PRL secretion, indicating the resumption of ovarian activity. Because the return of menstruation and fertility is usually delayed in women who breast-feed, it has been suggested that breast-feeding acts as a natural birth spacer or "nature's own contraceptive" [40]. In those societies where breast-feeding is the sole source of nutrition for the baby, *lactational amenorrhea* (postpartum infertility) may last for 2 to 3 years [28]. The duration of the period between birth and the onset of a menstrual cycle in the mother is probably a function of the frequency and duration of suckling. Although breast-feeding usually delays conception, it cannot do so indefinitely and women can become pregnant before the breast-feeding infant is weaned.

Breast-feeding is associated with a very significant prevention of infant morbidity and mortality throughout the world, and yet the duration, if not the incidence of breast-feeding, continues to decline worldwide. Nevertheless, the contraceptive effect of breast-feeding continues to make a substantial impact on fertility control worldwide [28].

HORMONAL CONTRACEPTION

The common contraceptive drugs in clinical use for women contain estrogens or progestogens, either singly or in a variety of combinations and concentrations. The estrogens are usually synthetic derivatives of ethinyl estradiol (Fig. 19.9). The progestogens are usually 19-nortestosterone or 17-hydroxyprogesterone derivatives such as norethindrone (Fig. 19.9). The *combination contraceptive preparations* contain an estrogen and a progestogen and are often administered daily for 20 days and stopped for 5 days, during

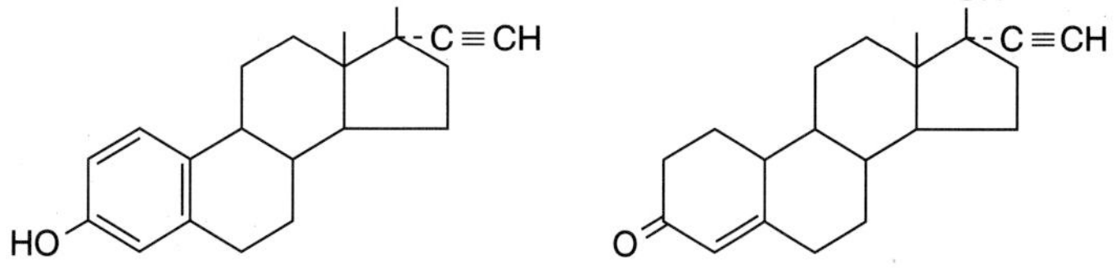

Figure 19.9 Examples of structures of two common contraceptive steroids, an estrogen, ethinyl estradiol, and a progestogen, norethindrone.

which time withdrawal uterine bleeding (menses) occurs. Through a combined negative feedback to the hypothalamus (and pituitary?) LH and FSH secretions are suppressed. There is an absence of an LH-FSH surge, and the failure of a follicular phase rise in FSH secretion results in lack of ovarian follicular development. Endogenous blood levels of E_2 remain low due to suppression of LH and FSH secretion.

Progestogens administered alone have complex effects that relate to the dosage. Besides suppression of gonadotropin secretion and inhibition of follicular development, cervical mucus composition is modified, which may prevent sperm entry into the uterine cavity. In addition, endometrial histology may be altered and thus interfere with implantation of the ovum should fertilization occur.

Some contraceptive steroid regimes consist of estrogens administered alone for a number of days (usually 15) followed by a progestogen for several days (usually 5). These *sequential contraceptive preparations* simulate to some degree the normal sequence of ovarian steroid secretion. A large dose of an estrogen has been used with some success as a postcoital contraceptive [46]. Silastic steroid-impregnated devices that provide a slow delivery of a steroid are available as contraceptive depot preparations. Even intrauterine devices (IUDs) impregnated with progestogens have been reported to provide significant contraceptive action.

Superactive agonistic analogs of GnRH have been developed for potential use in hypogonadal men and women. These stimulatory analogs have been discovered to exert paradoxical inhibitory effects on pituitary-gonadal function in both sexes. Postovulatory administration of these stimulatory analogs may have a luteolytic effect in women. The effects of these GnRH analogs may be mediated at the level of the pituitary, to cause a down-regulation of gonadotropin GnRH receptors, and also at the level of the gonad through some unknown action.

Pregnancy Termination.   Increased plasma progesterone concentrations are responsible for the lack of ovulation during pregnancy, presumably operating, via negative feedback, on the hypothalamus-pituitary LH release system. This inhibitory effect of progesterone is the basis of current oral contraceptives, which contain a synthetic progesterone analog (a progestin). RU 486, a steroid with high affinity for the progesterone receptor, is the first available active antiprogesterone (Fig. 19.10). It has been used successfully as a medical alternative for early pregnancy interruption, and it also has other potential applications in medicine [3, 4].

When progesterone enters the target cell, it binds to a nuclear protein receptor and, in the process, it changes the shape of the receptor and frees an associated heat shock protein (see Chap. 4). This allows the receptor-hormone complex to bind to the hormone response elements on the DNA. That step, in turn, alters the DNA so that the genes controlled by progesterone can be transcribed. RU 486, like progesterone, binds to the receptor but does not release the heat shock protein. Indeed, the heat shock protein may become even more tightly bound to the receptor. As a result, the receptor is unable to bind to the hormone response elements, and no transcription of the DNA takes place. In addition, since RU 486 occupies the receptors, it prevents progesterone from binding to them, and therefore prevents any physiological events that depend on progesterone, such as the maintenance of pregnancy (Fig. 19.11) [3, 4].

Anti-hormone

Figure 19.10   Structure of RU 486, a synthetic progesterone-antagonist.

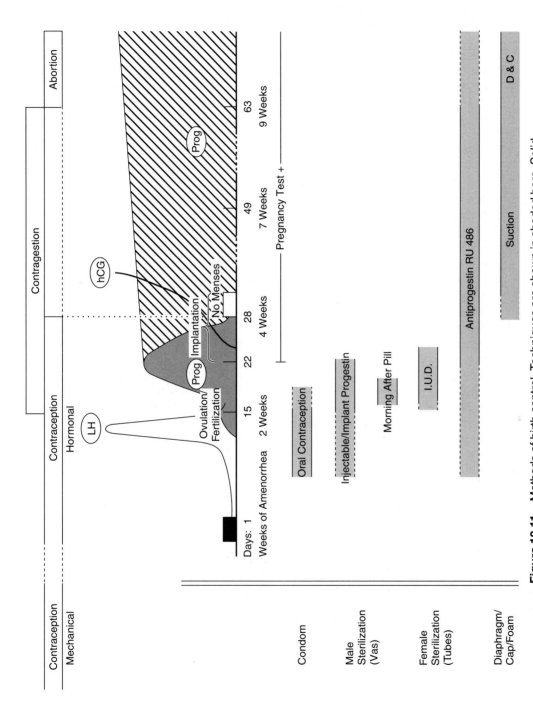

Figure 19.11 Methods of birth control. Techniques are shown in shaded bars. Solid lines indicate the times when a method is most efficient; for mechanical conception no time-dependency is indicated. Dotted lines show when the method might also have some effect. LH = luteinizing hormone; HCG = human chorionic gonadotrophin; prog = progesterone; IUD = intra-uterine device; D & C = dialation and curettage. (From Etienne-Emile Baulieu, with permission. "RU486: a compound that gets itself talked about." *Human Reproduction,* vol 9 (Suppl. 1), pp 1–6, 1994.)

Birth control techniques range from methods preventing fertilization to the interruption of pregnancy at various stages. Figure 19.11 shows the overlapping categories of several methods (classified as contraception, contragestion, and abortion) and their periods of efficacy, measured from the last menses. Common terms can be ambiguous. Contraception is usually understood to mean preventing fertilization, but specialists also use it to mean the period of time lasting until implantation is complete. To many biologists and theologians, abortion might mean any maneuver after fertilization; to practitioners, it takes place only after implantation. Most birth control techniques can work in several ways. Even some oral contraceptives do not always block ovulation; for example, they can alter the endometrium and may prevent implantation, which is a post-ovulatory effect. The figure shows contragestion from day 15, when fertilization takes place, and it spans the time of other post-ovulatory methods.

MENOPAUSE

The onset of menopause results from a loss in the cyclic activity of the ovary, which is believed to be caused by a failure at the level of the ovary to respond to gonadotropins. This is due in part to a depletion in the number of available follicles for growth. Fertility begins to decline about 10 years before the menopause and by age 50 most primary follicles have been lost. There appears to be no relationship between the age of onset of menopause and the age of the onset of menarche. Also, the number of children born or the age at the time of birth of the first child does not appear to be related to the age of menopause [29]. The nutritional status of the individual may, however, influence the onset of menopause. The age of menopause varies in different countries: 49.8 for white North Americans; 51.4 in the Netherlands; 44 or younger in the Punjab, New Guinea, and Central Africa. It appears that the onset of menopause is getting later.

As women approach menopause, there may be a striking increase in serum FSH levels, relative to those of LH. Eventually, as estradiol secretion falls to low levels, both FSH and LH concentrations rise and remain elevated, apparently due to the removal of the negative steroid feedback mechanism characteristic of active ovarian function. The premenopausal rise in FSH secretion may relate to the progressive loss of inhibin, whose role is postulated to exert a negative feedback control of pituitary FSH secretion. Progressive loss of ovarian follicles and their maturation would be expected to reduce the production of inhibin.

Many studies in animals have shown how the declining activity of the ovary is the primary cause of a reduced fertility in older females [2, 10]. Rising hypothalamic thresholds to the feedback actions of steroids are also age-related in rats. Similar situations might arise in women at the onset of the menopause, but it is not easy to design studies to clarify this situation. An opportunity to do so has been reported, based on analyses of hypothalamic GnRH function in 12 women of various ages between 27 and 64, who had been previously oophorectomized. Oophorectomy had been done between 10 months and several years before the study, and none of the women had taken oral steroids or injected estrogens for 30 days or more before the onset of the analysis. Plasma samples were collected every 10 minutes between 08.00 and 13.00 hours for assays of PRL, E_2, FSH, and LH. Estradiol levels were low, and mean levels of gonadotropins, together with their pulse frequency and pulse amplitude, did not differ in two groups of women between 27 and 49 years of age and 52 and 64 years of age, respectively. The calculations were the same whether chronological age or age after menarche was used for comparisons and despite varying intervals after the oophorectomy was performed.

The pattern of GnRH activity thus appears to be similar in the hypothalamus of young or aging women, and the rising levels of LH in postmenopausal women also display a pulse frequency similar to that of cyclic women in the follicular phase, that is, one pulse every 60–90 minutes. The inherent hypothalamic pulse mechanism does not seem to be affected by age, although it is possible that pituitary sensitivity to GnRH might increase after the menopause or oophorectomy, as the inhibitory effects of sex steroids or inhibition are withdrawn. It was concluded, therefore, that ovarian failure is the main consequence of reproductive aging in women [1].

In the absence of gonadal estrogens in the body during menopause, it is not unexpected that a number of physiological changes take place. The uterus, an estrogen-dependent organ, becomes smaller and the endometrium atrophic. Atrophic vaginitis as well as vaginal dryness may occur, but these changes can be reversed by exogenous estrogens applied locally or given systemically. There is an increased risk of coronary thrombosis in postmenopausal women, reaching a level of risk similar to that of men.

During the *climacterium,* that period preceding termination of the reproductive period, some women experience episodic sensations of heat (menopausal flushes/flashes), usually involving the face and neck and upper part of the chest, which may be associated with profuse sweating. There is a synchrony between these menopausal flushes and pulses of LH secretion. These flushes are not correlated with significant similar secretions of FSH, PRL, or catecholamines. The flushes are not caused by LH secretion per se, as they occur in hypophysectomized women. Apparently a suprapituitary mechanism involving GnRH secretion is involved. It has been suggested that these flushes may be a manifestation of a classical withdrawal syndrome, mediated through changes in neurons sensitive to estrogens. A central adrenergic mechanism may be involved as α-adrenergic agonists provide some symptomatic relief.

After the menopause there is a reduction in the cortical thickness and the tensile strength of bones, resulting from an increase in loss of mineral content. *Postmenopausal osteoporosis* can be prevented by estrogen administration, but this depends on how soon after menopause estrogen replacement therapy begins. Estrogens prevent osteoporosis and its most serious medical consequence, hip fracture. Estrogens also lower the risk of coronary heart disease. Estrogens reduce the risk of cardiovascular disease, probably through their beneficial effects on lipid metabolism [17]. Because death rates from coronary heart disease among American women are four times those from endometrial and breast cancers combined, estrogen's benefits could far outweigh any carcinogenic potential [11].

Given estrogen's high benefit-to-risk ratio in this setting, the therapeutic challenge is to identify the individuals for estrogen replacement therapy who are at increased risk for unwanted, adverse effects. Once these women are identified, the remainder can use estrogen replacement therapy so that they can continue to enjoy the same quality of life they experienced before menopause. Thus to avoid the recognized problems of estrogen deficiency, it has been suggested that nearly all women should begin a lifelong course of estrogen replacement therapy during the perimenopausal period [11].

Unopposed long-term estrogen therapy increases the risk of developing endometrial hyperplasia, endometrial cancer, and possibly breast cancer as well [7, 16, 33]. The risk of developing endometrial cancer has been reduced by combining a progestin with the estrogen. Although some progestins may reverse the cardioprotective effect of estrogens, those with minimal androgenicity appear less likely to do so. Hormone replacement therapy that combines estrogen with a progestin of minimal androgenicity is thus a rational alternative to unopposed estrogen therapy [17].

Menopause and Libido.   Women appear to show a decline in libido after the menopause, but there is considerable debate whether such changes are intrinsic or due to influences of the sexual partner or society. Changes in the female reproductive tract such as reduction in the thickness of the vaginal epithelium and decreases in vaginal secretions due to reductions in estrogen secretion might also be expected to affect female sexual responses. Although there have been many clinical trials of postmenopausal estrogen replacement, very few studies have assessed sexual function objectively. Contradictory results exist in behavior studies that have been published. It has been reported that estrogen replacement enhanced libido, sexual activity, and orgasmic capacity but also that estrogen replacement did not change coital frequency, coital satisfaction, or frequency of masturbation. The data is even more difficult to interpret because it is not possible to determine whether the effects of estrogen replacement are being mediated at the level of the reproductive tract or the central nervous system [43].

PATHOPHYSIOLOGY

Because of the complexity of the female reproductive system, the cyclic nature of ovarian hormone production and secretion, and the fact that the growth and development of a number of organs, in particular the uterus and mammary glands, are dependent on ovarian hormone secretion, it is not surprising that a large number of pathological states are attributable to endocrine dysfunctions. The pregnant state, dependent on a multitude of hormonal events unique to the female, is vulnerable to endocrine dysfunctions that can endanger the life of both the fetus and mother.

Hyperprolactinemia.   The most common example of pituitary hypersecretion of a hormone involves PRL [35]. Not only does hyperprolactinemia lead to *galactorrhea* (excess milk production), but amenorrhea and anovulation are complicating sequelae of excessive PRL secretion. Breast engorgement due to excessive lactogenesis usually results from excessive PRL secretion from a pituitary adenoma (prolactinoma). The etiology of the prolactinoma is uncertain but could result from a failure of hypothalamic release of PRL-inhibiting factor, thus leading to lactotroph hyperplasia and eventual adenoma formation. The onset of galactorrhea may date to a normal postpartum lactation that fails to be discontinued (Chiari-Frommel syndrome).

Suckling of the breasts is the normal stimulus to PRL secretion. It appears that stimuli that increase afferent impulses in the neuroendocrine reflex pathway leading to PRL secretion, such as surgery, trauma, tight-fitting garments, or continued breast manipulation, may lead to galactorrhea (neurogenic galactorrhea-amenorrhea). The amenorrhea that accompanies the galactorrhea probably results from PRL inhibition of hypothalamic GnRH secretion and a subsequent block of the ovulatory surge of gonadotropins. In addition elevated plasma PRL levels are directly inhibitory to ovarian estrogen production, which may also be, in part, responsible for the accompanying amenorrhea. Women with increased PRL levels and a resulting decreased estrogen production may experience bone demineralization and associated incidence of clinical bone fractures. Bromocryptine, a dopamine receptor agonist, is effective in establishing normal estrogen levels and ovulatory menstrual cycles in most hyperprolactinemic women [35].

Hormones and Breast Cancer.   The early observation that oophorectomy may effect a rapid remission of advanced breast cancer in some premenopausal women provided evidence that some human breast cancers may depend on sex steroids for their continued proliferation [5, 19, 25, 41, 44, 48]. Hypophysectomy and adrenalectomy are a means of hormone deprivation through endocrine ablation, but unfortunately not all women respond favorably to such radical treatment. This is because only 25% to 30% of human breast cancers are hormone dependent and therefore responsive to endocrine manipulation. Patients with hormone-dependent cancers may, however, be favorable candidates for endocrine therapy. It is important therefore to distinguish those women with such hormone-responsive cancers. It has been demonstrated that the quantitative determination of the estrogen receptor (estrophilin) content of an excised tumor specimen often provides useful information as to the best type of therapy for the patient with advanced breast cancer. Tumors that contain low or negligible amounts of estrophilin rarely respond to endocrine ablation or other hormone therapy (e.g., antiestrogen administration), whereas patients with receptor-rich cancers often benefit from endocrine treatment.

Early onset, long-lasting, ovulatory cycle function seems to increase the risk of breast cancer [18, 19]. Several studies on a number of populations and different ethnic groups have shown that women who have had an early menarche are at a greater risk of developing breast cancer than those who have had a late menarche. There has been, and in some countries still is, a secular trend in an earlier age at menarche, being most evident in countries in which the age at menarche has been high. In these countries also the breast cancer risk has been relatively low and is now increasing.

It has been reported that a physiological way to reduce breast cancer risk might exist. Subjects who had participated in organized athletic activity while in college had a lower lifetime occurrence rate of breast cancer than their nonathletic classmates. It was suggested that this might be dependent on endocrine mechanisms. The athletes in all age groups had a later age of menarche than the reference nonathlete group in this study. In a number of studies it has been shown that strenuous physical activity may lead to extensive delay in the onset of menarche [48].

Cigarette smoking is associated with several diseases of major importance in women. Notably, smokers appear to have an increased risk of cardiovascular disease and osteoporosis and a decreased risk of breast and endometrial cancer. Hormonal mechanisms, particularly an antiestrogenic effect of smoking in women, have been postulated as mediators of these differences in risk. This hypothesis is supported by the observation in several studies that cigarette smoking is also associated with changes in fertility and earlier menopause. In one study, cigarette smokers had significantly higher mean plasma levels of the adrenal androgens dehydroepiandrosterone sulfate and androstenedione than nonsmokers. These results suggest that the possible decreased risk of breast and endometrial cancer associated with cigarette smoking may not be mediated solely through lower levels of endogenous estrogen, at least in postmenopausal women, and they raise questions about the role of androgens in disease mechanisms in older populations. The higher levels of adrenal androgens and their consistent relation to smoking in both men and women suggested that more attention should be focused on the role of the androgens, or at least of the androgen-estrogen balance, in older populations [23].

REFERENCES

[1] Alexander, S. E., S. Aksel, J. M. Hazelton, R. R. Yeoman, and S. M. Gilmore. 1990. Hypothalamic function and the menopause. *Amer. J. Obstet. Gynecol.* 162:446.

[2] Avis, N. E., P. A. Kaufert, M. Luck, S. M. McKinlay, and K. Vass. 1993. The evolution of menopausal symptoms. *Baillière's Clin. Endocrinol. Metab.* 7:17–32.

[3] Baulieu, E.-E. 1989. Contragestion and other clinical applications of RU 486, an antiprogesterone at the receptor. *Science* 245:1351–7.

[4] ———. 1991. The antisteroid RU486. Its cellular and molecular mode of action. *TEM* 2:233–9.

[5] Bernstein, L., and R. K. Ross. 1993. Endogenous hormones and breast cancer risk. *Epidemiol. Rev.* 15:48–65.

[6] Bidart, J.-M., and D. Bellet.1993. Human chorionic gonadotropin. Molecular forms, detection, and clinical implications. *TEM* 4:285–90.

[7] Brinton, L. A., and C. Schairer. 1993. Estrogen replacement therapy and breast cancer risk. *Epidemiol. Rev.* 15:66–79.

[8] Bryant-Greenwood, G. D. 1991. Human decidual and placental relaxin. *Reprod. Fertil. Develop.* 3:385–9.

[9] Chen, F., and D. Puett. 1992. A single amino acid residue replacement in the β subunit of human chorionic gonadotropin results in the loss of biological activity. *J. Mol. Endocrinol.* 8:87–9.

[10] Eskin, B. A., ed. 1980. *The menopause.* New York: Masson Publishing Co.

[11] Ettinger, B. 1988. Estrogen replacement therapy symposium. *Obstet. Gynecol.* 72: 1S–5; 12S–7; 315–6.

[12] Fevold. H., F. L. Hisaw, and R. K. Meyer. 1930. The relaxative hormone of the corpus luteum. Its purification and concentration. *J. Am. Chem. Soc.* 52:3340–48.

[13] Fuchs, A.-R., L. Cubile, M. Y. Dawood, and F. S. Jorgensen. 1984. Release of oxytocin and prolactin by suckling in rabbits throughout lactation. *Endocrinology* 114:462–9.

[14] Garfield, R. E., S. Sims, and E. E. Daniel. 1977. Gap junctions: their presence and necessity in myometrium during parturition. *Science* 198:958–9.

[15] Gershengorn, M. C., B. E. Marcus-Samuels, and E. Geras. 1979. Estrogens increase the number of thyrotropin-releasing hormone receptors on mammotropic cells in culture. *Endocrinology* 105:171–6.

[16] Habel, L. A., and J. L. Stanford. 1993. Hormone receptors and breast cancer. *Epidemiol. Rev.* 15:209–18.

[17] Harlap, S. 1992. The benefits and risks of hormone replacement therapy: An epidemiologic overview. *Amer. J. Obstet. Gynecol.* 166:1986–92.

[18] Henderson, B. E. 1989. The cancer question: an overview of recent epidemiologic and retrospective data. *Amer. J. Obstet. Gynecol.* 151:1859–64.

[19] Henderson, B. E., R. K. Ross, and M. C. Pike. 1993. Hormonal chemoprevention of cancer in women. *Science* 259:633–8.

[20] Hsueh, A. J. W., and N. C. Ling. 1979. Effect of an antagonistic analog of gonadotropin releasing hormone upon ovarian granulosa cell function. *Life Sci.* 25:1223–30.

[21] Jameson, J. L., and A. N. Hollenberg. 1993. Regulation of chorionic gonadotropin gene expression. *Endocr. Rev.* 15:203–21.

[22] Jones, G. S. 1990. Corpus luteum: composition and function. *Fertil. Steril.* 54:21–6.

[23] Khaw, K.-T., S. Tazuke, and E. Barrett-Connor. 1988. Cigarette smoking levels of adrenal androgens in postmenopausal women. *New Engl. J. Med.* 318:1705–9.

[24] Koldovsky, O., and W. Thornburg. 1987. Hormones in milk. *J. Pediat. Gastroenter. Nutr.* 6:172–96.

[25] Malone, K. E., J. R. Daling, and N. S. Weiss. 1993. Oral contraceptives in relation to breast cancer. *Epidemiol. Rev.* 15:80–97.

[26] Marshall, J. M. 1981. Effects of ovarian steroids and pregnancy of adrenergic nerves of uterus and oviduct. *Amer. J. Physiol.* 240:C165–74.

[27] McFarland, K. C., R. Sprengel, H. S. Phillips, M. Kohler, N. Rosemblit, K. Nikolics, D. L. Segaloff, and P. H. Seeburg. 1989. Lutropin-choriogonadotropin receptor: an unusual member of the G protein-coupled receptor family. *Science* 245:494–9.

[28] McNeilly, A. S. 1993. Lactational amenorrhea. *Endocrinol. Metab. Clin. N. Amer.* 22:59–73.

[29] Merzenich, H., H. Boeing, and J. Wahrendorf. 1993. Dietary fat and sports activity as determinants for age at menarche. *Amer. J. Epidemiol.* 138:217–24.

[30] Nathanielsz, P. W., and T. J. McDonald. 1991. *Amer. J. Obstet. Gynecol.* (Sept. 15).

[31] Nikitovitch-Winer, M. B., and J. W. Everett. 1959. Histologic changes in grafts of rat pituitary on the kidney and upon retransplantation under the diencephalon. *Endocrinology* 65:357.

[32] Ormandy, C. J., and R. S. Sutherland. 1993. Mechanisms of prolactin receptor regulation in mammary gland. *Mol. Cell. Endocrinol.* 9:C1–6.

[33] Pike, M. C., D. V. Spicer, L. Dahmoush, and M. F. Press. 1993. Estrogens, progestogens, normal breast cell proliferation, and breast cancer risk. *Epidemiol. Rev.* 15:17–35.

[34] Rillema, J. A. 1994. Development of the mammary gland and lactation. *TEM* 5:149–54.

[35] Sarapura, V., and W. D. Schlaff. 1993. Recent advances in the understanding of the pathophysiology and treatment of hyperprolactinemia. *Curr. Opin. Obstet. Gynecol.* 5:360–7.

[36] Segaloff, D. L., and M. Ascoli. 1993. The lutropin/choriogonadotropin receptor . . . 4 years later. *Endocr. Rev.* 14:324–47.

[37] Sherwood, O. D., and V. E. Crnekovic. 1979. Development of a homologous radioimmunoassay for rat relaxin. *Endocrinology* 104:893–7.

[38] Sherwood, O. D., V. E. Crnekovic, W. L. Gordon, and J. E. Rutherford. 1980. Radioimmunoassay of relaxin throughout pregnancy and during parturition in the rat. *Endocrinology* 107:691–8.

[39] Sherwood, O. D., S. J. Downing, M. L. Guico-Lamm, J. J. Hwang, M. B. O'Day-Bowman, and P. A. Fields. 1993. The physiological effects of relaxin during pregnancy: studies in rats and pigs. *Oxford Rev. Reprod. Biol.* 15:143–89.

[40] Short, R. V. 1976. Lactation—the central control of reproduction. In Ciba Foundation Symposium 45, *Breast-feeding and the mother.* Excerpta Medica pp. 73–86. Amsterdam: Elsevier North-Holland, Inc.

[41] Stanford, J. L., and D. B. Thomas. 1993. Exogenous progestins and breast cancer. *Epidemiol. Rev.* 15:98–107.

[42] Stefaneanu, L., K. Kovacs, R. V. Lloyd, B. W. Scheithauer, W. F. Young, Jr., T. Sano, and L. Jin. 1992. Pituitary lactotrophs and somatotrophs in pregnancy: a correlative in situ hybridization and immunocytochemical study. *Virchows Archiv. B Cell Pathol.* 62:291–6.

[43] Steger, R. W., and J. J. Peluso. 1987. Sex hormones in the aging female. *Endocrinol. Metab. Clin. N. Amer.* 16:1027–43.

[44] Thomas, D. B. 1993. Oral contraceptives and breast cancer. *JNCI* 85:359–64.

[45] Thorburn, G. D., S. A. Hollingworth, and S. B. Hooper. 1991. The trigger for parturition in sheep: fetal hypothalamus or placenta? *J. Develop. Physiol.* 15:71–9.

[46] Van Look, P. F. A, and H. von Hertzen. 1993. Emergency contraception. *Brit. Med. Bull.* 49:158–70.

[47] Van Tienhoven, A. 1968. *Reproductive physiology.* Philadelphia: W.B. Saunders Company.

[48] Vihko, R. K., and D. L. Apter. 1986. The epidemiology and endocrinology of the menarche in relation to breast cancer. *Cancer Surveys* 5:561–71.

20 Endocrine Role of the Pineal Gland

*The evidence is convincing that the pineal gland (epiphysis cerebri) is involved in the control of reproductive processes of certain mammals, possibly even humans. Clinical evidence reveals that children with parenchymal pinealomas may be delayed in their sexual development, whereas destructive (nonparenchymal) pinealomas are often associated with precocious puberty [18]. However, the detailed mechanisms by which the pineal affects reproductive processes are unclear. It is generally believed that the pineal secretes a hormone that has antigonadotropic properties. A vast amount of experimental data indicates **melatonin**, an indoleamine, as the pineal antigonadotropin [47]. Circulating melatonin levels are elevated at night in essentially all vertebrates as a result of increased synthesis and release from the pineal gland. This increase serves as the "hormonal signal of night" and is used to coordinate daily and seasonal rhythms with the day/night cycle. The melatonin signal therefore is essential for survival in many seasonally breeding animals [19].*

This chapter summarizes the vast but sometimes conflicting literature on the role of the pineal in mammalian reproductive physiology. In addition the pineal as an endocrine organ controlling other physiological processes is discussed. A number of monographs are available that provide further information on the anatomy, biochemistry, and physiology of this intriguing endocrine organ and its hormone, melatonin [2, 5, 42, 45].

PINEAL DEVELOPMENT AND MORPHOLOGY

The human pineal gland arises as a median evagination of the diencephalic roof of the embryonic brain. In most mammals the pineal gland moves away from the roof of the third ventricle and loses connection with the brain, except for a thin stalk. The adult human pineal (epiphysis) is a pine-cone-shaped organ, a shape that suggested the organ's name (Fig. 20.1) The pineal is innervated by postganglionic fibers originating from the *superior cervical ganglia*; the pineal is therefore an effector organ of the autonomic nervous system [47]. The pineal parenchymal cells, pinealocytes, are derived from the ependymal lining of the epithalamus; both light and dark parenchymal cells can be distinguished in the mammalian pineal. The dark cells contain pigment granules of an unknown nature, as well as glycogen deposits of undefined physiological significance. Since distinction is based only on a difference in electron density of the cytoplasm, the "light" and "dark" pinealocytes may only reflect differences in the functional stage of the same cell type that may be manifested as a differential susceptibility to the fixative [16]. Fibroblasts and glial cells make up the rest of glandular mass, which, in humans, is about 170 to 175 mg in average weight.

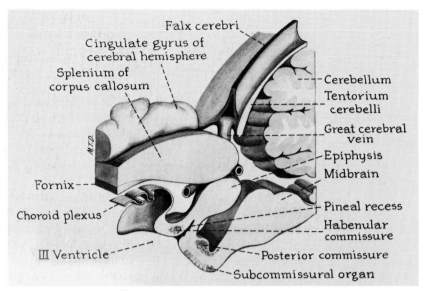

Figure 20.1 The human pineal gland (epiphysis) and its anatomical relation to the diencephalic roof. (From Wurtman, Axelrod, and Kelly [47], with permission).

Calcification of the human pineal begins during the second decade of life, and by 60 years 70% of all pineal glands may be at least partly calcified. Nevertheless, there is no evidence that calcification signals a loss of function; on the contrary, biochemical studies indicate no change in biochemical activity of the pineal with age.

THE MELATONIN HYPOTHESIS

Early anatomists held various views on the physiological function of the pineal in the human. This unique unpaired structure that lies deeply recessed under the cerebral hemispheres of the brain drew their attention and speculation. The philosopher Descartes considered it as the "seat of the soul."

Historical Perspective

The possible physiological significance of the pineal was first recognized by Heubner who noted precocious sexual maturity in a young boy whose pineal was destroyed by a tumor. Holmgren noted that the cells of the pineal gland of an elasmobranch were sensorylike in nature: the pinealocytes resembled the sensory cells of the retina. Because some reptiles possess a prominent "third eye," the pineal of mammals, including humans, was considered a vestige of this primitive visual organ. The observation that the human pineal may become calcified at an early age further consolidated thought that the pineal was, indeed, a vestigial organ and therefore of little physiological consequence. A monograph by Kitay and Altschule [18] described, however, some remarkable clinical correlations with pineal dysfunction. The evidence clearly revealed that the pineal might in some way be related to reproductive function in humans.

McCord and Allen made the interesting observation that bovine pineal extracts added to the water in which tadpoles swam caused the larvae to blanch, that is, to become very light in color or even transparent [22]. This interesting pigmentary effect was duly appreciated by the dermatologist Aaron Lerner, who was searching for a factor which might be responsible for vitiligo (white patches of skin) in humans. He was able to isolate and determine the structure of a pineal substance, an indoleamine, which he named melatonin. This

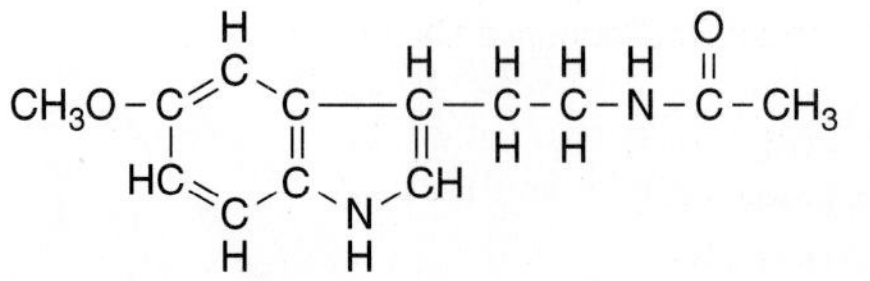

Figure 20.2 The structure of melatonin (N-acetyl-5-methoxytryptamine).

was a momentous event in the history of pineal research as this unique molecule of pineal origin could now be readily synthesized and made available for a variety of physiological studies. Melatonin, N-acetyl-5-methoxytryptamine (Fig. 20.2), proved to have potent effects on integumental pigmentation in some animals, but not humans, as will be discussed. Most important, however, this indoleamine was shown to have antigonadal effects on the mammalian reproductive system.

Profound changes in gonadal function are observed in many animals when they are exposed to continuous light or darkness. Maturation of the gonads of rodents, for example, is delayed when these animals are maintained under conditions of continuous darkness. This effect can be prevented by pinealectomy (epiphysectomy). In contrast, continuous light leads to the early onset of sexual development and to a more rapid increase in gonadal weight; constant light also causes a reduction in size and function of the pineal gland. Pineal ablation in young rodents usually leads to accelerated gonadal maturation, and these developmental effects can be reduced by injections of pineal extracts. Melatonin, like pineal extracts, administered to young rodents also results in a delay of gonadal maturation. These observations are consistent with a hypothesis that photic cues received by an animal in some way affect pineal release of melatonin, which then has an antigonadal action. The "melatonin hypothesis" has thus emerged. Other evidence that further relates to this hypothesis will be examined.

Animal Studies

From studies on the hamster the role of the pineal in mammalian reproductive processes has been further elucidated [29]. Changes in length of the daily photoperiod are especially important in controlling gonadal activity in the hamster, *Mesocricetus auratus,* which in its natural habitat breeds seasonally and hibernates. The reproductive organs of the hamster are extremely sensitive to the influence of environmental lighting and to the activity of the pineal gland. In the male, short photoperiods or blinding lead to gonadal atrophy with complete loss of testicular spermatogenic activity. The gonads may be reduced to only 20% of their normal size. The accessory organs (seminal vesicles and coagulating glands) also atrophy, indicating a loss of support by gonadal androgens. These atrophic effects result from decreased secretion of FSH and LH from the pituitary. Pinealectomy prevents gonadal regression in hamsters maintained on nonstimulatory short days. In the female the data are less clear, but there is a decrease in uterine weight, apparently due to decreased estrogen production in response to short photoperiods or blinding. Plasma gonadotropin levels of female golden hamsters on short days are decreased relative to that of females exposed to long days.

There is a daily rhythm of pineal melatonin synthesis in the hamster, a rhythm influenced by environmental lighting [29]. Superior cervical ganglionectomy, however, abolishes the rhythm of pineal melatonin production. There is evidence that melatonin is the hamster antigonadotropic hormone. The mechanism of antigonadotropic action has been determined through some ingenious experiments. There appears to be a short day-induced increase in the sensitivity of the hypothalamopituitary axis to the negative feedback effect of steroid hormones. On short days castrated male hamsters are much more sensitive to the negative feedback effects of exogenous testosterone (as determined by measurements of serum gonadotropin levels) than are animals exposed to long days. This increased sensitivity is blocked or reduced by pinealectomy. Thus the short-day-induced increase in sensitivity of the hamster hypothalamo-hypophysial axis to testosterone feedback is mediated, at least in part, by the pineal gland.

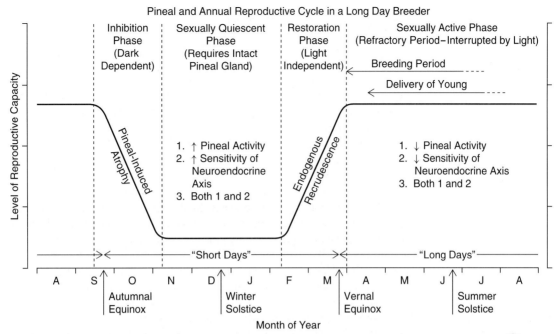

Figure 20.3   The role of the pineal in the annual reproduction cycle of a long-day breeder, the hamster. (From Reiter [29], with permission.)

Blinding does not cause permanent inhibition of testicular or ovarian function in the hamster. There is a spontaneous recrudescence of the gonads to the normal adult condition in hamsters that have been blinded for about 27 weeks. This could help explain what normally happens under hibernating conditions. Hamsters are reproductively competent when they emerge from their burrows in the spring. The spontaneous onset of the gonadal refractory condition appears to be a single occurrence, not a cyclical phenomenon, as the recrudesced gonads of blinded hamsters remain large indefinitely. In other species (ewe, starling), however, there is evidence for both a spontaneous onset and termination of reproductive activity that occurs cyclically with a period of about a year (i. e., circannually).

It is unclear why the gonads of blinded or hibernating hamsters spontaneously become activated. The hypothalamo-hypophysial-gonadal axis may become refractory to the pineal antigonadotropic hormone. It has been shown that exogenous melatonin injections cause testicular regression in pinealectomized hamsters regardless of the photoperiod. Injections of melatonin during the early part of the day, however, are often ineffective in causing gonadal atrophy in intact hamsters. Also, in the presence of continuously elevated levels of melatonin (in animals carrying implants of melatonin) pinealectomized animals are rendered insensitive to daily injections of the hormone. Thus the continuous exposure to melatonin renders the target tissue relatively unresponsive to this hormone. It may therefore be important that melatonin be released rhythmically from the pineal, rather than continuously, to be physiologically effective.

These observations leave little doubt that the pineal, through the action of its antigonadotropic hormone, melatonin, is a key component in the control of reproductive processes in this mammal (Fig. 20.3). There is evidence that the pineal functions in a similar role in some other mammals and some nonmammalian species.

PINEAL INDOLEAMINE BIOSYNTHESIS

The biochemistry of pineal indoleamine biosynthesis is well documented [43, 47]. Indoleamine biosynthesis involves use of the amino acid, tryptophan, which is converted to 5-hydroxytryptophan by the enzyme tryptophan hydroxylase (Fig. 20.4). The enzyme

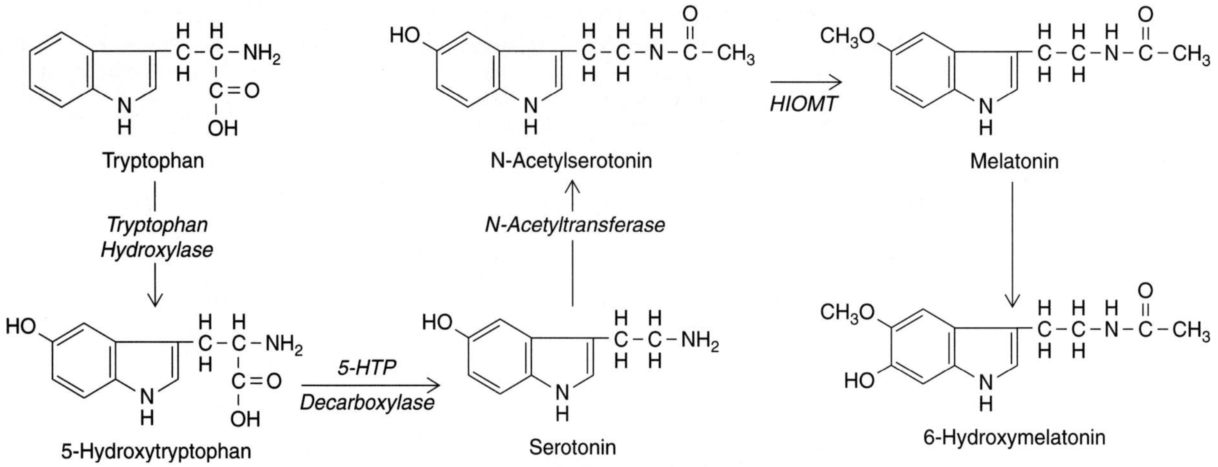

Figure 20.4   Pathway of melatonin biosynthesis and metabolism within the pineal gland.

5-hydroxytryptophan decarboxylase acts on 5-hydroxytryptophan to form 5-hydroxytryptamine (5-HT, *serotonin*), which is converted to *N*-acetylserotonin by the action of *N*-acetyltransferase. The *N*-acetylserotonin produced is O-methylated by hydroxyindole-O-methyltransferase (HIOMT) to form *N*-acetyl-5-methoxytryptamine (melatonin). It is believed that the increase in *N*-acetylserotonin concentration acts by a mass action effect to enhance the production of melatonin. Pineal melatonin biosynthesis is mainly controlled by *N*-acetyltransferase activity, which may be the rate-limiting event in the production of this indoleamine. Others argue, however, that HIOMT activity may be of prime importance to melatonin biosynthesis. Melatonin is then metabolized in the liver to 6-hydroxymelatonin by melatonin hydroxylase and converted to a sulfate or to a glucuronide for urinary excretion.

Although acetylation to *N*-acetylserotonin is a necessary step in the biosynthesis of melatonin, deamination of serotonin by monoamine oxidase can also occur in the pineal. The deaminated product may be either oxidized to 5-hydroxyindoleacetic acid or reduced to 5-hydroxytryptophol. The latter compounds can then become O-methylated by HIOMT to give 5-methoxyindole acetic acid and 5-methoxytryptophol.

Effect of Light on Pineal Indoleamine Biosynthesis

Melatonin synthesis within the rat pineal is dramatically affected by photic cues received by the lateral eyes. At night there is an increase in the activity of *N*-acetyltransferase, which is 10- to nearly 100-fold greater than values in the light. The concentration of *N*-acetylserotonin is subsequently increased to values 10 to 30 times greater than those observed under day conditions. HIOMT activity is also increased, which results in elevated levels of pineal melatonin. Pineal enzyme activities are rapidly depressed by light. Pineal serotonin levels reveal marked diurnal changes, with highest levels noted during the daylight hours. Serotonin levels are depressed after darkness, probably because serotonin is the substrate for *N*-acetyltransferase action and is therefore converted to *N*-acetylserotonin. Reversal of external lighting conditions reverses the rhythm of pineal enzyme activity and indoleamine biosynthesis. Thus a daily diurnal rhythm of pineal biosynthetic activity is observed and is controlled by the normal day-to-day changes in natural lighting. This diurnal fluctuation of pineal enzyme activity and melatonin synthesis is lost under conditions of continuous illumination. The rhythm is, however, maintained, though diminished, in animals kept in the dark. Some central nervous system (CNS) site may be responsible for producing a cyclic signal that is responsible for the persistence of pineal rhythmicity. The daily rhythm of pineal

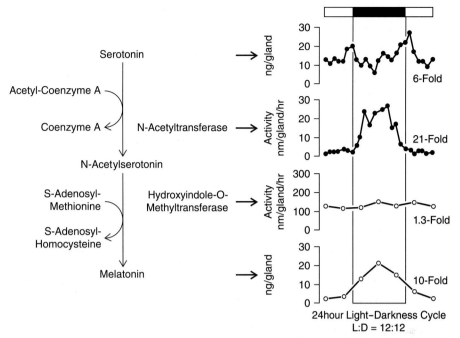

Figure 20.5 Pathway for serotonin conversion to melatonin in the pineal gland. Daily measurements over a 24-hour period of serotonin content. *N*-acetyltransferase activity (NAT), hydroxyindole-O-methyltransferase activity (HIOMT), and melatonin content in chick pineals were made. The bar at the top of the graph represents the 24-hour lighting regimen in which the birds were held (L:D 12:12 hour of light in alternation with 12 hour of dark). The daily change in melatonin is believed to be a consequence of the daily change in NAT. The numbers (x-fold) on the graph are the ratio of peak to nadir values. (Modified from Binkley [6], with permission.)

indoleamine biosynthesis in the bird [4, 6] is depicted in Fig. 20.5 and has also been carefully documented in the rat.

CNS Pathway in the Control of Pineal Indoleamine Biosynthesis

The role of the CNS in the control of pineal indoleamine biosynthesis in mammals has been determined by a variety of surgical techniques [14]. Melatonin is synthesized in response to norepinephrine released from postganglionic neurons from the superior cervical ganglia. Thus the pineal is considered to be a *neuroendocrine transducer*, like the adrenal chromaffin tissue, as neural input to these organs is converted into an endocrine output [47]. Postganglionic stimulation of pinealocytes depends on the absence of light activation of the retina of the lateral eyes. Light information perceived by the eyes is conveyed to the suprachiasmatic nuclei of the brain by way of a retinohypothalamic pathway [23]. The pineal gland, in essence, is the intermediary between the external photoperiod and internal milieu. The pineal gland is the site at which information about light and dark is translated, or transduced, into a chemical messenger [30, 31, 32]. There is also a suggestion that pineal melatonin biosynthesis may be affected by the electromagnetic spectrum [35].

Neuronal circuits from the suprachiasmatic nuclei convey information via the medial forebrain bundle to the upper thoracic spinal cord and then out to the superior cervical ganglia. From these ganglia the postganglionic neurons proceed to innervate the pineal. Disruption of this neural pathway anywhere between the lateral eyes and the

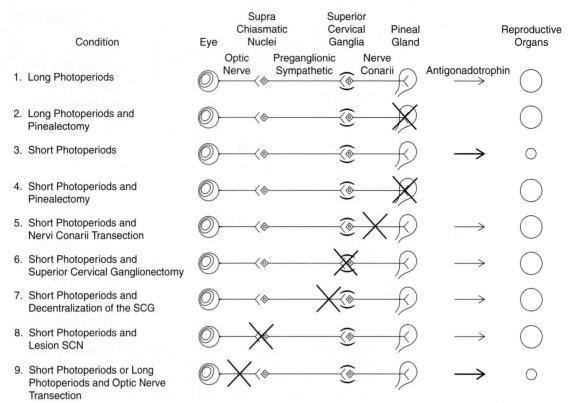

Figure 20.6 Surgical procedures that eliminate or exaggerate pineal antigonadotropic activity in mammals. The **X**s represent removal of the organ or surgical transection of a fiber tract. The thickness of the arrows indicates the antigonadotropic capability of the pineal gland. The phrase preganglionic sympathetic fibers refers to a multitude of neurons that intervene between the suprachiasmatic nuclei (SCN) and the superior cervical ganglia (SCG). Decentralization of the SCG refers to separating the SCG from their connections with the central nervous system. (From Reiter [29], with permission.)

suprachiasmatic nuclei stimulates pineal indoleamine biosynthesis. Removal of the superior cervical ganglia (ganglionectomy) or decentralization of the ganglia, on the other hand, abolishes the rhythms of indoleamine biosynthesis. Lesions of the medial forebrain bundle also block pineal *N*-acetyltransferase rhythms, as do lesions of the suprachiasmatic nuclei. A summary of the surgical procedures is provided (Fig. 20.6). These data suggest that the suprachiasmatic nuclei may be the CNS site responsible for generation of the nocturnal activity of pineal indoleamine biosynthesis in mammals. The circadian oscillatory activity of the cells of the suprachiasmatic nuclei may be entrained to the daily photoperiod.

Intracellular Control of Pineal Indoleamine Biosynthesis

Norepinephrine released from superior cervical postganglionic neurons interacts with pinealocyte β-adrenoceptors, which leads to an increase in pineal cAMP production. Elevation of this intracellular second messenger results in conversion of tryptophan to serotonin and then serotonin to *N*-acetylserotonin. This response is mimicked by $(Bu)_2$cAMP or theophylline, a phosphodiesterase inhibitor, which elevates pineal cAMP levels. Norepinephrine, but not $(Bu)_2$cAMP, increases uptake of tryptophan into pinealocytes. The neurotransmitter therefore has a twofold effect: it increases intracellular levels of the substrate, tryptophan, as well as cAMP, whose action is to enhance enzymatic utilization of

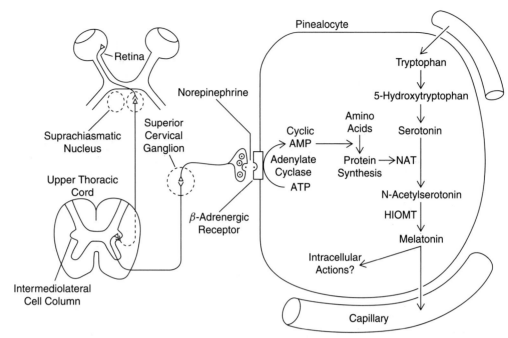

Figure 20.7 CNS pathway and mechanisms controlling pineal indole metabolism in mammals. (From Karasak and Reiter, "Morpho-functional aspects of the mammalian pineal gland." *Microscopy Res. and Tech.* 21:136–57. ©1992 John Wiley & Sons, Inc. Used by permission of Wiley-Liss, Inc, a subsidiary of John Wiley & Sons, Inc.)

the substrate for melatonin biosynthesis. Injection of propranolol, a β-adrenoceptor antagonist, just before the onset of darkness, inhibits the nighttime rise in pineal *N*-acetyltransferase activity, as does reserpine, a drug that depletes adrenergic neurons of catecholamines. A single dose of isoproterenol, a β-adrenoceptor agonist, administered during the day causes an immediate increase in pineal *N*-acetyltransferase activity. Electrical stimulation of the superior cervical ganglia causes a rapid increase in the concentration of cAMP in the pineal gland of rats. These experimental manipulations clearly reveal the role of noradrenergic postganglionic neurons in the control of pineal biosynthetic activity. A summary depicting the CNS pathways and mechanisms controlling pineal function is given (Fig. 20.7).

MELATONIN SECRETION AND CIRCULATION

Melatonin is present in the plasma and urine of all animals studied, including humans, and pinealectomy reduces the circulating levels of the indoleamine in experimental animals. As for pineal melatonin, plasma levels of melatonin of humans and other animals (sheep, pig, rat, cow, donkey, camel, chicken, salmon, lizard) are highest at mid-dark and lowest at midlight periods (Fig. 20.8) [46]. In addition to the daily melatonin rhythm in blood and urine of primates there is a diurnal melatonin rhythm in primate cerebrospinal fluid (CSF) [36]. Night peak values are 2 to 15 times higher than day values. This increase occurs soon after lights are turned off, and the decrease toward day values occurs rapidly after lights are turned on again (Fig. 20.9). The changes in CSF melatonin concentrations appear to reflect daily changes in plasma melatonin concentrations. It is not clear, however, whether melatonin is secreted into the CSF only, into the plasma only, or into both [46]. A 24-hour rhythm in the concentration of CSF melatonin suggests the possibility that the CSF may be an important route of communication between the pineal gland and other parts of the brain.

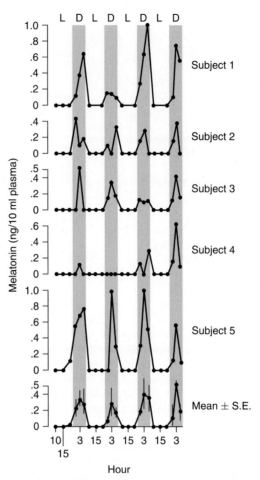

Figure 20.8 Diurnal plasma melatonin levels in humans. Note the nocturnal elevation during four consecutive cycles in five adult male subjects. (From Vaughan, Meyer, and Reiter [46], *Journal of Clinical Endocrinology and Metabolism*, vol. 42, pp. 752–764. © 1976 J. B. Lippincott Publishing Company, used by permission.)

HIOMT activity is present in some blood cells, the Harderian gland [7], and the retina, and melatonin may also be synthesized in other extrapineal sites, such as the hypothalamus, retina, and GI tract. These sites may theoretically assume some functional significance following pinealectomy.

SITE OF ACTION OF MELATONIN

There is evidence for brain, pituitary, and peripheral antigonadotropic actions of melatonin [24]. The evidence for a CNS effect is derived from the following information. Pinealectomy leads to increased motor and EEG activity, whereas melatonin administration reduces spontaneous motor activity, promotes sleep with slow EEG activity, and prolongs the duration of barbiturate-induced sleep. Melatonin may modify CNS neurotransmitter function as increased levels of gamma aminobutyric acid (GABA) and serotonin have been noted in the brain after melatonin administration. Melatonin implants into the medial preoptic and suprachiasmatic and retrochiasmatic areas of the mouse brain elicit complete gonadal regression. Using in vitro autoradiography, in combination with a high

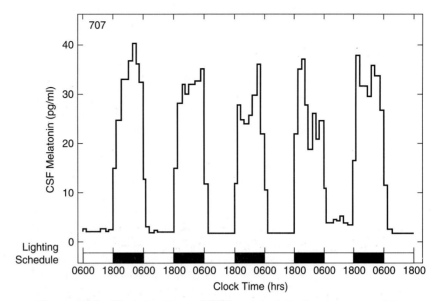

Figure 20.9 Diurnal pattern of CSF melatonin in the rhesus monkey. An individual animal was studied for 6 consecutive days and CSF was collected every 90 minutes. (From Reppert et al. [36], with permission. © 1979 American Roentgen Ray Society. Williams & Wilkins Company.)

affinity radioligand (2-[^{125}I]melatonin), melatonin binding sites have been reliably and repeatedly identified in the SCN and, as originally reported, in the median eminence region of the mammalian hypothalamus [30, 31, 32]. Melatonin may mediate its hypothalamic effect by inhibition of gonadotropin-releasing hormone (GnRH) synthesis and secretion.

PINEAL RHYTHMS AND BIOLOGICAL CLOCKS

The pineal gland synthesizes melatonin in response to photic information received from the lateral eyes. Because of the rapid response of the epiphysial-synthesizing machinery and the short half-life of the released product, melatonin, circulating levels of the indoleamine may be an accurate reflection of the amount of photic input to the lateral eyes. The pineal may therefore provide a mechanism for the measurement of the duration of the dark and light periods. Thus in animals whose reproductive patterns fit into a specific seasonal scheme the pineal may play a pivotal role in the control of their gonadal function [17]. Indeed, it is the pineal gland, an end organ of the visual system, that translates the photoperiodic visual message into a chemical signal. The pineal gland, in essence, is the intermediary between the external photoperiod and internal milieu. The pineal gland is the site at which light and dark information is translated, or transduced, into a chemical messenger. Melatonin is the "chemical expression of darkness" [31, 34].

In mammals light information is first perceived by photoreceptor elements of the lateral eyes; this information is then relayed through a retinohypothalamic pathway to the suprachiasmatic nuclei (SCN). A rhythm of *N*-acetyltransferase activity is, however, maintained in blinded animals kept in constant lighting or in normal animals in continuous darkness. It is suggested that the signal generator is an oscillator (*biological clock*) with a period of about 24 hours that only transmits a signal to the pineal gland periodically. The pineal rhythm is truly circadian in nature. Circadian rhythms have, by definition, periods of about 24 hours. They persist ("free-run") under constant conditions, with respect to principal environmental time cues (Zeitgebers), and are thus endogenous rhythms rather than driven ones (e.g., those that are repeatedly stimulated by a cyclically changing environment). They are entrained by light and temperature cycles and, in some cases, by other less prominent time cues. Entrainment normally serves to synchronize these not-quite-24-hour biological rhythms to the precise daily rhythm of the environment. Biological clocks are synchronized or entrained by periodically recurring environmental stimuli [44]. The SCN contain an endogenous circadian clock that generates a rhythm of pineal melatonin synthesis with a periodicity of slightly greater than 24 hours; restricting the cycle to precisely 24 hours is the function of the prevailing light to dark environment [31, 32]. Although more than one mammalian circadian clock may exist, the SCN is considered the master oscillatory system [48].

The SCN shows striking circadian glucose utilization. Its ablation eliminates overt behavioral rhythmicity and rhythmic electrical activity in the brain. Tissue explants containing the SCN continue to express circadian electrical rhythms in vitro. Circadian rhythmicity can be restored to SCN-lesioned arrhythmic hosts by implantation of fetal brain tissue containing SCN cells. The pacemaker role of the SCN in a mammalian circadian system was tested by neural transplantation from a mutant strain of hamster that shows a short circadian period. Small neural grafts from the suprachiasmatic region restored circadian rhythms to arrhythmic animals whose own nucleus had been ablated. The restored rhythms always exhibited the circadian period of the donor genotype regardless of the direction of the transplant, mutant to wild type (or vice versa), or genotype of the host. Rhythmicity was apparent 6 to 7 days after transplantation. Immunocytochemical analysis indicated that neural connections had been made between graft and host brain. The basic period of the overt circadian rhythm, therefore, is determined by cells of the suprachiasmatic region [28].

In female rats blinded early in pregnancy the circadian rhythms remain as they were at the time the rats were blinded. It was discovered that rat fetuses show their mothers' extrinsic day-night cycles [20]. These observations indicate that animal fetuses have functioning biological clocks that are set by their mother. The fetal clock is unaffected when the mother rat's pineal is removed, suggesting that melatonin of pineal origin does not set the fetal biological clock [44].

Chronobiology: Rhythms of Life. Chronobiology deals with the rhythmic patterns that occur in all forms of life. Virtually all organisms exhibit approximately daily (circadian) cycles. In human beings, prominent rhythms are found in blood pressure, circulatory pulse, body core temperature, and surface temperature, and in chemical variables of blood, urine, and tissues. For medicine, this new science may clarify the relationships of rhythms to prediction, prevention, diagnosis, and treatment of diseases. Several decades of research worldwide have established that medical diagnoses can be subject to a much higher proportion of false positives (e.g., office hypertension) and false negatives (e.g., odd-hour hypertension) when only single samples are taken at arbitrary times of the day, instead of taking rhythms into account. Radiation, chemotherapy, and other treatments have been shown to have markedly different efficacy and safety depending upon the pattern of administration within the day [12, 39].

Melatonin for the Control of Seasonal Reproductive Cycles. Manipulating the reproductive cycle of photoperiodic species in the laboratory can be accomplished by turning on and off a light switch at the desired time of day. In those photoperiodic species in which the breeding season in nature is confined to only a very limited time of year, reproductive activity in the laboratory can be initiated in any month by careful control of the light cycle prior to and during the induction of reproductive function.

Following confirmation of the link between pineal function and seasonality, coupled with the availability of sufficient quantities of melatonin for experimental procedures, melatonin was routinely administered to many mammalian species with a view to manipulating seasonal rhythms. Research groups from Australia, the United States, and Britain simultaneously demonstrated that daily (late afternoon) administration of supplementary melatonin to ewes in midsummer substituted for short photoperiodic conditions and advanced the onset of breeding activity. It was shown that continuous melatonin treatment by implant methods also simulated short day length to induce early reproductive activity in both ewes and rams. Such sustained elevations of plasma melatonin might be physiologically perceived as a "super-short" day. If melatonin treatment can effectively induce those seasonal responses associated with short photoperiod, it has an obvious commercial application in all sheep-producing countries, whether its primary intention is for early lambing, improved fecundity, or a combination of both [26].

PATHOPHYSIOLOGY

Two contrasting types of pinealoma are associated with precocious or delayed sexual maturation [40]. Parenchymal pinealomas, which consist of an enlarged mass of pinealocytes, are associated with delayed puberty. Destructive pinealomas, which consist of non-parenchymal tissue (e.g., connective tissue), are associated with enhanced precocious development of sexual maturation. The interpretation of these clinical observations is as follows. An overactive pineal (parenchymal pinealoma) secretes an excess of a factor that is inhibitory to gonadal development. In the absence of this factor, because of destruction of the pineal, the antigonadotropin is absent and the individual experiences a precocious development of the gonads [41]. Pineal tumors are rare in the female, but about one-third of all males below the age of sexual maturation who have pineal tumors undergo precocious puberty [18].

Hypogonadism in Humans.   Although the association has not been unequivocally established, a number of recent reports suggest that melatonin may influence human reproductive function. Some patients with hypothalamic hypogonadism have unusually high plasma melatonin concentrations, suggesting that increased pineal activity may be involved in the pathogenesis of this condition. Some boys with delayed puberty have elevated daytime plasma melatonin concentrations, and more than half of the children with precocious sexual development have plasma melatonin concentrations lower than those of age-matched normal children. These data suggest that melatonin may be responsible for pathologic conditions of the human reproductive system [27].

There are at least two reports showing that women suffering from hypothalamic amenorrhea have abnormally high nocturnal melatonin levels. Hypothalamic amenorrheic subjects are characterized by decreased GnRH pulsability, a change readily induced by melatonin. Likewise, women with this condition are typically anovulatory, a condition that could also be mediated by melatonin since it is known to be capable of suppressing the ovulatory hormone surges required for the rupture of ovarian follicles and shedding of the ova. In addition to an augmented melatonin secretion at night, the duration of elevated nocturnal melatonin is also prolonged in women with hypothalamic amenorrhea. Either the higher levels or the increased duration of elevated melatonin levels could account for the suppression of reproductive physiology in these women [32].

Melatonin Effects on Humans.   Melatonin has been injected into humans on and off over the last 20 years to determine the effects, if any, of the indoleamine on bodily function. It is hoped that therapeutic applications directed toward correcting abnormalities of circadian rhythms will be discovered. Melatonin administered orally may advance the time of self-rated "fatigue" or actual sleep. Melatonin may also cause an advance in the endogenous rhythm of melatonin secretion. Based upon these observations melatonin has been administered to attempt to alleviate jet-lag following long transmeridian flights. It has been claimed that the results support the concept that melatonin secretion works as an endogenous synchronizer, preventing loss of synchrony among the multitude of bodily rhythms [7, 25].

Although the phase-shifting effect of melatonin has improved sleep in subjects whose circadian system is desynchronized, this effect is considered separate from the more immediate hypnotic effects reported for melatonin. Melatonin can produce short-term hypnotic effects without concurrent shifts in the circadian system. Thus, it is unlikely that the short-term hypnotic effects of melatonin are related to immediate phase shifts of the circadian system. Current research suggests that melatonin administration increases the likelihood of sleep when the inclination for sleep is low, but not when it is high. This can be interpreted as a mild hypnotic effect or, alternatively, as evidence that melatonin functions as a sleep propensity modulator [9].

While melatonin can be shown to improve the sleep-wake pattern in free-running blind subjects, it is still not clear whether this effect is mediated by an hypnotic or circadian mechanism [37, 38]. Experimental studies of the phase-shifting effects of melatonin suggest a phase-response curve consistent with the proposition outlined above. There is evidence that melatonin can produce significant phase advances when administered in the late afternoon and early evening at doses that will be largely eliminated prior to the subsequent sleep period. This suggests that the improvement in sleep following evening administration may reflect the hypnotic effects, while afternoon melatonin administration is more likely to be related to circadian effects [19].

The Pineal Gland (Melatonin) and Aging.   Because of its exclusive nighttime synthesis, melatonin has come to be known as the "chemical expression of darkness" [31] and as the "Dracula of the endocrine system." At birth the circadian melatonin rhythm in mammals is absent. In the rodent pineal the cycle becomes apparent postnatally shortly after the postganglionic sympathetic nerves grow into the developing gland. In newborn humans, a melatonin rhythm in the blood is not discernible until 3–4 months of age, after which it seems to develop rapidly until one year of age. Prepubertal mammals exhibit a robust circadian melatonin rhythm. As humans undergo sexual maturation there is claimed to be a significant drop in nocturnal melatonin levels, a change that may be permissive to pubertal development. After adulthood is achieved, virtually all mammals continue to exhibit a 24 hour melatonin rhythm with low and high values being associated with day and night, respectively [32].

In recent years, melatonin has been implicated as an antiaging hormone [11]. Indeed, the hypothesis has been put forward that "aging is secondary to pineal failure." According to this hypothesis, aging is a syndrome of a relative melatonin deficiency accompanied by a diminished melatonin/5HT ratio, which is detrimental to neurophysiology and causally related to the aging process. Dietary restriction clearly increases the life span of a variety of animals; likewise the procedure also tends to preserve pineal melatonin rhythm. The conservation of the melatonin rhythm in food-restricted animals is particularly interesting since, typically, prolonged food restriction depresses the function of virtually every other endocrine organ; yet the melatonin cycle responds in an opposite manner, that is, it is maintained. The question then arises, is the prolonged life span experienced by food-restricted animals related to greater melatonin availability? Only a few data relate to the ability of melatonin to influence the duration of survival, but the correlations are positive. When mice were given melatonin in their drinking water, they lived noticeably longer (20%) that is, from a mean of 752±80 days in nonmelatonin treated mice to a mean of 931±80 days in mice given melatonin every night. The contrary expectation would be that pinealectomized animals, with the resulting melatonin deficiency, may die at an earlier age than pineal intact animals; such studies have not been performed [33].

Thus the pineal gland, via its hormone melatonin, may somehow, either directly or indirectly, delay aging itself or inhibit age-related disease processes. Because of these findings, melatonin has been classified as an antiaging hormone and as a juvenile hormone. If, in fact, these well-based predictions are finally unequivocally verified, the pineal gland could be known as the veritable "fountain of youth." The data accumulated to date might justify serious consideration that supplemental melatonin may be beneficial during aging [33].

The Pineal Gland and Cancer. Melatonin alters the firing rate of the gonadotropin-releasing hormone (GnRH) pulse frequency generator in the hypothalamus, thus reducing pituitary secretion of gonadotropins and PRL and, indirectly, the secretion of estrogens by the gonads. In mammals, melatonin has been shown to delay puberty, suppress ovulation and reduce gonadal steroidogenesis. The incidence of estrogen-related cancers in the female is directly correlated with the age of menarche (first menstruation). In other words, the earlier the onset of menstrual cycles the more years a woman is exposed to estrogens (which are known to be carcinogenic). The hypothesis has been advanced that blind women, particularly those blind since childhood, may have a low risk of breast cancer due to increased melatonin secretion from the pineal gland [8].

OTHER PROPOSED ROLES OF THE PINEAL

The pineal has been suggested to affect almost every endocrine gland in the body, as well as many other physiological activities [21]. The pineal may, like its diencephalic hypothalamic counterpart, the pituitary, function in the control of a large number of physiological processes. A few of the more recognized roles of the pineal will be described.

Ocular Melatonin

Melatonin is present in the retina of many animals as are the enzymes N-acetyltransferase (NAT) and HIOMT, and serotonin is converted to melatonin in the eye in vitro. Like the pineal, ocular NAT activity shows a daily light-dark cycle that can be modified by environmental lighting [6]. Ocular melatonin probably gets into the bloodstream, as rhythms of circulating melatonin are often still present after pinealectomy.

Melatonin synthesis by the eye might serve some endocrine role, or melatonin may act locally to regulate some ocular function. For example, the normal cyclic shedding of the outer retinal segment of the rat is blocked by reserpine treatment that also abolishes the circadian rhythm of indoleamine biosynthesis. Melatonin may therefore regulate the cyclic metabolism of photoreceptor cells. In addition the photoreceptors of some poikilotherms are retracted during periods of bright illumination, an event facilitated by melatonin. Pigment migration within retinal melanocytes also occurs in response to photic cues in some species. Pinealectomy abolishes this response, whereas melatonin has the opposite effect. Melatonin may therefore play an important role in retinal light sensitivity and visual acuity in some vertebrates.

The Pineal and the Circadian System of Birds

In the bird, as in mammals, the activity of the enzymes responsible for melatonin synthesis (NAT and HIOMT) and the amount of melatonin in the pineal gland are enhanced in darkness and depressed in light. Serum levels of melatonin are increased in birds during dark periods. Even after blinding, changes in pineal indoleamine biosynthesis occur in response to environmental lighting. The thin skull of birds may allow light to penetrate directly to the pineal. In addition a circadian rhythm of pineal melatonin synthesis occurs in isolated pineals maintained in organ culture in the absence of light; these isolated pineals are directly light sensitive [4, 5, 6].

In the sparrow *Passer domesticus* the pineal gland is essential for persistence of the circadian locomotor rhythm under conditions of constant darkness. Removal of the pineal results in arrhythmic locomotor activity. Pinealectomized sparrows will nevertheless still entrain to light-dark cycles and reveal other signs that are partially indicative of a circadian system. The free-running rhythm of locomotor activity is not abolished by disruption of the neural input to the pineal or its neural output. Most interestingly, rhythmicity can be restored to pinealectomized birds by the implantation of a donor pineal to the anterior chamber of the eye. The transplanted pineal transfers the phase of the donor bird's rhythm to the host. The avian pineal therefore seems to be coupled to other components of the circadian system by an endocrine, rather than a neural, mechanism [4, 5].

It has been suggested that the avian pineal contains a self-sustained oscillator that produces a rhythmic hormonal output. Furthermore, it is believed that circadian fluctuations of this hormone entrain a damped oscillator located elsewhere in the body, which in turn drives the locomotor activity. In this model each oscillator would have separate access to environmental light cycles. Locomotor and other behaviors of pinealectomized birds would be determined exclusively by the damped oscillator, but would be unable to free run (in the absence of light cues) because the self-sustained oscillator is lacking. Restoration of the damped oscillator to its normal state can be re-established by cyclic hormonal output from a transplanted pineal [4, 5].

The continuous administration of melatonin reduces the total amount of perch-hopping activity in sparrows, an effect reversed to normal after cessation of melatonin treatment. The evidence suggests that the pineal, through its product melatonin, may play a role in both the timing and the amount of activity expressed throughout the activity and resting cycle in birds. Pinealectomy abolishes the normal circadian rhythm of body temperature in constant darkness and also alters significantly the amplitude of body temperature rhythms entrained to light cycles. There is evidence that the pineal gland may influence thermoregulatory behavior and physiology in some reptiles and mammals. In some birds reproductive activity is clearly related to photoperiodic events, but the pineal gland and melatonin have not been implicated in the control of such activity.

The Photosensitive Pineal of Poikilotherms

In the mammal light information is received through the lateral eyes and conveyed through the CNS to control pineal melatonin synthesis. As discussed at the outset of this chapter, cells of the pineal of certain poikilotherms of amphibians, reptiles, and teleosts were shown to be sensory in structure and function (Fig. 20.10). The morphology of these cells resembles that of the retinal photoreceptors of the lateral eyes. In addition electrophysiological recordings indicate that these pineal sensory elements are directly photosensitive and are apparently activated in the absence of light to synthesize and release

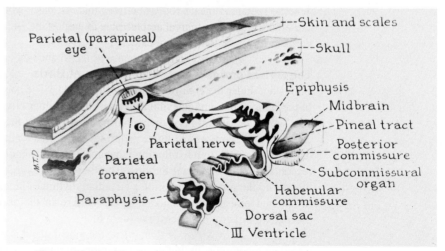

Figure 20.10   The lizard pineal gland and its anatomical relation to the diencephalic roof. (From Wurtman, Axelrod, and Kelly [47], with permission.)

melatonin. As in mammals there is a diurnal rhythm of plasma melatonin in poikilotherms (fishes, lizards) that is totally or partially abolished by pinealectomy, but other sources of melatonin may also exist.

Infant rats do not require lateral eyes for the cyclic nocturnal fall in their pineal serotonin levels [49]. This drop in pineal serotonin can, however, be inhibited by continuous illumination. Thus these young rodents appear to see even though their eyelids are closed. If, however, the heads of these animals are completely covered with black hoods, there is a decrease in pineal 5-HT levels. There is evidence that the pinealocytes of newborn rats contain photoreceptor organelles as do poikilothermic vertebrates. Thus in their ontogeny these cells recapitulate their phylogeny relative to the structure of these elements.

From a comparative evolutionary standpoint it is interesting that the earliest pineal systems (cyclostomes, elasmobranch and teleost fishes, amphibians, reptiles, and birds) are directly photosensitive [13]. In all these vertebrates the pineal synthesizes and releases melatonin in the absence of light. There is also evidence that the pineal glands of these animals are not directly controlled by nervous input. In adult mammals, on the other hand, the same biochemical events take place in the pineal cells in the absence of light, but the pinealocytes are regulated via photic cues received initially by the lateral eyes. Photostimulation of the lateral eyes results in neural information that is then conveyed to the pinealocytes. Even in their ontogeny the pinealocytes of both birds and mammals, at least in those few studied, possess photosensitive sensory cells. Thus there has been a gradual transformation from a directly photosensitive sensory system to an indirectly regulated system (in mammals), controlled through the nervous system by information received from the lateral eyes. Nevertheless, the evidence is clear that the pineal glands of all vertebrates, whether directly photoreceptive or not, are actively engaged in the biosynthesis of indoleamines.

Pineal/Melatonin Control of Chromatophores

The discovery of McCord and Allen [22] that bovine pineal glands contain a factor that causes tadpoles to lighten in color was ultimately responsible for the search and elucidation of the structure of melatonin. There is now evidence that melatonin controls color change in certain poikilothermic vertebrates, at least at certain developmental stages. When amphibian larvae are placed in the dark they rapidly become lighter in color. This body-blanching response is eliminated by pinealectomy but is mimicked when melatonin is added to the water in which larvae swim [45]. Melatonin-induced lightening of amphibian larvae is due to the direct effect of the indoleamine on melanosome aggregation within dermal melanophores (Chap. 8). There is strong experimental evidence that the body-blanching response of larval amphibians, as well as that of cyclostomes to darkness, is due to melatonin release from the pineal [1].

The normal background response or larval and adult amphibians to a light- or dark-colored background is controlled by the presence or absence of circulating levels of MSH and is not under the control of the pineal gland [1]. The control of chromatic responses by the pineal gland and melatonin in other vertebrates has not been studied in depth. Melanophores of certain species of fishes and reptiles do respond to melatonin, but this need not necessarily imply that the indoleamine plays any normal role in the control of chromatic behavior in these vertebrates.

MELATONIN MECHANISMS OF ACTION

The receptor for melatonin has now been cloned from the pigment cells (melanophores) of the skin of frogs [10]. The membrane receptor is a member of the G protein-linked receptor superfamily. Researchers now want to clone the receptor from the mammalian body. It might be expected that tissue from the brain, in particular the suprachiasmatic nucleus ("the body clock"), would be the richest source of the receptor. Drug makers may find the receptor useful for screening drugs to treat jet lag or sleep disorders (see discussion earlier in this chapter) [34].

There is evidence that melatonin mediates its cytoskeletal actions by intracellular interactions with calmodulin [3]. The high affinity binding of melatonin to CaM suggests that the hormone is able to modulate all activity by intracellularly binding to CaM at physiological concentrations. Antagonism of CaM by melatonin affects microtubular polymerization and thus cytoskeletal structure. Since the structures of melatonin and CaM are phylogenetically well preserved, CaM-melatonin interaction probably represents a major mechanism for cellular synchronization in animal physiology [3].

The fact that melatonin is extraordinarily effective in reversing the darkening (melanosome-dispersing) action of MSH is of broader significance than melatonin's immediate chromatic effect. Although there is strong evidence that melatonin is the mammalian pineal antigonadotropin, less information exists as to its locus of action. There is only meager information relative to the putative hypothalamic neurons, pituitary cells, or gonadal cells on which the indoleamine may mediate its action. Thus, because the cellular site of action is unknown, the mechanism of melatonin action has not been easily studied. The melanophores of some frogs, lizards, and fishes, however, provide model systems for deriving some information on melatonin mechanisms of action and have been used as a bioassay for the indoleamine. The cellular mechanisms by which chemical messengers work are generally similar between species. Therefore, it might be expected that studies of melatonin actions on integumental melanophores may be applicable to other cellular systems including those of humans. From a study of many structural analogs of melatonin, it was determined that a methoxy group on the fifth carbon atom of the indole nucleus is necessary for melanosome aggregation (skin lightening) within melanophores [15]. The *N*-acetyl group, on the other hand, is necessary for binding of melatonin to its receptor. This can be demonstrated by the use of *N*-acetyltryptamine, which lacks intrinsic agonistic (lightening) activity but is competitively inhibitory to the actions of melatonin. The tryptamine nucleus and the 5-methoxy and *N*-acetyl groups are therefore essential for complete activity of melatonin. The proposed structural requirements of the melatonin receptor of frog skin melanophores in terms of binding site affinity and intrinsic agonistic activity are shown (Fig. 20.11).

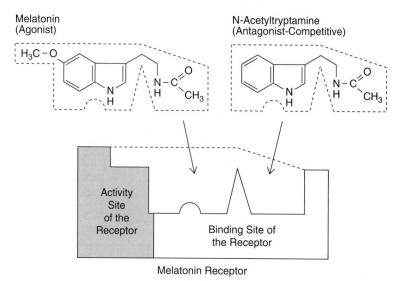

Figure 20.11   Schematic representation of the melatonin receptor based on structure-function studies of melatonin-related analogs. (Reprinted with permission from Heward and Hadley [15], *Life Sciences,* vol. 17, pp. 1167–1178. © 1975 Pergamon Press, Ltd.)

REFERENCES

[1] Bagnara, J. T., and M. E. Hadley, 1970. Endocrinology of the amphibian pineal. *Amer. Zool.* 10:201–16.

[2] Bartness, T. J., and B. D. Goldman. 1989. Mammalian pineal melatonin: a clock for all seasons. *Experientia* 45:939–45.

[3] Benitez-King, G., and F. Anton-Tay. 1993. Calmodulin mediates melatonin cytoskeletal effects. *Experientia* 49:635–41.

[4] Binkley, S. 1988. The pineal: endocrine and nonendocrine function. Prentice Hall Endocrinology Series. Englewood Cliffs: Prentice Hall Publishing Co., Inc.

[5] ———. 1993. Structures and molecules involved in generation and regulation of biological rhythms in vertebrates and invertebrates. *Experientia* 49:648–53.

[6] Binkley, S. A. 1979. Pineal rhythms in vivo and in vitro. *Comp. Biochem. Physiol.* 64A:201–206.

[7] Claustrat, B., J. Brun, and G. Chazot. 1990. Melatonin in humans, neuroendocrinological and pharmacological aspects. *Nucl. Med. Biol.* 27:625–32.

[8] Coleman, M. P. and R. J. Reiter. 1992. Breast cancer, blindness and melatonin. *Eur. J. Cancer* 28:501–3.

[9] Dawson, D., and N. Encel. 1993. Melatonin and sleep in humans. *J. Pineal Res.* 15:1–12.

[10] Ebisawa, T., S. Karne, M. R. Lerner, and S. M. Reppert. 1994. Expression cloning of a high-affinity melatonin receptor from *Xenopus* dermal melanophores. *Proc. Natl. Acad. Sci. USA* 91:6133–7.

[11] Grad, B. R., and R. Rozencwaig. 1993. The role of melatonin and serotonin in aging: up date. *Psychoneuro-endocrinology* 18:283–95.

[12] Halberg, F., E. Bakken, G. Cornelissen, J. Halberg, E. Halberg, and P. Delmore. 1988. Blood pressure assessment in a broad chronobiologic perspective. In *Heart Brain & Brain Heart,* eds. H. Refsum, J. A. Sulg, and K. Rasmussen, pp. 142–62. Berlin: Springer-Verlag.

[13] Hastings, M. H., G. Vance, and E. Maywood. 1989. Some reflections on the phylogeny and function of the pineal. *Experientia* 45:903–9.

[14] Herbert, J. 1989. Neural systems underlying photoperiodic time measurement: a blueprint. *Experientia* 45:965–72.

[15] Heward, C. B., and M. E. Hadley. 1975. Structure-activity relationships of melatonin and related indoleamines. *Life Sci.* 17:1167–78.

[16] Karasek, M., and R. J. Reiter. 1992. Morphofunctional aspects of the mammalian pineal gland. *Microscopy Res. Tech.* 21:136–57.

[17] Kauppila, A., A. Kivela, A. Pakarinen, and O. Vakkuri. 1987. Inverse seasonal relationship between melatonin and ovarian activity in humans in a region with a strong seasonal contrast in luminosity. *J. Clin. Endocrinol. Metab.* 65:823–8.

[18] Kitay, J. I., and D. Altschule. 1954. *The pineal gland.* Cambridge, Mass.: Harvard University Press.

[19] Klein, D. C., P. H. Roseboom, S. J. Donohue, and B. L. Marrs. 1992. Evolution of melatonin as a night signal: contribution from a primitive photosynthetic organism. *Mol. Cell. Neurosci.* 3:181–3.

[20] Kolata, G. 1985. Finding biological clocks in fetuses. *Science* 230:929–30.

[21] Maestroni, G. J. M. 1993. The immunoneuroendocrine role of melatonin. *J. Pineal Res.* 14:1–10.

[22] McCord, C. P., and F. P. Allen. 1917. Evidence associating pineal gland function with alterations in pigmentation. *J. Exp. Zool.* 23:207–24.

[23] Moore, R. Y. 1978. The innervation of the mammalian pineal gland. *Prog. Reprod. Biol.* 4:1–29.

[24] Morgan, P. J., and L. M. Williams. 1989. Central melatonin receptors: implications for a mode of action. *Experientia* 45:955–65.

[25] Petrie, K., J. V. Conaglen, L. Thompson, and K. Chamberlain. 1989. Effect of melatonin on jet lag after long haul flights. *Br. Med. J.* 298:705–7.

[26] Poulton, A. L. 1988. The proposed use of melatonin in controlled sheep breeding. *Aust. J. Biol. Sci.* 41:87–96.

[27] Puig-Domingo, M., S. M. Webb, J. Serrano, M.-A. Peinado, R. Corcoy, J. Ruscalleda, R. J. Reiter, and A. De Leiva. 1992. Melatonin-related hypogonadotropic hypogonadism. *New Eng. J. Med.* 1356–9.

[28] Ralph, M. R., R. G. Foster, F. C. Davis, and M. Menaker. 1990. Transplanted suprachiasmatic nucleus determines circadian period. *Science* 247:975–8.

[29] Reiter, R. J. 1978. Interaction of photoperiod, pineal and seasonal reproduction as exemplified by findings in the hamster. *Prog. Reprod. Biol.* 4:169–90.

[30] ———. 1991a. Neuroendocrine effects of light. *Intern. J. Biometerol.* 35:169–75.

[31] ———. 1991b. Melatonin: the chemical expression of darkness. *Mol. Cell. Endocrinol.* 79:C153–8.

[32] ———. 1991c. Pineal melatonin: cell biology of its synthesis and of its physiological interactions. *Endocr. Rev.* 12:151–80.

[33] ———. 1992. The ageing pineal gland and its physiological consequences. *BioEssays* 14:169–75.

[34] ———. 1993. The melatonin rhythm: both a clock and a calendar. *Experientia* 49:654–64.

[35] Reiter, R. J. and A. Lerchel. 1993. Regulation of mammalian pineal melatonin production by the electromagnetic spectrum. In *Melatonin: biosynthesis, physiological effects, and clinical applications*, eds. H.-S. Yu, and R. J. Reiter. pp. 107–27. Boca Raton: CRC Press.

[36] Reppert, S. M., J. Perlow, L. Tamarkin, and D. C. Klein. 1979. A diurnal rhythm in primate cerebrospinal fluid. *Endocrinology* 104:295–301.

[37] Sack, R. L., and A. J. Lewy. 1992. Human circadian rhythms: Lessons from the blind. *Ann. Med.* 25:303–5.

[38] Sack, R. L., A. J. Lewy, M. L. Blood, J. Stevenson, and L. D. Keith. 1991. Melatonin administration to blind people: phase advances and entrainment. *J. Biol. Rhythms* 6:249–61.

[39] Scheving, L. E., F. Halberg, and C. F. Ehret. 1987. *Chronobiotechnology and chronobiological engineering.* The Netherlands: Martinus Nijhoff.

[40] Silman, R. 1992. Melatonin: the clinical perspective in man. *Biochem. Soc. Trans.* 20:315–7.

[41] Sizonenko, P. C. 1989. Physiology of puberty. *J. Endocrinol. Invest.* 12:49–63.

[42] Stumpf, W. E. 1988. The endocrinology of sunlight and darkness: complementary roles of vitamin D and pineal hormones. *Naturwissenschaften* 75:247–51.

[43] Sugden, D. 1989. Melatonin biosynthesis in the mammalian pineal gland. *Experientia* 45:922–32.

[44] Turek, F. W. 1985. Circadian neural rhythms in mammals. *Annu. Rev. Physiol.* 47:49–64.

[45] Underwood, H. 1990. The pineal and melatonin: regulators of circadian function in lower vertebrates. *Experientia* 46:120–8.

[46] Vaughan, G. M., G. G. Meyer, and R. J. Reiter. 1978. Evidence for a pineal-gonad relationship in the human. *Prog. Reprod. Biol.* 4:191–223.

[47] Wurtman. R. J., J. Axelrod, and D. E. Kelly. 1968. *The pineal.* New York: Academic Press, Inc.

[48] Zucker, I. 1976. Light, behavior, and biologic rhythms. *Hosp. Pract.* 11(10):83–91.

[49] Zweig, M., S. H. Snyder, and J. Axelrod. 1966. Evidence for a nonretinal pathway of light in the pineal gland of newborn rats. *Proc. Natl. Acad. Sci.* 56:515–20.

Neurohormones

21

Classically, the endocrine system was separated from the nervous system based on its supposed different physiological role. The brain, in particular the hypothalamus, however, can be considered an endocrine organ as it synthesizes and secretes a large number of chemical messengers. Most interesting has been the discovery that many and possibly all classical peptide hormones are also found within the brain and other nervous tissues [25, 26]. For example, the gastrointestinal peptides cholecystokinin and substance P are found in the brain, as are α-MSH and ACTH, hormones of the pituitary. A number of peptides isolated and characterized from mammalian brain and GI tract (e.g., TRH, somatostatin, and substance P) have been found to be chemically similar, in some cases identical, to peptides present in amphibian skin. It is not surprising that certain peptides originally discovered in amphibian skin are present within mammalian tissues, including the brain.

Pearse formulated a unifying concept, the APUD hypothesis, which postulates that neurons and endocrine cells producing peptide hormones share common cytochemical and ultrastructural features. APUD, an acronym for "amine content and/or precursor uptake and decarboxylation," describes common features of neurons and endocrine cells. It is believed that both these cell types share a common embryonic origin, in that they are derived from the neuroectoderm. Therefore the ability of a neuron, a pituitary cell, or a skin cell to produce a peptide hormone is due to their derivation from a "neuroendocrine-programmed" ectoblast. This concept of a common cellular embryological origin may therefore provide a reasonable explanation for the observation that peptide hormones are common to both the CNS as well as the pituitary gland and to such peripheral organs as the GI tract and skin.

THE NEUROHORMONES: A REVIEW

Neurohormones, as the term denotes, are chemical messengers synthesized and secreted by nerve cells. Some neural messengers are relatively small molecules such as amino acids (glycine, glutamate) or molecules derived thereof, for example, serotonin, norepinephrine, and dopamine. Acetylcholine, histamine, and catecholamines such as dopamine and norepinephrine, are biogenic amines that were the earliest of the neurohormones to be studied in detail. The inhibitory amino acids, GABA (gamma amino butyric acid) and glycine, were later shown to function within the brain as neurohormones. Glutamate (derived from glutamic acid) is a stimulatory amino acid derivative that plays a major role in central nervous system function. Peptides, molecules consisting of two or more amino acids of a defined primary sequence, were then discovered to function as messengers within the nervous system. Most recently, to the wonderment or disbelief of many, several gases are now believed to function as chemical messengers of neural origin (discussed later in this chapter).

Neurohormones are released and delivered to their target cells by several routes. They can be released into a synaptic cleft to rapidly activate both pre- and postsynaptic membranes. This neurocrine route of delivery transfers information from neurons to adjacent neurons, muscle cells, or secretory (glandular) cells. Hormones released into a synaptic cleft to activate postsynaptic receptors are referred to as neurotransmitters. Neurohormones can also be released from less-specialized sites along the neuron to activate receptors on nearby cells. By this route of delivery the actions of the neurohormones are considered to be less rapid than transynaptic transduction, and the actions are considered to be neuromodulatory. In other words, neurohormones acting as neuromodulators modify adjacent neuronal activity, such as neurotransmission by neurotransmitters. It will be noted in this chapter that opiate peptides mediate their inhibitory action by such a mechanism.

Some brain hormones are released by nerves into a specific vascular bed to regulate hormone secretion from a nearby gland. For example, a number of peptide hormones are synthesized within parvocellular neurons to be released into the hypophysial portal system and carried to the pituitary gland where they either stimulate or inhibit hormone secretion from the hypophysis. These hypophysiotropic hormones (hypophysiotropins) of hypothalamic origin are delivered by a so-called neuroendocrine route of delivery (see Chap. 6). Other peptide hormones are released into the systemic circulation from larger, magnocellular neurons, to exert their actions on target cells at a great distance away (mammary glands, kidneys). Both parvocellular and magnocellular neurons are neurosecretory cells that deliver their hormones by a neuroendocrine (nerve to blood) route of delivery (see Chap. 7).

The diverse anatomical distribution of a particular peptide hormone implies that the hormone might regulate a variety of physiological functions. Within the nervous system peptide hormones function as neurotransmitters or neuromodulators or both, depending on their particular distribution or method of delivery within the tissue. To function as a neurotransmitter, a peptide hormone should fulfill certain criteria:

(1) it should be synthesized within neurons and concentrated in presynaptic terminals;
(2) it should be released by presynaptic stimulation;
(3) it should have specific high-affinity, saturable, and reversible binding sites on postsynaptic membranes;
(4) it should be metabolically degraded by nervous tissue; and
(5) it should evoke a postsynaptic potential.

Most criteria would apply to neuromodulatory peptides of nervous system origin.

Not all neuromodulators are neurohormones. Gonadal and adrenal steroid hormones and thyroid hormones are released from their endocrine glands to regulate a variety of functions, one of which is to provide a feedback inhibition of CNS neural activity. For example, testicular androgens regulate sexual behavior by modulating the activity of specific hypothalamic neurons (see Chap. 16). Although steroid hormones are known to interact with intracellular receptors to activate slower genomic mechanisms of transcription and translation, there is increasing evidence that several steroid hormones interact with the neuronal plasmalemma to evoke rapid neural actions [2, 38]. The nature and roles of a few of the numerous neurohormones found within the brain and peripheral nervous system will be described.

GASES AS NEURAL MESSENGERS (NEUROHORMONES)

Oxygen is essential for aerobic life, and displacement of its binding to the heme molecule by other gaseous oxides, such as nitric oxide (NO) and carbon monoxide (CO), has generally been seen only from a view of cytotoxicity. Experimental evidence now clearly implicates these gaseous chemical messengers in roles as neurohormones.

Nitric Oxide as Neurohormone. Work by the Solomon Snyder group suggests that NO in low concentrations acts as a neurotransmitter, carrying nerve impulses from one cell to another [44]. Interest in NO developed after it had been identified as the mysterious "endothelial relaxing factor," which is released by endothelial cells and causes blood vessels to dilate. Snyder decided to take a look at NO in the brain, but assaying for it directly would have been hopeless, because of its instability. So, instead, he and his colleagues looked for the synthase enzyme [6].

Within the brain, NO synthase occurs exclusively in neurons. Nitric oxide fulfills many of the classical criteria for a neurotransmitter. It is made in nerve cells and inhibiting its synthesis can block nerve stimulation. Unlike other neurotransmitters, however, which are made in advance and stored in small vesicles until needed, NO is made and produced immediately. It does not act through a conventional membrane receptor the way other neurotransmitters do. Instead, nitric oxide's "receptor" is the iron bound to enzymes, including guanylyl cyclase, which synthesizes cGMP, an important regulator of cellular activities. Stimulation of nerve cells by the excitatory neurotransmitter, glutamate, causes Ca^{2+} to move into cells. Then calcium ions, working in conjunction with the regulatory protein, calmodulin, turn on the synthesis of NO (derived from arginine in its conversion to citrulline), which in turn diffuses to adjacent cells where it activates guanylyl cyclase, resulting in the appropriate physiological response (Fig. 21.1). NO synthase has been localized to rat penile neurons innervating the corpora cavernosa and to neuronal plexuses in the adventitial layer of penile arteries. Small doses of NO-synthase inhibitors abolish electrophysiologically induced penile erections. These results establish NO as a physiologic mediator of erectile function [9, 24].

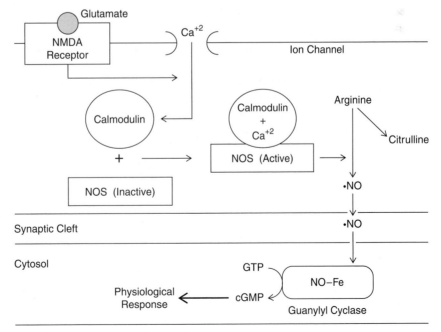

Figure 21.1 Proposed mechanism of NO (nitric oxide) production and role as a neurohormone. NOS, nitric oxide synthase. (Courtesy of Carrie Haskell-Luevano.)

Carbon Monoxide as Neurohormone. The discovery that NO can act as a physiological chemical messenger led to the notion that other such molecules might also function in a neurohormonal role. There is now convincing evidence that carbon monoxide (CO) may also be a candidate neurohormone [5]. Like NO, CO also activates the soluble form of guanylate cyclase. CO is formed by the action of the enzyme heme oxygenase. By in situ hybridization in brain slices, the discrete neuronal localization of mRNA for the constitutive form of heme oxygenase throughout the brain was demonstrated [50]. The localization was essentially the same as that for the soluble form of guanylate cyclase mRNA. A potent and selective inhibitor of heme oxygenase depleted endogenous cGMP. Other supporting evidence includes: (1) the chemical interaction of CO with the heme molecule, (2) the correlation between heme oxygenase activity and cGMP levels, and (3) evidence that CO can modulate cGMP levels in systemic organ preparations [32]. Therefore, CO, like NO, may be a physiologic regulator of cGMP and function as a neurohormone.

THE ENDORPHINS

In 1965 C.H. Li discovered a peptide in the pituitary of cattle and named it β-lipotropin. This so-called *lipotropic peptide*, β-LPH, named for its action on adipose tissue, was considered for many years to be a hormone in search of a function. With the discovery of endogenous morphinelike peptides in the brain, β-LPH may at last have an identified function. Opiate receptors have been discovered in the brain and have been pharmacologically characterized by their interaction with opiate agonists and antagonists such as morphine and naloxone, respectively (Fig. 21.2). Because it is reasonable to conclude that such highly specific receptors have not evolved to interact with exogenous opiate alkaloids, it was suggested that endogenous opiatelike substances might exist as natural ligands for the identified opiate receptors. Two peptides possessing opiatelike activity were isolated from bovine brain tissue as pentapeptides, differing only at the C-terminus (Fig. 21.3), possessing either leucine or methionine at that position. These peptides are referred to as *enkephalins,* and methionine enkephalin was recognized to be identical to an amino acid sequence within a larger peptide of the pituitary, β-LPH (Fig. 21.4) [8].

Endorphins are the class of substances isolated from the brain and pituitary gland that exhibit opiatelike activity. It was also discovered that the pituitary contains an endogenous opioid with a molecular weight greater than the enkephalins. This peptide was isolated, sequenced, and found to correspond to the 61–91 sequence of bovine β-LPH (Fig. 21.4). This β-endorphin, as well as the enkephalins and other more recently discovered endorphins, are under intense study as possible candidates for the body's own antipain (analgesic) hormones. Indeed, these peptides do appear to play such a role; therefore β-LPH might be considered to function as a prohormone for the production of at least some of these endorphins.

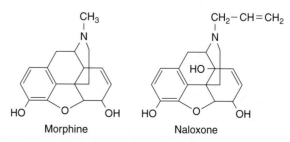

Figure 21.2 Structures of an opiate receptor agonist (morphine) and antagonist (naloxone).

OH
CH3
S
CH2
CH2
CH2
H
H
CH2
NH2–CH–CO–NH–CH–CO–NH–CH–CO–NH–CH–CO–NH–CH–COOH
Tyr
Gly
Gly
Phe
Met
Methionine Enkephalin
OH
CH3
HC–CH3
CH2
CH2
H
H
CH2
NH2–CH–CO–NH–CH–CO–NH–CH–CO–NH–CH–CO–NH–CH–COOH
Tyr
Gly
Gly
Phe
Leu
Leucine Enkephalin

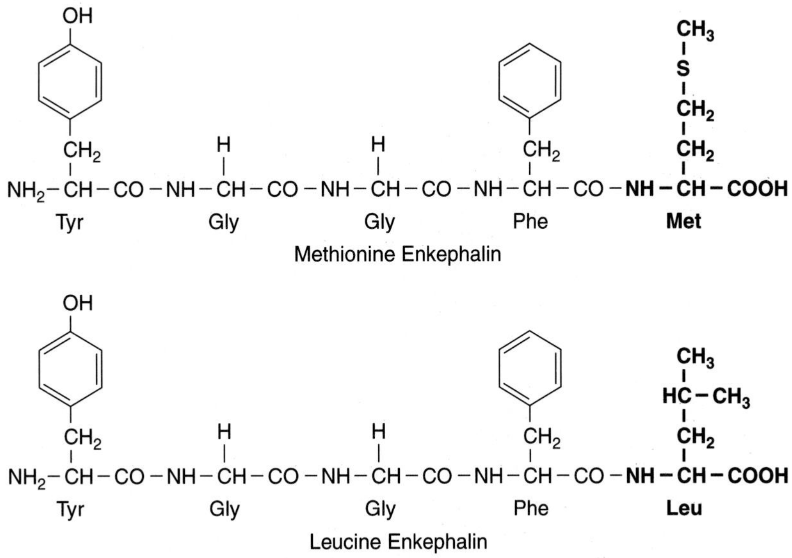

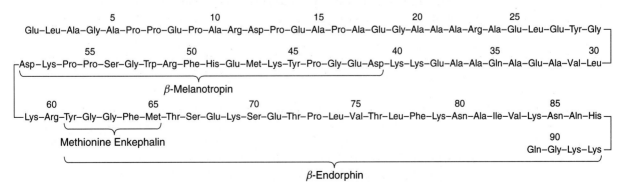

Figure 21.3 Structures of Met- and Leu-enkephalins.

Source, Synthesis, Chemistry, and Metabolism

Opiate drugs such as morphine affect the perception of pain, consciousness, motor control, and autonomic function by interacting with specific receptors expressed throughout the central and peripheral nervous systems. The endogenous ligands of these opiate receptors have been identified as a family of more than 20 opioid peptides that derive from the three precursor proteins, pro-opiomelanocortin, proenkephalin, and prodynorphin. Although the opioid peptides belong to a class of molecules distinct from the opiate alkaloids, they share common structural features, including a positive charge juxtaposed with an aromatic ring that is required for interaction with the receptor [16, 37].

Pituitary β-LPH is found in both the pars distalis and pars intermedia in association with ACTH. Corticotrophs and melanotrophs of the pars distalis and pars intermedia, respectively, of the pituitary produce a large molecular weight (31,000 daltons) protein that contains the sequence of β-LPH and ACTH. The term *pro-opiomelanocortin* (POMC) was suggested for this protein that appears to be the common precursor for β-endorphin and corticotropin. POMC is found within secretory granules of corticotrophs of the pars distalis and the granules of secretory cells (melanotrophs) of the pars intermedia. The precursor protein serves as a prohormone for ACTH production in the pars distalis; in the pars intermedia enzymatic activity results in cleavage of POMC to yield α-MSH (see Fig. 8.4). The complete amino acid sequence of bovine POMC has been reported.

5 10 15 20 25
Glu–Leu–Ala–Gly–Ala–Pro–Pro–Glu–Pro–Ala–Arg–Asp–Pro–Glu–Ala–Pro–Ala–Glu–Gly–Ala–Ala–Ala–Arg–Ala–Glu–Leu–Glu–Tyr–Gly
55 50 45 40 35 30
Asp–Lys–Pro–Pro–Ser–Gly–Trp–Arg–Phe–His–Glu–Met–Lys–Tyr–Pro–Gly–Glu–Asp–Lys–Lys–Glu–Ala–Ala–Gln–Ala–Glu–Ala–Val–Leu
β-Melanotropin
60 65 70 75 80 85
Lys–Arg–Tyr–Gly–Gly–Phe–Met–Thr–Ser–Glu–Lys–Ser–Glu–Thr–Pro–Leu–Val–Thr–Leu–Phe–Lys–Asn–Ala–Ile–Val–Lys–Asn–Aln–His
Methionine Enkephalin
90
Gln–Gly–Lys–Lys
β-Endorphin

Figure 21.4 Structure of bovine β-lipotropin illustrating the sequences of Met-enkephalin, β-endorphin, and β-MSH.

Tyr–Gly–Gly–Phe–Leu–Arg–Arg–Ile–Arg–Pro–Lys–Leu–Lys–Trp–Asp–Asn–Gln

Figure 21.5   Primary structure of porcine dynorphin.

The so-called lipotropic activity of β-LPH is a common property of β-LPH and other melanotropic peptides since they possess structural similarities. There is no clear evidence, however, that any one of the peptides plays a normal physiological role in affecting adipose tissue lipolysis. It is unclear whether β-endorphin or its metabolic products present within corticotrophs or melanotrophs of the pituitary play any hormonal role or are only necessary byproducts of ACTH and α-MSH secretion. Although β-MSH has been localized to the pars intermedia, this peptide (see Fig. 8.1), which is present within the structure of β-LPH (Fig. 21.4), is an artifact of extraction. There is no evidence that β-MSH is secreted from the pars intermedia other than as a component of β-LPH (see Chap. 8).

Although there is no evidence that β-endorphin of pituitary origin serves any physiologically relevant humoral role, another opioid peptide, dynorphin, has been isolated from the posterior pituitary. This heptadecapeptide contains Leu-enkephalin as its NH$_2$-terminal sequence (Fig. 21.5). The potency of this peptide is greater than that of any other known endogenous opiatelike peptide, but the peptide's physiological role is undetermined. Cells that stain immunocytochemically for dynorphin are found within specific sites within the hypothalamus and myenteric plexus of the gut. Within the pituitary the peptide is specifically localized to the neurohypophysis. Dynorphin and vasopressin occur in the same hypothalamic magnocellular neurons of rats; their synthesis, however, appears to be under separate genetic control. Dynorphin is not present within oxytocin-containing neurons.

A number of independent endorphin pathways in the brain have been delineated: a β-endorphin system with a single cell group in the hypothalamus and long axons innervating midbrain and limbic structures, and two enkephalin systems with multiple cell groups throughout the spinal cord and brainstem, which possess relatively short axons. The immunocytochemical mapping of Leu- and Met-enkephalins suggests that the two pentapeptides occur in completely separate nerve cells in neural pathways that differ considerably anatomically. The relative proportions of Met- and Leu-enkephalin vary between different brain regions and also between different species, further demonstrating the existence of separate populations of Met- and Leu-enkephalin nerves. Many areas of the brain that are rich in enkephalins correspond to areas closely associated with dopaminergic, noradrenergic, serotonergic, and substance P-containing neuronal systems (Fig. 21.6). Many enkephalin-containing neurons appear to be short interneurons.

Outside the CNS there is a rich enkephalinergic innervation of the GI tract, and there is evidence that enkephalins may also be contained in various autonomic nerves and ganglion cells and in mucosal cells of the stomach. Present evidence suggests that β-LPH, ACTH, and β-endorphin sequences occur within the same neurons in the brain and that POMC may therefore also function as a prohormone for β-endorphin, α-MSH, or ACTH production within the CNS. The enkephalins, on the other hand, are derived from different, precursors; "big" forms of both Met-enkephalin and Leu-enkephalin have been discovered. The amino acid sequence of these peptides differs from that of β-LPH, suggesting separate precursors for β-endorphin and each of the enkephalins.

Physiological Roles

The physiological roles of the identified opioid systems are not fully elucidated. The endorphins are found in high concentrations in brain areas involved in pain transmission, respiration, motor activity, pituitary hormone secretion, and mood. The suggestion of a relationship between the endorphins and ACTH secretion is intriguing as behavioral studies indicate that stress increases the concentrations of endorphins in blood and brain, with parallel changes in pain threshold. Histochemical localization also suggests that the opioid substances may have important relations to noradrenergic and dopaminergic systems.

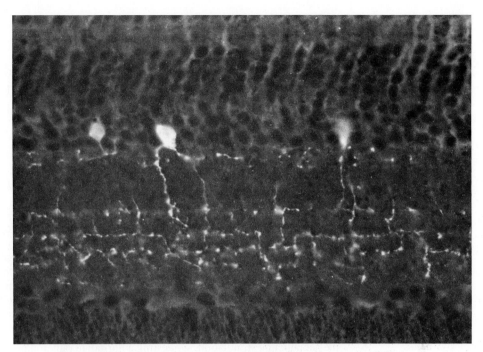

Figure 21.6 Immunocytochemical localization of Leu-enkephalin to an amacrine cell of the avian retina. (From Brecha, Karten, and Laverack [7], with permission.)

Analgesic Function. The most clearly understood action of an endorphin is in the spinal cord where small enkephalin-containing neurons impinge on the terminals of peripheral sensory nerve cells that convey pain information to the spinal cord. These primary afferent neurons contain (and release) another peptide known as substance P. Substance P (Arg-Pro-Lys-Pro-Gln-Gln-Phe-Phe-Gly-Leu-Met-NH$_2$) has been immunocytochemically localized to sensory pain fibers of the dorsal root ganglia. The higher concentration of SP in dorsal root neurons compared to ventral root nerves suggests that SP is the neurotransmitter released by the central terminals of primary afferent sensory fibers. SP has an excitatory action on single neural units in the dorsal horn of the spinal cord. The units excited by SP are among those excited by noxious cutaneous simulation; SP causes an enhancement of the responses of these nociceptive (pain-sensing) units to noxious stimulation.

Met-enkephalin blocks the release of SP from nerve terminals of sensory pain fibers, and the effect of the endorphin is antagonized by naloxone (an opiate antagonist). The distribution of opiate receptors closely parallels that of SP neurons, and the SP neurons contain binding sites (receptors) for the enkephalins. Thus enkephalin-containing neurons within the dorsal horn may inhibit release of SP from dorsal root sensory neurons and thereby inhibit pain transmission to the brain (Fig. 21.7). There is evidence that another major site of enkephalin modulation of the nociceptive information transfer in the dorsal horn is on the projection neurons themselves [26]. The relationship between enkephalins and SP may be the physiological basis for the postulated "pain gate." This gate in the spinal cord lets pain impulses perceived and transmitted by sensory neurons through to the brain. Prevention of SP release by enkephalin may be what closes the gate (Fig. 21.7)

One fascinating finding suggests that endorphins and their receptors can affect acupuncture-induced analgesia. For example, the firing rate of cells in the spinal cord is greatly increased in response to painful stimuli. Acupuncture suppressed this increased electrical activity, but this acupuncture effect was completely blocked by the specific opiate antagonist, naloxone. The acupuncture effect was slow in onset and it long outlasted

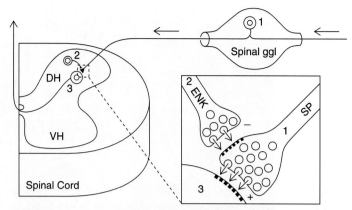

Figure 21.7 Schematic illustration of the hypothetical interaction between (1) substance P-containing (pain-conveying?) primary afferents, and (2) enkephalin interneurons in the dorsal horn (DH). The third neuron represents a pathway ascending to higher centers. (VH means ventral horn.) (In *Advances in pharmacology and therapeutics,* ed. S. Simon, pp. 131–42. © 1979 New York: Pergamon Press, Inc. [26].)

the acupuncture stimulation, suggesting a hormonal rather than a direct neuronal response. Acupuncture and electroacupuncture have also been shown to be reversed by opiate antagonists; experiments suggest that the opioid system may play a role in placebo analgesia, which is effective in about 30% of the population. A study in Beijing, China, indicates that electroacupuncture in rats causes an analgesia that involves release of opioid peptides. Using radioimmunoassays it was found that low-frequency electroacupuncture led to release of enkephalins into spinal perfusates, while high-frequency electroacupuncture resulted in the release of a dynorphin. These results were confirmed by experiments in which the injection of antibodies against enkephalin or dynorphin was shown to block electroacupuncture analgesia [43].

Several studies have implicated an endogenous opiate system in human behavior specifically related to pain and psychiatric disorders. It was found that stimulation of the periaqueductal gray matter of the brain produces naloxone-reversible analgesia in patients suffering from intractable pain. This response was accompanied by an increase in ventricular endorphinlike activity. These data support the findings that basal levels of endogenous opioids in the CSF of patients with persistent pain are depressed. These observations suggest, as do the animal studies cited earlier, that analgesic brain stimulation may result in the release of an endogenous opiatelike substance. Preliminary trials have suggested that β-endorphin itself produces significant pain relief when administered to terminal cancer patients. These results offer the possibility that with further well-controlled clinical trials a more detailed understanding of the mechanisms of pain and pain relief may be achieved.

Endorphins as Possible Adrenomedullary Hormones. Stressful stimuli often elicit marked neurogenic stimulation of the adrenal medulla. Many forms of stress also induce significant analgesia that can be partially blocked by naloxone. A large number of enkephalin-containing peptides are present in mammalian adrenal chromaffin tissue. They are stored within chromaffin granules and are cosecreted in response to the same stimuli that induce catecholamine secretion. Denervation of the rat adrenal increases the amounts of enkephalin and enkephalin-containing polypeptides in the gland. These peptides may all derive from a pro-enkephalin through proteolysis. One such peptide (peptide E) contains within its structure both the met and Leu-enkephalin sequences (Fig. 21.8). This peptide is 30 times more potent than Met-enkephalin. It is suggested that free enkephalins may not be the physiologically relevant end product derived from pro-enkephalin but,

```
1          5              10             15             20             25
Tyr–Gly–Gly–Phe–Met–Arg–Arg–Val–Gly–Arg–Pro–Glu–Trp–Trp–Met–Asp–Tyr–Gln–Lys–Arg—Tyr–Gly–Gly–Phe–Leu
```

Figure 21.8 Primary structure of bovine peptide E derived from adrenal chromaffin tissue. The sequences of Met- and Leu-enkephalin within the peptide are indicated [28].

rather, that peptide E and other adrenal enkephalin-containing peptides may serve as unique physiological regulatory substances [28]. Specifically, it has been suggested that adrenomedullary enkephalins may contribute to the attenuation of pain during life-threatening stress.

Control of Pituitary Hormone Secretion. There is evidence that opioid peptides may play a physiological role in controlling the release of pituitary hormones [39]. For example, in the pig-tailed monkey the concentration of β-endorphin is more than 100 times greater in the hypophysial blood than in the peripheral plasma. Intravenous injection of opioid peptides causes the release of PRL, GH, AVP, and MSH. These peptides are, however, inhibitory to FSH and LH secretion, and these endorphin effects on pituitary hormone release are reversed by naloxone. Opioid peptides and antagonists are without any effect on isolated pituitaries, suggesting that their effects are mediated at the level of the hypothalamus. The simplest interpretation is that endogenous opioid peptides inhibit dopaminergic (or noradrenergic) pathways that normally control some pituitary hormone secretions. Prolactin secretion from the adenohypophysis is normally inhibited by a PRL-inhibiting factor that apparently is dopamine (see Chap. 5). Endorphin inhibition of dopamine secretion would therefore result in PRL secretion. These results demonstrate that the release of PRL under physiological conditions can be reduced by blockade of opiate receptors, which further suggests that endogenous endorphins participate tonically in the regulation of PRL hormone secretion. Likewise, β-endorphin inhibition of dopamine or norepinephrine secretion from median eminence catecholaminergic neurons (which are stimulatory to hypothalamic gonadotropin-releasing hormone neurons) would account for the inhibition of FSH and LH secretion that follows central administration of an endorphin. Opiate receptor antagonists, as expected, stimulate gonadotropin secretion, suggesting that GnRH secretion is under tonic inhibition by an exogenous endorphin.

Role in Reproductive Physiology. A synthetic analog of Met-enkephalin inhibits copulatory behavior in sexually active male rats; its action is prevented by naloxone, a specific inhibitor of opioid receptors. Naloxone itself induces copulatory behavior in inactive male rats, which suggests that endorphins normally exert a tonic inhibition of copulatory behavior. These observations provide strong evidence that endorphins may be important in the regulation of sexual behavior [19].

Mechanisms of Action

Endorphins modify the excitability of a variety of neurons in the central nervous system. Microiontophoresis of Met-enkephalin onto single neurons in the rat brainstem shows that endorphin's predominant action is to suppress the firing rate of spontaneously active neurons. Similar effects are obtained with the narcotic agonists morphine and etorphine; their actions and those of Met-enkephalin are blocked by iontophoretically applied naloxone. Endorphins and opiate narcotics inhibit spontaneously responsive cells in the cortex, brainstem, caudate nucleus, and thalamus. In the hippocampus, however, pyramidal cells are usually excited and are also naloxone sensitive. Opiate receptors are apparently localized presynaptically on some nerve fibers, and endorphins may reduce the release of dopamine and other neurotransmitters by an action on these receptors. A major function of an endorphin therefore may be to mediate presynaptic inhibition on a variety of neuronal systems in the central nervous system [26]. The presynaptic effects of endorphins or opiate narcotics on neuronal activity would depress or excite neurons depending on whether the presynaptic neurons are excitatory or inhibitory to the neurons being monitored electrophysiologically. Thus *disinhibition* of an active neuron that is inhibitory to a quiescent neuron would result in excitation of this latter neuron. Although opiate receptors mediate neuronal inhibition in most brain regions, the ultimate action of exogenous opiates on a given region may depend on regional cytological relationships.

Endorphins interact with opiate receptors as shown by their ability to displace radiolabeled narcotic agonists and antagonists from the receptors. Opiate receptors fall into a number of distinct classes as characterized by pharmacological and biochemical methods. Classical pharmacological studies have defined three classes of opioid receptors: δ, μ, and k, that differ in their affinity for various opioid ligands and in their anatomical distribution. The δ receptors bind with the greatest affinity to enkephalins and have a more discrete distribution in the brain than either μ or k receptors, with high concentrations in the basal ganglia and limbic regions. Although morphine interacts principally with μ receptors, peripheral administration of this opiate induces release of enkephalins. Thus enkephalins may mediate part of the physiological response to morphine, presumably by interaction with δ receptors. The specific anatomical localizations suggest that the different types of receptors mediate different physiological functions [16]. The so-called mu receptors (μ) may mediate analgesic actions, whereas delta receptors (δ) may preferentially regulate emotional behavior. The μ and δ receptors are regulated by Met- and Leu-enkephalins, respectively. Dynorphin appears to be a specific endogenous ligand for the kappa (κ) subclass of opioid receptor. Thus the opiates, like adrenergic, cholinergic, and dopaminergic agonists, initiate their broad spectrum of diverse physiological actions by interaction with multiple receptor types. This provides some hope that opiate drugs might be developed that possess morphinelike analgesic actions but lack addictive effects. Despite pharmacological and physiological heterogeneity, the three types of opioid receptors inhibit adenylyl cyclase, increase K^+ conductance, and inactivate Ca^{2+} channels through a pertussis toxin-sensitive mechanism (see Chap. 4). These results and others suggest that opioid receptors belong to the large family of cell surface receptors that signal through G proteins [16].

Pathophysiology

In studies on a neuroblastoma hybrid cell line grown in tissue culture, it was found that continuous exposure to opiates resulted initially in decreased cAMP production. With time, more of the opiate agonist was required to decrease cAMP production to the original levels produced by the opiate; the cells had apparently become *tolerant* to the actions of the drug. It was found that the cells synthesized more adenylate cyclase and, upon removal of the opiate from the cells, cAMP levels rose dramatically and responded excessively to other hormonal stimulation. This excessive production of cAMP may represent the biochemical correlate of withdrawal symptoms noted in humans taken off opiate drugs. There is evidence that opiate drugs and peptides also mediate their actions on nervous tissue through stimulation of cGMP production.

Classical *tolerance* and *dependence* develop in rodents continuously infused with endorphins. The animals are also cross dependent on morphine. This might be expected, as the receptors for opiate drugs and peptides are identical. It has been suggested that heroin addicts, at some stage in their addiction, may suffer from an endorphin deficiency. Excess target tissue hormones (e.g., cortisol) are known to exert a negative feedback to hypothalamic production of releasing hormones (i.e., CRH). Possibly the production of brain or pituitary endorphins is shut off in a similar manner due to feedback inhibition by opiate drugs. Addicts then might be suffering from a true hormone (endorphin) deficiency [48].

According to the catecholamine theory of schizophrenia, psychosis results from the overproduction of dopamine and therefore overstimulation of dopaminergic receptors

[10]. There is evidence that endorphins affect certain CNS dopaminergic pathways. The opiate antagonist, naloxone, alters some schizophrenic symptoms. This observation might support the hypothesis that endorphins may be involved in some schizophrenic symptomatology.

Neurohormonal/Neuroanatomical Correlates of Addictive Drugs. The mesolimbic system of the brain appears to be a neural center responsible for receiving signals that lead to euphoric (pleasant) feelings that can become addictive. When the mesolimbic system is stimulated certain neurons release dopamine (DA). This neurotransmitter stimulates postsynaptic neuronal membranes, and a signal is generated that leads to a feeling of euphoria, conditioning an animal to seek out substances causing the sensation again. Cocaine and related addictive drugs block the reuptake of DA at the nerve terminals, thus prolonging its action and enhancing its euphoric effects. Nicotine also works on these same dopaminergic neurons. Nicotine, however, acts by stimulating the release of DA rather than by inhibiting its reuptake, as does cocaine. But the effects are the same, a pleasant, euphoric sensation [35], a pleasurable habit hard to kick.

BRAIN HORMONES AND BEHAVIOR

Neurohormones regulate all aspects of behavior including sexual behaviors (mating, maternal, aggressive) and behaviors related to fluid and food consumption. The role of cholecystokinin in feeding behavior will be described as just one example of the role of neurohormones in the control of behavior [3, 40].

Cholecystokinin and Feeding Behavior

Most members of a species grow to an average weight characteristic of the group. It is proposed that certain brain centers control appetite (consummatory) behavior. Humoral and neural cues may interact with these neural centers to stimulate or inhibit feeding behavior. The relation of food intake to caloric needs is an example of one of the body's major homeostatic mechanisms.

Bilateral destruction of the ventral medial hypothalamus (VMH) produces a dramatic increase in food intake (hyperphagia). Destruction of the lateral hypothalamic nuclei, on the other hand, inhibits feeding (aphagia), which may lead to severe, long-lasting anorexia. Electrical stimulation of the VMH inhibits feeding behavior, whereas electrical stimulation of the LH initiates eating. During hunger and the onset of feeding, electrical activity of the LH increases, whereas that of the VMH decreases. Norepinephrine infused into the medial or the lateral hypothalamus initiates or inhibits ingestive behavior. It was originally proposed that a satiety center (within the VMH) is tonically inhibitory (through noradrenergic neurons) to a feeding center (within the lateral hypothalamus) and that the presence or absence of humoral or local neural cues inhibitory or stimulatory to the satiety center would affect feeding-center activity. There is evidence that neural afferents deriving from both the VMH, as well as the LH, reciprocally affect the activity of the other area of the hypothalamus.

Cells within the VMH and LH may function as glucoreceptors by monitoring blood glucose levels to control food intake. Glucoreceptive neural units have been demonstrated by electrophysiological methods to be present in the VMH and LH. A nonmetabolizable glucose compound, 2-deoxy-D-glucose (2-DG), which blocks the intracellular use of glucose and therefore causes glucoprivation, stimulates feeding when injected intracisternally. The 2-DG-induced feeding response is blocked if animals are pretreated with the α-adrenoceptor antagonist phentolamine. These observations and other evidence suggest that central glucoreceptors may be noradrenergic neurons or that these glucostats mediate their actions indirectly through such neurons.

Other humoral or neural cues may also control the activity of the putative hypothalamic satiety and feeding centers. Partially digested food, chyme, released into the duodenum of the small intestine from the stomach, triggers the release of several GI hormones that regulate the release of pancreatic digestive enzymes and the motility of the digestive tract (see Chap. 10). Specific metabolic substrates of the chyme, such as proteins, lipids, carbohydrates, or degradative products thereof, also interact with cellular receptors of the gut epithelium to activate specific GI hormone secretions. Besides local effects on gastrointestinal activity, these metabolic substrates or GI hormones may provide cues that inform the animal of its short-term metabolic status. The food intake of a hungry rat, for example, is reduced if the rat's blood is mixed with blood from a recently fed rat, but not if too much time has elapsed between feeding and the blood transfusion.

Cholecystokinin (CCK) is released from the duodenum in response to certain factors present in the chyme in the stomach. CCK stimulates gallbladder contraction, secretion of pancreatic enzymes, and numerous other GI functions. There is now evidence that CCK may also function as a satiety signal [40]. Systemic injections of CCK inhibit food intake in the rat and the rhesus monkey in a dose-related manner. In humans a consistent dose-response relationship has not been noted, although rapid intravenous injection of CCK does reduce food intake. CCK (synthetic octapeptide), in a dose-dependent manner, also prolongs the intermeal interval in the rat by considerably delaying the start of the next meal. This is important since a CCK-satiety hypothesis would suppose that elevation of CCK in the plasma as an animal eats would inhibit feeding; as long as the level of CCK in the blood remains high, food intake would be expected to be inhibited.

The C-terminal octapeptide of CCK is inhibitory to food intake (but not water intake), and some analogs of CCK are more potent than the native peptide on such CCK-mediated responses as gallbladder contraction and pancreatic enzyme secretion. These peptides are also more effective in reducing food intake; thus a common CCK receptor is implicated in the control of satiety and GI function. Cerulean, a decapeptide isolated from the skin of a frog, shares a very similar C-terminal sequence with CCK (see Fig. 10.15), and it is also effective in altering food intake.

If CCK plays a role as a humoral factor controlling food intake, where is its site of action? The effects of systemically injected CCK are abolished by vagotomy specifically, (a division of the gastric branch of the vagus nerve), suggesting that vagal afferents may provide important satiety cues to the hypothalamus [17]. Nevertheless, there is convincing evidence for a central site of action of CCK or a structurally-related peptide. Injections of CCK into the cerebral ventricles inhibit feeding in sheep. The ineffectiveness of systemically injected CCK compared to the satiety effects of the peptide at much lowered concentrations when administered intracerebroventricularly suggests that CCK acts on CNS structures involved in food intake [12]. This is further substantiated by the observation that injections of anti-CCK sera into the cerebral ventricles stimulate feeding in sheep. Rats with lesions in the VMH show reduced sensitivity to cerulean, whereas rats with lateral hypothalamic damage exhibit heightened sensitivity to the peptide. Microinjections of cerulean into the VMH, but not into the LH, limit feeding. In addition tritiated cerulean is selectively bound to tissue in the VMH. Systemic injections or local application of CCK-related peptides activate neural units within the LH; the particular response elicited is influenced by the nutritional state of the animal. A peptide closely related immunologically to CCK-octapeptide, the C-terminal 8-amino-acid sequence of CCK, is present within the brain where it is localized to specific neurons. A peptide similar to CCK-4 (the COOH-terminal tetrapeptide of CCK) has also been described as being localized to specific brain areas. Feeding responses elicited by hypothalamic infusions of norepinephrine are blocked by CCK administered either intraperitoneally or to NE-sensitive hypothalamic sites. In addition, systemic administration of CCK releases NE within the hypothalamus. A tentative hypothesis is that CCK released by the GI tract or afferent vagal neurons is stimulatory to noradrenergic neurons of the VMH which, through the release of norepinephrine, are inhibitory to the lateral hypothalamic feeding centers.

NEUROENDOCRINOLOGY OF EXTRINSIC SENSORY PERCEPTION

Extrinsic stimuli such as light (or its absence), taste, and smell are intercepted by receptors, which then, through transduction mechanisms, transfer those sensory cues to the brain to be perceived (decoded). It might at first seem extraordinary, although not unexpected, that light (photons) and molecules affecting smell (odorants) and taste (tastants) are interpreted by receptors; these receptors then, as for most hormones, transduce a signal resulting in membrane depolarization or hyperpolarization and/or in second-messenger production. The transduction pathways involved in sensory perception will be detailed [33].

Taste (Gustatory) Transduction

Taste cells respond to a variety of chemical stimuli: certain ions are perceived as salty (Na^+) or sour (H^+); other small molecules are recognized as sweet (sugars) and bitter (alkaloids). Interaction of chemical substances with membrane components (receptors) of these taste bud cells results, either directly or indirectly, in depolarization or hyperpolarization of these electrically excitable cells with resulting stimulation or inhibition, respectively, of transsynaptic afferent taste bud fibers and information flow to the brain (Fig. 21.9).

Salty Taste. Na^+ causes taste cell depolarization via entry of Na^+ ions through apical Na^+ channels. The taste cell Na^+ channels are voltage-independent and can be blocked by the diuretic, amiloride (Fig. 21.9).

Sour Taste. Sourness is a measurement of the proton concentration (acidity) of a solution. In mammalian taste cells H^+ ions exert their effects by blocking K^+ or Na^+ entry via the apical Na^+ channel involved in salt taste, with resulting cellular hyperpolarization (Fig. 21.9).

Sweet and Bitter Tastes. These tastes are transduced by second-messenger mediated pathways. Sweet stimuli from binding of sugar molecules to specific receptors are coupled to G-proteins ($\alpha\beta\gamma$). Activation of this pathway leads to adenylate cyclase

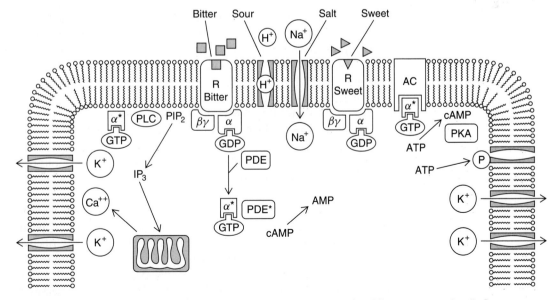

Figure 21.9 Transduction mechanisms for different taste stimuli. See text for details. (From Margolskee [33], with permission. *Bioessays* 15:645–50, 1993.)

generation of cAMP, which activates protein kinase A (PKA) and leads to phosphorylation and closure of basolateral K^+ channels. K^+ channel closure leads to taste cell depolarization. Bitter substances are believed to bind to specific receptors (R_{bitter}) that are also coupled to G-proteins. Two bitter transduction mechanisms are proposed. In one pathway, a G protein activates phospholipase C (PLC), which generates inositol 1,4,5-triphosphate (IP_3). IP_3 causes Ca^{2+} release from internal stores, which leads to neurotransmitter release on to gustatory afferents. A second proposed pathway for bitter perception (transduction) involves a G protein activation of cAMP phosphodiesterase (PDE) to decrease intracellular cAMP. This would lead to hyperpolarization of taste cells via decreased phosphorylation of basolateral K^+ channels (Fig. 21.9).

A new G protein α subunit (α-gustducin) has been identified and cloned from lingual tissue. Gustducin mRNA is specifically expressed in taste buds, since it is not expressed in nonsensory portions of the tongue, and is also not expressed in other tissues. α-Gustducin most closely resembles the G-protein α subunit of rods and cones, transducin. This suggests that gustducin's role in taste transduction may be analogous (see below) to that of transducin in visual transduction.

Taste perception as discussed above (Fig. 21.9) may involve: (1) permeation of apical ion channels (salt), a stimulus influx; (2) blockage of ion channels (sour); (3) direct activation of channels; or (4) binding to receptors linked to second messengers. Whatever the mechanism the final result of these interactions is the modulation of transmitter release onto gustatory afferent neurons [20].

Olfactory Transduction

Humans can distinguish about 10,000 different odors. The question raised is "how does the nose know?" [6] A present hypothesis based upon experimental data is that the receptors for odorant molecules are typical seven-membrane spanning elements that interact with odorant ligands just as these receptors interact with hormones. There may be up to 1000 or more such membrane receptors specifically localized to the membranes of the olfactory epithelium. To discriminate among the multitude of possible odorants each cell may possess two or more such receptors that, when simultaneously stimulated, provide the information ("cross-talk") for the detection of a particular smell. Activation of two or more receptors on an olfactory neuron would provide the diversity on the level of one neuron-type per smell [4]. Receptor interaction then involves activation of the α subunit of a trimeric G protein that is commonly associated with other sensory ligands (including hormones). Odorants are known to cause olfactory neurons to produce cAMP. This cyclic nucleotide may then activate a gated ion channel. Transmembrane depolarization would then transmit information along the olfactory sensory neuron to the brain (Fig. 21.10).

Rhodopsin and Phototransduction: A Model for
G Protein-Linked Receptors

Rhodopsin is the receptive substance of rods and cones that responds to a photic stimulus and transduces the signal into a physiological response (as described above) [15, 21, 22, 23, 30, 41]. As in most other hormonal ligands (except steroid and thyroid hormones), this receptor (rhodopsin) consists of seven transmembrane helices with an N-terminal extracellular and an internal C-terminal segment (Figure 21.11). Bovine rhodopsin is a 348-amino-acid membrane protein that contains a light-sensitive chromophore, 11-cis retinal. This 11-cis retinal is bound as a protonated Schiff base to the ε-amino group of lysine 296; upon reception of a photon of light, 11-cis retinal is photoisomerized to its all-trans conformation. The activated chromophore now functions as does a hormonal ligand to cause a positional change in some component of the rhodopsin transmembrane helices. As noted in Fig. 21.11, the conformational change in rhodopsin now allows access of the intracellular receptor loops to a trimeric G protein. This binding allows GTP to replace GDP on

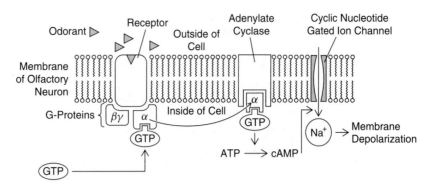

Figure 21.10 Mechanisms of odorant-induced sensory transduction within olfactory neurons. (Modified from Barinaga [4].)

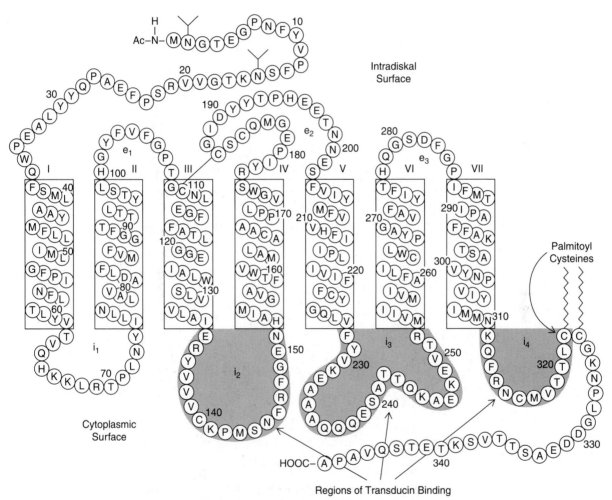

Figure 21.11 Model for rhodopsin topography. Here the 348-amino acid sequence of bovine rhodopsin is shown in its orientation in the disk membrane. Its amino terminal sequence, bearing oligosaccharide chains on Asn 2 and 15, is exposed to the intradiskal membrane surface. The polypeptide chain traverses the lipid bilayer seven times (helices I–VII), exposing loops e_1–e_3 to the inside surface of the disk membrane and loops i_1–i_4 and the carboxyl terminus to the intracellular or cytoplasmic surface. The putative loop i_4 would be formed by the insertion of palmitoyl cysteines into the lipid bilayer. Loops i_2, i_3, and i_4 are shown as sites of interaction with transducin. (From Hargrave et al. [21], with permission. *Bioessays* 15:43–50, 1993.)

the α subunit (transducin), and this allows the subunit to detach from the $\beta\gamma$ subunit. One photoisomerized rhodopsin activates hundreds of molecules of transducin within a fraction of a second [30]. Transducin is then available to activate a cGMP phosphodiesterase (as noted in Fig. 21.12). This is reminiscent of the role of the $G\alpha_s$ subunit in the activation of adenylate cyclase (see Chap. 4).

As described for the β-adrenoceptor (see Chap. 14), the intracellular terminal segment of rhodopsin becomes phosphorylated (Fig. 21.11) by a protein kinase (in this case, a rhodopsin kinase). Phosphorylation of photoexcited rhodopsin does not completely prevent it from activating transducin. However, this initial phosphorylation allows the binding of a protein, arrestin (as for the β-adrenoceptor), to rhodopsin, and formation of this complex prevents further activation of transducin [23]. Subsequent to dephosphorylation of the rhodopsin by a phosphatase, 11-cis retinal can bind to the rhodopsin to again participate in the phototransduction process. Figure 21.12 depicts the receptor/transduction events in a photoreceptor.

Alterations in the primary structure of rhodopsin can lead to defects in vision. For example, proper folding of rhodopsin requires two cysteines (110 and 187) that form a disulfide bridge (Fig. 21.11). A natural human mutation in one of these cysteines leads to a loss of visual pigmentation in red cone cells, resulting in color blindness. The importance of the N-terminal extracellular chain of rhodopsin is noted by the finding that a point mutation of Pro[23] to His is shown to be a cause of the retinal degenerative disease, retinitis pigmentosa [13]. Substitution of Glu for Lys[296] results in alteration of the normal bind-

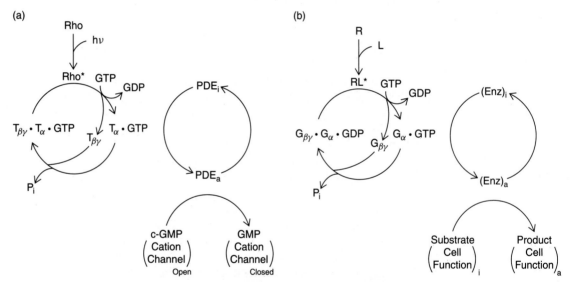

Figure 21.12 Function of the receptor rhodopsin as an example of a general mechanism for G protein-coupled receptors. (A) Rhodopsin (Rho) in rod cells of the retina is activated (Rho*) by light. Rho* activates the G protein, transducin ($T_{\alpha\beta\gamma}$), causing the subunit T_α to exchange its bound GDP for GTP, which causes it to dissociate from subunits $T_{\beta\gamma}$. The T_α GTP complex causes inactive cGMP-phosphodiesterase (PDE$_i$) to become activated (PDE$_a$). PDE hydrolyzes cGMP, which in high concentration keeps the plasma membrane cation channel open. The channel closes at lowered concentrations of cGMP. (B) The more generalized scheme shows a receptor (R) binding to a ligand (L) to form the activated receptor ligand complex, RL*. This complex activates the cellular $G\alpha$ that is specific for it, forming $G\alpha$-GTP. Generally the $G\alpha$-GTP influences the activity of a target enzyme whose substrate or product influences a function in its particular differentiated cell. (From Hargrave and Mcdowell [23], with permission. *FASEB J.* 6:2323–31, 1992.)

ing of 11-cis retinal to rhodopsin, again resulting in a form of retinitis pigmentosa. Examples of related defects in hormone receptors and their natural ligands will be discussed next in a general discussion of endocrine-related pathophysiology.

NEUROENDOCRINE PATHOPHYSIOLOGY

Disorders of endocrine origin can relate to any one of the following aspects of hormone action [27, 46, 47, 51]:

(1) hormone biosynthesis and/or secretion,
(2) hormone circulation and/or metabolism,
(3) hormone receptor interaction,
(4) hormone receptor signaling (transduction),
(5) post-receptor (e.g., second messenger) actions,
(6) termination of hormone action.

A few examples of defects in the temporal pathways of hormone production and action are provided.

Hormone Biosynthesis and/or Secretion

Hormones can be produced in excessive or inadequate amounts as in hypercortisolism (Cushing's disease) or hypocortisolism (Addison's disease). In Type-1 (juvenile/childhood) diabetes mellitus there is a lack of insulin due to loss of the β-cells of the pancreatic islets, often due to cytotoxic antibodies, or quite possibly to a virus. In familial central (neurogenic) diabetes insipidus there is a failure of hypothalamic magnocellular neurons to produce vasopressin (AVP), which is required to prevent excessive water loss. In Parkinson's disease there may be destruction or dysfunction of the neurons that synthesize and secrete dopamine, a neurotransmitter. On the other hand, in the biogenic amine theory of schizophrenia, there may be an excess of dopamine production and/or availability leading to alterations in behavior that are usually associated with the condition. Recently a defect(s) in the dopamine (D_2) receptor is being implicated.

Nutrition can account for some examples of hormone deficiency. Inadequate iodide intake, would for example, prevent thyroid hormone production by the thyroid gland, which leads to endemic hypothyroidism, to development of goiter, and to cretinism in the young child (see Chap. 13). Goitrogens found in some edible plants also inhibit thyroid hormone production, again leading to goiter. Failure to obtain vitamin D (cholecalciferol) from the diet (in the absence of adequate sunlight on the skin) can lead to nutritional rickets, resulting from a lack of formation of the hormonal form of vitamin D $(1,25\text{-}(OH_2)D_3)$ (see Chap. 9).

In the biosynthesis of a peptide hormone there may be alterations in the primary sequence, due to mutations in the DNA (gene) coding for the peptide. In familial (genetic) hyperinsulinemia, for example, there may be an incorrect residue at one of the two dibasic sequences of the proinsulin molecule, thus preventing cleavage of the prohormone into the functional form of insulin. A single-base mutation leading to an amino substitution at either position 24 or 25 of the β-chain of insulin results in a totally defective hormone, again with resulting development of diabetes mellitus. Homozygous mutations in the thyroid stimulating hormone (TSH) β or luteinizing hormone (LH) β subunits cause hypothyroidism and hypogonadism, respectively. Mutations in the β subunit result in failure of heterodimerization with the α subunit, which is necessary for receptor interaction and activation (see Chap. 13). In the adrenal glands or gonads there may be one or more defective enzymes that are necessary to convert precursor substrates into active steroid hormones. A defect in the desmolase system (side-chain cleavage enzymes), for example, prevents the use of cholesterol for steroid biosynthesis (congenital adrenal lipoidal hyperplasia); this would be fatal at or soon after birth. Other defects in any one of the numerous enzymes required for steroid hormone biosynthesis can lead to failure in cortisol or aldosterone production in the adrenal cortex or to a deficiency of testicular androgen or ovarian estrogen production.

Tumors of endocrine origin may account for many of the cases of hormone overproduction and subsequent hyperfunction. In Conn's syndrome an adrenocortical tumor secreting aldosterone is responsible for the hypertension due to hyperaldosteronism. Hyperaldosteronism can also result indirectly from oversecretion of the renin-secreting cells of the kidney, either due to a tumor of these cells or to their hypersecretion of renin due to an unknown (idiopathic) cause. Hypertension of adrenal origin can also relate to a tumor (pheochromocytoma) of the adrenomedullary (chromaffin tissue) that secretes excessive amounts of epinephrine and/or norepinephrine. A gastrinoma secreting excessive levels of gastrin can have grave consequences on the GI tract, most notably severe gastric ulcers. An insulinoma secreting excessive amounts of insulin causes severe hypoglycemia, which becomes rapidly fatal due to glucose deprivation to the brain. Hyperplastic growth of the thyroid gland can lead to severe thyrotoxicosis, wherein the tumorous tissue must be surgically removed or eradicated by other means (radioiodine therapy). Stimulatory antibodies to thyroid cell TSH receptors also lead to enhanced T_4 and T_3 production resulting in thyrotoxicosis (e.g., Graves' disease).

Ectopic Hormone Secretion.   Hormones released from endocrine/or nonendocrine tissue found at an abnormal anatomical site can lead to hypersecretion with resulting hyperfunction related to the hormone. For example, in the *syndrome of inappropriate antidiuretic hormone (vasopressin) secretion*, the hypertension developing from the hypervolemia as a result of excess water retention is due to AVP secretion from a neoplasm of ectopic origin. Excess secretion of cortisol from an "oat-cell carcinoma" of the lung is the etiological basis for the hypercortisolism of Cushing's disease of ectopic origin.

An association of acromegaly to extrapituitary neoplasmic secretion of a substance with GH-releasing activity was documented by several research groups [31]. Subsequently, the isolation and structural identification of the STH-releasing hormone (somatocrinin) was determined from the different pancreatic tumors. Somatocrinin was then extracted from the human hypothalamus and found to be identical to the peptide isolated from the pancreatic tumors. The discovery of somatocrinin presents a unique example where a hormone was isolated and sequenced first from an ectopic source (pancreas), rather than from the tissue normally producing the hormone.

Hormone Circulation and Metabolism

Thyroid hormones and most steroid hormones circulate bound to one or more binding proteins. These binding proteins provide a ready reserve of the hormones. Mutations in the binding proteins for thyroid hormones (thyroxine-binding globulin, albumin, thyroxine-binding prealbumin) may result in low levels of bound thyroid hormones in the serum. Excess production or altered forms of the binding proteins can also cause hyperthyroxinemia by binding excess amounts of thyroid hormone.

Cortisol binds as readily as does aldosterone to mineralocorticoid receptors. However, although cortisol has ready access to the mineralocorticoid receptor, it is normally metabolized intracellularly in aldosterone target cells by 11 β-hydroxysteroid dehydrogenase to cortisone, which is biologically inactive. In the *syndrome of apparent mineralocorticoid excess* there is a decreased intracellular conversion of cortisol to cortisone. The apparent "mineralocorticoid excess" is therefore, in reality, due to the abnormal glucocorticoid activation of mineralocorticoid receptors.

Hormone-Receptor Interaction

A great number of endocrinopathies relate to alterations in the cellular receptors necessary for hormone binding and subsequent physiological response. Receptor defects can be at the level of the plasma membrane for most hormones or they can be cytoplasmic where most receptors for thyroid and steroid hormones are localized. Dwarfism is a particularly interesting example of such receptor dysfunction (see Chap. 12). Growth hormone released by the pituitary (see Chap. 5) binds to and activates hepatic GH receptors leading to somatomedin (insulinlike growth factor I, IGF-I) biosynthesis and release. IGF-I interacts with numerous target tissue (e.g., cartilage, adipose tissue) receptors to stimulate bodily growth. Of course, an absence of pituitary GH secretion can lead to dwarfism (hypopituitary dwarfism). Failure of GH to bind to hepatic receptors, however, leads to what is referred to as Laron dwarfism, or as in an African tribe, pygmyism. Defects (deletions or missense substitutions of amino acids) in the primary structure of the receptor have been demonstrated. It is to be expected that defects in IGF-I receptors would result in end-organ resistance to the growth factor, resulting again in dwarfism. Numerous mutations in the insulin receptor have been documented (see Table 11.1), and they account for many of the causes of insulin resistance such as Leprechaunism and Type A insulin resistance (see Chap. 11).

Hypothyroidism can result from thyroid-stimulating hormone (TSH, thyrotropin) receptor defects at the level of the thyroid gland. Failure of TSH activation of thyroid gland receptors leads to diminished production of thyroid hormones (T_4 and T_3). Defects in peripheral T_4/T_3 receptors lead to end-organ resistance and, again, to the symptoms of hypothyroidism; in the child, this defect leads to cretinism, whereas in the adult this leads to myxedema (see Chap. 13).

Congenital insensitivity to ACTH has been described as a familial form of Addison's disease. A point mutation in the ACTH receptor associated with familial ACTH resistance has now been demonstrated. A single base mutation at position 74 converting serine to isoleucine may be responsible for the hormone-insensitive receptor. This defect leads to hypocortisolism [11].

Defects in the primary sequence of the androgen receptor lead to the syndromes of androgen resistance, most often resulting in varying degrees of male pseudo-hermaphroditism (see Chap. 16, 17). Mutations in the receptor can occur at the site for androgen occupancy (see Fig. 17.8) or in the area of the receptor required for binding to the DNA hormone response element (HRE) (see Fig. 17.9). In either case, the absence of androgen action leads to feminization of the male phenotype. Hypocalcemic vitamin D-resistance rickets results in a rare form of the disease (childhood osteomalacia/rickets) that is unresponsive to treatment with 1 α,25-dihydroxyvitamin D_3 (1 α,25(OH)$_2$cholecalciferol) due to receptor defects. A variety of mutations have been identified in different kindreds, including amino acid substitutions in the zinc-finger DNA-binding domains of the receptor (see Fig. 9.16) [27].

Other examples of defective ligand-activated transcription factors (steroid and thyroid hormone receptors) account for disorders related to glucocorticoid (cortisol) and mineralocorticoid (aldosterone) inactivity with resulting hypofunctions (e.g., hypocortisolism and hypoaldosteronism, respectively).

Hormone-Receptor Signal Transduction

For many membrane hormone receptors, hormone-receptor interaction results in a cascade of temporal events culminating in a particular cellular response. As noted previously, receptor signal transduction by many membrane receptors involves the participation of G proteins (Fig. 21.13). The α subunit, in particular, is responsible for activating or inhibiting a particular enzyme event, usually leading to stimulation or inhibition of second-messenger formation. Posttranslational modification of $G\alpha_s$ subunits by bacterial exotoxins were the

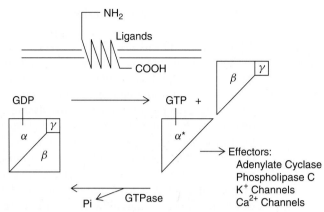

Figure 21.13 G-proteins are heterotrimeric proteins, composed of α, β, and γ subunits. The functional specificity of each G protein is due to the α subunit, which differs from one G-protein to another. The α subunit contains the GDP/GTP binding site and has intrinsic GTPase activity. Receptor occupancy causes conformational changes of the α subunit leading the displacement of bound GDP by GTP. After GTP binding, G-proteins undergo a dissociation reaction resulting in free $\beta\gamma$-dimer and active α-GTP complex, which is effective in regulating the activity of intracellular effectors (e.g., adenylate cyclase). GTPase activity intrinsic to the α subunit causes hydrolysis of α-GTP to α-GDP, thus ensuring turn-off of the reaction. (From Spada et al., [45], with permission. *Frontiers in Neuroendocrinology* 14:214–32, 1993. Raven Press, Inc.)

first examples of G protein alterations associated with disease. Cholera toxin, for example, irreversibly activates the α-stimulatory ($G\alpha_s$) subunit in certain cells of the gastrointestinal tract. Cholera toxin catalyzes the ADP ribosylation of residue Arg[201] of α_s, resulting in constitutive activation due to a marked reduction of the intrinsic GTPase activity of the G-protein subunit. (Reduced GTPase activity results in continued activation of the α_s subunit by GTP.) This leads to overproduction of cAMP and excessive water secretion from gastrointestinal mucosa cells leading to watery diarrhea, dehydration, and most often, death. Pertussis toxin riboxylates a cysteine residue four amino acids from the carboxy-terminus of $\alpha_{i/o}$ subunits, resulting in an uncoupling of these G proteins from their receptors. Inhibition of the action of these inhibitory G-protein subunits results in a continuous uninhibited cellular response. The actions of these toxins are therefore responsible for some of the clinical manifestations of *Vibrio cholerae* and *Bordetta pertussis* infection.

Mutations in the $G\alpha_s$ subunit have been identified in somatotroph adenomas [45]. These mutations inhibit GTP hydrolysis and therefore result in continuous constitutive activation of the subunit leading to excess cAMP formation. Enhanced cyclic nucleotide formation leads to excess GH secretion and to the condition of acromegaly in the adult or to gigantism in the child. cAMP is also stimulatory to somatotroph hypertrophy and hyperplasia leading to somatotroph adenoma (tumor) formation (Fig. 21.14). These mutations are somatic rather than inherited and therefore are tissue specific.

For a given defect in a G-protein coupled pathway, the extent of the manifestations will generally be determined by the cellular distribution of the affected component. Defects can be manifested in a single cell type (see examples below) and cause a focal disorder, whereas defects in more generally expressed component (e.g., β-adrenergic receptors) may be widely expressed.

The McCune-Albright syndrome (MAS) is characterized by several distinguishing characteristics, including multiple endocrinopathies. The molecular basis for MAS is a mutation in $G\alpha_s$ that results in the constitutive activation of adenylate cyclase in affected

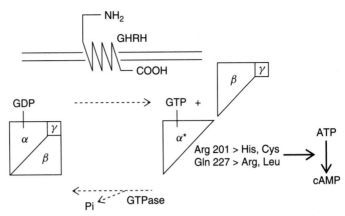

Figure 21.14 Single amino acid substitutions replacing Arg 201 with either Cys, His, or Gln 227 with either Arg or Leu in the α subunit of Gs have been identified in one-third of GH-secreting adenomas. Both mutations lead to the constitutive activation of adenylyl cyclase and cAMP formation by inhibiting GTPase activity. Therefore the mutations stabilize the α subunit in its active conformation, mimicking the effect of specific extracellular growth factors, such as GHRH. (From Spada et al., [45], with permission. *Frontiers in Neuroendocrinology* 14:214–32, 1993. Raven Press, Inc.)

tissues (as in somatotroph hyperplasia discussed above). The mutation occurs during early (postzygotic) embryogenesis and therefore patients with MAS are mosaic [42]. In MAS there is promotion of autonomous function and clonal expansion of cells carrying the mutation. These mutations in $G\alpha_s$ have therefore been characterized as oncogenes, termed *gsp1* [51]. *Ras* is also a GTPase that is structurally related to the G-proteins. Ras proteins are involved in the control of cell growth and development. Somatic mutations in some *ras* genes have been identified in a number of different human malignancies, including tumors of the endocrine system [27]. Recently the *ras* oncogene has been identified in one prolactinoma characterized by unusual invasiveness.

As noted in Chap. 4, the importance of G proteins is emphasized by the fact that a Nobel Prize in Physiology/Medicine was awarded to two American researchers, Gilman and Rodbell, for their discoveries and studies of these signal transduction proteins.

Post Receptor/Transduction Defects

Pit-1 is a transcription factor whose expression is restricted to the pituitary gland. The protein is localized solely to somatotrophs, lactotrophs, and thyrotrophs. The possibility that mutations in the Pit-1 gene might lead to multiple pituitary hormone deficiency was first demonstrated in mice. Similarly, in humans, mutations inhibit the ability of Pit-1 to bind to specific promotor sequences and activate transcription of target genes. This results in the absence of somatotrophs, lactotrophs, thyrotrophs, and their associated peptide hormones [36].

SRY is the critical gene for an early step in male sex determination. Mutations in the SRY gene responsible for the production of testes-determining factor (TDF), a transcription factor, leads to a defect in the primary structure of TDF and results in genetic XY females. A single amino acid substitution in the transcription factor can, indeed, determine whether an individual will be female rather than male in appearance.

Termination of Hormone Action

As noted above, mutations of the $G\alpha_s$ protein involved in hormone signal transduction may result in cellular activation that can not be terminated. As discussed, this can also result when *Vibrio cholerae* or *B. pertussis* toxins irreversibly affect G-protein activity. An even more interesting example involving the secretion of parathormone (PTH) has been reported. A cell membrane Ca^{2+}-sensing receptor cDNA has been cloned from parathyroid glands. This cation-sensing receptor has been reported to be defective (missense mutations) in some individuals resulting in "familial" hypocalciuric hypercalcemia and severe neonatal hyperparathyroidism. The function of the receptor is apparently to sense the extracellular Ca^{2+} concentration of the intercellular space. High concentrations of Ca^{2+} are inhibitory to PTH secretions. In the absence of a functional Ca^{2+}-sensing receptor the cells secrete excessive amounts of PTH and the resulting hyperparathyroidism causes excessive bone mineral resorption and Ca^{2+} retention, thus producing the symptoms of severe hypercalcemia and hypocalciuria (see Chap. 9).

EVOLUTION OF HORMONES

It is known that peptides of identical or related primary structure are found in a wide variety of tissues. Originally, peptides, such as GI hormones, were isolated from the GI mucosa and their putative functions characterized. After determining of their primary structures, subsequent synthesis of these peptides allowed antibodies to be produced for radioimmunoassay and immunocytochemical studies. This then provided evidence for the localization of these peptides to the CNS and even to specific neurons within the brain and spinal cord. Thus new functions are suggested for these peptides in addition to the original roles classically ascribed [1].

New Theory of Hormones

It has been discovered that peptide hormones (or immunologically similar peptides) are present within tissues of flies, worms, protozoa, and even bacteria. It has been suggested that a primitive role of chemical messengers may have been as tissue growth factors [29]. They may have been released initially as intracellular chemical messengers to regulate cellular growth processes. Subsequently, their release into the extracellular environment may have provided a stimulus to their own growth or to other cells of the same cellular species. This point is well documented in the cellular slime mold.

The role of cAMP as an intracellular messenger of hormone action in vertebrates is well established [18]. This cyclic nucleotide is also an intermediate in the action of some insect hormones. Most interesting was the discovery that cAMP is used in communication in cellular slime molds and in that capacity serves as the initial stimulus for amoeboid movement and subsequent morphogenesis [14, 34, 49]. *Dictyostelium discoideum* is a cellular slime mold that passes through a number of distinctive stages in its life cycle. Initially, spores germinate to yield irregularly shaped, solitary, amoeboid cells that live on microorganisms usually available on the forest floor. During this stage the individual cells grow and divide by binary fission. When food sources are depleted, the starving amoebae mass together in response to periodic pulses of chemical attractant and form multicellular aggregates. The cells initially begin moving in a pulsatile manner toward a central point and then form pulsating streams of aggregating cells. Aggregation is initiated by a small number of cells that release an attractant, originally known as *acrasin*. Eventually it was discovered that acrasin was identical to cAMP. In response to cAMP, cells move toward the cyclic nucleotide and, in the process, release their own pulse of cAMP. After releasing or responding to cAMP, the cells appear insensitive to the nucleotide for several minutes, apparently because it is destroyed by a membrane cAMP phosphodiesterase. When a new pulse of cAMP arrives, the cells respond again; thus the amoebae migrate in pulsatile steps in response to alternations in sensitivity to the attractant.

Cyclic AMP apparently interacts with cellular receptors of the amoebae, because slime molds that fail to respond to cAMP do not bind radiolabeled cAMP. The starvation stimulus apparently induces the formation of cAMP receptor proteins in the plasma membrane of amoebae, which allows them to recognize the aggregation signal. The actual mechanism of cAMP perception is not understood, but it is possible that the amoebae compute the difference in concentration of cAMP from the front to the back of the cells and thereby sense the presence of a gradient of the nucleotide. Other theories are equally attractive [34]. Movement, per se, involves activation of contractile proteins on the side of the cells that receive the signal to move. It is possible that cAMP may activate ion channels and elevate local intracellular levels of Ca^{2+}. Calmodulin or other intracellular Ca^{2+} receptors might then activate the contractile machinery required for amoeboid movement.

In its role as an extracellular chemical messenger cAMP functions in the classical sense as a pheromone. This might be considered a more primitive function of the cyclic nucleotide. Not all species of slime molds respond chemotactically to cAMP: other chemical attractants, possibly small peptides, may be used. It is possible that a large number of chemically diverse "communicational molecules" may be employed by microorganisms [34]. Studies of these chemical messengers may provide important insights into the role of similar molecules that may be important in directing morphogenic movements in early development of invertebrate and vertebrate species.

Early in evolution, cell-cell communication in multicellular organisms may have been effected by local hormones. Although a paracrine mechanism of communication might be envisioned as operative in "simple" multicellular organisms (e.g., *Volvox*), more rapid delivery of a local hormone to a more distant site may have necessitated cellular elongation (dendritogenesis and axonal development). This would have resulted in the evolution of the first neurons whose original secretions may have been purely paracrine/neurocrine in nature (see Fig. 10.5). Chemotactic orientation to a chemical gradient may have provided the initial stimulus to cellular elongation. Nerve growth factor, for example, provides the hormonal stimulus to directed growth of sympathetic neurons. The development of the complex structural element, the synapse, might be viewed as a later evolutionary acquisition. Release of a hormone into a synaptic cleft would have provided the mechanism for a more localized (efficient) delivery of the chemical messenger. Further evolution of the synapse may have involved localized membrane ion flow, rapid transmembrane electrical changes, and action potential transmission, features that characterize neurotransmitter mechanisms of action.

To mediate their actions hormones must be recognized by target cells. A variation of the old chicken-or-the-egg argument—what came first, the hormone or the receptor—is raised. Both hormones and receptors most likely evolved simultaneously. Even the most primitive of cells needed to "sense" the environment. Change in salinity is known to stimulate morphological changes in some single-celled organisms. Some cellular receptor substance must therefore be able to interact with and subsequently respond to changes in Na^+ or Cl^- concentration. Even in mammals, chemoreceptors detect changes in Na^+ concentration of the blood. Calmodulin, an intracellular Ca^{2+} receptor (see Chap. 4), may well represent a reasonable example of such a chemoreceptive protein.

Peptide hormones probably evolved from cellular proteins that originally served other functions. Enzymatic hydrolysis, both intracellularly and extracellularly, may have then yielded smaller biologically active sequences that evolved a hormonal function. Point mutations of DNA bases would have provided new protein species necessary for the evolutionary selection process. It might be expected that selection would have favored enhanced hormone-receptor interaction. Through mutational changes in the DNA, the hormones and their receptors would have evolved together to provide their sensitivity and selectivity. Stability of peptide structures may have involved post-translational modifications of the carboxy- and amino-terminal groups of some peptide hormones. Gene duplication followed by base mutations would have provided the means for hormonal structure variation and subsequent evolution of the various families of hormones (Fig. 21.15).

With the development of diverse tissue types, other forms of hormones may have evolved. Mesodermal tissues, for example, are the specific source of steroid hormones.

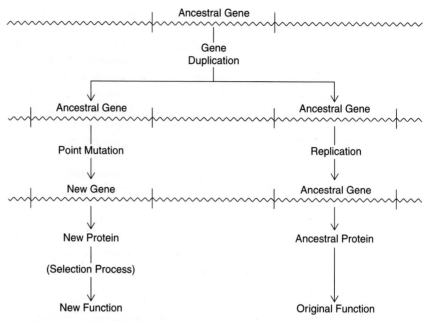

Figure 21.15 Scheme of peptide hormone evolution through gene duplication and base mutation.

But the ability to synthesize steroidlike structures is not restricted to animal tissues. Plants are able to produce vitamin D-like and estrogenic steroids [2]. Is it possible that their *raison d'etre* is to modify (adversely) physiological processes of animal tissues? For example, certain plant steroids may affect insect growth and development and cause egg maturation to occur at a seasonally inappropriate time.

From an evolutionary perspective it appears that ancestral molecules supplied the raw material on which evolutionary selective processes provided the present-day diversity of vertebrate hormones. Most important, these ancestral hormones often evolved to regulate species-specific physiological processes. The evolution of the terrestrial vertebrate from an aquatic habitat probably necessitated putting old hormones to new or additional uses or evolving new hormones. Conservation of water and Ca^{2+} may have become particularly important processes that required new hormonal control systems in the terrestrial habitat. The ancestral prolactin molecule antedated the evolutionary acquisition of mammary glands in the vertebrates. Melanotropins may have been particularly important hormones for certain species of animals where adaptive coloration was of survival value. In certain large groups of birds and many mammals MSH no longer appears to serve such a role. This is particularly evident in humans and birds, where the source of MSH, the pars intermedia, is lacking. However, in some mammals, including humans, MSH is present within the brain where it may function as a neurohormone to regulate other behavioral and physiological processes.

REFERENCES

[1]   Acher, R. 1993. Neurohypophysial peptide systems: processing machinery, hydro-osmotic regulation, adaptation and evolution. *Reg. Pept.* 45:1–13.

[2]   Agarwal, M. K. 1993. Receptors for mammalian steroid hormones in microbes and plants. *Fed. Europ. Biochem. Soc.* 322:207–10.

[3]   Baile, C. A., C. L. McLaughlin, and M. A. Della-Fera. 1986. Role of cholecystokinin and opioid peptides in control of food intake. *Physiol. Rev.* 66:172–234.

[4]   Barinaga, M. 1991. How the nose knows: olfactory receptor cloned. *Science* 252:209–10.

[5]   ———. 1993. Carbon monoxide: killer to brain messenger in one step. *Science* 259:309.

[6]   ———. 1994. Learning by diffusion: nitric oxide may spread memories. *Science* 263:466.

[7]   Brecha, N., H. J. Karten, and C. Laverack. 1979. Enkephalin-containing amacrine cells in the avian retina: immunohistochemical localization. *Proc. Natl. Acad. Sci. USA* 76:3010–4.

[8]   Browstein, M. J. 1993. A brief history of opiates, opioid peptides, and opioid receptors. *Proc. Natl. Acad. Sci. USA* 90:5391–3.

[9]   Burnett, A. L., C. J. Lwenstein, D. S. Bredt, T. S. K. Chang, and S. H. Snyder. 1992. Nitric oxide: a physiologic mediator of penile erection. *Science* 257:401–3.

[10]   Carlsson, A. 1988. The current status of the dopamine hypothesis of schizophrenia. *Neuropsychopharmacology* 1:179–86.

[11]   Clark, A. J. L., L. McLoughlin, and A. Grossman. 1993. Familial glucocorticoid deficiency associated with a point mutation in the adrenocorticotropin receptor. *Lancet* 341:461–2.

[12]   Della-Fera, M. A., and C. A. Baile. 1979. Cholecystokinin octapeptide: continuous picomole injections into the cerebral ventricles of sheep suppresses feeding. *Science* 206:471–3.

[13]   Deryja, T. P., T. L. McGee, E. Reichel, L. B. Hahn, et al. 1990. A point mutation of the rhodopsin gene in one form of retinitis pigmentation. *Nature* 343:364–6.

[14]   Devreotes, P. 1989. *Dictyostelium discoideum*: a model system for cell-cell interactions in development. *Science* 245:1054–8.

[15]   Dizhorr, A. M., S. Ray, S. Kumar, G. Niemi, M. Spencer, D. Brolley, K. A. Walsh, P. P. Philipov, J. B. Hurley, and L. Stryer. 1991. Recoverin: a calcium sensitive activator of retinol rod guanylate cyclase. *Science* 251:915–8.

[16]   Evans, C. J., D. E. Keith, Jr., H. Morrison, K. Magendzo, and R. H. Edwards. 1992. Cloning of a delta opioid receptor by functional expression. *Science* 258:1952–5.

[17]   Garlicki, J., P. K. Konturek, J. Majka, N. Kwiecien, and S. J. Kon Turek. 1990. Cholecystokinin receptors and vagal nerves in control of food intake in rats. *Amer. J. Physiol.* 258:E40–5.

[18]   Gerisch, G. 1987. Cyclic AMP and other signals controlling cell development and differentiation in *Dictyostelium*. *Annu. Rev. Biochem.* 56:853–79.

[19]   Gessa, G. L., E. Paglietti, and B. Pelligrini Quarantotti. 1979. Induction of copulatory behavior in sexually inactive rats by naloxone. *Science* 204:203–4.

[20]   Gilbertson, T .A. 1993. The physiology of vertebrate taste reception. *Curr. Opin. Neurobiol.* 3:532–9.

[21]   Hargrave, P. A., H. E. Hamm, and K. P. Hofmann. 1993. Interaction of rhodopsin with the G-protein transducin. *BioEssays* 15:43–50.

[22]   Hargrave, P. A. and J. H. McDowell. 1992a. Rhodopsin and phototransduction. *Intern. Rev. Cytol.* 137B:49–97.

[23]   ———. 1992b. Rhodopsin and phototransduction: a model system for G protein-linked receptors. *FASEB J.* 6:2323–31.

[24]   Hoffman, M. 1991. A new role for gases: neurotransmission. *Science* 252:1788.

[25]   Hökfelt, T. 1991. Neuropeptides in perspective. The last ten years. *Neuron* 7:867–79.

[26]   Hökfelt, T., O. Johansson, A. Ljungdahl, J. Lundberg, M. Schultzberg, L. Terenius, M. Goldstein, R. Elde, H. Steinbusch, and A. Verhofstad. 1979. Histochemistry of transmitter interactions-neural coupling and coexistence of transmitters. In *Advances in pharmacology and therapeutics*, ed. S. Simon, pp. 131–42.

[27]   Jameson, J. L., and A. N. Hollenberg. 1992. Recent advances in studies of the molecular basis for endocrine disease. *Horm. Metab. Res.* 24:201–9.

[28]   Kilpatrick, D. L., T. Taniguchi, B. N. Jones, A. S. Stern, J. E. Shively, J. Hullihan, S. Kimura, S. Stein, and S. Undenfriend. 1981. A highly potent 3200-dalton adrenal opioid peptide that contains both a [Met]- and [Leu]-enkephalin sequence. *Proc. Natl. Acad. Sci. USA* 78:3265–8.

[29]   Kolata, G. 1982. New theory of hormones proposed. *Science* 215:1383–84.

[30]   Lagnado, L., and D. Baylor. 1992. Signal flow in visual transduction. *Neuron* 8:995–1002.

[31]   Losa, M., J. Schopohl, and K. von Werder. 1993. Ectopic secretion of growth hormone-releasing hormone in man. *J. Endocrinol. Invest.* 16:69–81.

[32] Maines, M. D. 1993. Carbon monoxide: an emerging regulator of cGMP in the brain. *Mol. Cell. Neurosci.* 4:389–97.

[33] Margolskee, R. F. 1993. The molecular biology of taste transduction. *Bioessays* 15:645–50.

[34] Newell, P. C. 1977. How cells communicate: the system used by slime molds. *Endeavor* 1:63–8.

[35] Nowak, R. 1994. Nicotine scrutinized as FDA seeks to regulate cigarettes. *Science* 263:1555–6.

[36] Parks, J. S., E. Kinoshita, and R. W. Pfäffle. 1993. Pit-1 and hypopituitarism. *TEM* 4:81–5.

[37] Pasternak, G. W. 1993. Pharmacological mechanisms of opioid analgesics. *Clin. Neuropharmacol.* 16:1–18.

[38] Paul, S. M., and R. H. Purdy. 1992. Neuroactive steroids. *FASEB J.* 6:2311–22.

[39] Pechnick, R. N. 1993. Effects of opioids on the hypothalamo-pituitary-adrenal axis. *Annu. Rev. Pharmacol. Toxicol.* 32:353–82.

[40] Peikin, S. R. 1989. Role of cholecystokinin in the control of food intake. *Gastroenterol. Clin. N. Amer.* 18:757–75.

[41] Pfister, C., N. Bennett, F. Bruckert, P. Catty, A. Clerc, F. Pagés, and P. Deterre. 1993. Interactions of a G-protein with its effector and cGMP phosphodiesterase in the retina of rats. *Cell. Signaling* 5:235–51.

[42] Schwindinger, W. F., and M. A. Levine. 1993. McCune-Albright syndrome. *TEM* 4:238–42.

[43] Simon, E. J. 1991. Opioid receptors and endogenous opioid peptides. *Med. Res. Rev.* 11:357–74.

[44] Snyder, S. H. 1992. Nitric oxide: first in a new class of neurotransmitters? *Science* 257:494–6.

[45] Spada, A., L. Vallar, and G. Faglia. 1993. G-Proteins and hormonal signaling in human pituitary tumors: genetic mutations and functional alterations. *Front. Neuroendocrinol.* 14:214–32.

[46] Spiegel, A. M., A. M. Shenker, and L. S. Weinstein. 1992. Receptor-effector coupling by G proteins. Implications for normal and abnormal signal transduction. *Endocr. Rev.* 13:536–65.

[47] Spiegel, A. M., L. S. Weinstein, and A. Shenker. 1993. Abnormalities in G protein-coupled signal transduction pathways in human disease. *J. Clin. Invest.* 92:1119–25.

[48] Thomas, J. M., and B. B. Hoffman. 1987. Adenylate cyclase supersensitivity: a general means of cellular adaptation to inhibitory agonists? *Trends Pharmacol. Sci.* 3:308–11.

[49] Tomchik, K. J., and P. N. Devreotes. 1981. Adenosine 3′,5′-monophosphate waves in *Dictyostelium discoideum:* a demonstration by isotope dilution-fluorography. *Science* 212:443–6.

[50] Verma, A., D. J. Hirsch, C. E. Glatt, G. V. Ronnett, and S. H. Snyder. 1993. Carbon monoxide: a putative neural messenger. *Science* 259:381–4.

[51] Weinstein, L. S., and A. Shenker. 1993. G protein mutations in human disease. *Clin. Biochem.* 26:333–8.

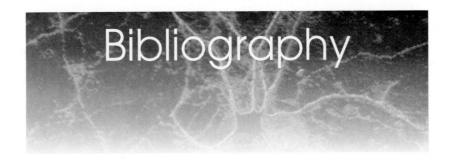
Bibliography

BOOKS AND MONOGRAPHS

BOLANDER, F. F. 1989. *Molecular endocrinology*. San Diego: Academic Press, Inc.

FREGLY, M. J., and W. G. LUTTGE. 1984. *Human endocrinology: an interactive text*. New York: Elsevier North-Holland, Inc.

FRIEDEN, E. H. 1976. *Chemical endocrinology*. New York: Academic Press, Inc.

FRIEDEN, E. H., and H. LIPNER. 1971. *Biochemical endocrinology of the vertebrates*. Englewood Cliffs, N.J.: Prentice-Hall Publishing Co., Inc.

GORBMAN, A., W. W. DICKHOFF, S. R. VIGNA, N. B. CLARK, and C. L. RALPH. 1983. *Comparative endocrinology*. New York: John Wiley and Sons, Inc.

JUBIZ, W. 1985. *Endocrinology: a logical approach for clinicians*. New York: McGraw-Hill Book Company.

KRIEGER, D. T., and J. C. HUGHES. 1980. *Neuroendocrinology. A hospital practice book*. Sunderland, MA: Sinauer Associates.

LAUFER, H., and R. G. H. DOWNER, eds. 1988. *Invertebrate endocrinology, vol. 2: Endocrinology of selected invertebrate types*. New York: Alan R. Liss, Inc.

LEE, J., and J. LAYCOCK. 1978. *Essential endocrinology*. New York: Oxford University Press.

METZ, R., and E. B. LARSON. 1985. *Blue book of endocrinology*. Philadelphia: W. B. Saunders Company.

NORMAN, A. W., and G. LITWACK. 1987. *Hormones*. Orlando, FL: Academic Press, Inc.

NORRIS, D. O. 1985. *Vertebrate endocrinology*, 2nd ed. Philadelphia: Lea & Febiger.

NORRIS, D. O., and R. E. JONES, eds. 1987. *Hormones and reproduction in fishes, amphibians, and reptiles*. New York: Plenum Press.

O'RIORDAN, J. L. H., P. G. MALAN, and R. P. GOULD. 1982. *Essentials of endocrinology*. Boston: Blackwell Scientific Publications, Inc.

PANG, P. K. T., and M. P. SCHREIBMAN, eds. 1987. *Vertebrate endocrinology, vol 2: Regulation of water and electrolytes*. San Diego: Academic Press, Inc.

PANG, P. K. T., and M. P. SCHREIBMAN, eds. 1987. *Vertebrate endocrinology, vol 3: Regulation of calcium and phosphate*. San Diego: Academic Press, Inc.

PANG, P. K. T., M. P. SCHREIBMAN, and A. GORBMAN, eds. 1986. *Vertebrate endocrinology, vol 1: Morphological considerations*. San Diego: Academic Press, Inc.

PAXTON, M. J. W. 1986. *Endocrinology*. Dubuque, Iowa: William C. Brown Company, Publishers.

RALPH, C. L. 1986. *Comparative endocrinology: developments and directions*. New York: Alan R. Liss, Inc.

WILLIAMS, R. H. 1981. *Textbook of endocrinology*. 6th ed. Philadelphia: W. B. Saunders Company.

MAJOR ENDOCRINOLOGY JOURNALS

Acta Endocrinologica (Acta Endocrinol.)
Advances in Cyclic Nucleotide Research (Advan. Cyclic Nucl. Res.)
Annals d'Endocrinologie (Ann. d'Endocrinol.)

Baillière's Clinical Endocrinology and Metabolism (Baillière's Clin. Endocr. Metab.)
Clinical Endocrinology (Clin. Endocrinol.)
Endocrine Reviews (Endocr. Rev.)
Endocrine Journal (Endocr. J.)
Endocrine Pathology (Endocr. Pathol.)
Endocrine Research (Endocr. Res.)
Endocrine Research Communications (Endocr. Res. Commun.)
Endocrinologica Japonica (Endocrinol. Jpn.)
Endocrinology
Experimental and Clinical Endocrinology (Exp. Clin. Endocrinol.)
Frontiers in Neuroendocrinology
General and Comparative Endocrinology (Gen. Comp. Endocrinol.)
Growth Factors
Hormone Research (Horm. Res.)
Hormones and Behavior (Horm. Behav.)
Hormone and Metabolism Research (Horm. Metab. Res.)
Journal of Endocrinology (J. Endocrinol.)
Journal of Clinical Endocrinology and Metabolism (J. Clin. Endocrinol. Metab.)
Journal of Neuroendocrinology (J. Neuroendocr.)
Journal of Endocrinological Investigation (J. Endocrinol. Invest.)
Molecular and Cellular Endocrinology (Mol. Cell. Endocrinol.)
Neuroendocrinology
Psychoneuroendocrinology
Regulatory Peptides (Reg. Pept.)
The Endocrinologist
Trends in Endocrinology and Metabolism (TEM)

ENDOCRINOLOGY-RELATED JOURNALS

Advances in Prostaglandin and Thromboxane Research
Advances in Steroid Biochemistry and Pharmacology
American Journal of Physiology (Amer. J. Physiol.)
Cell and Tissue Research (Cell Tissue Res.)
Clinical Investigation (Clin. Invest.)
Diabetes
Federation Proceedings (Fed. Proc.)
Journal of Biological Chemistry (J. Biol. Chem.)
Journal of Clinical Investigation (J. Clin. Invest.)
Journal of Cyclic Nucleotide Research (J. Cyclic Nucl. Res.)
Journal of Experimental Zoology (J. Exp. Zool.)
Journal of General Physiology (J. Gen. Physiol.)
Journal of Neurophysiology (J. Neurophysiol.)
Journal of Physiology (J. Physiol.)
Journal of Receptor Research (J. Receptor Res.)
Laboratory Investigation (Lab. Invest.)
Life Sciences (Life Sci.)
News in Physiological Sciences (NIPS)
Peptides
Proceedings of the National Academy of Sciences USA (PNAS)

SERIAL PUBLICATIONS

Annual Review of Biochemistry (Annu. Rev. Biochem.)
Annual Review of Medicine (Annu. Rev. Med.)
Annual Review of Neuroscience (Annu. Rev. Neurosci.)
Annual Review of Pharmacology and Toxicology (Annu. Rev. Pharmacol. Toxicol.)
Annual Review of Physiology (Annu. Rev. Physiol.)
Contemporary Endocrinology (formerly *The Year in Endocrinology)*
Physiological Reviews (Physiol. Rev.)
Recent Progress in Hormone Research (Rec. Prog. Horm. Res.)
Vitamins and Hormones (Vit. Horm.)

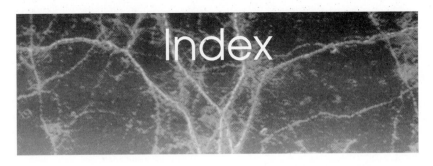

Index

Some Common Endocrine Abbreviations and Terminology

ACTH	Adrenocorticotropic hormone (corticotropin)
ADH	Antidiuretic hormone
ANF	Atrial natriuretic factor
ANS	Autonomic nervous system
APUD	Amine precursor uptake and decarboxylation
AVP	Arginine vasopressin
AVT	Arginine vasotocin
cAMP	Cyclic adenosine monophosphate (cyclic AMP)
CaM	Calmodulin
CaBP	Calcium-binding protein
CBG	Corticosteroid-binding globulin, transcortin
CCK	Cholecystokinin
cGMP	Cyclic guanosine monophosphate (cyclic GMP)
CNS	Central nervous system
COMT	Catechol-O-methyltransferase
CRH	Corticotropin-releasing hormone
CSF	Cerebral spinal fluid
DG	Diacylglycerol (or DAG)
DBH	Dopamine β-hydroxylase
DHT	Dihydrotestosterone
DIT	Diiodotyrosine
DOPA	Dihydroxyphenylalanine
EGF	Epidermal growth factor
FGF	Fibroblast growth factor
FSH	Follicle-stimulating hormone (follitropin)
GH	Growth hormone (somatotropin, STH)
GHRH	Growth hormone releasing hormone (somatocrinin)
GIP	Gastric inhibitory peptide
GRP	Gastrin-releasing peptide
GLP-1	Glucagonlike peptide 1
GnRH	Gonadotropin-releasing hormone (LH/FSH-RH)
GTP	Guanosine triphosphate
HCG	Human chorionic gonadotropin (choriogonadotropin)
HIOMT	Hydroxyindole-O-methyltransferase
hPL	Human placental lactogen
HRE	Hormone response element
5-HT	5-Hydroxytryptamine (serotonin)
IGFs	Insulinlike growth factors (I and II)